RN Adult Medical Surgical Nursing
Review Module Edition 9.0

CONTRIBUTORS

Sheryl Sommer, PhD, RN, CNE
VP Nursing Education & Strategy

Janean Johnson, MSN, RN
Nursing Education Strategist

Karin Roberts, PhD, MSN, RN, CNE
Nursing Education Coordinator

Sharon R. Redding, EdD, RN, CNE
Nursing Education Specialist and Content Project Coordinator

Lois Churchill, MN, RN
Nursing Education Specialist

Brenda Ball, MEd, BSN, RN
Nursing Education Specialist

Norma Jean Henry, MSN/Ed, RN
Nursing Education Specialist

Peggy Leehy, MSN, RN
Nursing Education Specialist

Pamela Roland, MSN, RN
Nursing Education Specialist

EDITORIAL AND PUBLISHING

Derek Prater
Spring Lenox
Michelle Renner
Mandy Tallmadge
Kelly Von Lunen

CONSULTANTS

Tracey Bousquet, BSN, RN
Pam DeMoss, MSN, RN
Carol J. Green, PhD, CNS, RN, CNE
Justina Higgins, RN, MSN, PLNC, HCE, CHC
Honey C. Holman, MSN, RN

Deb Johnson-Schuh, MSN, RN, CNE
Terri Lemon, DNP, MSN, RN
Tami J. Rogers, PhD(c), DVM, MSN, CNE
Julie Skrabal, RN, MSN
Virginia E. Tufano, EdD, MSN, RN

Intellectual Property Notice

Important Notice to the Reader

User's Guide

Welcome to the Assessment Technologies Institute® RN Adult Medical Surgical Nursing Review Module Edition 9.0. The mission of ATI's Content Mastery Series® review modules is to provide user-friendly compendiums of nursing knowledge that will:

- Help you locate important information quickly.

- Assist in your learning efforts.

- Provide exercises for applying your nursing knowledge.

- Facilitate your entry into the nursing profession as a newly licensed RN.

Organization

This review module is organized into units covering the foundations of nursing care (Unit 1), body systems and physiological processes (Units 2 to 13), and perioperative nursing care (Unit 14). Chapters within these units conform to one of three organizing principles for presenting the content.

- Nursing concepts

- Procedures (diagnostic and therapeutic)

- Systems disorders

Nursing concepts chapters begin with an overview describing the central concept and its relevance to nursing. Subordinate themes are covered in outline form to demonstrate relationships and present the information in a clear, succinct manner.

Procedures chapters include an overview describing the procedure(s) covered in the chapter. These chapters will provide you with nursing knowledge relevant to each procedure, including indications, interpretation of findings, nursing actions, and complications.

System disorders chapters include an overview describing the disorder(s) and/or disease process. These chapters may provide information on health promotion and disease prevention before addressing assessments, including risk factors, subjective data, and objective data. Next, you will focus on collaborative care, including nursing care, medications, interdisciplinary care, therapeutic procedures, surgical interventions, and care after discharge. Finally, you will find complications related to the disorder, along with nursing actions in response to those complications.

Application Exercises

Questions are provided at the end of each chapter so you can practice applying your knowledge. The Application Exercises include NCLEX-style questions, such as multiple-choice and multiple-select items, and questions that ask you to apply your knowledge in other formats, such as by using an ATI Active Learning Template. After the Application Exercises, an answer key is provided, along with rationales for the answers.

NCLEX® Connections

To prepare for the NCLEX-RN, it is important for you to understand how the content in this review module is connected to the NCLEX-RN test plan. You can find information on the detailed test plan at the National Council of State Boards of Nursing's Web site: https://www.ncsbn.org/. When reviewing content in this review module, regularly ask yourself, "How does this content fit into the test plan, and what types of questions related to this content should I expect?"

To help you in this process, we've included NCLEX Connections at the beginning of each unit and with each question in the Application Exercises Answer Keys. The NCLEX Connections at the beginning of each unit will point out areas of the detailed test plan that relate to the content within that unit. The NCLEX Connections attached to the Application Exercises Answer Keys will demonstrate how each exercise fits within the detailed content outline.

These NCLEX Connections will help you understand how the detailed content outline is organized, starting with major client needs categories and subcategories and followed by related content areas and tasks. The major client needs categories are:

- Safe and Effective Care Environment
  - Management of Care
  - Safety and Infection Control
- Health Promotion and Maintenance
- Psychosocial Integrity
- Physiological Integrity
  - Basic Care and Comfort
  - Pharmacological and Parenteral Therapies
  - Reduction of Risk Potential
  - Physiological Adaptation

An NCLEX Connection might, for example, alert you that content within a unit is related to:

- Reduction of Risk Potential
  - Diagnostic Tests
    - Monitor the results of diagnostic testing and intervene as needed.

QSEN Competencies

As you use the review modules, you will note the integration of the Quality and Safety Education for Nurses (QSEN) competencies throughout the chapters. These competencies are integral components of the curriculum of many nursing programs in the United States and prepare you to provide safe, high-quality care as a newly licensed RN. Icons appear to draw your attention to the six QSEN competencies:

- Safety: The minimization of risk factors that could cause injury or harm while promoting quality care and maintaining a secure environment for clients, self, and others.

- Patient-Centered Care: The provision of caring and compassionate, culturally sensitive care that addresses clients' physiological, psychological, sociological, spiritual, and cultural needs, preferences, and values.

- Evidence-Based Practice: The use of current knowledge from research and other credible sources, on which to base clinical judgment and client care.

- Informatics: The use of information technology as a communication and information-gathering tool that supports clinical decision-making and scientifically based nursing practice.

- Quality Improvement: Care related and organizational processes that involve the development and implementation of a plan to improve health care services and better meet clients' needs.

- Teamwork and Collaboration: The delivery of client care in partnership with multidisciplinary members of the health care team to achieve continuity of care and positive client outcomes.

Icons

Icons are used throughout the review module to draw your attention to particular areas. Keep an eye out for these icons:

 This icon is used for NCLEX connections.

 This icon is used for content related to safety and is a QSEN competency. When you see this icon, take note of safety concerns or steps that nurses can take to ensure client safety and a safe environment.

 This icon is a QSEN competency that indicates the importance of a holistic approach to providing care.

 This icon, a QSEN competency, points out the integration of research into clinical practice.

 This icon is a QSEN competency and highlights the use of information technology to support nursing practice.

 This icon is used to focus on the QSEN competency of integrating planning processes to meet clients' needs.

 This icon highlights the QSEN competency of care delivery using an interprofessional approach.

This icon indicates that a media supplement, such as a graphic, animation, or video, is available. If you have an electronic copy of the review module, this icon will appear alongside clickable links to media supplements. If you have a hardcopy version of the review module, visit www.atitesting. com for details on how to access these features.

Feedback

ATI welcomes feedback regarding this review module. Please provide comments to: comments@atitesting.com.

TABLE OF CONTENTS

APPENDIX **Active Learning Templates**

UNIT 1   Foundations of Nursing Care for Adult Clients

CHAPTERS

› Health, Wellness, and Illness
› Emergency Nursing Principles and Management

NCLEX® CONNECTIONS

When reviewing the chapters in this unit, keep in mind the relevant sections of the NCLEX® outline, in particular:

Client Needs: Health Promotion and Maintenance

› Relevant topics/tasks include:
  » Health and Wellness
    › Encourage client participation in appropriate behavior modification programs related to health and wellness.
  » Health Promotion/Disease Prevention
    › Educate the client on actions to promote/maintain health and prevent disease.

Client Needs: Physiological Adaptation

› Relevant topics/tasks include:
  » Hemodynamics
    › Intervene to improve the client's cardiovascular status.
  » Illness Management
    › Educate the client about managing illness.
  » Medical Emergencies
    › Apply knowledge of pathophysiology when caring for a client experiencing a medical emergency.

chapter 1

Overview

- Health and wellness combine to form a state of optimal physical functioning and a feeling of emotional and social contentment. Wellness involves the ability to adapt emotionally and physically to a changing state of health and environment.
- Illness is an altered level of functioning in response to a disease process. Disease is a condition that results in the physiological alteration in the composition of the body.
- Nurses must understand the variables affecting health/wellness/illness and how they relate to a client's health needs.

Health and Wellness

- Aspects of health and wellness
  - Physical – able to perform activities of daily living
  - Emotional – adapts to stress; expresses and identifies emotions
  - Social – interacts successfully with others
  - Intellectual – effectively learns and disseminates information
  - Spiritual – adopts a belief that provides meaning to life
  - Occupational – balances occupational activities with leisure time
  - Environmental – creates measures to improve standards of living and quality of life
- A client's state of health and wellness is constantly changing and adapting to a continually fluctuating external and internal environment.
  - The external environment
    - Social – crime versus safety, poverty versus prosperity, and peace versus social unrest
    - Physical – access to health care, sanitation, availability of clean water, and geographic isolation
  - The internal environment includes cumulative life experiences, cultural and spiritual beliefs, age, developmental stage, gender, and other support systems.
- The level of health and wellness is unique to each individual and relative to the individual's usual state of functioning.
  - For example: A person with rheumatoid arthritis who has a strong support system and positive outlook may consider himself healthy while functioning at an optimal level with minimal pain.

- Variables
  - Modifiable – may be changed, such as smoking, nutrition, health education and awareness, sexual practices, and exercise
  - Nonmodifiable – cannot be changed, such as gender, age, developmental level, and genetic traits
- Desired outcomes are to obtain and maintain optimal state of wellness and function.
  - Can be achieved through health education and positive action (smoking cessation, weight loss, seeking health care)
- The health/wellness/illness continuum is an assessment tool that is used to measure the level of wellness to premature death.
  - It may be useful as an assessment guide or tool to set goals and find ways to improve the client's state of health or to have the client return to a previous state of health, which may include an illness within optimal wellness. The health care professional can assist the client to see at what point he is at on the continuum and seek ways to move toward optimal wellness.
  - At the center of the continuum is the client's normal state of health.
  - Level of health/illness is assessed in comparison to the norm for a client.
  - The range of health to illness runs from optimal wellness to severe illness.
  - The degree of wellness is relative to the usual state of wellness for a client and is achieved through awareness, education, and personal growth.

Illness

- Response to disease may be influenced by:
  - Degree of physical changes as a result of the disease process.
  - Perceptions by self and others of the disease, which may be influenced by various reliable and unreliable sources of information, such as friends, magazines, TV, and the Internet.
  - Cultural values and beliefs.
  - Denial or fear of illness.
  - Social demands, time constraints, economic resources, and health care access.

Nursing Care

- Evaluate the health needs of a client and create strategies to meet those needs.
- Health/wellness assessment
  - Physical assessment
  - Evaluating health perceptions
  - Identifying risks to health/wellness
  - Identifying access to health care

- Identifying obstacles to compliance and adherence
  - Perceptions of illness – awareness of the severity of the illness
  - Confidence in the provider
  - Belief in the prescribed therapy
    - For example: A person who has had a negative experience with the health care system may not trust the health care provider and may not follow the advice and comply with the treatment prescribed.
  - Availability of support systems
  - Family role and function (One member of the family may be the family caregiver and may neglect caring for him/herself.)
  - Financial restrictions that may lead to prioritized health care (e.g., prescription medication or a parent may seek medical care for children, but not for herself)
- Health promotion and disease prevention – Use health education and awareness to reduce risk factors and promote health care.
- Interventions:
  - Provide resources to strengthen coping abilities.
  - Encourage use of support systems during times of illness and stress.
  - Identify obstacles to health and wellness and create strategies to reduce these obstacles.
  - Identify ways to reduce health risks and improve compliance.
  - Develop health education methods to improve health awareness and reduce health risks.

APPLICATION EXERCISES

1. A nurse is caring for an older adult client who has a new diagnosis of type 2 diabetes mellitus and reports difficulty following the diet and remembering to take the prescribed medication. Which of the following are appropriate actions by the nurse? (Select all that apply.)

_____ A. Ask the dietitian to assist with meal planning.

_____ B. Contact the client's support system.

_____ C. Assess for age-related cognitive awareness.

_____ D. Encourage the use of a daily medication dispenser.

_____ E. Provide educational materials for home use.

2. A nurse in a health care clinic is evaluating the level of wellness for clients using the health/wellness/illness continuum tool. Which of the following clients is measured at the center of the continuum?

A. A college student who has influenza

B. An older adult who is newly diagnosed with type 2 diabetes mellitus

C. A new mother who has a urinary tract infection

D. A young male who has a long history of well-controlled rheumatoid arthritis

3. A nurse is evaluating clients at a health fair for modifiable variables affecting health and wellness. The nurse identifies which of the following as a modifiable variable? (Select all that apply.)

_____ A. A male who smokes on social occasions

_____ B. A female with a BMI of 28

_____ C. An adult with alopecia

_____ D. An adolescent with Trisomy 21

_____ E. An infant with reflux

4. A nurse is caring for a client who was just told she has breast cancer and the nurse evaluates the client's response. Which of the following statements by the client reflects a lack of understanding of an illness perspective?

    A. "I have no family history of breast cancer."

    B. "I need a second opinion; there is no lump."

    C. "I am glad we live in the city near several large hospitals."

    D. "I will schedule surgery next week, over the holidays."

5. A nurse in a clinic is caring for a client who continues to smoke despite numerous attempts to quit and has a family history of cardiovascular disease. Which nursing interventions should the nurse use to meet the health needs of this client? Use the ATI Active Learning Template: Basic Concept to complete this item. Include the following:

    A. Related Content: One statement.

    B. Underlying Principles: One statement.

    C. Nursing Interventions: Minimum of 4.

APPLICATION EXERCISES KEY

1. A. **CORRECT:** The nurse provides resources to strengthen coping abilities by asking the dietician to assist the client with meal planning. This will improve client compliance.

   B. **CORRECT:** The nurse can contact members of the client's support system and encourage the client to use this support during times of illness and stress to improve compliance.

   C. INCORRECT: Assessing the client for age-related cognitive awareness is important but it is not an appropriate intervention that enhances the client's compliance.

   D. **CORRECT:** The nurse encourages the use of a daily medication dispenser to reduce health risks and improve medication compliance by the client.

   E. **CORRECT:** The nurse provides educational materials to the client to improve health awareness and reduce health risks after discharge.

    NCLEX® Connection: Physiological Adaptations, Alterations in Body Systems

2. A. INCORRECT: The client who has influenza is measured on the continuum by the level of health to illness in comparison to the norm for the client.

   B. INCORRECT: The client who is newly diagnosed with type 2 diabetes mellitus is measured by the level of health to illness in comparison to the norm for the client.

   C. INCORRECT: The client who has a urinary tract infection is measured on the continuum by the level of health to illness in comparison to the norm for the client.

   D. **CORRECT:** The client with well-controlled rheumatoid arthritis is measured at the center of the continuum, which is the client's normal state of health.

    NCLEX® Connection: Health Promotion and Maintenance, Developmental Stages and Transitions

3. A. **CORRECT:** The nurse identifies smoking as a modifiable variable that can be changed by providing the client with educational materials and information on smoking cessation.

   B. **CORRECT:** The nurse identifies a BMI of 28 as a modifiable variable that can be changed by providing the client with educational materials and information on weight reduction and exercising.

   C. INCORRECT: The nurse identifies alopecia as a nonmodifiable variable because alopecia is a genetic disorder.

   D. INCORRECT: The nurse identifies Trisomy 21 as a nonmodifiable variable because Trisomy 21 is genetic in origin.

   E. **CORRECT:** The nurse identifies reflux as a modifiable variable that may be changed by providing the parents with step-by-step educational information about the infant's treatment.

    NCLEX® Connection: Health Promotion and Maintenance, Health Promotion/Disease Prevention

4. A. INCORRECT: The client's lack of a family history of cancer may influence the client's response to the new diagnosis, but it does not reflect a lack of understanding of an illness perspective.

    B. **CORRECT:** The client's statement of denial reflects a lack of understanding of the illness perspective and may influence the client's acceptance of the diagnosis.

    C. INCORRECT: Access to health care resources may influence the client's response to the new diagnosis, but it does not reflect a lack of understanding of an illness perspective.

    D. INCORRECT: Time constraints may influence a client's response to the diagnosis, but it does not reflect a lack of understanding of an illness perspective.

    Ⓝ NCLEX® Connection: Health Promotion and Maintenance, Health Screening

5. *Using the ATI Active Learning Template: Basic Concept*

    A. Related Content
    - Identifying obstacles for compliance and adherence

    B. Underlying Principles
    - Health promotion and disease prevention are influenced by many factors that a nurse should address for a client success.

    C. Nursing Interventions
    - Provide the client with resources to strengthen coping abilities.
    - Encourage use of support systems (e.g. family, support group).
    - Identify ways to improve compliance.
    - Develop health education methods to reduce health risks.
    - Identify the client's obstacles to health and wellness.
    - Create strategies to reduce the client's obstacles.

    Ⓝ NCLEX® Connection: Health Promotion and Maintenance, High Risk Behaviors

chapter 2

Overview

- Emergency nursing principles are the guidelines that nurses follow to assess and manage emergency situations for a client or multiple clients.
- Nurses must have the ability to identify emergent situations and rapidly assess and intervene when life-threatening conditions exist. Emergent conditions are common to all nursing environments.
- Emergency nursing principles
  - Triage
  - Primary survey
  - Airway/cervical spine, breathing, circulation, disability, and exposure/environmental control (ABCDE)
  - Poisoning
  - Rapid response team
  - Cardiac emergency
  - Postresuscitation

Triage

- Triage Under Usual Conditions
  - Triage ensures that clients with the highest acuity needs receive the quickest treatment.
  - Clients are categorized based upon their acuity. One example of a triage framework is the Emergent, Urgent, Nonurgent model.
    - Emergent triage indicates a life- or limb-threatening situation.
    - Urgent triage indicates that the client should be treated soon, but that the risk posed is not life-threatening.
    - Nonurgent cases generally can wait for an extended length of time without serious deterioration.
  - Emergency departments often implement the five-level system to include resuscitation and minor level.
    - Resuscitation triage requires immediate treatment to prevent death.
    - Minor triage is a non-life-threatening condition requiring simple evaluation and management of care.

- Triage Under Mass Casualty Conditions
  - This is a military form of triage that is implemented with a focus of achieving the greatest good for the greatest number of people.
  - Classifications
    - Emergent or Class I – identified with a red tag indicating an immediate threat to life
    - Urgent or Class II – identified with a yellow tag indicating major injuries that require immediate treatment
    - Nonurgent or Class III – identified with a green tag indicating minor injuries that do not require immediate treatment
    - Expectant or Class IV – identified with a black tag indicating one who is expected and allowed to die

Primary Survey

- A primary survey is a rapid assessment of life-threatening conditions. It should take no longer than 60 seconds to perform.
- The primary survey should be completed systematically so conditions are not missed.
- Standard precautions – gloves, gowns, eye protection, face masks, and shoe covers – must be worn to prevent contamination with bodily fluids.
- The ABCDE principle guides the primary survey.

ABCDE Principle

- Emergency care is guided by the principle of ABCDE.
- Airway/Cervical Spine
  - This is the most important step in performing the primary survey. If a patent airway is not established, subsequent steps of the primary survey are futile.
  - If a client is awake and responsive, the airway is open.
  - If a client's ability to maintain an airway is lost, it is important to inspect for blood, broken teeth, vomitus, or other foreign materials in the airway that may cause an obstruction.
  - If the client is unresponsive without suspicion of trauma, the airway should be opened with a head-tilt/chin-lift maneuver.
    - This is the most effective manual technique for opening a client's airway.
    - Do NOT perform this technique on clients who have a potential cervical spine injury.
    - The nurse should assume a position at the head of the client, place one hand on his forehead, and place the other hand on his chin. His head should be tilted while his chin is lifted superiorly. This lifts the tongue out of the laryngopharynx and provides for a patent airway.
  - If the client is unresponsive with suspicion of trauma, the airway should be opened with a modified jaw thrust maneuver.
    - The nurse should assume a position at the head of the client, and place both hands on either side of the client's head. Locate the connection between the maxilla and the mandible. Lift the jaw superiorly while maintaining alignment of the cervical spine.

- ○ Once the airway is opened, it should be inspected for blood, broken teeth, vomitus, and secretions. If present, obstructions should be cleared with suction or a finger-sweep method.

- ○ The open airway can be maintained with airway adjuncts, such as an oropharyngeal or nasopharyngeal airway.

- ○ A bag valve mask with a 100% oxygen source is indicated for clients who need additional support during resuscitation.

- ○ A nonrebreather mask with 100% oxygen source is indicated for clients who are spontaneously breathing.

- • Breathing

  - ○ Once a patent airway is achieved, the presence and effectiveness of breathing should be assessed.

  - ○ Breathing assessment

    - ▪ Auscultation of breath sounds

    - ▪ Observation of chest expansion and respiratory effort

    - ▪ Notation of rate and depth of respirations

    - ▪ Identification of chest trauma

    - ▪ Note position of trachea

    - ▪ Assess for jugular vein distention

  - ○ If a client is not breathing or is breathing inadequately, manual ventilation should be performed by a bag valve mask with supplemental oxygen or mouth-to-mask ventilation until a bag valve mask can be obtained.

- • Circulation

  - ○ Once adequate ventilation is accomplished, circulation is assessed.

  - ○ Nurses should assess heart rate, blood pressure, and perfusion.

  - ○ Nurses should consider cardiac arrest, myocardial dysfunction, and hemorrhage as precursors to shock and leading to ineffective circulation.

  - ○ Interventions geared toward restoring effective circulation

    - ▪ CPR

    - ▪ Assess for external bleeding

      - ▫ Hemorrhage control (Apply direct pressure to visible, significant external bleeding; apply a tourniquet distal to a traumatic amputation.)

    - ▪ Obtain IV access using large-bore IV catheters inserted into the antecubital fossa of both arms.

    - ▪ Infuse IV fluids such as lactated Ringer's and 0.9% normal saline and/or blood.

  - ○ Shock may develop if circulation is compromised. Shock is the body's response to inadequate tissue perfusion and oxygenation. It manifests with an increased heart rate and hypotension and may result in tissue ischemia and necrosis.

  - ○ Interventions to alleviate shock include the following:

    - ▪ Administer oxygen.

    - ▪ Apply pressure to bleeding that is obvious.

    - ▪ Elevate the client's feet to shunt blood to vital organs.

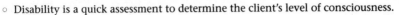

- Administer IV fluids and blood products as ordered.
- Monitor vital signs.
- Remain with the client and provide reassurance and support for anxiety.
- Disability
  - Disability is a quick assessment to determine the client's level of consciousness.

  - The AVPU mnemonic is useful.
    - A – Alert
    - V – Responsive to voice
    - P – Responsive to pain
    - U – Unresponsive
  - The Glasgow Coma Scale is another widely used method.
    - Components include eye opening, verbal response, and motor response.
    - A low score of 3 indicates a client who is totally unresponsive, and a high score of 15 indicates a client who is within normal limits neurologically.
  - Neurologic assessment must be repeated at frequent intervals to assure immediate response to any change.
- Exposure
  - The nurse removes the client's clothing for a complete physical assessment.
  - Clothing is always removed during a resuscitation situation to assess for additional injuries or those related to chemical and thermal burns involving the clothing.
  - Evidence such as clothing, bullets, drugs, or weapons may need to be preserved.
  - Hypothermia is a primary concern for clients. Hypothermia leads to vasoconstriction and impaired oxygenation.
  - To prevent hypothermia:
    - Remove wet clothing from the client.
    - Cover the client with blankets or use a heat lamp to provide additional warmth.
    - Increase the temperature of the room.
    - Infuse warmed IV fluids as prescribed.

Poisoning

- Poisoning is exposure to a toxic agent.
  - Medications, illicit drugs, ingestion of a toxic agent
  - Environmental (e.g., pollutants, snake and spider bites)
- Poisoning is considered a medical emergency and requires rapid management therapy.
  - Obtain a client history to identify the toxic agent.
  - Implement supportive care.
  - Determine type of poison.

- ○ Prevent further absorption of the toxin.
- ○ Extract or remove the poison.
- ○ Administer antidotes when necessary.
  - ▪ Antivenin based on the type and severity of a snake bite within 4 to 12 hr.
  - ▪ For ingested poison, three procedures are available: activated charcoal, gastric lavage and aspiration, or whole-bowel irrigation. (Syrup of ipecac is no longer recommended.)
- • Interventions to manage the clinical status of the client exposed to or who ingested a toxic agent:
  - ○ Provide measures for respiratory support (oxygen, airway management, mechanical ventilation).
  - ○ Monitor compromised circulation (resulting from excess perspiration, vomiting, diarrhea).
  - ○ Restore fluids with IV fluid therapy.
  - ○ Monitor blood pressure, cardiac monitoring, ECG.
  - ○ Assess for tissue edema every 15 to 30 min if bitten by a snake or spider.
  - ○ Administer opioid medications for pain due to snake or spider bite.
  - ○ Monitor ABGs, blood glucose levels, coagulation profile.
  - ○ Administer IV diazepam (Valium) if seizures occur.
  - ○ Reverse heroin and other opiate toxicity with naloxone (Narcan).
  - ○ Implement dialysis and an exchange blood transfusion as a nonpharmacologic technique to remove toxic agents.

Rapid Response Team

- • A group of critical care experts (ICU nurse, respiratory therapist, a critical care provider, hospitalist).
- • Responds to an emergency call from nurses or family members when a client exhibits indications of a rapid decline.
- • Provides early recognition and response before a respiratory or cardiac arrest or stroke occurs.
- • Policies and procedures are established in a health care setting.
- • Training for personnel is provided about criteria for calling for assistance when a client's condition changes toward a crisis situation.
- • SBAR (Situation, Background, Assessment, Recommendation) communication techniques are used for contacting the team and documentation of event.
- • Implement follow-up, education, and sharing of stories for participants after the call.
- • Discuss information to identify system failures (not recognizing a crisis, lack of adequate communication, failure in the plan of care).
- • Retrieve more information from www.ihi.org.

Cardiac Emergency

- Cardiac arrest – the sudden cessation of cardiac function caused most commonly by ventricular fibrillation or ventricular asystole.
- Ventricular fibrillation (VF) – a fluttering of the ventricles causing loss of consciousness, pulselessness, and no breathing. This requires collaborative care to defibrillate immediately using ACLS protocol.
- Pulseless ventricular tachycardia (VT) – an irritable firing of ectopic ventricular beats at a rate of 140 to 180/min. The client over time will become unconscious and deteriorate into VF.
- Ventricular asystole – a complete absence of electrical activity and ventricular movement of the heart. The client is in complete cardiac arrest and requires implementation of BLS and ACLS protocol.
- Pulseless electrical activity (PEA) – a rhythm that appears to have electrical activity but is not sufficient to stimulate effective cardiac contractions and requires implementation of BLS and ACLS protocol.

Emergency Nurse Certifications

- Basic Life Support (BLS), Advanced Cardiac Life Support (ACLS), and Pediatric Advanced Life Support (PALS) are certifications required for nurses practicing in United States emergency departments.
  - BLS involves a hands-on approach for assessment and management to restore airway, breathing, and circulation.
  - ACLS builds on the BLS assessment and management skills to include advanced concepts.
    - Cardiac monitoring for special resuscitation rhythms
    - Invasive airway management
    - Electrical therapies (defibrillation or cardioversion)
    - Obtaining IV access
    - Administration of IV antidysrhythmic medications
    - Management of the client postresuscitation
  - PALS is built on the BLS protocol for neonatal and pediatric assessment and management skills to include advanced concepts for resuscitation of children.
- Certification courses are based on evidence-based practice management theory, and the basic concepts and techniques for cardiopulmonary resuscitation (CPR).
- Retrieve the current BLS and ACLS guidelines from the American Heart Association (AHA) at www.americanheart.org.
- AHA ACLS Protocols
  - VF or pulseless ventricular tachycardia (VT)
    - Initiate the CPR components of BLS.
    - Defibrillate according to BLS guidelines.
    - Establish IV access.
    - Administer IV antidysrhythmic medications according to ACLS guidelines.
      - Epinephrine 1 mg IV push every 3 to 5 min or vasopressin 40 units IV x 1 only (switch to epinephrine if no response)

- Consider the following medications:
  - Amiodarone hydrochloride (Cordarone)
  - Lidocaine hydrochloride (Xylocaine)
  - Magnesium sulfate
  - Procainamide (Procan SR)
  - Vasopressin
- Pulseless electrical activity (PEA)
  - Initiate the CPR components of BLS.
  - Defibrillate according to BLS guidelines.
  - Establish IV access.
  - Consider the most common causes.
    - 5 H's
      - Hypovolemia
      - Hypoxia
      - Hydrogen ion accumulation, resulting in acidosis
      - Hyperkalemia or hypokalemia
      - Hypothermia
    - 5 T's
      - Toxins (accidental or deliberate drug overdose)
      - Tamponade (cardiac)
      - Tension pneumothorax
      - Thrombosis (coronary)
      - Thrombosis (pulmonary)
  - Administer epinephrine 1 mg IV push every 3 to 5 min.
- Asystole
  - Initiate the CPR components of BLS.
  - Defibrillate according to BLS guidelines.
  - Establish IV access.
  - Begin immediate transcutaneous pacing, if possible.
  - Give epinephrine 1 mg push every 3 to 5 min.
  - Consider ceasing resuscitation if asystole persists.

Postresuscitation

- Pharmacological Management
  - Medication therapy following a successful cardiac arrest includes IV medications that cause a catecholamine adrenergic agonist's effect.
  - Catecholamine adrenergic agonists cannot be taken by the oral route, do not cross the blood-brain barrier, and have a short duration of action.
  - Medications include epinephrine, dopamine, and dobutamine.
  - These medications respond to an identifiable receptor and produce specific effects.

RECEPTORS	SITE/RESPONSE
Alpha$_1$	› Activation of receptors in arterioles of skin, viscera and mucous membranes, and veins lead to vasoconstriction.
Beta$_1$	› Heart stimulation leads to increased heart rate, increased myocardial contractility, and increased rate of conduction through the atrioventricular (AV) node. › Activation of receptors in the kidney leads to the release of renin.
Beta$_2$	› Activation of receptors in the arterioles of the heart, lungs, and skeletal muscles lead to vasodilation. › Bronchial stimulation leads to bronchodilation. › Activation of receptors in uterine smooth muscle causes relaxation. › Activation of receptors in the liver cause glycogenolysis. › Skeletal muscle receptor activation leads to muscle contraction.
Dopamine	› Activation of receptors in the kidney cause the renal blood vessels to dilate.

Emergency Medications

RECEPTORS	PHARMACOLOGICAL ACTION	THERAPEUTIC USE
Epinephrine (Adrenaline)		
› Alpha$_1$	› Vasoconstriction	› Slows absorption of local anesthetics › Manages superficial bleeding › Reduces congestion of nasal mucosa › Increases blood pressure
› Beta$_1$	› Increases heart rate › Strengthens myocardial contractility › Increases rate of conduction through the AV node	› Treatment of AV block and cardiac arrest
› Beta$_2$	› Bronchodilation	› Asthma
Dopamine (Intropin)		
› Dopamine	› Low dose – dopamine (2 to 5 mcg/kg/min) › Renal blood vessel dilation	› Shock › Heart failure
› Beta$_1$	› Moderate dose – dopamine (5 to 10 mcg/kg/min) › Renal blood vessel dilation › Increases: » Heart rate » Myocardial contractility » Rate of conduction through the AV node » Blood pressure	
› Beta$_1$ › Alpha$_1$	› High dose – dopamine (>10 mcg/kg/min) › Renal blood vessel vasoconstriction › Increases: » Heart rate » Myocardial contractility » Rate of conduction through the AV node » Blood pressure » Vasoconstriction	
Dobutamine (Dobutrex)		
› Beta$_1$	› Increases: » Heart rate » Myocardial contractility » Rate of conduction through the AV node	› Heart failure

Adverse Effects: Nursing Interventions and Client Education

ADVERSE EFFECTS	NURSING INTERVENTIONS/CLIENT EDUCATION
Epinephrine (Adrenaline)	
› Vasoconstriction from activation of alpha$_1$ receptors in the heart can lead to hypertensive crisis.	› Provide the client with continuous cardiac monitoring. › Report changes in the client's vital signs to the provider.
› Beta$_1$ receptor activation in the heart can cause dysrhythmias. Beta$_1$ receptor activation also increases the workload of the heart and oxygen demand, leading to the development of angina.	› Provide the client with continuous cardiac monitoring. › Monitor the client closely for dysrhythmias, change in heart rate, and chest pain. › Monitor for hyperglycemia in diabetic clients. › Notify the provider if the client experiences dysrhythmias, an elevated heart rate, or chest pain, and treat per protocol.
Dopamine (Intropin)	
› Beta$_1$ receptor activation in the heart can cause dysrhythmias. Beta$_1$ receptor activation also increases the workload of the heart and oxygen demand, leading to the development of angina.	› Provide the client with continuous cardiac monitoring. › Monitor the client closely for dysrhythmias, change in heart rate, and chest pain. › Notify the provider of signs of dysrhythmias, elevated heart rate, and chest pain, and treat per protocol. › Monitor for urinary output less than 30 mL/hr. › Do not confuse dopamine with dobutamine.
› Necrosis can occur from extravasation of high doses of dopamine.	› Infuse dopamine into the central line. Monitor the IV site carefully. › Discontinue the infusion at first sign of irritation.
Dobutamine (Dobutrex)	
› Increased heart rate	› Provide the client with continuous cardiac monitoring. › Report changes in the client's vital signs to the provider. › Monitor for urinary output less than 30 mL/hr. › Do not confuse dobutamine with dopamine.

Contraindications/Precautions

- Pregnancy Risk Category C – epinephrine, dopamine, dobutamine
- These medications are contraindicated in clients who have tachydysrhythmias and ventricular fibrillation.
- Use cautiously in clients who have hyperthyroidism, angina, history of myocardial infarction, hypertension, and diabetes mellitus.

Medication/Food Interactions: Nursing Interventions and Client Education

MEDICATION/FOOD INTERACTIONS	NURSING INTERVENTIONS/CLIENT EDUCATION
› MAOIs promote the release of norepinephrine from sympathetic nerves and thereby prolong and intensify the effects of epinephrine and can cause a hypertensive crisis.	› Avoid the use of MAOIs in clients who are receiving epinephrine.
› Tricyclic antidepressants block the uptake of epinephrine, which will prolong and intensify the effects of epinephrine.	› Clients taking these medications concurrently may need a lower dose of epinephrine.
› General anesthetics can cause the heart to become hypersensitive to the effects of epinephrine, which leads to dysrhythmias.	› Perform continuous ECG monitoring of the client. › Notify the provider if the client experiences chest pain, dysrhythmias, or an elevated heart rate.
› Alpha-adrenergic blocking agents, such as phentolamine, block action at alpha receptors. They do not interact with dobutamine.	› Phentolamine may be used to treat epinephrine toxicity.
› Beta-adrenergic blocking agents, such as propranolol, block the action at beta receptors.	› Propranolol may be used to treat chest pain and dysrhythmias.
› Diuretics promote the beneficial effect of dopamine.	› Monitor the client for therapeutic effects.

Nursing Interventions and Client Education

- Medications must be administered by continuous IV infusion.
- Use IV pump to control infusion.
- Titrate dosage based on the client's blood pressure (BP) response and/or heart rate response (these drugs affect heart rate and BP).

- Stop the infusion at the first sign of infiltration. Extravasation can be treated with a local injection of an alpha-adrenergic blocking agent, such as phentolamine.
- Assess/monitor the client for chest pain. Notify the provider if the client experiences chest pain.
- Provide continuous ECG monitoring. Notify the provider if the client experiences tachycardia or dysrhythmias.

APPLICATION EXERCISES

1. A nurse on a medical-surgical unit is caring for a group of clients. The nurse should notify the rapid response team for which of the following clients?

   A. Client who has an ulceration of the right heel whose blood glucose is 300 mg/dL

   B. Client who reports right calf pain and shortness of breath

   C. Client who has blood on a pressure dressing in the femoral area following a cardiac catheterization

   D. Client who has dark red coloration of left toes and absent pedal pulse

2. A nurse is caring for a client who has ingested a toxic agent. Which of the following actions should the nurse plan to take? (Select all that apply.)

   _____ A. Induce vomiting.

   _____ B. Instill activated charcoal.

   _____ C. Perform a gastric lavage with aspiration.

   _____ D. Administer syrup of ipecac.

   _____ E. Complete a whole-bowel irrigation.

3. A nurse in the emergency department is caring for a client who fell through the ice on a pond and is unresponsive and breathing slowly. Which of the following are appropriate actions by the nurse? (Select all that apply.)

   _____ A. Remove wet clothing.

   _____ B. Maintain normal room temperature.

   _____ C. Apply warm blankets.

   _____ D. Apply a heat lamp.

   _____ E. Infuse warmed IV fluids.

4. A nurse in the emergency department is assessing a client who is unresponsive. The client's partner states, "He was pulling weeds in the yard and dropped to the ground." Which of the following techniques should the nurse use to open the client's airway?

   A. Head-tilt, chin-lift

   B. Modified jaw thrust

   C. Hyperextension of the head

   D. Flexion of the head

5. A nurse is reviewing the common emergency management protocol for clients during a cardiac emergency. Which of the following is an appropriate action by the nurse?

    A. Administer IV dobutamine (Dobutrex).

    B. Administer IV dopamine (Intropin).

    C. Administer IV epinephrine (Adrenaline).

    D. Administer IV atropine (Atropair).

6. A nurse in the emergency department (ED) is implementing triage using the five-level system. Use the ATI Active Learning Template: Basic Concept to complete this item.

    A. Related Content: Describe the five levels of the ED triage system.

    B. Underlying Principles: Define each of the five triage levels.

    C. Nursing Interventions: Describe a client who meets the criteria for each of the five triage levels.

APPLICATION EXERCISES KEY

1.   A. INCORRECT: The nurse should notify the provider. The situation does not indicate the beginning of a rapid decline in the client's condition.

B. **CORRECT:** Using the priority-setting framework of urgent vs. nonurgent, the nurse should call the rapid response team because the signs indicate the beginning of a rapid decline in the client's condition.

C. INCORRECT: This assessment does not indicate the beginning of a rapid decline in the client's condition at this time. The nurse should reassess the client and notify the provider if the bleeding increases.

D. INCORRECT: The nurse should notify the provider. The situation does not indicate the beginning of a rapid decline in the client's condition.

   Ⓝ NCLEX® Connection: Physiological Adaptations, Medical Emergencies

2.   A. INCORRECT: Vomiting places the client at risk for aspiration.

B. **CORRECT:** This is an appropriate action by the nurse because activated charcoal adsorbs drugs and other chemicals, and the charcoal does not pass into the bloodstream.

C. **CORRECT:** This is an appropriate action by the nurse because gastric lavage with aspiration removes the toxic substance when the instilled fluid is suctioned from the gastrointestinal tract.

D. INCORRECT: Administering syrup of ipecac induces vomiting, which increases the client's risk for aspiration.

E. **CORRECT:** This is an appropriate action by the nurse because a solution of polyethylene glycol with electrolytes is ingested or administered through an nasogastric tube, and the toxic agent and solution are eliminated from the bowels.

   Ⓝ NCLEX® Connection: Physiological Adaptations, Medical Emergencies

3.   A. **CORRECT:** This is an appropriate action by the nurse because the body temperature can rise more quickly when heat is applied to dry skin.

B. INCORRECT: The nurse should increase the temperature of the room to help return the client to a normal body temperature.

C. **CORRECT:** This is an appropriate action by the nurse because the client's body temperature can rise more quickly when warm blankets are applied.

D. **CORRECT:** This is an appropriate action by the nurse because the client's body temperature can rise more quickly when a heat lamp is safely applied.

E. **CORRECT:** This is an appropriate action by the nurse because the client's body temperature can rise more quickly when warmed IV fluids are infused.

   Ⓝ NCLEX® Connection: Physiological Adaptations, Medical Emergencies

4.   A. **CORRECT:** The nurse should open the client's airway by the head-tilt, chin-lift because the client is unresponsive without suspicion of trauma.

   B. INCORRECT: The nurse should not open the client's airway with the modified jaw thrust because this method is used for a client who is unresponsive with suspected traumatic neck injury.

   C. INCORRECT: The nurse should not open the client's airway with hyperextension of the head because hyperextension of the head can close off the airway and cause injury.

   D. INCORRECT: The nurse should not open the client's airway with flexion of the head because flexion of the head does not open the airway.

    NCLEX® Connection: Physiological Adaptations, Medical Emergencies

5.   A. INCORRECT: Administering dobutamine during a cardiac emergency is not an appropriate action by the nurse because this medication is administered during the postresuscitation phase.

   B. INCORRECT: Administering dopamine during a cardiac emergency is not an appropriate action by the nurse because this medication is administered during the postresuscitation phase.

   C. **CORRECT:** Administering epinephrine during a cardiac emergency is an appropriate action by the nurse because it increases heart rate, improves cardiac output, and promotes bronchodilation.

   D. INCORRECT: Administering atropine during a cardiac emergency is not appropriate action by the nurse because the medication is no longer used during the crisis period.

    NCLEX® Connection: Physiological Adaptations, Medical Emergencies

6. *Using the ATI Active Learning Template: Basic Concept*

A. Related Content

- Resuscitation
- Emergent
- Urgent
- Nonurgent
- Minor

B. Underlying Principles

- Resuscitation – The client needs immediate treatment to prevent death.
- Emergent – The client requires time sensitive treatment that is a life or limb-threatening situation.
- Urgent – The client requires treatment but the situation is not life-threatening.
- Nonurgent – The client is able to wait for a period of time without immediate treatment.
- Minor – The client requires simple evaluation and minor management of care.

C. Nursing Interventions

- Resuscitation: A client who is experiencing a myocardial infarction, stroke, pulmonary emboli, or drug overdose.
- Emergent: A client who has sustained a traumatic amputation, head or neck injury, snake or spider bite.
- Urgent – A client who has a kidney stone, gallbladder colic, or fracture.
- Nonurgent – A client who has a bladder infection, laceration, or infected toe.
- Minor – A client who has an upper respiratory infection, minor cut, or backache.

Ⓝ NCLEX® Connection: Physiological Adaptations, Medical Emergencies

Nursing Care of Clients with Neurosensory Disorders

SECTIONS

› Diagnostic and Therapeutic Procedures
› Central Nervous System Disorders
› Sensory Disorders
› Neurologic Emergencies

NCLEX® CONNECTIONS

When reviewing the chapters in this unit, keep in mind the relevant sections of the NCLEX® outline, in particular:

Client Needs: Basic Care and Comfort	Client Needs: Pharmacological and Parenteral Therapies	Client Needs: Reduction of Risk Potential
› Relevant topics/tasks include: » Nonpharmacological Comfort Interventions › Assess the client's need for pain management and intervene as needed using non-pharmacological comfort measures. » Mobility/Immobility › Assess the client for mobility, gait, strength, and motor skills. » Nutrition and Oral Hydration › Assess the client's ability to eat.	› Relevant topics/tasks include: » Adverse Effects/ Contraindications/Side Effects/Interactions › Provide information to the client on common side effects/adverse effects/ potential interactions of medications and when to notify the provider. » Expected Actions/Outcomes › Evaluate the client's use of medications over time. » Pharmacological Pain Management › Use pharmacological measures for pain management, as needed.	› Relevant topics/tasks include: » Diagnostic Tests › Compare the client's diagnostic findings with pretest results. » Potential for Complications of Diagnostic Tests/ Treatments/Procedures › Intervene to prevent potential neurological complications. » Therapeutic Procedures › Apply knowledge of related nursing procedures and psychomotor skills when caring for clients undergoing therapeutic procedures.

chapter 3

Overview

- Neurologic assessment and diagnostic procedures are used to evaluate neurologic function by testing indicators such as mental status, motor functioning, electrical activity, and intracranial pressure.
- Neurologic assessment and diagnostic procedures that nurses should be knowledgeable about include:
  - Cerebral angiogram
  - Cerebral computed tomography (CT) scan
  - Electroencephalography (EEG)
  - Glasgow Coma Scale (GCS)
  - Intracranial pressure (ICP) monitoring
  - Lumbar puncture (spinal tap)
  - Magnetic resonance imaging (MRI) scan
  - Positron emission tomography (PET) and single-photon emission computed tomography (SPECT) scans
  - Radiography (x-ray)

Cerebral Angiogram

- A cerebral angiogram provides visualization of the cerebral blood vessels.
  - Digital subtraction angiography "subtracts" the bones and tissues from the images, providing x-rays with only the vessels apparent.
  - The procedure detects defects, narrowing, or obstruction of arteries or blood vessels in brain.
  - The procedure is performed within the radiology department because iodine-based contrast dye is injected into an artery during the procedure.
- Indications
  - A cerebral angiogram is used to assess the blood flow to and within the brain, identify aneurysms, and define the vascularity of tumors (useful for surgical planning). It may also be used therapeutically to inject medications that treat blood clots or to administer chemotherapy.

- Preprocedure
  - If the client is pregnant, a determination of the risks to the fetus versus the benefits of the information obtained by this procedure should be made.
  - Nursing Actions
    - Instruct the client to refrain from consuming food or fluids for 4 to 6 hr prior to the procedure.
    - Assess for allergy to shellfish or iodine, which would require the use of a different contrast media. Any history of bleeding or taking anticoagulant medication requires additional considerations and additional monitoring to ensure clotting after the procedure.
    - Assess BUN and serum creatinine to determine kidney's ability to excrete the dye.
    - Ensure that the client is not wearing any jewelry.
    - A mild sedative for relaxation is occasionally administered prior to and during the procedure and vital signs are continuously monitored during the procedure.
  - Client Education
    - Instruct the client about the importance of not moving during the procedure and about the need to keep the head immobilized.
    - Instruct the client to void immediately before the test.
    - Instruct the client about a metallic taste in the mouth, a warm sensation over the face, jaw, tongue, lips, and behind the eyes from the dye injected during procedure.
- Intraprocedure
  - The client is placed on a radiography table, where the client's head is secured.
  - A catheter is placed into an artery (usually in the groin or the neck), dye is injected, and x-ray pictures are taken.
  - Once all pictures are taken, the catheter is removed and a arterial closure device is used or pressure is held over the artery to control bleeding by thrombus formation sealing the artery.
- Postprocedure
  - Nursing Actions
    - The area is closely monitored to ensure that clotting occurs.
    - Movements are restricted depending on the type of procedure used to seal the artery to prevent rebleeding at the catheter site.
- Complications
  - Bleeding
    - There is a risk for bleeding or hematoma formation at the entry site.
    - Nursing Actions
      - Check the insertion site frequently.
      - Check the affected extremity distal to the puncture site for adequate circulation (e.g., color, temperature, pulses, and capillary refill).
      - If bleeding does occur, apply pressure over the artery and notify the provider.

Cerebral Computed Tomography (CT) Scan

- A CT scan provides cross-sectional images of the cranial cavity. A contrast media may be used to enhance the images.

- Indications

  ○ A CT scan can be used to identify tumors and infarctions, detect abnormalities, monitor response to treatment, and guide needles used for biopsies.

- Preprocedure

  ○ If the client is pregnant, a determination of the risks to the fetus versus the benefits of the information obtained by this procedure should be made.

  ○ Nursing Actions

    ▪ If contrast media and/or sedation is expected:

      □ Instruct the client to refrain from consuming food or fluids for at least 4 hr prior to the procedure.

      □ Assess for allergy to shellfish or iodine, which would require the use of a different contrast media.

      □ Assess renal function (BUN and creatinine), because contrast media is excreted by the kidneys.

    ▪ Because this procedure is performed with the client in a supine position, placing pillows in the small of the client's back may assist in preventing back pain. The head must be secured to prevent unnecessary movement during the procedure.

    ▪ Ensure that the client's jewelry is removed prior to this procedure. In general, clients wear a hospital gown to prevent any metals from interfering with the x-rays.

- Intraprocedure

  ○ The client must lie supine with the head stabilized during the procedure.

  ○ Although CT scanning is painless, sedation may be provided.

- Postprocedure

  ○ Nursing Actions

    ▪ There is no follow-up care associated with a CT scan.

    ▪ If contrast media is injected, monitor for allergic reaction and changes in kidney function.

    ▪ If sedation is administered, monitor the client until stable.

Electroencephalography (EEG)

- This noninvasive procedure assesses the electrical activity of the brain and is used to determine if there are abnormalities in brain wave patterns.

- Indications

  ○ EEGs are most commonly performed to identify and determine seizure activity, but they are also useful for detecting sleep disorders and behavioral changes.

- Preprocedure
  - Nursing Actions
    - Review medications with the provider to determine if they should be continued prior to this procedure.
  - Client Education
    - Instruct the client to wash his hair prior to the procedure and eliminate all oils, gels, and sprays.
    - If indicated, instruct the client to be sleep-deprived because this provides cranial stress, increasing the possibility of abnormal electrical activity, such as seizure potentials, occurring during the procedure.
      - Increased electrical activity may be stimulated with exposure to bright flashing lights, or by requesting the client to hyperventilate for 3 to 4 minutes.
- Intraprocedure
  - The procedure generally takes 1 hr.
  - There are no risks associated with this procedure.
  - With the client resting in a chair or lying in bed, small electrodes are placed on the scalp and connected to a brain wave machine or computer.
  - Electrical signals produced by the brain are recorded by the machine or computer in the form of wavy lines. This documents brain activity.
  - Notations are made when stimuli are presented or when sleep occurs. (Flashes of light or pictures may be used during the procedure to assess the client's response to stimuli.)
  - An EEG provides information about the ability of the brain to function and highlights areas of abnormality.
- Postprocedure
  - Client Education
    - Instruct the client that normal activities may be resumed.

Glasgow Coma Scale (GCS)

- This assessment concentrates on neurologic function and is useful to determine the level of consciousness and monitor response to treatment. The GCS is reported as a number, which allows health care providers to immediately determine if neurologic changes have occurred.
- Indications
  - GCS scores are helpful in determining changes in the level of consciousness for clients with head injuries, space occupying lesions or cerebral infarctions, and encephalitis. This is important because complications related to neurologic injuries may occur rapidly and require immediate treatment.

- Interpretation of Findings
  - The best possible GCS score is 15. In general, total scores of the GCS correlate with the degree or level of coma.
  - Less than 8 – Associated with severe head injury and coma
  - 9 to 12 – Indicate a moderate head injury
  - Greater than 13 – Reflect minor head trauma
- Procedure
  - The GCS is calculated by using appropriate stimuli (a painful stimulus may be necessary) and then assessing the client's response in three areas.
    - Eye opening (E) – The best eye response, with responses ranging from 4 to 1
      - 4 = Eye opening occurs spontaneously.
      - 3 = Eye opening occurs secondary to voice.
      - 2 = Eye opening occurs secondary to pain.
      - 1 = Eye opening does not occur.
    - Verbal (V) – The best verbal response, with responses ranging from 5 to 1
      - 5 = Conversation is coherent and oriented.
      - 4 = Conversation is incoherent and disoriented.
      - 3 = Words are spoken, but inappropriately.
      - 2 = Sounds are made, but no words.
      - 1 = Vocalization does not occur.
    - Motor (M) – The best motor response, with responses ranging from 6 to 1
      - 6 = Commands are followed.
      - 5 = Local reaction to pain occurs.
      - 4 = There is a general withdrawal to pain.
      - 3 = Decorticate posture (adduction of arms, flexion of elbows and wrists) is present.
      - 2 = Decerebrate posture (abduction of arms, extension of elbows and wrists) is present.
      - 1 = Motor response does not occur.
  - Responses within each subscale are added, with the total score quantitatively describing the client's level of consciousness. E + V + M = Total GCS
    - In critical situations, where head injury is present and close monitoring is required, subscale results may also be documented. Thus, a GCS may be reported as either a single number, indicating the sum of the subscales (3 to 15), or as 3 numbers, one from each subscale result, and the total (E3 V3 M4 = GCS 13). This allows providers to determine specific neurologic function.
    - Intubation limits the ability to use GCS summed scores. If intubation is present, the GCS may be reported as two scores, with modification noted. This is generally reported as "GCS 5t" (with the t representing the intubation tube).

Intracranial Pressure (ICP) Monitoring

- An ICP monitor is a device inserted into the cranial cavity that records pressure and is connected to a monitor that shows a picture of the pressure waveforms.

  ○ Monitoring ICP facilitates continual assessment and is more precise than vague clinical manifestations.

  ○ The insertion procedure is always performed by a neurosurgeon in the operating room, emergency department, or critical care unit. This procedure is rarely used unless the client is comatose, so there is minimal need for pain medication and preprocedural teaching.

- Three Basic Types of ICP Monitoring Systems

  ○ Intraventricular catheter (also called a ventriculostomy)

    ▪ A fluid-filled catheter is inserted into the anterior horn of the lateral ventricles (most often on the right side) through a burr hole. The catheter is connected to a sterile drainage system with a three-way stopcock that allows simultaneous monitoring of pressures by a transducer connected to a bedside monitor and drainage of CSF.

  ○ Subarachnoid screw or bolt

    ▪ A special hollow, threaded screw or bolt is placed into the subarachnoid space through a twist-drill burr hole in the front of the skull, behind the hairline. The bolt is connected by fluid-filled tubing to a transducer leveled at the approximate location of the lateral ventricles.

  ○ Epidural or subdural sensor

    ▪ A fiber-optic sensor is inserted into the epidural space through a burr hole. The fiber-optic device measures changes in the amount of light reflected from a pressure-sensitive diaphragm in the catheter tip. The cable is connected to a precalibrated monitor that displays the numerical value of ICP. This method of monitoring is noninvasive because the device does not penetrate the dura.

- Indications

  ○ ICP monitoring is useful for early identification and treatment of increased intracranial pressure. Clients who are comatose and/or have GCS scores of 8 are candidates for ICP monitoring.

  ○ Client Presentation

    ▪ Symptoms of increased ICP include severe headache, deteriorating level of consciousness, restlessness, irritability, dilated or pinpoint pupils, slowness to react, alteration in breathing pattern (Cheyne Stokes respirations, central neurologic hyperventilation, apnea), deterioration in motor function, and abnormal posturing (decerebrate, decorticate, flaccidity).

- Interpretation of Findings

  ○ Normal ICP is 10 to 15 mm Hg. Persistent elevation of ICP extinguishes cerebral circulation, which will result in brain death if not treated urgently.

- Preprocedure

  ○ The head is shaved around the insertion location. The site is then cleansed with an antibacterial solution.

- Intraprocedure
  - ○ Local anesthetic can be used to numb the area if the client's GCS indicates some level of consciousness (GCS 8 to 11).
  - ○ Insertion and care of any ICP monitoring device requires surgical aseptic technique to reduce the risk for CNS infection.
- Postprocedure
  - ○ Nursing Actions
    - Maintain system integrity at all times. There is a risk of serious, life-threatening infection.
    - Inspect the insertion site at least every 24 hr for redness, swelling, and drainage. Change the sterile dressing covering the access site per facility protocol.
    - ICP monitoring equipment must be balanced and recalibrated per facility protocols.
    - After the insertion procedure, observe ICP waveforms, noting the pattern of waveforms and monitoring for increased ICP (a sustained elevation of pressure above 15 mm Hg).
    - Assess the client's clinical status and monitor routine and neurologic vital signs every hour as needed.
- Complications
  - ○ Infection and bleeding
    - The insertion and maintenance of an ICP monitoring system can cause infection and bleeding.
    - Nursing Actions
      - □ Follow strict surgical aseptic technique.
      - □ Perform sterile dressing changes per facility protocol.
      - □ Keep drainage systems closed.
      - □ Limit monitoring to 3 to 5 days.
      - □ Irrigate the system only as needed to maintain patency.

Lumbar Puncture (Spinal Tap)

- A lumbar puncture is a procedure during which a small amount of cerebrospinal fluid (CSF) is withdrawn from the spinal canal and then analyzed to determine its constituents.
- Indications
  - ○ This procedure is used to detect the presence of certain diseases (multiple sclerosis, syphilis, meningitis), infection, and malignancies. A lumbar puncture may also be used to reduce CSF pressure, instill a contrast medium or air for diagnostic tests, or administer medication or chemotherapy directly to spinal fluid.

- Preprocedure
  - ○ The risks versus the benefits of a lumbar puncture should be discussed with the client prior to undertaking this procedure.
    - ▪ A lumbar puncture may be associated with rare but serious complications, especially when performed in the presence of increased ICP (brain herniation).
    - ▪ Lumbar punctures for clients with bleeding disorders or taking anticoagulants may result in bleeding that compresses the spinal cord.
  - ○ Nursing Actions
    - ▪ Ensure that all the client's jewelry has been removed and that the client is wearing only a hospital gown.
    - ▪ Instruct the client to void prior to the procedure.
    - ▪ Clients should be positioned to stretch the spinal canal. This may be done by having the client assume a "cannonball" position while on one side or by having the client stretch over an overbed table if sitting is preferred.
- Intraprocedure
  - ○ The area of the needle insertion is cleansed, and a local anesthesia is injected.
  - ○ This is not a painful procedure; there should be little need for pain or relaxing medication other than the local anesthesia.
  - ○ The needle is inserted and the CSF is withdrawn, after which the needle is removed.
  - ○ A manometer may be used to determine the opening pressure of the spinal cord, which is useful if increased pressure is a consideration.
- Postprocedure
  - ○ CSF is sent to the pathology department for analysis.
  - ○ Nursing Actions
    - ▪ Monitor the puncture site. The client should remain lying for several hours to ensure that the site clots and to decrease the risk of a post-lumbar puncture headache, caused by CSF leakage.
  - ○ Client Education
    - ▪ Once stable, advise the client that normal activities may be resumed.
- Complications
  - ○ CSF leakage
    - ▪ If clotting does not occur to seal the dura puncture site, CSF may leak, resulting in a headache and increasing the potential for infection.
  - ○ Nursing Action
    - ▪ Encourage the client to lie flat in bed, provide fluids for hydration, and administer pain medication.
    - ▪ Prepare the client for an epidural blood patch to seal off the hole in the dura if the headache persists.

Magnetic Resonance Imaging (MRI) Scan

- An MRI scan provides cross-sectional images of the cranial cavity. A contrast media may be used to enhance the images.
  - Unlike CT scans, MRI images are obtained using magnets, thus the consequences associated with radiation are avoided. This makes this procedure safer for women who are pregnant.
  - The use of magnets precludes the ability to scan a client who has an artificial device (pacemakers, surgical clips, intravenous access port). If these are present, shielding may be done to prevent injury.
  - MRI-approved equipment must be used to monitor vital signs and provide ventilator/oxygen assistance to clients undergoing MRI scans.
- Indications
  - MRI scans may be used to detect abnormalities, monitor response to treatment, and guide needles used for biopsies.
  - MRIs are capable of discriminating soft tissue from tumor or bone. This makes the MRI scan more effective at determining tumor size and blood vessel location.
- Preprocedure
  - Nursing Actions
    - Assess for allergy to shellfish or iodine, which would require the use of a different contrast media.
    - Ensure that the client's jewelry is removed prior to this procedure. The client should wear a hospital gown to prevent any metals from interfering with the magnet.
    - If sedation is expected, the client should refrain from food or fluids for 4 to 8 hr prior to the procedure.
    - Determine if the client has a history of claustrophobia and explain the tight space and noise.
    - Question the client about any implants containing metal (e.g., pacemaker, orthopedic joints, artificial heart valves, intrauterine devices, aneurysm clips).
    - Health care providers (and family members) who are in the scanning area while the magnet is on must remove all jewelry, pagers, and phones to prevent damage to themselves or the magnet.
    - Because this procedure is performed with the client in a supine position, placing pillows in the small of the client's back may assist in preventing back pain. The head must be secured to prevent unnecessary movement during the procedure.
- Intraprocedure
  - The client must lie supine with the head stabilized.
  - MRI scanning is noisy, and earplugs or sedation may be provided.
- Postprocedure
  - Nursing Actions
    - No follow-up care is required after an MRI scan.
    - If contrast media is injected, monitor the site to ensure that clotting has occurred and monitor for any signs of an allergic reaction.
    - If sedation is administered, monitor the client until stable.

PET and SPECT Scans

- PET and SPECT scans are nuclear medicine procedures that produce three-dimensional images of the head. These images can be static (depicting vessels) or functional (depicting brain activity).
  - A glucose-based tracer is injected into the blood stream prior to the PET scan. This initiates regional metabolic activity, which is then documented by the PET scanner. A radioisotope is used for SPECT scanning.
  - A CT scan may be performed after a PET/SPECT scan, as this provides information regarding brain activity and pathological location (e.g., brain injury, death, neoplasm).
- Indications
  - A PET/SPECT scan capture of regional metabolic is most useful in determining tumor activity and/or response to treatment. PET/SPECT scans are also able to determine the presence of dementia, indicated by the inability of the brain to respond to the tracer.
- Preprocedure
  - PET/SPECT scans use radiation, thus the risk/benefit consequences to any client who may be pregnant must be discussed.
  - Nursing Actions
    - Assess for a history of diabetes mellitus. While this condition does not preclude a PET/SPECT scan, alterations in the client's medications may be necessary to avoid hyperglycemia or hypoglycemia before and after this procedure.
- Intraprocedure
  - While the pictures are being obtained, the client must lie flat with the head restrained.
  - This procedure is not painful and sedation is rarely necessary.
- Postprocedure
  - Nursing Actions
    - If radioisotopes are used, assess for allergic reaction.
    - There is no follow-up care after a PET/SPECT scans.
    - Because the tracer is glucose based and short acting (less than 2 hr), it is broken down within the body as a sugar, not excreted.

Radiography (X-Ray)

- An x-ray uses electromagnetic radiation to capture images of the internal structures of an individual.
  - A structure's image is light or dark relative to the amount of radiation the tissue absorbs. The image is recorded on a radiograph, which is a black and white image that is held up to light for visualization. Some are recorded digitally and are available immediately.
  - X-rays must be interpreted by a radiologist, who documents the findings.
- Indications
  - X-ray examinations of the skull and spine can reveal fractures, curvatures, bone erosion and dislocation, and possible soft tissue calcification, all of which can damage the nervous system.

- Preprocedure
  - Nursing Actions
    - There is no special preprocedure protocol for x-rays that do not use contrast. X-rays are often the first diagnostic tool used after an injury (rule out cervical fracture in head trauma), and they can be done without any preparation.
    - Determine if female clients are pregnant.
    - Ensure that the client's jewelry is removed and that no clothes cover the area.
  - Client Education
    - Explain that the amount of radiation used in contemporary x-ray machines is very small.
- Intraprocedure
  - Client Education
    - Instruct the client to remain still during the procedure.
- Postprocedure
  - Nursing Actions
    - No postprocedure care is required.
  - Client Education
    - Inform the client when results will be available.

APPLICATION EXERCISES

1. A nurse is caring for a client post-lumbar puncture who reports a throbbing headache when sitting upright for meals. Which of the following are appropriate actions by the nurse? (Select all that apply.)

           A. Use the Glasgow Coma Scale when assessing the client.

  X   B. Assist client to eat meals while lying flat in bed.

  X   C. Administer an opioid medication.

  X   D. Encourage client to increase fluid intake.

           E. Place client in a "cannonball" position.

2. A nurse is caring for a client who experienced a traumatic head injury and has an intraventricular catheter (ventriculostomy) for ICP monitoring. The nurse should monitor the client for which of the following complications related to the ventriculostomy?

A. Headache

(B.) Infection

C. Aphasia

D. Hypertension

3. A nurse is assessing a client for changes in the level of consciousness using the Glasgow Coma Scale. The client opens his eyes when spoken to, speaks incoherently, and moves his extremities when pain is applied. Which of the following is the correct scoring by the nurse using the Scale that indicates the client has a moderate head injury?

A. E2 + V3 + M5 = 10

(B.) E3 + V4 + M4 = 11

C. E4 + V5 + M6 = 15

D. E2 + V2 + M4 = 8

4. A nurse is developing a plan of care for a client who is scheduled for a cerebral angiogram with contrast dye. Which of the following statements by the client should the nurse report to the provider? (Select all that apply.)

_____ A. "I think I may be pregnant."

_____ B. "I take Coumadin."

_____ C. "I take antihypertensive medication."

_____ D. "I am allergic to shrimp."

_____ E. "I am allergic to latex."

5. A nurse is providing education to a client who is to undergo an electroencephalogram (EEG) the next day. Which of the following information should the nurse include in the teaching?

A. "Do not wash your hair the morning of the procedure."

B. "Try to stay awake most of the night prior to the procedure."

C. "The procedure will take approximately 15 minutes."

D. "You will need to lie flat for 4 hours after the procedure."

6. A nurse is developing a plan of care for a client who is scheduled for a magnetic resonance imaging (MRI) scan with contrast dye. What should be included in the plan of care? Use the ATI Active Learning Template: Diagnostic Procedure to complete this item. Include the following:

A. Procedure Name: A definition of this diagnostic test.

B. Nursing Actions: Identify three preprocedure actions, one intraprocedure action, and one postprocedure action.

APPLICATION EXERCISES KEY

1. A. INCORRECT: The Glasgow Coma Scale is used to assess a client's level of consciousness.

    B. **CORRECT:** The prone position may relieve a headache following a lumbar puncture.

    C. **CORRECT:** Administering an opioid medication for a client's report of headache pain is an appropriate action by the nurse.

    D. **CORRECT:** Maintaining positive fluid balance may relieve a headache following a lumbar puncture.

    E. INCORRECT: The cannonball position is appropriate for the client undergoing the procedure of lumbar puncture, but it is not used to relieve a client's headache following the procedure.

     NCLEX® Connection: Reduction of Risk Potential, Potential for Complications of Diagnostic Tests/ Treatments/Procedures

2. A. INCORRECT: The nurse should monitor a client who has increased ICP for a headache, but a headache does not indicate a complication directly related to the ventriculostomy.

    B. **CORRECT:** The nurse should monitor a client with a ventriculostomy for infection, which is a complication. Strict asepsis should be used to avoid this life-threatening condition, which may result in meningitis.

    C. INCORRECT: The nurse should monitor a client who has increased ICP for aphasia related to the head injury, but this not a complication directly related to the ventriculostomy.

    D. INCORRECT: The nurse should monitor a client who has increased ICP for hypertension, but this is not a complication directly related to the ventriculostomy.

     NCLEX® Connection: Reduction of Risk Potential, Potential for Complications of Diagnostic Tests/ Treatments/Procedures

3. A. INCORRECT: The client's score reflects moderate head injury. However, the calculation is incorrect. E2 represents eyes opening secondary to pain, V3 represents verbal response with words spoken inappropriately, and M5 represents motor response to pain with a local reaction.

    B. **CORRECT:** The client's score is calculated correctly, indicating moderate head injury. E3 represents opening eyes secondary to voice stimulation, V4 represents verbal conversation that is incoherent and disoriented, and M4 represents motor response as a general withdrawal to pain.

    C. INCORRECT: The client's score is calculated incorrectly, reflecting a minor head injury. E4 represents eyes opening spontaneously, V5 represents verbal conversation as coherent and oriented, and M6 is a motor response with comments that follow a reaction to pain.

    D. INCORRECT: The client's score is calculated incorrectly, reflecting a severe head injury and coma. E2 represents eyes opening secondary to pain, V2 represents verbal response by the client making sounds but speaking no words, and M4 is a motor response with a general withdrawal to pain.

     NCLEX® Connection: Reduction of Risk Potential, Diagnostic Tests

4. A. **CORRECT:** The client's statement of possible pregnancy should be reported to the provider because the contrast dye may place the fetus at risk.

B. **CORRECT:** The client taking Coumadin should be reported to the provider due to the potential for bleeding following the angiogram.

C. INCORRECT: The nurse understands there is no contraindication related to contrast dye for a client who is taking antihypertensive medication.

D. **CORRECT:** A client's report of allergy to shrimp, which is a shellfish, should be reported to the provider due to a potential allergic reaction to the contrast dye.

E. INCORRECT: There is no contraindication related to contrast dye for a client who has an allergy to latex.

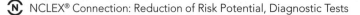 NCLEX® Connection: Reduction of Risk Potential, Diagnostic Tests

5. A. INCORRECT: Teaching should include washing hair on the morning of the procedure to remove oils, gels, and sprays, which may affect the EEG readings.

B. **CORRECT:** The nurse should teach the client to remain awake most of the night to provide cranial stress and increase the possibility of abnormal electrical activity.

C. INCORRECT: The nurse should inform the client that the procedure will take approximately 1 hr.

D. INCORRECT: The nurse should teach the client that normal activity can resume immediately following the procedure.

NCLEX® Connection: Reduction of Risk Potential, Therapeutic Procedures

6. *Using the ATI Active Learning Template: Diagnostic Procedure*

A. Procedure Name
- Magnetic Resonance Imaging (MRI) Scan relies on magnetic field to take multiple images of the body.

B. Nursing Actions
- Preprocedure
  - Remove all client jewelry.
  - Determine if the client has claustrophobia.
  - Question the client concerning implants containing metal.
  - Question the client regarding allergies.
- Intraprocedure
  - Stabilize the client's head
- Postprocedure
  - Monitor for allergic reaction to the contrast dye during the MRI.

NCLEX® Connection: Reduction of Risk Potential, Diagnostic Tests

UNIT 2 NURSING CARE OF CLIENTS WITH NEUROSENSORY DISORDERS
SECTION: DIAGNOSTIC AND THERAPEUTIC PROCEDURES

CHAPTER 4 Pain Management

Overview

- Effective pain management includes the use of pharmacological and nonpharmacological pain management therapies. Invasive therapies such as nerve ablation may be appropriate for intractable cancer-related pain.

- Clients have a right to adequate assessment and management of pain. Nurses are accountable for the assessment of pain. The nurse's role is that of an advocate and educator for effective pain management.

- Nurses have a priority responsibility for the continual assessment of the client's pain level and to provide individualized interventions. They should assess the effectiveness of the interventions 30 to 60 min after implementation.

- Assessment challenges may occur with clients who are cognitively impaired or on a ventilator.

- Undertreatment of pain is a serious health care problem. Consequences of undertreatment of pain include physiological and psychological components.

  ○ Acute/chronic pain can cause anxiety, fear, and depression.

  ○ Poorly managed acute pain may lead to chronic pain syndrome.

Physiology of Pain

- Transduction is the conversion of painful stimuli to an electrical impulse through peripheral nerve fibers (nociceptors).

- Transmission occurs as the electrical impulse travels along the nerve fibers, where neurotransmitters regulate it.

- The pain threshold is the point at which a person feels pain.

- Pain tolerance is the amount of pain a person is willing to bear.

SUBSTANCES THAT INCREASE PAIN TRANSMISSION AND CAUSE AN INFLAMMATORY RESPONSE		SUBSTANCES THAT DECREASE PAIN TRANSMISSION AND PRODUCE ANALGESIA
› Substance P	› Bradykinin	› Serotonin
› Prostaglandins	› Histamine	› Endorphins

- Perception or awareness of pain occurs in various areas of the brain, with influences from thought and emotional processes.

- Modulation occurs in the spinal cord, causing muscles to contract reflexively, moving the body away from painful stimuli.

Pain Categories

ACUTE PAIN

› Acute pain is protective, temporary, usually self-limiting, and resolves with tissue healing.
› Physiological responses (sympathetic nervous system) are fight-or-flight responses (tachycardia, hypertension, anxiety, diaphoresis, muscle tension).
› Behavioral responses include grimacing, moaning, flinching, and guarding.
› Interventions include treatment of the underlying problem.

CHRONIC PAIN

› Chronic pain is not protective. It is ongoing or recurs frequently, lasting longer than 6 months and persisting beyond tissue healing.
› Physiological responses do not usually alter vital signs, but clients may have depression, fatigue, and a decreased level of functioning.
› Psychosocial implications may lead to disability.
› Chronic pain may not have a known cause, and it may not respond to interventions.
› Management aims at symptomatic relief.
› Chronic pain can be malignant or nonmalignant.

NOCICEPTIVE PAIN

› Nociceptive pain arises from damage to or inflammation of tissue other than that of the peripheral and central nervous systems.
› It is usually throbbing, aching, and localized.
› This pain typically responds to opioids and nonopioid medications.
› Types of nociceptive pain include:
  » Somatic – in bones, joints, muscles, skin, or connective tissues.
  » Visceral – in internal organs such as the stomach or intestines. It can cause referred pain in other body locations separate from the stimulus.
  » Cutaneous – in the skin or subcutaneous tissue.

NEUROPATHIC PAIN

› Neuropathic pain arises from abnormal or damaged pain nerves.
› It includes phantom limb pain, pain below the level of a spinal cord injury, and diabetic neuropathy.
› Neuropathic pain is usually intense, shooting, burning, or described as "pins and needles."
› This pain typically responds to adjuvant medications (antidepressants, antispasmodic agents, skeletal muscle relaxants).

- Risk factors for undertreatment of pain include the following:
  - Cultural and societal attitudes
  - Lack of knowledge
  - Fear of addiction
  - Exaggerated fear of respiratory depression

- Populations at risk for undertreatment of pain include the following:
  - Infants
  - Children
  - Older adults
  - Clients who have substance use disorder
- Causes of acute and chronic pain include the following:
  - Trauma
  - Surgery
  - Cancer (tumor invasion, nerve compression, bone metastases, associated infections, immobility)
  - Arthritis
  - Fibromyalgia
  - Neuropathy
  - Diagnostic or treatment procedures (injection, intubation, radiation)
- Factors that affect the pain experience include the following:
  - Age
    - Infants cannot verbalize or understand their pain.
    - Older adult clients may have multiple pathologies that cause pain and limit function.
  - Fatigue, which can increase sensitivity to pain.
  - Genetic sensitivity, which can increase or decrease pain tolerance.
  - Cognitive function.
    - Clients who are cognitively impaired may not be able to report pain or report it accurately.
  - Prior experiences, which can increase or decrease sensitivity depending on whether clients obtained adequate relief.
  - Anxiety and fear, which can increase sensitivity to pain.
  - Support systems that are present and can decrease sensitivity to pain.
  - Culture, which may influence how clients express pain or the meaning they give to pain.

Assessment/Data Collection

- According to noted pain experts Margo McCaffery and Chris Pasero, pain is whatever the person experiencing it says it is, and it exists whenever the person says it does. The client's report of pain is the most reliable diagnostic measure of pain. Self-report using standardized pain scales is useful for clients over the age of 7 years. Specialized pain scales are available for use with younger children.
- Assess and document pain (the fifth vital sign) frequently.
- Use a symptom analysis to obtain subjective data.

DESCRIPTION	QUESTIONS
› Use anatomical terminology and landmarks to describe location.	› Ask, "Where is your pain? Does it radiate anywhere else?" Ask clients to point to the location.
› Quality refers to how the pain feels: sharp, dull, aching, burning, stabbing, pounding, throbbing, shooting, gnawing, tender, heavy, tight, tiring, exhausting, sickening, terrifying, torturing, nagging, annoying, intense, or unbearable.	› Ask, "What does the pain feel like?" Give more than two choices ("Is the pain throbbing, burning, or stabbing?").
› Intensity, strength, and severity are "measures" of the pain. Use visual analog scales (description scale, number rating scale) to measure pain, monitor pain, and evaluate the effectiveness of interventions.	› Ask the following questions: » "How much pain do you have now?" » "What is the worst/best the pain has been?" » "Rate your pain on a scale of 0 to 10."
› Timing – onset, duration, frequency	› Ask the following questions: » "When did it start?" » "How long does it last?" » "How often does it occur?" » "Is it constant or intermittent?"
› Setting – how the pain affects daily life or how activities of daily living (ADLs) affect the pain	› Ask the following questions: » "Where are you when the symptoms occur?" » "What are you doing when the symptoms occur?" » "How does the pain affect your sleep?" » "How does the pain affect your ability to work and do your job?"
› Document associated symptoms (fatigue, depression, nausea, anxiety).	› Ask, "What other symptoms do you have when you are feeling pain?"
› Aggravating/relieving factors	› Ask the following questions: » "What makes the pain better?" » "What makes the pain worse?" » "Are you currently taking any prescription, herbal, or over-the-counter medications?"

M View Video: Pain Assessment

- Objective Data
  - Behaviors complement self-report and assist in pain assessment of nonverbal clients.
    - Facial expressions (grimacing, wrinkled forehead), body movements (restlessness, pacing, guarding)
    - Moaning, crying
    - Decreased attention span
- Blood pressure, pulse, and respiratory rate increase temporarily with acute pain. Eventually, increases in vital signs will stabilize despite the persistence of pain. Therefore, physiologic indicators may not be an accurate measure of pain over time.

Nonpharmacological Pain Management

- Cutaneous (skin) stimulation – transcutaneous electrical nerve stimulation (TENS), heat, cold, therapeutic touch, and massage
  - Interruption of pain pathways
  - Cold for inflammation
  - Heat to increase blood flow and to reduce stiffness
- Distraction
  - Includes ambulation, deep breathing, visitors, television, and music
- Relaxation
  - Includes meditation, yoga, and progressive muscle relaxation
- Imagery
  - Focusing on a pleasant thought to divert focus
  - Requires an ability to concentrate
- Acupuncture – vibration or electrical stimulation via tiny needles inserted into the skin and subcutaneous tissues at specific points
- Reduction of pain stimuli in the environment
- Elevation of edematous extremities to promote venous return and decrease swelling

Pharmacological Interventions

- Analgesics are the mainstay for relieving pain. The three classes of analgesics are nonopioids, opioids, and adjuvants.
- Nonopioid analgesics (acetaminophen, nonsteroidal anti-inflammatory drugs [NSAIDs], including salicylates) are appropriate for treating mild to moderate pain.
  - Be aware of the hepatotoxic effects of acetaminophen. Clients who have a healthy liver should take no more than 4 g/day. Make sure clients are aware of opioids that contain acetaminophen, such as hydrocodone bitartrate 5 mg/acetaminophen 500 mg (Vicodin).
  - Monitor for salicylism (tinnitus, vertigo, decreased hearing acuity).
  - Prevent gastric upset by administering the medication with food or antacids.
  - Monitor for bleeding with long-term NSAID use.

- Opioid analgesics, such as morphine sulfate, fentanyl (Sublimaze), and codeine, are appropriate for treating moderate to severe pain (postoperative pain, myocardial infarction pain, cancer pain).
  - Managing acute severe pain with short-term (24 to 48 hr) around-the-clock administration of opioids is preferable to following a PRN schedule.
  - The parenteral route is best for immediate, short-term relief of acute pain. The oral route is better for chronic, nonfluctuating pain.
  - Consistent timing and dosing of opioid administration provide consistent pain control.
  - It is essential to monitor and intervene for adverse effects of opioid use.
    - Constipation – Use a preventative approach (monitoring of bowel movements, fluids, fiber intake, exercise, stool softeners, stimulant laxatives, enemas).
    - Orthostatic hypotension – Advise clients to sit or lie down if symptoms of light-headedness or dizziness occur. Instruct clients to avoid sudden changes in position by slowly moving from a lying to a sitting or standing position. Provide assistance with ambulation.
    - Urinary retention – Monitor I&O, assess for distention, administer bethanechol (Urecholine), and catheterize.
    - Nausea/vomiting – Administer antiemetics, advise clients to lie still and move slowly, and eliminate odors.
    - Sedation – Monitor level of consciousness and take safety precautions. Sedation usually precedes respiratory depression.
    - Respiratory depression – Monitor respiratory rate prior to and following administration of opioids (especially for clients who are opioid-naïve). Initial treatment of respiratory depression and sedation is generally a reduction in opioid dose. If necessary, slowly administer diluted naloxone (Narcan) to reverse opioid effects.
- Adjuvant analgesics enhance the effects of nonopioids, help alleviate other symptoms that aggravate pain (depression, seizures, inflammation), and are useful for treating neuropathic pain.
  - Adjuvant medications include:
    - Anticonvulsants: carbamazepine (Tegretol)
    - Antianxiety agents: diazepam (Valium)
    - Tricyclic antidepressants: amitriptyline (Elavil)
    - Antihistamine: hydroxyzine (Vistaril)
    - Glucocorticoids: dexamethasone (Decadron)
    - Antiemetics: ondansetron (Zofran)
- Patient-controlled analgesia (PCA) is a medication delivery system that allows clients to self-administer safe doses of opioids.
  - Small, frequent dosing ensures consistent plasma levels.
  - Clients have less lag time between identified need and delivery of medication, which increases their sense of control and may decrease the amount of medication they need.
  - Morphine and hydromorphone (Dilaudid) are typical opioids for PCA delivery.
  - Clients should let the nurse know if using the pump does not control the pain.
  - To prevent inadvertent overdosing, the client is the only person who should push the PCA button.

- Other strategies for effective pain management include the following:

  ○ Taking a proactive approach by giving analgesics before pain becomes too severe. It takes less medication to prevent pain than to treat pain.

  ○ Instructing clients to report developing or recurrent pain and not wait until pain is severe (for PRN pain medication).

  ○ Explaining misconceptions about pain.

  ○ Helping clients reduce fear and anxiety.

  ○ Creating a treatment plan that includes both nonpharmacological and pharmacological pain-relief measures.

- Strategies specific for relieving chronic pain include the above interventions, plus:

  ○ Administering long-acting or controlled-release opioid analgesics (including the transdermal route).

  ○ Administering analgesics around the clock rather than PRN.

Complications and Nursing Implications

- Undertreatment of pain is a serious complication and may lead to increased anxiety with acute pain and depression with chronic pain. Assess clients for pain frequently, and intervene as appropriate.

- Sedation, respiratory depression, and coma can occur as a result of overdosing. Sedation always precedes respiratory depression.

  ○ Identify high-risk clients (older adult clients, clients who are opioid-naïve).

  ○ Carefully titrate doses while closely monitoring respiratory status.

  ○ Stop the opioid and give the antagonist naloxone (Narcan) if respiratory rate is below 8/min and shallow, or the client is difficult to arouse.

  ○ Identify the cause of sedation.

  ○ Use a sedation scale in addition to a pain rating scale to assess pain, especially when administering opioids.

APPLICATION EXERCISES

1. A nurse is assessing the pain level of a client who has come to the emergency department reporting severe abdominal pain. The nurse asks the client whether he has nausea and has been vomiting. The nurse is assessing which of the following?

    A. Presence of associated symptoms

    B. Location of the pain

    C. Pain quality

    D. Aggravating and relieving factors

2. A nurse is assessing a client who is reporting pain despite analgesia. The nurse can best assess the intensity of the client's pain by

    A. asking what precipitates the pain.

    B. questioning the client about the location of the pain.

    C. offering the client a pain scale to measure his pain.

    D. using open-ended questions to identify the sensation.

3. A nurse is obtaining a history from a client who has pain. The nurse's guiding principle throughout this process should be that

    A. some clients exaggerate their level of pain.

    B. pain must have an identifiable source to justify the use of opioids.

    C. objective data are essential in assessing pain.

    D. pain is whatever the client says it is.

4. A nurse is caring for a client who is receiving morphine via a patient-controlled analgesia (PCA) infusion device after abdominal surgery. Which of the following statements indicates that the client knows how to use the device?

    A. "I'll wait to use the device until it's absolutely necessary."

    B. "I'll be careful about pushing the button so I don't get an overdose."

    C. "I should tell the nurse if the pain doesn't stop after I use this device."

    D. "I will ask my son to push the dose button when I am sleeping."

5. A nurse is monitoring a client who is receiving opioid analgesia for adverse effects of the medication. Which of the following effects should the nurse anticipate? (Select all that apply.)

_____ A. Urinary incontinence

_____ B. Diarrhea

_____ C. Bradypnea

_____ D. Orthostatic hypotension

_____ E. Nausea

6. A nurse on a medical-surgical unit is reviewing with a group of nursing students the various types of pain the clients on the unit have. Use the ATI Active Learning Template: Basic Concept to complete this item. Include under Underlying Principles: list the four different types of pain, their definitions, and characteristics.

APPLICATION EXERCISES KEY

1. A. **CORRECT:** Nausea and vomiting are common symptoms clients have when they are in pain.

   B. INCORRECT: The location of the pain is where the client feels the pain.

   C. INCORRECT: Pain quality is what the pain feels like, such as throbbing and dull.

   D. INCORRECT: Aggravating and relieving factors are what might make the pain better or worse.

   Ⓝ NCLEX® Connection: Pharmacological and Parenteral Therapies, Pharmacological Pain Management

2. A. INCORRECT: Assessment of pain triggers will provide valuable information to help select pain-control interventions, but it does not provide information about the intensity of pain.

   B. INCORRECT: Identification of the location of the client's pain provides valuable information to help select pain-control interventions, but it does not provide information about the intensity of pain.

   C. **CORRECT:** A pain scale can help the client measure the amount of pain he has and its intensity.

   D. INCORRECT: Asking open-ended questions is important in pain assessment, but it does not provide for consistent quantification of pain intensity.

   Ⓝ NCLEX® Connection: Pharmacological and Parenteral Therapies, Pharmacological Pain Management

3. A. INCORRECT: A misconception about pain is that clients exaggerate their pain level.

   B. INCORRECT: Clients can have pain without being able to identify the source.

   C. INCORRECT: Objective data are not always present when clients have pain.

   D. **CORRECT:** Pain is a subjective experience, and the client is the best source of information about it.

   Ⓝ NCLEX® Connection: Pharmacological and Parenteral Therapies, Pharmacological Pain Management

4. A. INCORRECT: The client may use the device when he begins to feel pain. It will help prevent unnecessary worsening of the pain and more doses of analgesia to relieve it.

    B. INCORRECT: A feature of PCA devices is the timing control or lockout mechanism, which enforces a preset minimum interval between medication doses. This safety feature is one means of preventing an overdose because the client cannot self-administer another dose of medication until that time interval has passed.

    C. **CORRECT:** PCA is a method of delivering pain medication through an electronic infusion device that allows the client to self-administer pain medication on an as-needed basis. If the client is not achieving adequate pain control, he should let the nurse know so that she can initiate a reevaluation of the client's pain management plan.

    D. INCORRECT: The client is the only one who should operate the PCA pump. In situations where the client is not able to do so, the provider may authorize a nurse or a family member to operate the pump.

    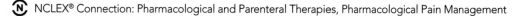 NCLEX® Connection: Pharmacological and Parenteral Therapies, Pharmacological Pain Management

5. A. INCORRECT: Urinary retention, not urinary incontinence, is a common adverse effect of opioid analgesia.

    B. INCORRECT: Constipation, not diarrhea, is a common adverse effect of opioid analgesia.

    C. **CORRECT:** Respiratory depression, which causes respiratory rates to drop to dangerously low levels, is a common adverse effect of opioid analgesia.

    D. **CORRECT:** Dizziness or light-headedness when changing positions is a common adverse effect of opioid analgesia.

    E. **CORRECT:** Nausea and vomiting are common adverse effects of opioid analgesia.

    NCLEX® Connection: Pharmacological and Parenteral Therapies, Pharmacological Pain Management

6. *Using the ATI Active Learning Template: Basic Concept*
   - Underlying Principles
     - Acute Pain
       - Definition: protective, temporary, usually self-limiting, resolves with tissue healing
       - Physiological responses: tachycardia, hypertension, anxiety, diaphoresis, muscle tension
       - Behavioral responses: grimacing, moaning, flinching, guarding
     - Chronic Pain
       - Definition: not protective; ongoing or recurs frequently, lasts longer than 6 months, persists beyond tissue healing, can be malignant or nonmalignant
       - Physiological responses: no change in vital signs, depression, fatigue, decreased level of functioning, disability
     - Nociceptive Pain
       - Definition: arises from damage to or inflammation of tissue other than that of the peripheral and central nervous systems, is usually throbbing, aching, localized; pain typically responds to opioids and nonopioid medications
       - Types of nociceptive pain:
       - Somatic – in bones, joints, muscles, skin, or connective tissues
       - Visceral – in internal organs such as the stomach or intestines, can cause referred pain
       - Cutaneous – in skin or subcutaneous tissue
     - Neuropathic Pain
       - Definition: arises from abnormal or damaged pain nerves (phantom limb pain, pain below the level of a spinal cord injury, diabetic neuropathy), usually intense, shooting, burning, or "pins and needles"
       - Physiological responses to adjuvant medications (antidepressants, antispasmodic agents, skeletal muscle relaxants).

   Ⓝ NCLEX® Connection: Pharmacological and Parenteral Therapies, Pharmacological Pain Management

chapter 5

Overview

- Meningitis is an inflammation of the meninges, which are the membranes that protect the brain and spinal cord.

- Viral, or aseptic, meningitis is the most common form of meningitis and commonly resolves without treatment.

- Fungal meningitis is common in clients who have AIDS.

- Bacterial, or septic, meningitis is a contagious infection with a high mortality rate. The prognosis depends on how quickly care is initiated.

- There are three vaccines for different pathogens that cause bacterial meningitis. One is available for high-risk populations, such as residential college students.

Health Promotion and Disease Prevention

- *Haemophilus influenzae* type b (Hib) vaccine – Ensure infants receive vaccine for bacterial meningitis on schedule.

- Pneumococcal polysaccharide vaccine (PPSV) – Vaccinate adults who are immunocompromised, who have a chronic disease, who smoke cigarettes, or who live in a long-term care facility. CDC guidelines should be followed for revaccination. Give one dose to adults older than 65 years of age who have not previously been vaccinated nor have history of disease.

- Meningococcal vaccine (MCV4) (*Neisseria meningitidis*) – Ensure that adolescents receive the vaccine on schedule and prior to living in a residential setting in college. Individuals in other communal living conditions (military) also should be immunized.

  - Client Education

    - Use an insect repellent when risk of being bitten by a mosquito exists.

Assessment

- Risk Factors

  - Viral meningitis

    - Viral illnesses such as the mumps, measles, herpes, and arboviruses (West Nile).

    - There is no vaccine against viral meningitis.

  - Fungal Meningitis

    - Fulminant fungal-based infection of the sinuses are from the organism *Cryptococcus neoformans*.

- ○ Bacterial meningitis
  - Bacterial-based infections, such as otitis media, pneumonia, or sinusitis, in which the infectious micro-organism is *Neisseria meningitidis*, *Streptococcus pneumoniae*, or *Haemophilus influenzae*
  - Immunosuppression
  - Invasive procedures, skull fracture, or penetrating head wound (direct access to cerebrospinal fluid)
  - Overcrowded or communal living conditions
- Subjective Data
  - ○ Excruciating, constant headache
  - ○ Nuchal rigidity (stiff neck)
  - ○ Photophobia (sensitivity to light)
- Objective Data
  - ○ Physical Assessment Findings
    - Fever and chills
    - Nausea and vomiting
    - Altered level of consciousness (confusion, disorientation, lethargy, difficulty arousing, coma)
    - Positive Kernig's sign (resistance and pain with extension of the client's leg from a flexed position)
    - Positive Brudzinski's sign (flexion of extremities occurring with deliberate flexion of the client's neck)

M View Videos
  › Positive Kernig's Sign   › Positive Brudzinski's Sign

- Hyperactive deep tendon reflexes
    - Tachycardia
    - Seizures
    - Red macular rash (meningococcal meningitis)
    - Restlessness, irritability
  - ○ Laboratory Tests
    - Urine, throat, nose, and blood culture and sensitivity
      - □ Perform culture and sensitivity of various body fluids to identify possible infectious bacteria and an appropriate broad-spectrum antibiotic. Not definitive for meningitis but can guide initial selection of antimicrobial.
    - CBC
      - □ Elevated WBC count

○ Diagnostic Procedures

- Cerebrospinal fluid (CSF) analysis

  □ CSF analysis is the most definitive diagnostic procedure. CSF is collected during a lumbar puncture performed by the provider.

  □ Results indicative of meningitis

    ▸ Appearance of CSF – cloudy (bacterial) or clear (viral)

    ▸ Elevated WBC

    ▸ Elevated protein

    ▸ Decreased glucose (bacterial)

    ▸ Elevated CSF pressure

  □ New enteroviral diagnostic test, called counterimmunoelectrophoresis (CIE), can be done on CSF to determine whether infectious agent is viral or protozoa. This diagnostic study is also indicated if the client has received antibiotics before the CSF was collected.

- CT scan and MRI

  □ A CT scan or an MRI may be performed to identify increased intracranial pressure (ICP) and/or an abscess.

Patient-Centered Care

- Nursing Care

  ○ Isolate the client as soon as meningitis is suspected.

  ○ Maintain isolation precautions per hospital policy.

  - This should be droplet precautions, which require a private room. Droplet precautions should continue until antibiotics have been administered for 24 hr and when oral and nasal secretions are no longer infectious.

  - Standard precautions are implemented for all clients who have meningitis. Clients who have bacterial meningitis should remain on droplet precautions continuously.

  ○ Implement fever-reduction measures, such as a cooling blanket, if necessary.

  ○ Report meningococcal infections to the public health department.

  ○ Decrease environmental stimuli.

  - Provide a quiet environment.

  - Minimize exposure to bright light (natural and electric).

  ○ Maintain bed rest with the head of the bed elevated to 30°.

  ○ Monitor the client for increased intracranial pressure (ICP).

  - Tell the client to avoid coughing and sneezing, which increase ICP.

  ○ Maintain client safety, such as seizure precautions.

  ○ Replace fluid and electrolytes as indicated by laboratory values.

  ○ Older adult clients are at an increased risk for secondary complications, such as pneumonia.

- Medications
  - Ceftriaxone (Rocephin) or cefotaxime (Claforan) in combination with vancocin (Vancomycin)
    - Antibiotics given until culture and sensitivity results are available. Effective for bacterial infections.
  - Phenytoin (Dilantin)
    - Anticonvulsants given if ICP increases or client experiences a seizure.
  - Decadron (dexamethasone)
  - Corticosteroid, may improve outcome in adults if given before first dose of antibiotic
  - Acetaminophen (Tylenol), ibuprofen (Motrin)
    - Analgesics for headache and/or fever – nonopioid to avoid masking changes in the level of consciousness.
  - Ciprofloxacin (Cipro), rifampin (Rifadin), or ceftriaxone (Rocephin)
    - Prophylactic antibiotics given to individuals in close contact with the client.

Complications

- Increased ICP (possibly to the point of brain herniation)
  - Meningitis can cause ICP to increase.
  - Nursing Actions
    - Monitor for signs of increasing ICP (decreased level of consciousness, pupillary changes, impaired extraocular movements).
    - Provide interventions to reduce ICP (positioning and avoidance of coughing and straining).
    - Mannitol can be administered via IV.
- Syndrome of inappropriate antidiuretic hormone (SIADH)
  - SIADH can be a complication of meningitis by abnormal stimulation to the hypothalamic area of the brain, causing excess secretion of antidiuretic hormone (vasopressin).
  - Nursing Actions
    - Monitor for signs and symptoms (dilute blood, concentrated urine).
    - Provide interventions, such as the administration of demeclocycline (Declomycin) and restriction of fluid.
- Septic emboli (leading to disseminated intravascular coagulation or cardiovascular accident)
  - Septic emboli can form during meningitis and travel to other parts of the body, particularly the hands and feet.
  - Development of gangrene will necessitate an amputation.

 View Image: Gangrenous Toe

  - Nursing Actions
    - Monitor circulatory status of extremities and coagulation studies.
    - Report any alterations immediately to the provider.

APPLICATION EXERCISES

1. A nurse is assessing a client who reports severe headache and a stiff neck. The nurse's assessment reveals positive Kernig's and Brudzinski's signs. Which of the following actions should the nurse perform first?

    A. Administer antibiotics

    B. Implement droplet isolation precautions

    C. Initiate IV access

    D. Decrease bright lights

2. A nurse is assessing for the presence of Brudzinski's sign in a client who has suspected meningitis. Which of the following are appropriate actions by the nurse when performing this technique? (Select all that apply.)

    _____ A. Place client in supine position.

    _____ B. Flex client's hip and knee.

    _____ C. Place hands behind the client's neck.

    _____ D. Bend client's head toward chest.

    _____ E. Straighten the client's flexed leg at the knee.

3. A nurse is reviewing the health record of a student newly admitted to a university and living in a dormitory. The health record indicates the student requires follow-up immunizations. Which of the following organisms should the nurse plan to vaccinate the student against?

    A. *Streptococcus pneumoniae*

    B. *Neisseria meningitidis*

    C. *Bartonella henselae*

    D. *Rickettsia rickettsii*

4. A nurse is planning care for a client who has meningitis and is at risk for increased intracranial pressure (ICP). Which of the following are appropriate nursing actions? (Select all that apply.)

_____ A. Implement seizure precautions.

_____ B. Perform neurological checks four times a day.

_____ C. Administer morphine for the report of neck and generalized pain.

_____ D. Turn off room lights and television.

_____ E. Monitor for impaired extraocular movements.

_____ F. Encourage the client to cough frequently.

5. A nurse is planning care for a client who has bacterial meningitis. Which of the following actions should the nurse include in the plan of care? (Select all that apply.)

_____ A. Monitor for bradycardia.

_____ B. Provide an emesis basin at the bedside.

_____ C. Administer antipyretic medication as prescribed.

_____ D. Perform a skin assessment.

_____ E. Keep the head of the bed flat.

6. A nurse is reviewing the plan of care for a client who has meningococcal meningitis. What medication can the nurse anticipate the provider will prescribe? Use the ATI Active Learning Template: Systems Disorder to complete this item. Include the following:

A. Description of Disease Process: Define meningococcal meningitis.

B. Medications: Identify four medications, their actions, and the reason for administration.

C. Potential Complications: Describe two complications of meningitis.

APPLICATION EXERCISES KEY

1. A. INCORRECT: The nurse should administer antibiotics as early as possible to stop the micro-organisms from multiplying, but this is not the priority action.

   B. **CORRECT:** When using the urgent vs. nonurgent approach to care, the nurse determines the priority action is to place the client in droplet precaution isolation when meningitis is suspected to prevent spread of the disease to others.

   C. INCORRECT: The nurse should initiate IV access as early as possible to allow IV medication and fluid administration, but this is not the priority action.

   D. INCORRECT: The nurse should decrease bright lights because of the client's sensitivity to light, but this is not the priority action.

    NCLEX® Connection: Safety and Infection Control, Standard Precautions/Transmission-Based Precautions/Surgical Asepsis

2. A. **CORRECT:** The nurse should place the client in supine position when assessing for Brudzinski's sign.

   B. INCORRECT: The nurse should flex the client's hip and knee when assessing for Kernig's sign but not Brudzinski's sign.

   C. **CORRECT:** The nurse should place her hands behind the client's neck when assessing for Brudzinski's sign, in order to flex the client's neck.

   D. **CORRECT:** The nurse should bend the client's head toward the chest when assessing for Brudzinski's sign; it is a positive if the client reports pain.

   E. INCORRECT: The nurse should straighten the client's flexed leg at the knee when assessing for Kernig's sign but not Brudzinski's sign.

    NCLEX® Connection: Reduction of Risk Potential, Diagnostic Tests

3. A. INCORRECT: The nurse should not plan to administer a vaccine against *Streptococcus pneumoniae* because the immunization is not recommended for this population group.

   B. **CORRECT:** The nurse should plan to administer a vaccine against *Neisseria meningitidis* because it is recommended that college students living in close proximity be immunized to against meningitis.

   C. INCORRECT: The nurse should not plan to administer a vaccine against *Bartonella henselae* because there is no vaccine available against this organism.

   D. INCORRECT: The nurse should not plan to administer a vaccine for *Rickettsia rickettsii* because there is no vaccine available against this organism.

   NCLEX® Connection: Safety and Infection Control, Standard Precautions/Transmission-Based Precautions/Surgical Asepsis

4.   A. **CORRECT:** It is an appropriate nursing action to implement seizure precautions for a client who is at risk for increased ICP.

   B. INCORRECT: This is not an appropriate nursing action because the nurse should perform neurological checks at least every 1 to 2 hr for a client who is at risk for ICP.

   C. INCORRECT: This is not an appropriate nursing action because the nurse should avoid administering opioids to a client who is at risk for ICP. Opioids can mask changes in the client's level of consciousness.

   D. **CORRECT:** This is an appropriate nursing action because the bright lights and flickering television can increase neuron stimulation and cause a seizure when a client is at risk for increased ICP.

   E. **CORRECT:** This is an appropriate nursing action because impaired extraocular movement can indicate increased ICP.

   F. INCORRECT: This is not an appropriate nursing action because encouraging the client to cough frequently can cause increased ICP.

   Ⓝ NCLEX® Connection: Physiological Adaptations, Alterations in Body Systems

5.   A. INCORRECT: The nurse should plan to monitor for tachycardia when a client has meningitis.

   B. **CORRECT:** The nurse should provide an emesis basin at the bedside because the client who has meningitis may have nausea and vomiting.

   C. **CORRECT:** The nurse should plan to administer antipyretic medication for fever to a client who has meningitis.

   D. **CORRECT:** The nurse should perform a skin assessment to determine whether the client has a red macular rash associated with meningococcal meningitis.

   E. INCORRECT: The nurse should elevate the head of the client's bed 30° to promote venous drainage from the head and prevent increased intracranial pressure (ICP).

   Ⓝ NCLEX® Connection: Physiological Adaptations, Illness Management

6. *Using the ATI Active Learning Template: Systems Disorder*

A. Description of Disease Process
- Meningococcal meningitis is a bacterial infection that causes an inflammation of the meninges, the membranes that protect the brain and spinal cord. Clients who are in communal living conditions (military, college dormitories) should be immunized.

B. Medications
- Decadron (dexamethasone) – a corticosteroid used to decrease inflammation. Administer before the first dose of antibiotics.
- Ceftriaxone (Rocephin) with vancocin (Vancomycin) – antibiotics administered to treat the infection.
- Acetaminophen (Tylenol) – an antipyretic used to treat a fever.
- Administer phenytoin (Dilantin) – an anticonvulsant given to prevent the client from experiencing a seizure when at risk of ICP.

C. Potential Complications
- Increased intracranial pressure (ICP), which can lead to seizures, coma, and death.
- Syndrome of inappropriate antidiuretic hormone (SIADH), which is due to pressure from inflammation abnormally stimulating the hypothalamus, causing increased secretion of antidiuretic hormone (vasopressin).

Ⓝ NCLEX® Connection: Physiological Adaptations, Illness Management

chapter 6

Overview

- Seizures are abrupt, abnormal, excessive and uncontrolled electrical discharge of neurons within the brain that may cause alterations in the level of consciousness and/or changes in motor and sensory ability and/or behavior.

- Epilepsy is the term used to define a syndrome characterized by chronic recurring abnormal brain electrical activity.

- The International Classification of Epileptic Seizures uses three broad categories to describe seizures: generalized, partial or focal/local, and unclassified or idiopathic.

Assessment

- Risk Factors

  - Genetic predisposition – Absence seizures are more common in children and tend to occur in families.

  - Acute febrile state – particularly among infants and children younger than the age of 2 years

  - Head trauma – May be early or late onset (up to 9 months) and incidence is increased when the head trauma includes a skull fracture.

  - Cerebral edema – especially when it occurs acutely and seizure activity tends to disappear when the edema is successfully treated

  - Abrupt cessation of antiepileptic drugs (AEDs) – as a rebound activity

  - Infection – if intracranial, a result of increased intracranial pressure; if systemic, a result of the persistent febrile state

  - Metabolic disorder – a result of insufficient or excessive chemicals within the brain such as occurs with hypoglycemia or hyponatremia

  - Exposure to toxins – especially those associated with pesticides, carbon monoxide, and lead poisoning

  - Brain tumor – if benign, seizures caused by the increased bulk associated with the tumor; if malignant, associated with the ability of the brain tissue to function

  - Hypoxia – results in a decreased oxygen level of the brain; necessary for neuronal activity

  - Acute drug and alcohol withdrawal – dehydration that accompanies withdrawal, creating a toxic level of the drug in the body

  - Fluid and electrolyte imbalances – results in abnormal levels of nutrients required for neuronal function

- ○ With older adult clients, increased seizure incidence is associated with cerebrovascular diseases.
- ○ Triggering Factors
  - Increased physical activity
  - Excessive stress
  - Hyperventilation
  - Overwhelming fatigue
  - Acute alcohol ingestion
  - Excessive caffeine intake
  - Exposure to flashing lights
  - Specific chemicals, such as cocaine, aerosols, and inhaling glue products
- Subjective and Objective Data
  - ○ Generalized seizure
    - A generalized seizure is also called a tonic-clonic seizure (previously referred to as a grand mal seizure).
    - It may begin with an aura (alteration in vision, smell, hearing, or emotional feeling).
    - A generalized seizure begins for only a few seconds with a tonic episode (stiffening of muscles) and loss of consciousness.
    - A 1- to 2-min clonic episode (rhythmic jerking of the extremities) follows the tonic episode.
    - Breathing may stop during the tonic phase and become irregular during the clonic phase.
    - Cyanosis can accompany breathing irregularities.
    - Biting of the cheek or tongue can occur during clonic phase.
    - Incontinence can also accompany a seizure.
    - During the postictal phase, a period of confusion and sleepiness follows the seizure.
    - Tonic seizure
      - □ During a seizure, only the tonic phase is experienced.
      - □ The seizure usually lasts 30 seconds to several minutes.
      - □ A loss of consciousness occurs.
      - □ This type of seizure is much less common than a tonic-clonic seizure.
    - Clonic seizure
      - □ Only the clonic phase is experienced.
      - □ The seizure lasts several minutes.
      - □ During this type of seizure, the muscles contract and relax.
      - □ This type of seizure is much less common than a tonic-clonic seizure.
    - Absence seizure
      - □ Absence seizures are most common in children.
      - □ The seizure consists of a loss of consciousness lasting a few seconds.

- □ This type of seizure is associated with blank staring.
- □ Seizure activity also may include unconscious, involuntary behavior associated with eye fluttering, smacking of the lips, and picking at clothes called automatisms.
- □ Baseline neurological function is resumed after seizures, with no apparent sequelae.
  - ▪ Myoclonic seizure
    - □ Myoclonic seizures consist of brief jerking or stiffening of the extremities, which may be symmetrical or asymmetrical.
    - □ This type of seizure lasts for seconds.
  - ▪ Atonic or akinetic seizure
    - □ Atonic or akinetic seizures are characterized by a few seconds in which muscle tone is lost.
    - □ The seizure is followed by a period of confusion.
    - □ The loss of muscle tone frequently results in falling.
- ○ Partial or focal/local seizure
  - ▪ Complex partial seizure
    - □ Complex partial seizures have associated automatisms (behaviors that the client is unaware of, such as lip smacking or picking at clothes).
    - □ The seizure can cause a loss of consciousness for several minutes.
    - □ Amnesia may occur immediately prior to and after the seizure.
  - ▪ Simple partial seizures
    - □ Consciousness is maintained throughout simple partial seizures.
    - □ Seizure activity may consist of unusual sensations, a sense of déjà vu, autonomic abnormalities, such as changes in heart rate and abnormal flushing, unilateral abnormal extremity movements, pain or offensive smell.
- ○ Unclassified or idiopathic seizures do not fit into other categories. These types of seizures account for half of all seizures activities and occur for no known reason.
- ○ Laboratory Tests
  - ▪ Should include alcohol and illicit drug levels, HIV testing, and, if suspected, screen for the presence of excessive toxins.
- ○ Diagnostic Procedures
  - ▪ Electroencephalogram (EEG)
    - □ An EEG records electrical activity and may identify the origin of seizure activity.
  - ▪ Magnetic resonance imaging (MRI), computed tomography imaging (CT)/computed axial tomography (CAT) scan, positron emission tomography (PET) scan, cerebrospinal fluid (CSF) analysis, skull x-ray, can all be used to identify or rule out potential causes of seizures.

Collaborative Care

- Nursing Care

> **M** View Video: Seizure Precautions

- During a seizure:
  - Protect the client's privacy and the client from injury (move furniture away, hold head in lap if on the floor).
  - Position client to provide a patent airway.
  - Be prepared to suction oral secretions.
  - Turn the client to the side to decrease the risk of aspiration.
  - Loosen restrictive clothing.
  - Do not attempt to restrain the client.
  - Do not attempt to open jaw or insert airway during seizure activity (may damage teeth, lips, and tongue). Do not use padded tongue blades.
  - Document onset and duration of seizure and client findings/observations prior to, during, and following the seizure (level of consciousness, apnea, cyanosis, motor activity, incontinence).
- Post seizure:
  - The postictal phase of the seizure episode.
  - Maintain the client in a side-lying position to prevent aspiration and to facilitate drainage of oral secretions.
  - Check vital signs.
  - Assess for injuries.
  - Perform neurological checks.
  - Allow the client to rest if necessary.
  - Reorient and calm the client (may be agitated or confused).
  - Institute seizure precautions including placing the bed in the lowest position and padding the side rails to prevent future injury.
  - Determine if client experienced an aura, which can possibly indicate the origin of seizure in the brain.
  - Try to determine possible trigger (fatigue).
- Medications
  - Administer prescribed antiepileptic drugs (AED), such as phenytoin (Dilantin).
    - Nursing Considerations
      - Initial goal is to control seizure activity using only one medication. If the chosen medication is not effective, either the dose is increased, or another medication is added or substituted.
      - Therapeutic levels are determined by blood tests. These are performed on a routine schedule to ensure compliance and effectiveness of the medication.

- Medications should be taken at the same time every day to enhance effectiveness.
- Be aware of drug-drug adverse effects and drug-food adverse effects. These are specific to the medication.
- Allergic reactions to these medications are rare, yet may occur immediately or late in therapy. If allergic, another medication may be substituted.
- Some antiepileptic medications cause oral gum overgrowth. Routine oral hygiene and dental visits can minimize this side effect.
- When using phenytoin, specific instructions should include avoidance of oral contraceptives, as this medication decreases their effectiveness. Warfarin (Coumadin) should also not be given with this medication, as phenytoin may decrease absorption and increase metabolism of oral anticoagulants.

- Teamwork and Collaboration
  - Refer client to a social service to aid in obtaining medications if cost will affect the client's ability to adhere to the medication routine.
  - If employment is affected by seizure activity, refer to social agencies for financial support and vocational evaluation.
  - If seizure activity affects a school-age child's performance in the classroom, this condition should be reported to the disability office, which can develop specialized interventions or facilitate an Individualized Education Program (IEP).
  - Discrimination on the basis of epilepsy is illegal in all states.

- Surgical Interventions
  - Surgical interventions include placement of a vagal nerve stimulator and excision of the portion of the brain causing the seizures for intractable seizures.
  - Vagal nerve stimulator

 View Image: Vagal Nerve Stimulator

- The vagal nerve stimulator is a device implanted into the left chest wall and connected to an electrode placed on the left vagus nerve.
- This procedure is performed under general anesthesia.
- The device is then programmed to administer intermittent stimulation of the brain via stimulation of the vagal nerve, at a rate specific to the client's needs.
- Client Education
  - In addition to routine stimulation, the client may initiate vagal nerve stimulation by holding a magnet over the implantable device, at the onset of seizure activity. This either aborts the seizure, or lessens its severity.
  - Avoid diagnostic procedure such as MRI, ultrasound diathermy, the use of microwave ovens, and shortwave radios.

○ Surgical removal or interruption of brain tissue causing seizure activity

■ Requires an open craniotomy that may be performed with the client awake, in an effort to ensure that only abnormal brain tissue is destroyed.

■ EEG monitoring or brain stimulation activities are done during this lengthy procedure to identify the abnormal brain tissue.

■ Anterior temporal lobe resection may also be undertaken to treat refractory complex partial seizures.

■ These procedures have associated morbidities, including infection, loss of cerebral function, and a lack of success in preventing seizures.

■ Nursing Actions

□ Provide client education regarding seizure management.

▸ The importance of monitoring AED levels and maintaining therapeutic medication levels.

▸ Possible medication interactions (decreased effectiveness of oral contraceptives).

□ Encourage the client to wear a medical identification tag at all times.

□ Instruct the client to research the driving laws for individuals with a history of seizures in his state. Some states restrict or limit the driving of an individual with a recent history of seizures.

Complications

- Status epilepticus

○ This is prolonged seizure activity occurring over a 30-min time frame. The complications associated with this condition are related to decreased oxygen levels, inability of the brain to return to normal functioning, and continued assault on neuronal tissue. This acute condition requires immediate treatment to prevent loss of brain function, which may become permanent.

○ The usual causes are withdrawal from drugs or alcohol, sudden withdrawal from antiepileptic medication, head injury, cerebral edema, infection, and fever.

○ Nursing Actions

■ Maintain an airway, provide oxygen, establish IV access, perform ECG monitoring, and monitor pulse oximetry and ABG results.

■ As prescribed, administer a loading dose of diazepam (Valium) or lorazepam (Ativan) followed by a continuous infusion of phenytoin (Dilantin).

APPLICATION EXERCISES

1. A nurse is assessing a client who has a seizure disorder. The client reports he thinks he is about to have a seizure. Which of the following actions should the nurse implement? (Select all that apply.)

_____X_____ A. Provide privacy.

_____X_____ B. Ease the client to the floor if standing.

_____X_____ C. Move furniture away from the client.

_____X_____ D. Loosen the client's clothing.

_____X_____ E. Protect the client's head with padding.

_____ F. Restrain the client.

2. A nurse is caring for a client who just experienced a generalized seizure. Which of the following actions should the nurse perform first?

(A.) Keep the client in a side-lying position.

B. Monitor the client's vital signs.

C. Reorient the client to the environment.

D. Check the client for injuries.

3. A nurse is providing discharge instructions to a female client who has a prescription for phenytoin (Dilantin). Which of the following information should the nurse include?

A. Consider taking oral contraceptives when on this medication.

B. Watch for receding gums when taking the medication.

(C.) Take the medication at the same time every day.

D. Provide a urine sample to determine therapeutic levels of the medication.

4. A nurse is reviewing trigger factors that can cause seizures with a client who has a new diagnosis of generalized seizures. Which of the following information should the nurse include in this review? (Select all that apply.)

_X_ A. Overwhelming fatigue should be avoided.

_X_ B. Caffeinated products should be removed from the diet.

_X_ C. Looking at flashing lights should be limited.

_____ D. Aerobic exercise may be performed.

_____ E. Episodes of hypoventilation should be limited.

_____ F. Use of aerosol hairspray is recommended.

5. A nurse is completing discharge teaching to a client who has seizures and received a vagal nerve stimulator to decrease seizure activity. Which of the following information should the nurse include in the teaching?

A. The use of a microwave to heat food is permitted.

B. Inform a provider to order only a MRI when a scan is needed.

C. Place a magnet over the implantable device when an aura occurs.

D. The use of ultrasound diathermy for pain management is recommended.

6. A nurse is planning care for a client who is experiencing status epilepticus. Which concepts should the nurse include in the plan of care? Use the ATI Active Learning Template: Basic Concept to complete this item. Include the following:

A. Related Content: Define the condition.

B. Underlying Principles: Describe four possible causes.

C. Nursing Interventions: Describe five actions during a seizure.

APPLICATION EXERCISES KEY

1. A. **CORRECT:** The nurse should implement privacy to minimize the client's embarrassment.

    B. **CORRECT:** The nurse should ease the client to the floor to prevent falling.

    C. **CORRECT:** The nurse should move the furniture away from the client to prevent injury.

    D. **CORRECT:** The nurse should loosen the client's clothing to minimize restriction of movement.

    E. **CORRECT:** The nurse should protect the client's head from injury by placing the client's head in her lap or using a pillow or blanket under the head during a seizure.

    F. INCORRECT: The nurse should not restrain the client, which may cause an injury or more seizure activity.

    Ⓝ NCLEX® Connection: Physiological Adaptations, Alterations in Body Systems

2. A. **CORRECT:** The greatest risk to the client is aspiration during the postictal phase. Therefore, the priority intervention is to keep the client in a side-lying position so secretions can drain from the mouth.

    B. INCORRECT: Monitoring vital signs to determine the stability of the client is important, but it is not the priority nursing action.

    C. INCORRECT: Reorienting the client to the environment because the client may feel confused after a seizure is important, but it is not the priority nursing action.

    D. INCORRECT: Checking the client for injuries that may of occurred from involuntary movement during the seizure is important, but it is not the priority nursing action.

    Ⓝ NCLEX® Connection: Physiological Adaptations, Alterations in Body Systems

3. A. INCORRECT: The nurse should not instruct the client to take oral contraceptives, because contraceptive effectiveness is decreased when taking phenytoin.

    B. INCORRECT: The nurse should instruct the client that phenytoin causes overgrowth of the gums.

    C. **CORRECT:** The nurse should instruct the client to take phenytoin at the same time every day to enhance effectiveness.

    D. INCORRECT: The nurse should instruct the client to have period blood tests to determine the therapeutic level of phenytoin.

    Ⓝ NCLEX® Connection: Pharmacological and Parenteral Therapies, Medication Administration

4.   A. **CORRECT:** The nurse should instruct the client to avoid overwhelming fatigue, which may trigger a seizure by stimulating abnormal electrical neuron activity.

  B. **CORRECT:** The nurse should instruct the client to remove caffeinated products from the diet, which may trigger a seizure by stimulating abnormal electrical neuron activity.

  C. **CORRECT:** The nurse should instruct the client to refrain from looking at flashing lights, which may trigger a seizure by stimulating abnormal electrical neuron activity.

  D. INCORRECT: The nurse should instruct the client to decrease physical activity, which may help to avoid triggering a seizure.

  E. INCORRECT: The nurse should instruct the client to limit excess hyperventilation, which may trigger a seizure by stimulating abnormal electrical neuron activity.

  F. INCORRECT: The nurse should instruct the client to avoid using aerosol hairspray, which may trigger a seizure by stimulating abnormal electrical neuron activity.

   NCLEX® Connection: Physiological Adaptations, Alterations in Body Systems

5.   A. INCORRECT: The client should be instructed to avoid using a microwave, which may affect the stimulator.

  B. INCORRECT: The client should be instructed to inform his providers about the stimulator, which would be affected if an MRI were performed.

  C. **CORRECT:** The client should be instructed to hold a magnet over the implantable device when an aura occurs so as to decrease seizure activity.

  D. INCORRECT: The client should be instructed to avoid the use of ultrasound diathermy for pain management because of its effect on the stimulator.

   NCLEX® Connection: Reduction of Risk Potential, Therapeutic Procedures

6.   *Using the ATI Active Learning Template: Basic Concept*

  A. Related Content

   • Status epilepticus is prolonged seizure activity occurring over a 30-min period.

  B. Underlying Principles: Seizures may be related to

   • Withdrawal from alcohol

   • Withdrawal from antiepileptic medication

   • Infection

   • Fever

  C. Nursing Interventions

   • Maintain a patent airway

   • Perfom ECG monitoring

   • Review ABG results

   • Establish IV access

   • Administer lorazepam (Ativan)

   NCLEX® Connection: Physiological Adaptations, Alterations in Body Systems

chapter 7

Overview

- Parkinson's disease (PD) is a progressively debilitating disease that grossly affects motor function. It is characterized by four primary symptoms: tremor, muscle rigidity, bradykinesia (slow movement), and postural instability. These symptoms occur due to overstimulation of the basal ganglia by acetylcholine.

- The secretion of dopamine and acetylcholine in the body produce inhibitory and excitatory effects on the muscles respectively.

- Overstimulation of the basal ganglia by acetylcholine occurs because degeneration of the substantia nigra results in decreased dopamine production. This allows acetylcholine to dominate, making smooth, controlled movements difficult.

- Treatment of PD focuses on increasing the amount of dopamine or decreasing the amount of acetylcholine in a client's brain.

- As PD is a progressive disease, there are 5 stages of involvement.

  - Stage 1 – Unilateral shaking or tremor of one limb.

  - Stage 2 – Bilateral limb involvement occurs, making walking and balance difficult.

  - Stage 3 – Physical movements slow down significantly, affecting walking more.

  - Stage 4 – Tremors may decrease but akinesia and rigidity make day-to-day tasks difficult.

  - Stage 5 – Client unable to stand or walk, is dependent for all care, and may exhibit dementia.

Assessment

- Risk Factors

  - Onset of symptoms between age 40 to 70

  - More common in men

  - Genetic predisposition

  - Exposure to environmental toxins and chemical solvents

  - Chronic use of antipsychotic medication

- Subjective Data

  - Report of fatigue

  - Report of decreased manual dexterity over time

- Objective Data

   View Video: Assessment Findings with Parkinson's Disease

  - ○ Physical Assessment Findings
    - Stooped posture
    - Slow, shuffling, and propulsive gait
    - Slow, monotonous speech
    - Tremors/pill-rolling tremor of the fingers
    - Muscle rigidity (e.g. rhythmic interruption, mildly restrictive, or total resistance to movement)
    - Bradykinesia/akinesia
    - Masklike expression
    - Autonomic symptoms (orthostatic hypotension, flushing, diaphoresis)
    - Difficulty chewing and swallowing
    - Drooling
    - Dysarthria
    - Progressive difficulty with ADLs
    - Mood swings
    - Cognitive impairment (dementia)
  - ○ Laboratory Tests
    - There are no definitive diagnostic procedures.
    - Diagnosis is made based on symptoms, their progression, and by ruling out other diseases.

Patient-Centered Care

- Nursing Care
  - ○ Administer the client's medications at prescribed times.
    - Monitor medication effectiveness and make recommendations for changes in dosage and time of administration to provide best coverage.
  - ○ Monitor swallowing and maintain adequate nutrition. Consult speech and language therapist to assess swallowing if the client demonstrates a risk for choking.
    - Consult the client's dietitian for appropriate diet.
    - Document the client's weight at least weekly.
    - Keep a diet intake log.
    - Encourage fluids and document intake.
    - Provide smaller, more frequent meals.
    - Add commercial thickener to thicken food.
    - Provide supplements as prescribed.

- ○ Maintain client mobility for as long as possible.

  - Encourage exercise, such as yoga (may improve mental status as well).
  - Encourage use of assistive devices as disease progresses.
  - Encourage range-of-motion (ROM) exercises.
  - Teach the client to stop occasionally when walking to slow down speed and reduce risk for injury.
  - Pace activities by providing rest periods.
  - Assist the client with ADLs as needed (hygiene, dressing).
- ○ Promote client communication for as long as possible.
  - Teach the client facial muscle strengthening exercises.
  - Encourage the client to speak slowly and to pause frequently.
  - Use alternate forms of communication as appropriate.
  - Refer client to a speech-language pathologist.
- ○ Monitor client's mental and cognitive status
  - Observe for signs of depression and dementia.
  - Provide a safe environment (no throw rugs, encourage the use of an electric razor).
  - Assess personal and family coping with the client's chronic, degenerative disease.
  - Provide a list of community resources (support groups) to the client and the client's family.
  - Refer the client to a social worker or case manager as condition advances (financial issues, long-term home care, and respite care).
- Medications
  - ○ May take several weeks of use before improvement of symptoms is seen.
  - ○ While the client is taking a combination of medications, maintenance of therapeutic medication levels is necessary for adequate control.
  - ○ Dopaminergics
    - When given orally, medications, such as levodopa (Dopar), are converted to dopamine in the brain, increasing dopamine levels in the basal ganglia.
    - Dopaminergics may be combined with carbidopa (Sinemet) to decrease peripheral metabolism of levodopa requiring a smaller dose to make the same amount available to the brain. Side effects are subsequently less.
    - Due to medication tolerance and metabolism, the client's dosage, form of medication, and administration times must be adjusted to avoid periods of poor mobility.
    - Nursing Considerations
      - □ Monitor for the "wearing-off" phenomenon and dyskinesias (problems with movement), which can indicate the need to adjust the dosage or time of administration or the need for a medication holiday.

- ○ Dopamine agonists
  - Dopamine agonists, such as bromocriptine (Parlodel), ropinirole (Requip), and pramipexole (Mirapex), activate release of dopamine. May be used in conjunction with a dopaminergic for better results.
  - Nursing Considerations
    - □ Monitor for orthostatic hypotension, dyskinesias, and hallucinations.

- ○ Anticholinergics
  - Anticholinergics, such as benztropine (Cogentin) and trihexyphenidyl (Artane), help control tremors and rigidity
  - Nursing Considerations
    - □ Monitor for anticholinergic effects (dry mouth, constipation, urinary retention, acute confusion).
- ○ Catechol O-methyltransferase (COMT) inhibitors
  - COMT inhibitors, such as entacapone (Comtan), decrease the breakdown of levodopa making more available to the brain as dopamine. Can be used in conjunction with a dopaminergic and dopamine agonist for better results.
  - Nursing Considerations
    - □ Monitor for dyskinesia/hyperkinesia when used with levodopa.
    - □ Assess for diarrhea.
    - □ Dark urine is a normal finding.
- ○ Antivirals
  - Antivirals, such as amantadine (Symmetrel), stimulate release of dopamine and prevent its reuptake.
  - Nursing Considerations
    - □ Monitor for swollen ankles and discoloration of the skin.
    - □ Client may also experience atropine-like effects.
- • Teamwork and Collaboration
  - ○ Since PD is a degenerative, neurological disorder, long-term treatment and care must be accommodated.
  - ○ During the later stages of the disorder, the client will need referrals to and support from such disciplines as speech therapists, occupational therapists, physical therapists, and social service, culminating with placement in a long-term care facility.
- • Surgical Interventions
  - ○ Stereotactic pallidotomy
    - Strict eligibility criteria generally includes those who have not responded to other therapies.
    - Stereotactic pallidotomy is the destruction of a small portion of the brain within the globus pallidus through the use of brain imaging and electrical stimulation.
    - Target area is identified with a CT scan or an MRI.
    - Mild electrical stimulation is provided through a burr hole to a target area.
    - Client is assessed for a decrease in tremors and muscle rigidity.

- When a decrease is elicited, a temporary lesion is formed and the client is reassessed.
- If symptomatic relief is demonstrated (e.g., alleviation of tremors and rigidity), a permanent lesion is made.
- Nursing Actions
  - Assess for a neurological impairment and brain hemorrhage postoperatively.
- Deep brain stimulation
  - An electrode is implanted in the thalamus.
  - A current is delivered through an implanted pacemaker type of generator.
  - The goal of the current is to interfere with electrical conduction in tremor cells decreasing tremors.
  - Nursing Actions
    - Monitor for infection, brain hemorrhage, or strokelike symptoms.
  - Client Education
    - The client will need to be instructed on how to use a magnet to adjust the current.
    - The battery to the magnet will need to be replaced every few years.
- Client Outcomes
  - The client's medication will be scheduled so the "wearing-off" phenomenon does not occur.
  - The client will ambulate safely through the use of assistive devices.
  - The client will maintain adequate hydration and nutrition via appropriate diet and thickened liquids.

Complications

- Aspiration pneumonia
  - As PD advances in severity, alterations in chewing and swallowing will worsen, increasing the risk for aspiration.
  - Nursing Actions
    - Use swallowing precautions to decrease the risk for aspiration.
    - Develop individual dietary plan based on the speech therapist's recommendations.
    - Have a nurse in attendance when the client is eating.
    - Encourage the client to eat slowly and chew thoroughly before swallowing.
    - Feed the client in an upright position and have suction equipment on standby.
- Altered cognition (dementia, memory deficits)
  - Clients in advanced stages of PD may exhibit altered cognition in the form of dementia and memory loss.
  - Nursing Actions
    - Acknowledge the client's feelings.
    - Provide for a safe environment.
    - Develop a comprehensive plan of care with the family, client, and interprofessional team.

APPLICATION EXERCISES

1. A nurse is caring for a client who displays signs of stage 3 Parkinson's disease. Which of the following actions should the nurse include in the plan of care?

    A. Recommend a community support group.

    B. Integrate a daily exercise routine.

    C. Provide a walker for ambulation.

    D. Consultation with a dietitian.

2. A nurse is developing a plan of care for the nutritional needs of a client who has stage 4 Parkinson's disease. Which actions should the nurse include in the plan of care? (Select all that apply.)

    _____ A. Provide three large balanced meals daily.

    _____ B. Record diet and fluid intake daily.

    _____ C. Document weight every other week.

    _____ D. Add thickener to liquids.

    _____ E. Offer nutritional supplements between meals.

3. A nurse is reinforcing teaching with a client who has Parkinson's disease and has received a prescription for bromocriptine (Parlodel). Which of the following instructions should the nurse include in the teaching?

    A. Rise slowly when standing.

    B. Increase carbohydrate intake.

    C. Limit exposure to heat.

    D. Report any skin discoloration.

4. A nurse is assessing a client for manifestations of Parkinson's disease. Which of the following are expected findings? (Select all that apply.)

    _____ A. Decreased vision

    _____ B. Pill-rolling tremor of the fingers

    _____ C. Shuffling gait

    _____ D. Drooling

    _____ E. Bilateral ankle edema

    _____ F. Lack of facial expressions

5. A nurse is caring for a client who has Parkinson's disease and displays signs of bradykinesia. Which of the following is an appropriate action by the nurse?

    A. Allow client extra time for verbal responses to questions.

    B. Complete passive range-of-motion exercises.

    C. Provide an alternate form of communication.

    D. Assist with hygiene as needed.

6. A nurse is preparing a plan of care for a client who has a new diagnosis of Parkinson's disease. Which of the following considerations should the nurse include in the plan of care? Use the ATI Active Learning Template: Systems Disorder to include the following:

    A. Description of Disorder/Disease Process: One statement.

    B. Potential Complications: Identify four.

    C. Collaborative Care – Nursing Care: Describe six nursing actions.

    D. Collaborative Care – Client Outcomes: Identify four (e.g., the client will...).

APPLICATION EXERCISES KEY

1. A. INCORRECT: The client/family should be involved in a community support group at the onset of the disease process to enhance coping mechanisms.

    B. INCORRECT: The client should be doing daily exercises with the onset of the disease process to promote mobility and independence for as long as possible.

    C. **CORRECT:** The client should use a walker for ambulation in stage 3 of Parkinson's disease because movement slows down significantly and gait disturbances occur.

    D. INCORRECT: The client should have a consultation with the dietitian at the onset of the disease process in order to maintain adequate nutrition.

     NCLEX® Connection: Safety and Infection Control, Accident/Error/Injury Prevention

2. A. INCORRECT: The nurse should plan to provide small frequent meals during the day to maintain adequate nutrition.

    B. **CORRECT:** The nurse should record the client's diet and fluid intake daily to assess for dietary needs and to maintain adequate nutrition and hydration.

    C. INCORRECT: The nurse should document the client's weight weekly to identify weight loss and intervene to maintain the client's weight.

    D. **CORRECT:** The nurse should provide thickener to liquids to prevent aspiration due to pharyngeal muscle involvement, which makes swallowing difficult.

    E. **CORRECT:** The nurse should offer nutritional supplements between meals to maintain the client's weight.

     NCLEX® Connection: Basic Care and Comfort, Nutrition and Oral Hydration

3.   A.   **CORRECT:** Orthostatic hypotension is a common adverse effect of bromocriptine. Therefore, rising slowly when standing up will decrease the risk of dizziness and lightheadedness.

     B.   INCORRECT: The client should increase fiber in the diet because an adverse effect of bromocriptine is constipation.

     C.   INCORRECT: The client should limit exposure to cold because an adverse effect of bromocriptine is Raynaud's phenomenon.

     D.   INCORRECT: Skin discoloration is not an adverse effect of bromocriptine.

     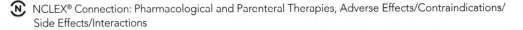 NCLEX® Connection: Pharmacological and Parenteral Therapies, Adverse Effects/Contraindications/ Side Effects/Interactions

4.   A.   INCORRECT: Decreased vision is not an expected finding in a client who has PD.

     B.   **CORRECT:** The client who has PD may manifest pill-rolling tremors of the fingers because of overstimulation of the basal ganglia by acetylcholine, making controlled movement difficult.

     C.   **CORRECT:** The client who has PD may manifest shuffling gait because of overstimulation of the basal ganglia by acetylcholine, making controlled movement difficult.

     D.   **CORRECT:** The client who has PD may manifest drooling because of overstimulation of the basal ganglia by acetylcholine, making the controlled movement of swallowing secretions difficult.

     E.   INCORRECT: Bilateral ankle edema is not an expected finding in a client who has PD, but may be an adverse effect of certain medications used for treatment.

     F.   **CORRECT:** The client who has PD may manifest a lack of facial expressions because of overstimulation of the basal ganglia by acetylcholine, making controlled movement difficult.

     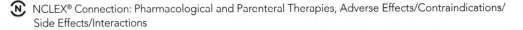 NCLEX® Connection: Physiological Adaptations, Pathophysiology

5.   A.   INCORRECT: The nurse should allow extra time for the client who has PD to express self verbally, but this is not related to bradykinesia.

     B.   INCORRECT: The nurse should encourage active, not passive, range-of-motion exercises to promote mobility in the client who has PD and is displaying bradykinesia.

     C.   INCORRECT: The nurse may provide an alternate form of communication for the client who has PD, but this is not related to bradykinesia.

     D.   **CORRECT:** Bradykinesia is abnormally slowed movement and is seen in clients who have PD. Therefore, the nurse should assist with hygiene as needed.

     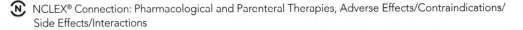 NCLEX® Connection: Reduction of Risk Potential, System Specific Assessments

6. *Using the ATI Active Learning Template: Systems Disorder*

   A. Description of Disorder/Disease Process

- Parkinson's disease is a debilitating condition that progresses to complete dependent care. The disease involves a decrease in dopamine production and an increase in secretion of acetylcholine causing resting tremor, slowed movement, and muscular rigidity.

   B. Potential Complications

- Aspiration due to pharyngeal muscle involvement making swallowing difficult

- Orthostatic hypotension, slow movement, and muscle rigidity

- Change in speech pattern: slow, monotonous speech

- Altered emotional changes that may include depression and fear

   C. Collaborative Care – Nursing Care

- Add thickener to liquids to prevent aspiration.

- Consult with a dietician about appropriate diet.

- Encourage periods of rest between activities.

- Allow adequate time to rise slowly from a sitting to standing position.

- Encourage slower speech when expressing thoughts.

- Observe for signs of depression and dementia.

   D. Collaborative Care – Client Outcomes

- The client will maintain weight by adequate fluid and nutrition intake.

- The client will have a safe environment by ambulating with assistive devices.

- The client will have an established routine medication schedule to prevent "wearing-off" effects of the medication.

- The client will have a support system to assist in coping with fears related to the disease process.

Ⓝ NCLEX® Connection: Physiological Adaptations, Illness Management

chapter 8

Overview

- Alzheimer's disease (AD) is a nonreversible type of dementia that progressively develops over many years. A special framework made up of seven stages has been designed to categorize the disease and its manifestations. The framework is based on three general stages: early stage, mid stage, and late stage.

- Dementia is defined as multiple cognitive deficits that impair memory and can affect language, motor skills, and/or abstract thinking.

- Some people die 4 to 6 years after diagnosis, but others can live with the disease for up to 20 years.

- AD is responsible for 60% of dementia cases in clients over 65 years of age. Manifestations may appear in clients in their 40s, which is referred to as presenile or early dementia, Alzheimer's type.

- Age is the number one known risk factor for AD, which usually occurs after the age of 65.

- AD is characterized by memory loss, problems with judgment, and changes in personality.

- Severe physical decline occurs along with deteriorating cognitive functions.

Assessment

- Risk Factors
  - Advanced age
  - Genetic predisposition, apolipoprotein E (ApoE)
  - Environmental agents (herpes virus, metal, or toxic waste)
  - Previous head injury
  - Sex (female)
- Subjective and Objective Data

ALZHEIMER'S STAGES	
STAGE	MANIFESTATIONS
› Stage 1: No impairment (Normal function)	› No memory problems
› Stage 2: Very mild cognitive decline (May be normal age-related changes or very early signs of AD)	› Forgetfulness, especially of everyday objects (eyeglasses or wallet) › No memory problems evident to provider, friends, or coworkers

ALZHEIMER'S STAGES	
STAGE	**MANIFESTATIONS**
› Stage 3: Mild cognitive decline (Problems with memory or concentration may be measurable in clinical testing or during a detailed medical interview)	› Mild cognitive deficits, including losing or misplacing important objects › Decreased ability to plan › Short-term memory loss noticeable to close relatives › Decreased attention span › Difficulty remembering words or names › Difficulty in social or work situations
› Stage 4: Moderate cognitive decline (Mild or early-stage AD; medical interview will detect clear-cut deficiencies)	› Personality changes – appearing withdrawn or subdued, especially in social or mentally challenging situations › Obvious memory loss › Limited knowledge and memory of recent occasions, current events, or personal history › Difficulty performing tasks that require planning and organizing (paying bills or managing money) › Difficulty with complex mental arithmetic
› Stage 5: Moderately severe cognitive decline (Moderate or mid-stage AD)	› Increasing cognitive deficits emerge › Inability to recall important details such as address, telephone number, or schools attended, but memory of information about self and family remains intact › Assistance with ADLs becomes necessary › Disorientation and confusion as to time and place
› Stage 6: Severe cognitive decline (Moderately severe or mid-stage AD)	› Memory difficulties continue to worsen › Loss of awareness of recent events and surroundings › May recall own name, but unable to recall personal history › Significant personality changes are evident (delusions, hallucinations, and compulsive behaviors) › Wandering behavior › Requires assistance with usual daily activities such as dressing, toileting, and other grooming › Normal sleep/wake cycle is disrupted › Increased episodes of urinary and fecal incontinence
› Stage 7: Very severe cognitive decline (Severe or late-stage AD)	› Ability to respond to environment, speak, and control movement is lost › Unrecognizable speech › General urinary incontinence › Inability to eat without assistance and impaired swallowing › Gradual loss of all ability to move extremities (ataxia)

Alzheimer's Association National Office (2013), Stages of Alzheimer's, retrieved Jan 23, 2013, from www.alz.org/alzheimers_disease_stages_of_alzheimers.asp.

- ○ Laboratory Tests
  - ▪ Genetic testing for the presence of apolipoprotein E can determine if late-onset dementia is due to AD.
- ○ Diagnostic Procedures
  - ▪ There is no definitive diagnostic procedure, except brain tissue examination upon death.
  - ▪ Magnetic resonance imaging (MRI), computed tomography (CT) imaging/computed axial tomography (CAT) scan, positron emission tomography (PET) scan, and electroencephalogram (EEG) may be performed to rule out other possible causes of findings.

Patient-Centered Care

- • Nursing Care
  - ○ Assess cognitive status, memory, judgment, and personality changes.
  - ○ Initiate bowel and bladder program with the client based on a set schedule.
  - ○ Encourage the client and family to participate in an AD support group.
  - ○ Provide a safe environment.
  - ○ Keep the client on a sleeping schedule and monitor for irregular sleeping patterns.
  - ○ Provide verbal and nonverbal ways to communicate with the client.
  - ○ Offer snacks or finger foods if the client is unable to sit for long periods of time.
  - ○ Check the client's skin weekly for breakdown.
  - ○ Provide cognitive stimulation.
    - ▪ Offer varied environmental stimulations, such as walks, music, or craft activities.
    - ▪ Keep a structured environment and introduce change gradually (client's daily routine or a room change).
    - ▪ Use a calendar to assist with orientation.
    - ▪ Use short directions when explaining an activity or care the client needs, such as a bath.
    - ▪ Be consistent and repetitive.
    - ▪ Use therapeutic touch.
  - ○ Provide memory training.
    - ▪ Reminisce with the client about the past.
    - ▪ Use memory techniques such as making lists and rehearsing.
    - ▪ Stimulate the client's memory by repeating the client's last statement.
  - ○ Avoid overstimulation. (Keep noise and clutter to a minimum and avoid crowds.)
  - ○ Promote consistency by placing commonly used objects in the same location and using a routine schedule.
    - ▪ Reality orientation (early stages)
    - ▪ Easily viewed clock and single-day calendar
    - ▪ Pictures of family and pets
    - ▪ Frequent reorientation to time, place, and person

- ○ Validation therapy (later stages)
  - ▪ Acknowledge the client's feelings.
  - ▪ Don't argue with the client; this will lead to the client becoming upset.
  - ▪ Reinforce and use repetitive actions or ideas cautiously.
- ○ Promote self-care as long as possible. Assist the client with activities of daily living as appropriate.
- ○ Speak directly to the client in short, concise sentences.
- ○ Reduce agitation (use calm, redirecting statements; provide a diversion).
- ○ Provide a routine toileting schedule.
- • Medications
  - ○ Most medications for clients who have dementia attempt to target behavioral and emotional problems, such as anxiety, agitation, combativeness, and depression.
  - ○ These medications include antipsychotics, antidepressants, and anxiolytics. Clients receiving these medications should be closely monitored for adverse effects.
  - ○ AD medications temporarily slow the course of the disease and do not work for all clients.
  - ○ Pharmacotherapeutics is based on the theory that AD is a result of depleted levels of the enzyme acetyltransferase, which is necessary to produce the neurotransmitter acetylcholine.
  - ○ Benefits for those clients who do respond to medication include improvements in cognition, behavior, and function.
  - ○ If a client fails to improve with one medication, a trial of one of the other medications is warranted.
  - ○ Donepezil (Aricept)
    - ▪ Prevents the breakdown of acetylcholine (ACh), which increases the amount of ACh available. This results in increased nerve impulses at the nerve sites.
    - ▪ Cholinesterase inhibitors help slow this process.
    - ▪ Nursing Considerations
      - ▫ Observe the client for frequent stools or upset stomach.
      - ▫ Monitor the client for dizziness and or headache. The client may feel lightheaded or have an unsteady gait.
      - ▫ Use caution when administering this medication to clients who have asthma or COPD.
- • Teamwork and Collaboration
  - ○ Refer the client and family to social services and case managers for possible adult day care facilities or long-term care facilities.
  - ○ Refer the client and family to the Alzheimer's Association and community outreach programs. This can include in-home care or respite care.
- • Therapeutic Procedures
  - ○ Alternative therapy
    - ▪ Estrogen therapy for women may prevent Alzheimer's disease, but it is not useful in decreasing the effects of pre-existing dementia.
    - ▪ Ginkgo biloba, an herbal product taken to increase memory and blood circulation, can cause a variety of side effects and medication interactions. If a client is using ginkgo biloba or other nutritional supplements, that information should be shared with health care providers.

- Care After Discharge
  - Refer to social services and case managers for long-term/home management.
  - Alzheimer's Association, community outreach programs and support groups
  - Client Education
    - Educate family/caregivers about illness, methods of care, and adaptation of the home environment.
    - Home safety measures to be implemented may include:
      - Removing scatter rugs.
      - Installing door locks that cannot be easily opened, and placing alarms on doors.
      - Keeping a lock on the water heater and thermostat, and keeping the water temperature tuned down to a safe level.
      - Providing good lighting, especially on stairs.
      - Installing handrails on stairs and marking step edges with colored tape.
      - Placing the mattress on the floor.
      - Removing clutter and clearing hallways for walking.
      - Securing electrical cords to baseboards.
      - Keeping cleaning supplies in locked cupboards.
      - Installing handrails in the bathroom, at bedside, and in the tub; placing a shower chair in the tub.
      - Having the client wear a medical identification bracelet if living at home with a caregiver.
      - Monitoring for improvement in memory and the client's quality of life.
    - Provide support for caregivers.
      - Determine teaching needs for the client, especially for family members, when the client's cognitive ability is progressively declining.
      - Review the resources available to the family as the client's health declines. Include long-term care options. A wide variety of home care and community resources, such as respite care, may be available to the family in many areas of the country, and these resources may allow the client to remain at home rather than in an institution.

APPLICATION EXERCISES

1. A nurse is providing teaching to the partner of an older adult client who has Alzheimer's disease and has a new prescription for donepezil (Aricept). Which of the following statements by the partner indicates the teaching is effective?

    A. "This medication should increase my husband's appetite."

    B. "This medication should help my husband sleep better."

    C. "This medication should help my husband's daily function."

    D. "This medication should increase my husband's energy level."

2. A nurse is making a home visit to a client who has AD. The client's partner states that the client is often disoriented to time and place, is unsteady on his feet, and has a history of wandering. Which of the following safety measures should the nurse review with the partner? (Select all that apply.)

    _____ A. Remove floor rugs.

    _____ B. Have door locks that can be easily opened.

    _____ C. Provide increased lighting in stairwells.

    _____ D. Install handrails in the bathroom.

    _____ E. Place the mattress on the floor.

3. A nurse is caring for a client who has AD and falls frequently. Which of the following actions should the nurse take first to keep the client safe?

    A. Keep the call light near the client.

    B. Place the client in a room close to the nurses' station.

    C. Encourage the client to ask for assistance.

    D. Remind the client to walk with someone for support.

4. A nurse working in a long-term care facility is planning care for a client in stage 5 of Alzheimer's disease. Which of the following interventions should be included in the plan of care?

    A. Use a gait belt for ambulation.

    B. Thicken all liquids.

    C. Provide protective undergarments.

    D. Assist with ADLs.

5. A nurse is caring for a client who has Alzheimer's disease. A family member of the client asks the nurse about risk factors for the disease. Which of the following should be included in the nurse's response? (Select all that apply.)

_____ A. Exposure to metal waste products

_____ B. Long-term estrogen hormone therapy

_____ C. Sustained use of vitamin E

_____ D. Previous head injury

_____ E. History of herpes infection

6. A nurse educator in a long-term care facility is providing a program to assistive personnel about caring for a client who has Alzheimer's disease. What should be included in this program? Use the ATI Active Learning Template: Systems Disorder to complete this item to include the following:

A. Nursing Care: Describe three nursing interventions for each of the following areas:
- Providing cognitive stimulation
- Providing memory training

APPLICATION EXERCISES KEY

1. A. INCORRECT: Donepezil does not affect appetite.

    B. INCORRECT: Donepezil does not affect sleep or sleep patterns.

    C. **CORRECT:** Donepezil helps slow the progression of AD and may help improve behavior and daily functions.

    D. INCORRECT: Donepezil does not affect energy levels.

    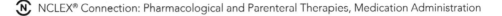 NCLEX® Connection: Pharmacological and Parenteral Therapies, Medication Administration

2. A. **CORRECT:** Removing floor rugs can decrease the client's risk of falling.

    B. INCORRECT: Easy-to-open door locks increase the risk for a client who wanders to get out of his home and get lost.

    C. **CORRECT:** Good lighting can decrease the risk for falling in dark areas, such as stairways.

    D. **CORRECT:** Installing handrails in the bathroom can be useful for the client to hold on to when his gait is unsteady.

    E. **CORRECT:** By placing the client's mattress on the floor, the client's risk of falling or tripping is decreased.

    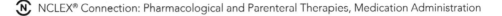 NCLEX® Connection: Safety and Infection Control, Home Safety

3. A. INCORRECT: Keeping the call light within the client's reach is an appropriate action, but not the first action because the client may not remember to use it.

    B. **CORRECT:** Using the safety and risk reduction priority-setting framework, placing the client in close proximity to the nurse's station for close observation is the first action the nurse should take.

    C. INCORRECT: Encouraging the client to ask for assistance is an appropriate action, but not the first action because the client may not remember to ask for assistance.

    D. INCORRECT: Reminding the client to walk with someone is an appropriate action, but not the first action because the client may not remember to call for assistance.

    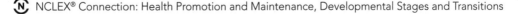 NCLEX® Connection: Health Promotion and Maintenance, Developmental Stages and Transitions

4. A. INCORRECT: Ambulation is affected as the client advances into stage 7 of Alzheimer's disease.

    B. INCORRECT: Impaired swallowing is a finding as the client advances into stage 7 of Alzheimer's disease.

    C. INCORRECT: The client in stages 6 and 7 of Alzheimer's disease experiences episodes of urinary and fecal incontinence.

    D. **CORRECT:** A client in Alzheimer's disease stage 5 requires assistance with ADLs as increasing cognitive deficits emerge.

    (N) NCLEX® Connection: Safety and Infection Control, Home Safety

5. A. **CORRECT:** Exposure to metal and toxic waste is a risk factor for Alzheimer's disease.

    B. INCORRECT: Long-term estrogen hormone therapy may prevent Alzheimer's disease.

    C. INCORRECT: Long-term use of vitamin E is not a risk factor for Alzheimer's disease.

    D. **CORRECT:** A previous head injury is a risk factor for Alzheimer's disease.

    E. **CORRECT:** A history of herpes infection is a risk factor for Alzheimer's disease.

    (N) NCLEX® Connection: Health Promotion and Maintenance, Health Promotion/Disease Prevention

6. *Using the ATI Active Learning Template: Systems Disorder*

    A. Nursing Care

    - Cognitive stimulation
        - Offer varied environmental stimulations such as walks, music, and craft activities.
        - Keep a structured environment. Introduce change slowly.
        - Use a calendar to assist with orientation.
        - Use short directions when explaining care to be provided, such as a bath.
        - Be consistent and repetitive.
        - Use therapeutic touch.
    - Memory training
        - Reminisce about the past.
        - Help the client make lists and rehearse.
        - Repeat the client's last statement to stimulate memory.

    (N) NCLEX® Connection: Health Promotion and Maintenance, Developmental Stages and Transitions

chapter 9

Overview

- Brain tumors occur in any part of the brain and are classified according to the cell or tissue of origin. Types of brain tumors include malignant gliomas (neuroglial cells), benign meningiomas (meninges), pituitary adenomas, and acoustic neuromas (acoustic cranial nerve).

- Supratentorial tumors occur in the cerebral hemispheres above the tentorium cerebelli. Those below the tentorium cerebelli, such as tumors of the brainstem and cerebellum, are classified as infratentorial tumors.

- Brain tumors apply pressure to surrounding brain tissue, resulting in decreased outflow of cerebrospinal fluid, increased intracranial pressure, cerebral edema, and neurological deficits. Tumors that involve the pituitary gland may cause endocrine dysfunction.

- Malignant brain tumors are associated with a high overall mortality rate.

- Primary malignant brain tumors originate from neuroglial tissue and rarely metastasize outside of the brain. Secondary malignant brain tumors are lesions that are metastases from a primary cancer located elsewhere in the body.

  ○ Cranial metastatic lesions are most common from breast, kidney, and gastrointestinal tract cancers.

- Benign brain tumors develop from the meninges or cranial nerves and do not metastasize. These tumors have distinct boundaries and cause damage either by the pressure they exert within the cranial cavity and/or by impairing the function of the cranial nerve.

Health Promotion/Disease Prevention

- There are no routine screening procedures to detect brain tumors.

Assessment

- Risk Factors
  ○ The cause is unknown, but several risk factors have been identified
    - Genetics
    - Environmental agents
    - Exposure to ionizing radiation
    - Exposure to electromagnetic fields
    - Previous head injury

- Subjective and Objective Data
  - Physical Assessment Findings
    - Dysarthria
    - Dysphagia
    - Positive Romberg sign
    - Positive Babinski's sign
    - Vertigo
    - Hemiparesis
    - Cranial nerve dysfunction (inability to discriminate sounds, loss of gag reflex, loss of blink response)
  - Manifestations specific to supratentorial brain tumors
    - Severe headache – worse upon awakening but improving over time
    - Visual changes (blurring, visual field deficit)
    - Seizures
    - Loss of voluntary movement or the inability to control movement
    - Change in cognitive function (memory loss, language impairment)
    - Change in personality, inability to control emotions
    - Nausea with or without vomiting
  - Manifestations specific to infratentorial brain tumors
    - Hearing loss or ringing in the ear
    - Facial drooping
    - Difficulty swallowing
    - Nystagmus, crossed eyes, or decreased vision
    - Autonomic nervous system (ANS) dysfunction
    - Ataxia or clumsy movements
    - Hemiparesis
    - Cranial nerve dysfunction (inability to discriminate sounds, loss of gag reflex, loss of blink response)

> **View Media**
> › Nystagmus (Animation)   › Testing for Romberg Sign (Video)
> › Babinski's Reflex (Video)

  - Laboratory Tests
    - CBC and differential to rule out anemia or malnutrition
    - Blood alcohol and toxicology screen to rule out these as possible causes of altered physical assessment findings
    - TB and HIV screening if social conditions warrant

- Diagnostic Procedures
  - X-ray, computed tomography (CT) imaging scan, magnetic resonance imaging (MRI), brain scan, position emission tomography (PET) scan, and cerebral angiography are used to determine the size, location, and extent of the tumor.
  - Cerebral biopsy – performed to identify cellular pathology
    - This procedure may be performed in the surgical suite or in a radiology specialty suite.
    - Diagnostic procedure may be used to guide the biopsy, such as a CT or MRI scan. Image guiding systems, which use CT or MRI scan information, may be used in the surgical suite.
    - A piece of cerebral tissue that appears abnormal on the CT/MRI scan is obtained. This tissue is then sent to pathology, where diagnostic tests are performed.
    - Benefit – Biopsy is minimally disruptive to the rest of the brain, provides a decreased recovery time and is not associated with the risks of an open craniotomy.
    - Negative – Biopsy does not remove or debulk the tumor, the diagnostic determination by pathology may be inconclusive (related to insufficient tissue), and a misdiagnosis can occur if the tumor contains many types of tissue or the specimen is taken from one site.
    - Client Education
      - Include specific instruction regarding medications.
        - If the client is on antiepileptic medications, these must be continued to prevent seizure activity.
        - If the client is on aspirin products, these should be discontinued at least 72 hr prior to the procedure to minimize the risk of intracerebral bleeding.
        - Other medications may be withheld prior to the procedure.
        - Normally, preprocedure activities may be resumed after the client recovers from the general anesthetic. Care of the incision should include keeping the area clean and dry. If sutures are in place, they need to be removed 1 to 7 days later. Driving or other dangerous activities should be avoided until follow-up appointment occurs and diagnosis is known.

Patient-Centered Care

- Nursing Care
  - Maintain airway (monitor oxygen levels, administer oxygen as needed, monitor lung sounds).
  - Monitor neurological status, in particular, assessing for changes in level of consciousness, neurological deficits, and occurrence of seizures.
  - Maintain client safety (assist with transfers and ambulation, provide assistive devices as needed).
  - Implement seizure precautions.
  - Administer medications as prescribed.
- Medications
  - Nonopioid analgesics are used to treat headaches.
    - Opioid medications are avoided because they tend to decrease the client's level of consciousness.

- Corticosteroids are used to reduce cerebral edema.
  - Corticosteroid medications quickly reduce cerebral edema and may be rapidly administered to maximize their effectiveness.
  - Chronic administration is used to control cerebral edema associated with the presence or treatment of benign or malignant brain tumors.
- Anticonvulsant medications are used to control or prevent seizure activity.
  - Anticonvulsant medications suppress the neuronal activity within the brain, which prevents seizure activity.
  - There are several classifications of antiepileptic medications, each specifically designed to treat specific seizure behavior.
- H_2-antagonists are used to decrease the acid content of the stomach, reducing the risk of stress ulcers.
  - H_2-antagonist medications are administered during acute or stressful periods, such as after surgery, at the initiation of chemotherapy, or during the first several radiation therapy treatments.
  - The impact of these treatments, together with the necessity of corticosteroids, places the client at risk for stress ulcers. This is primarily preventative treatment.
- Antiemetics are used if nausea with or without vomiting is present.
  - Nausea and vomiting may be present as a result of the increased intracranial pressure, the site of the tumor, or the treatment required.
  - These medications are administered as prescribed, and may be provided as a preventative intervention, especially when the treatment is associated with nausea and/or vomiting.
- Teamwork and Collaboration
  - Initiate appropriate referrals (social services, support groups, medical equipment, and physical, speech, and occupational therapy).
  - Treatments include steroids, surgery, chemotherapy, conventional radiation therapy, stereotactic radiosurgery, and clinical trials. Chemotherapy and/or conventional radiation therapy may be administered prior to surgery to reduce the bulk of the tumor, or after surgery to prevent tumor recurrence.
  - In most cases when the tumor is benign, surgery is a curative treatment. However, these tumors can regrow. Thus, radiation and/or chemotherapy may be provided to prevent recurrence.
  - Some tumors may be "malignant by location," meaning that while the pathology is benign, the location makes the mortality rate associated with them high.
  - In cases where the tumor is a metastatic lesion from a primary lesion elsewhere in the body, treatments are palliative in nature. These treatments may consist of surgery, radiation, and chemotherapy, in any combination, and are aimed at controlling intracerebral lesions.
- Surgical Interventions
  - Craniotomy – complete or partial resection of brain tumor through surgical opening in the skull
    - Nursing Actions
      - Preoperative
        - Explain the procedure to the client, answering all appropriate questions and providing emotional support.
        - Questions regarding the surgery and its outcomes should be written, in an effort to ensure all questions are answered.

▶ The client's significant other should be present to hear the responses and avoid miscommunication/misunderstanding.

▶ If the client is on aspirin, this medication needs to be stopped at least 72 hr prior to the procedure.

▶ If the client is taking alternative/complementary medications or receiving treatments, these should be made known to the provider.

▶ A living will and durable power for health care decisions should be completed.

▶ Medications should be administered as prescribed. An antianxiety or muscle relaxant medication can be administered, if requested, and provided by the provider.

▫ Postoperative

▶ Vital signs and neurological status should be closely monitored, including using the Glasgow Scale.

▶ Pain should be treated adequately.

▶ The head of the client should be elevated 30° and placed in a neutral position to prevent increased intracranial pressure.

▶ Straining activities (moving up in bed and attempting to have a bowel movement) should be avoided to prevent increased intracranial pressure. Postoperative bleeding and seizure activity are the greatest risks.

Complications

- Syndrome of inappropriate antidiuretic hormone (SIADH)

  ○ This is a condition where fluid is retained as a result of an overproduction of vasopressin or antidiuretic hormone (ADH) from the posterior pituitary gland.

  ○ The condition occurs when the hypothalamus has been damaged and can no longer regulate the release of ADH.

  ○ Treatment of SIADH consists of fluid restriction, administration of oral demeclocycline, and treatment of hyponatremia.

  ○ If SIADH is present, the client may be disorientated, report a headache, and/or vomit.

  ○ If severe or untreated, this condition may cause seizures and/or a coma.

- Diabetes insipidus (DI)

  ○ This is a condition where large amounts of urine are excreted as a result of a deficiency of ADH from the posterior pituitary gland.

  ○ The condition occurs when the hypothalamus has been damaged and can no longer regulate the release of ADH.

  ○ Treatment of DI consists of massive fluid replacement, careful attention to laboratory values, and replacement of essential nutrients as indicated.

APPLICATION EXERCISES

1. A nurse is caring for a client who is having surgery for the removal of an encapsulated acoustic tumor. Which of the following potential complications should the nurse monitor for postoperatively? (Select all that apply.)

_____ A. Increased intracranial pressure

_____ B. Hemorrhagic shock

_____ C. Hydrocephalus

_____ D. Hypoglycemia

_____ E. Seizures

2. A nurse is caring for a client who has just undergone a craniotomy for a supratentorial tumor. Which of the following postoperative prescriptions should the nurse clarify with the provider?

A. Dexamethasone (Decadron) 30 mg IV bolus BID

B. Morphine sulfate 2 mg IV bolus PRN every 2 hr for pain

C. Ondansetron (Zofran) 4 mg IV bolus PRN every 4 to 6 hr for nausea

D. Phenytoin (Dilantin) 100 mg IV bolus TID

3. A nurse is completing an assessment of a client who has increased intracranial pressure. Which of the following are expected findings? (Select all that apply.)

_____ A. Disoriented to time and place

_____ B. Restlessness and irritability

_____ C. Unequal pupils

_____ D. ICP 15 mm/Hg

_____ E. Headache

4. A nurse is reviewing a prescription for dexamethasone (Decadron) with a client who has an expanding brain tumor. Which of the following are appropriate statements by the nurse? (Select all that apply.)

_____ A. "It is given to reduce swelling of the brain."

_____ B. "You will need to monitor for low blood sugar."

_____ C. "You may notice weight gain."

_____ D. "Tumor growth will be delayed."

_____ E. "It can cause you to retain fluids."

5. A nurse is caring for a client who has a benign brain tumor. The client asks the nurse if he can expect this same type of tumor to occur in other areas of his body. Which of the following is an appropriate response by the nurse?

    A. "It can spread to breasts and kidneys."

    B. "It can develop in your gastrointestinal tract."

    C. "It is limited to brain tissue."

    D. "It probably started in another area of your body and spread to your brain."

6. A nurse is reviewing the health record of a client who has a malignant brain tumor and notes the client has a positive Romberg sign. Which of the following actions should the nurse take to assess for this sign?

    A. Stroke the lateral aspect of the sole of the foot.

    B. Ask the client to blink his eyes.

    C. Observe for facial drooping.

    D. Have the client stand erect with eyes closed.

7. A nurse is completing preoperative teaching for a client who has a brain tumor and will undergo a craniotomy. What should be included in the teaching? Use the ATI Active Learning Template: Therapeutic Procedure to complete this item to include the following sections:

    A. Description of Procedure

    B. Nursing Interventions: Describe three preoperative and three postoperative interventions.

APPLICATION EXERCISES KEY

1. A. **CORRECT:** A client who has had a craniotomy should be monitored postoperatively for increased ICP.

    B. INCORRECT: Although hypovolemic shock can occur secondary to SIADH, hemorrhagic shock is not a concern.

    C. **CORRECT:** Following a craniotomy, the client should be monitored for the development of hydrocephalus.

    D. INCORRECT: An alteration in glucose metabolism is not usually a postoperative concern after this surgery.

    E. **CORRECT:** Seizures is a postoperative complication that should be monitored following a craniotomy.

    Ⓝ NCLEX® Connection: Reduction of Risk Potential, System Specific Assessments

2. A. INCORRECT: Dexamethasone is given to prevent cerebral edema and has no CNS depressant effects.

    B. **CORRECT:** Narcotic analgesics should be avoided postoperatively due to their CNS depressant effects.

    C. INCORRECT: Ondansetron is prescribed to manage nausea and has no CNS depressant effects.

    D. INCORRECT: Phenytoin is prescribed to prevent seizures and has no CNS depressant effects.

    Ⓝ NCLEX® Connection: Pharmacological and Parenteral Therapies, Adverse Effects/Contraindications/ Side Effects/Interactions

3. A. **CORRECT:** Changes in level of consciousness are an early indicator of increased ICP.

    B. **CORRECT:** Increased ICP can cause behavior changes, such as restlessness and irritability.

    C. **CORRECT:** Unequal pupils indicates pressure on the oculomotor nerve secondary to increased ICP.

    D. INCORRECT: An ICP of 15 mm Hg is within the expected reference range.

    E. **CORRECT:** A headache is a manifestation of increased ICP.

    Ⓝ NCLEX® Connection: Reduction of Risk Potential, System Specific Assessments

4. A. **CORRECT:** Dexamethasone is a common steroid prescribed to reduce cerebral edema.

    B. INCORRECT: The client may experience hyperglycemia as an adverse effect of dexamethasone.

    C. **CORRECT:** Weight gain is an adverse effect of dexamethasone.

    D. INCORRECT: Dexamethasone does not affect tumor growth. It is given to prevent cerebral edema.

    E. **CORRECT:** Fluid retention is an adverse effect of dexamethasone.

    Ⓝ NCLEX® Connection: Pharmacological and Parenteral Therapies, Medication Administration

5.   A. INCORRECT: Metastases of a benign brain tumor do not occur.

     B. INCORRECT: Metastases of a benign brain tumor do not occur.

     C. **CORRECT:** Benign brain tumors develop from the meninges or cranial nerves and do not metastasize.

     D. INCORRECT: Benign brain tumors develop from the meninges or cranial nerves and are not secondary to other types of tumors.

      NCLEX® Connection: Physiological Adaptations, Alterations in Body Systems

6.   A. INCORRECT: Babinski's sign is elicited by stroking the lateral aspect of the sole of the foot.

     B. INCORRECT: Asking the client to blink his eyes assesses cranial nerve function and is not part of the Romberg test.

     C. INCORRECT: Observing for facial drooping assesses cranial nerve function and is not part of the Romberg test.

     D. **CORRECT:** A positive Romberg sign is indicated when a client loses his balance while attempting to stand erect with his eyes closed.

     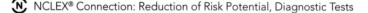 NCLEX® Connection: Reduction of Risk Potential, Diagnostic Tests

7.   *Using the ATI Active Learning Template: Therapeutic Procedure*
     A. Description of Procedure
        • A craniotomy is a surgical opening in the skull to expose brain tissue. It involves a complete or partial resection of the brain tumor.
     B. Nursing Interventions
        • Preoperative
           ○ Explain the procedure, answer appropriate questions, and provide emotional support.
           ○ Provide written explanations.
           ○ Include the client's partner in teaching.
           ○ Remind client to stop taking aspirin at least 72 hr prior to the procedure, if appropriate.
           ○ Review use of alternative/complementary therapies and report their use to the provider.
           ○ Review the need for a living will and durable power for health care decisions.
           ○ Administer medications (anxiolytics, muscle relaxants) as prescribed.
        • Postoperative
           ○ Monitor vital signs and neurological status to include use of Glasgow Scale.
           ○ Maintain client's head elevated to 30° and in a neutral position to prevent increased ICP.
           ○ Monitor for postoperative bleeding and seizures.
           ○ Prevent client performing any straining activities (moving up in bed, attempting to have a bowel movement).

      NCLEX® Connection: Reduction of Risk Potential, Therapeutic Procedures

chapter 10

Multiple Sclerosis, Amyotrophic Lateral Sclerosis, and Myasthenia Gravis

Overview

- Multiple sclerosis (MS), amyotrophic lateral sclerosis (ALS), and myasthenia gravis (MG) are neurological diseases that typically result in impaired and worsening function of voluntary muscles. While MS and ALS affect nerve cells in the brain and spinal cord, MG affects the neuromuscular junction.

- MS is an autoimmune disorder characterized by development of plaque in the white matter of the central nervous system (CNS). This plaque damages the myelin sheath and interferes with impulse transmission between the CNS and the body.

- ALS is a disease of the upper and lower motor neurons characterized by muscle weakness progressing to muscle atrophy and eventually paralysis and death. ALS does not involve autonomic changes, sensory alterations, or cognitive changes.

- MG is an autoimmune disorder characterized by antibody-mediated loss of acetylcholine receptors at the neuromuscular junction, interfering with communication between motor neurons and innervated muscles.

MULTIPLE SCLEROSIS

Overview

- MS follows several possible courses. The most common is relapsing and remitting.

  ○ The disease is marked by relapses and remissions that may or may not return the client to their previous baseline level of function. Overtime, the client may eventually progress to the point of quadriplegia.

- MS is a chronic disease with no known cure that progresses in severity over time. Initial findings may be so vague that diagnosis is not made for several years.

- Some forms of MS are aggressive and can shorten the lifespan. In most cases, life expectancy is not adversely affected by this disease.

Assessment

- Risk Factors

  ○ The onset of MS is typically between 20 and 40 years of age and occurs twice as often in women. The etiology of MS is unknown. There is a family history (first-degree relative) of MS in many cases.

  ○ Because MS is an autoimmune disease, there are factors that trigger relapses.

    ▪ Viruses and infectious agents

    ▪ Living in a cold climate

    ▪ Physical injury

    ▪ Emotional stress

- Pregnancy
- Fatigue
- Overexertion
- Temperature extremes
- Hot shower/bath

- Subjective and Objective Data
  - Fatigue – especially of the lower extremities
  - Pain or paresthesia
  - Diplopia, changes in peripheral vision, decreased visual acuity
  - Uhthoff's sign (a temporary worsening of vision and other neurological functions commonly seen in clients who have or are predisposed to MS, just after exertion or in situations where they are exposed to heat)
  - Tinnitus, vertigo, decreased hearing acuity
  - Dysphagia
  - Dysarthria (slurred and nasal speech)
  - Muscle spasticity
  - Ataxia and/or muscle weakness
  - Nystagmus
  - Bowel dysfunction (constipation, fecal incontinence)
  - Bladder dysfunction (areflexia, urgency, nocturia)
  - Cognitive changes (memory loss, impaired judgment)
  - Sexual dysfunction
  - Laboratory Tests – Cerebrospinal fluid analysis (elevated protein level and a slight increase in WBCs)
  - Diagnostic Procedures – Magnetic resonance imaging (MRI) reveals plaques of the brain and spine, which is most diagnostic.

Patient-Centered Care

- Nursing Care
  - Monitoring of
    - Visual acuity
    - Speech patterns – fatigue with talking
    - Swallowing
    - Activity tolerance
    - Skin integrity
  - MS is a potentially debilitating condition. Discuss client coping mechanisms and sources of support (family, friends, spiritual figures, support groups).
  - Encourage fluid intake and other measures to decrease the risk of developing a urinary tract infection. Assist the client with bladder elimination (intermittent self-catheterization, bladder pacemaker, Credé maneuver [placing manual pressure on abdomen over the bladder to expel urine]).

- Monitor cognitive changes and plan interventions to promote cognitive function (reorient the client, place objects used daily in routine places).

- Facilitate effective communication (dysarthria) using a communication board.

- Apply alternating eye patches to treat diplopia. Teach scanning techniques.

- Exercise and stretch involved muscles (avoid fatigue and overheating).

- Promote energy conservation by grouping cares and planning rest periods.

- Promote and maintain safe home and hospital environment to reduce the risk of injury (walk with wide base of support, assistive devices, skin precautions).

- Medications

  - Azathioprine (Imuran) and cyclosporine (Sandimmune)

    - Immunosuppressive agents are used to reduce the frequency of relapses.

    - Nursing Considerations

      - Monitor for long-term effects.

      - Be alert for manifestations of infection.

      - Assess for hypertension.

      - Assess for kidney dysfunction.

  - Prednisone

    - Corticosteroids are used to reduce inflammation in acute exacerbations.

    - Nursing Considerations – Monitor for increased risk of infection, hypervolemia, hypernatremia, hypokalemia, hyperglycemia, gastrointestinal bleeding, and personality changes.

  - Dantrolene (Dantrium), tizanidine (Zanaflex), baclofen (Lioresal), and diazepam (Valium)

    - Antispasmodics are used to treat muscle spasticity.

    - Intrathecal baclofen can be used for severe cases of MS.

    - Nursing Considerations

      - Observe for increased weakness.

      - Monitor for liver damage if on tizanidine or dantrolene.

    - Client Education

      - Report increased weakness and jaundice to provider.

      - Avoid stopping baclofen abruptly.

  - Interferon beta (Betaseron) – Immunomodulators are used to prevent or treat relapses.

  - Carbamazepine (Tegretol) – Anticonvulsants are used for paresthesia.

  - Docusate sodium (Colace) – Stool softeners are used for constipation.

  - Propantheline – Anticholinergics are used for bladder dysfunction.

  - Primidone (Mysoline) and clonazepam (Klonopin) – Beta-blockers are used for tremors.

- Teamwork and Collaboration

  - Plan for disease progression. Provide community resources and respite services for the client and family.

  - Consider referral to occupational and physical therapy for home environment assessment to determine safety and ease of mobility. Use adaptive devices to assist with activities of daily living.

  - Refer to speech language therapist for dysarthria and dysphagia.

AMYOTROPHIC LATERAL SCLEROSIS

Overview

- Amyotrophic lateral sclerosis (ALS) is a degenerative neurological disorder of the upper and lower motor neurons that results in deterioration and death of the motor neurons. This results in progressive paralysis and muscle wasting that eventually causes respiratory paralysis and death. Cognitive function is not usually affected.

- ALS is also known as Lou Gehrig's disease, after the professional baseball player who died of this disease in 1941.

- Death usually occurs due to respiratory failure within 3 to 5 years of the initial manifestations. The cause of ALS is unknown, and there is no cure.

- Health Promotion and Disease Prevention

  ○ Client Education – Genetic counseling is suggested for family members of clients who have ALS.

Assessment

- Risk Factors – ALS affects more men than women, often developing between the ages of 40 to 70.
- Subjective Data

  ○ Fatigue

  ○ Twitching and cramping of muscles

- Objective Data

  ○ Physical Assessment Findings

    ▪ Muscle weakness – usually begins in one part of the body

    ▪ Muscle atrophy

    ▪ Dysphagia

    ▪ Dysarthria

    ▪ Hyperreflexia of deep tendon reflexes

  ○ Laboratory Tests – Increased creatine kinase (CK-BB) level

  ○ Diagnostic Procedures

    ▪ Electromyogram (EMG) – Reduction in number of functioning motor units of peripheral nerves

    ▪ Muscle biopsy – Reduction in number of motor units of peripheral nerves and atrophic muscle fibers

Patient-Centered Care

- Nursing Care

  ○ Maintain a patent airway, and suction and/or intubate as needed.

  ○ Monitor ABGs, and administer oxygen, intermittent positive pressure ventilation, bilevel positive airway pressure, or mechanical ventilation as needed.

  ○ Keep the head of the bed at 45°; turn, cough, and deep breathe every 2 hr; and conduct incentive spirometry/chest physiotherapy.

○ Facilitate effective communication (dysarthria) with the use of a communication board or a speech language therapist referral.

○ Assess coping and depression.

○ Assess swallow reflex and ensure safety with oral intake. Thicken fluids as needed.

○ Meet nutritional needs for calories, fiber, and fluids. When no longer able to swallow, provide enteral nutrition as prescribed.

○ Use energy conservation measures.

○ Address the client's interest in the establishment of advance directives/living wills.

- Medications

  ○ Riluzole (Rilutek) is a glutamate antagonist that can slow the deterioration of motor neurons by decreasing the release of glutamic acid. It must be taken early in disease process, and will add approximately 2 to 3 months of life to the client's overall lifespan.

    ▪ Nursing Considerations

      □ Monitor liver function tests – hepatotoxic risk.

      □ Assess for dizziness, vertigo, and somnolence.

    ▪ Client Education

      □ Avoid drinking alcohol.

      □ Take medication at evenly spaced regular intervals (e.g., every 12 hr).

      □ Store medication away from bright light.

  ○ Baclofen (Lioresal), dantrolene sodium (Dantrium), diazepam (Valium)

    ▪ Antispasmodics are used to decrease spasticity.

- Teamwork and Collaboration

  ○ Initiate appropriate referrals (dietician, social service, physical therapy, occupational therapy, clinical psychologist) for extended care in the home or a long-term care facility as client's condition deteriorates.

  ○ Consider referral to a speech pathologist for speech and swallowing issues.

  ○ Consider hospice referral to provide support to the client and family coping with the terminal phase of the illness.

Complications

- Pneumonia can be caused by respiratory muscle weakness and paralysis contributing to ineffective airway exchange.

  ○ Nursing Actions – Assess respiratory status routinely and administer antimicrobial therapy as indicated.

- Respiratory failure may necessitate mechanical ventilation.

  ○ Nursing Actions – Assess respiratory status and be prepared to provide ventilatory support as needed per the client's advance directives.

MYASTHENIA GRAVIS

- Myasthenia gravis (MG) is a progressive autoimmune disease that produces severe muscular weakness. It is characterized by periods of exacerbation and remission. Muscle weakness improves with rest and worsens with increased activity.
- It is caused by antibodies that interfere with the transmission of acetylcholine at the neuromuscular junction.

Assessment

- Risk factors associated with rheumatoid arthritis, scleroderma, and systemic lupus erythematosus.
  - ○ Causes
    - ▪ Coexisting autoimmune disorder
    - ▪ Frequently associated with hyperplasia of the thymus gland
  - ○ Factors that trigger exacerbations
    - ▪ Infection
    - ▪ Stress, emotional upset, and fatigue
    - ▪ Pregnancy
    - ▪ Increases in body temperature (fever, sunbathing, hot tubs)
- Subjective Data
  - ○ Progressive muscle weakness
  - ○ Diplopia
  - ○ Difficulty chewing and swallowing
  - ○ Respiratory dysfunction
  - ○ Bowel and bladder dysfunction
  - ○ Poor posture
  - ○ Fatigue after exertion
- Objective Data
  - ○ Physical Assessment Findings
    - ▪ Impaired respiratory status (difficulty managing secretions, decreased respiratory effort)
    - ▪ Decreased swallowing ability
    - ▪ Decreased muscle strength, especially of the face, eyes, and proximal portion of major muscle groups
    - ▪ Incontinence
    - ▪ Drooping eyelids – unilateral or bilateral
  - ○ Diagnostic Procedures
    - ▪ Tensilon testing
      - □ Baseline assessment of the cranial muscle strength is done.
      - □ Edrophonium (Tensilon) is administered.
        - ▸ Medication inhibits the breakdown of acetylcholine, making it available for use at the neuromuscular junction. A positive test results in marked improvement in muscle strength that lasts approximately 5 min.

□ Nursing Actions

▸ Assist provider in administering this test.

▸ Observe for complications such as fasciculations around the eyes and face, as well as cardiac arrhythmias.

▸ Have atropine available, which is the antidote for edrophonium (bradycardia, sweating, and abdominal cramps).

□ Client Education

▸ Explain purpose of the test to the client.

▸ Encourage the client to follow the provider's directions in moving previously affected muscles.

▸ Discourage the client from demonstrating improvement by increasing effort, which could skew the test results.

▪ Electromyography

□ Shows the neuromuscular transmission characteristics of MG.

□ Decrease in amplitude of the muscle is demonstrated over a series of consecutive muscle contractions.

Patient-Centered Care

- Nursing Care

  ○ Assess and intervene as needed to maintain a patent airway (muscle weakness of diaphragm, respiratory, and intercostal muscles).

  ○ Use energy conservation measures. Allow for periods of rest.

  ○ Assess swallowing to prevent aspiration. Keep oxygen, endotracheal intubation, suctioning equipment, and a bag valve mask available at the client's bedside.

  ○ Provide small, frequent, high-calorie meals and schedule at times when medication is peaking.

  ○ Have the client sit upright when eating, and use thickener in liquids as necessary.

  ○ Apply a lubricating eye drop during the day and ointment at night if the client is unable to completely close his eyes. The client may also need to patch or tape his eyes shut at night to prevent damage to the cornea.

  ○ Encourage the client to wear a medical identification wristband or necklace at all times.

  ○ Administer medications as prescribed and at specified times.

- Medications

  ○ Anticholinesterase agents are the first line in therapy.

    ▪ Nursing Considerations

      □ Ensure that the medication is given at the specified time, usually four times a day.

      □ If periods of weakness are observed, discuss change in administration times with the provider.

      □ Use cautiously in clients who have a history of asthma or cardiac dysrhythmias.

- Client Education
  - Take with food to address gastrointestinal side effects.
  - Eat within 45 min of taking the medication to strengthen chewing and reduce the risk for aspiration.
  - Stress the importance of maintaining therapeutic levels and taking the medication at the same time each day.
- Pyridostigmine (Mestinon) and neostigmine (Prostigmin)
  - Used to increase muscle strength in the symptomatic treatment of MG. It inhibits the breakdown of acetylcholine and prolongs its effects.
  - Nursing Considerations
    - Assess the client for a history of seizures.
    - Use cautiously in clients who have a history of asthma and cardiovascular disease.
- Immunosuppressants such as prednisone and azathioprine (Imuran)
  - Immunosuppressants are given during exacerbations when pyridostigmine is not adequately effective.
  - Because MG is an autoimmune disease, immunosuppressants decrease the production of antibodies.
  - A corticosteroid, such as prednisone, is the first medication of choice. Cytotoxic medications, such as azathioprine (Imuran), are given if corticosteroids are ineffective.
  - Nursing Considerations
    - Monitor for infection.
    - Taper use gradually.
  - Client Education
    - Explain to the client the importance of slowly tapering off of a corticosteroid.
    - Tell the client to observe for manifestations of infection and take precautions against exposure to viruses and contaminants.

- IV immunoglobulins (IVIg) are used for acute management in clients who do not respond to the above treatments.
- Teamwork and Collaboration
  - Consult physical therapy for durable medical equipment needs.
  - Consult occupational therapy for assistive devices to facilitate ADLs.
  - Consult with a speech and language therapist if weakening of facial muscles impacts communication or swallowing.
- Therapeutic Procedures
  - Plasmapheresis removes circulating antibodies from the plasma. This is usually done several times over a period of days and may continue on a regular basis for some clients.
    - Nursing Actions
      - Preprocedure – Assess vital signs, laboratory values, and weight.
      - Intraprocedure
        - Assess for dizziness and hypotension.
        - Maintain the patency of shunts during the procedure (one is usually placed in each upper extremity).

- □ Postprocedure
  - ▸ Apply a pressure dressing.
  - ▸ Monitor for infection.
  - ▸ Assess laboratory findings.
  - ▸ Monitor for the possible complications of hypovolemia, hypokalemia, and hypocalcemia.
- ▪ Client Education – Instruct the client that the procedure will typically last 2 to 5 hr.
- Surgical Interventions
  - ○ Thymectomy – removal of the thymus gland is done to attain better control or complete remission.
    - ▪ May take months to years to see results due to the life of the circulating T cells.
  - ○ Nursing Actions
    - ▪ Postoperatively, monitor the client's respiratory status. Depending on the type of surgical procedure (transcervical using a video-assisted thoracoscope versus the open sternal approach), the client may be intubated and have a chest tube.
    - ▪ Ensure the client turns, coughs, and deep breathes every 2 hr.
    - ▪ Observe the client for findings of a pneumo- or hemothorax.

Complications

- Myasthenic crisis and cholinergic crisis
  - ○ Myasthenic crisis occurs when the client is experiencing a stressor that causes an exacerbation of MG, such as infection, or is taking inadequate amounts of cholinesterase inhibitor.
  - ○ Cholinergic crisis occurs when the client has taken too much cholinesterase inhibitor.
  - ○ The manifestations of both can be very similar (muscle weakness, respiratory failure).
  - ○ The client's highest risk for injury is due to respiratory compromise and failure.

Complications and Nursing Implications

MYASTHENIC CRISIS	CHOLINERGIC CRISIS
Undermedication	Overmedication
› Respiratory muscle weakness – mechanical ventilation	› Muscle twitching to the point of respiratory muscle weakness – mechanical ventilation
› Myasthenic findings (weakness, incontinence, fatigue)	› Cholinergic manifestations – hypersecretions (nausea, diarrhea, respiratory secretions) and hypermotility (abdominal cramps)
› Hypertension	› Hypotension
› Temporary decrease of findings with administration of Tensilon	› Tensilon has no positive effect on manifestations, and can actually worsen findings (more anticholinesterase – more cholinergic manifestations).
	› Manifestations decrease with the administration of an anticholinergic medication, such as atropine.
MIXED CRISIS	
› Clients may experience mixed crisis when myasthenic crisis is overtreated with anticholinesterase drugs.	
› Manifestations include dyspnea, dysphagia, dysarthria, restlessness, apprehension, salivation, and lacrimation.	

APPLICATION EXERCISES

1. A nurse is caring for a client admitted to the hospital with respiratory difficulty after being diagnosed with amyotrophic lateral sclerosis (ALS) approximately 1 year ago. Which of the following client findings should the nurse anticipate? (Select all that apply.)

_____ A. Loss of sensation

_____ B. Fluctuations in blood pressure

_____ C. Incontinence

_____ D. Ineffective cough

_____ E. Loss of cognitive function

2. A nurse is teaching a client who has ALS about a new prescription for riluzole (Rilutek). Which of the following instructions should the nurse give the client?

A. "Take this medication immediately prior to eating."

B. "Drink a glass of milk with the medication."

C. "Avoid consuming alcoholic beverages."

D. "Monitor your blood pressure daily."

3. A nurse is caring for a client who has myasthenia gravis (MG) and has developed drooping eyelids. Which of the following actions should the nurse take? (Select all that apply.)

_____ A. Apply lubricating eye drops.

_____ B. Encourage use of sunglasses.

_____ C. Support the head with pillows.

_____ D. Tape eyes closed at night.

_____ E. Provide for periods of rest during the day.

4. A nurse instructs a client who has MG about home care and the risk factors that can exacerbate the disease. Which of the following client statements indicates a need for further teaching?

A. "I should take my medication 45 min before meals."

B. "I have suction equipment at home in case I start to choke."

C. "I will soak in a warm bath every day."

D. "I ordered a medical identification bracelet to wear."

5. A nurse is beginning a physical assessment of a client who was recently diagnosed with multiple sclerosis (MS). Which of the following findings should the nurse expect? (Select all that apply.)

_____ A. Areas of paresthesia

_____ B. Involuntary eye movements

_____ C. Alopecia

_____ D. Increased salivation

_____ E. Ataxia

6. A nurse is providing education to family members of a client who has a new diagnosis of MS. What should be included in the teaching? Use the ATI Active Learning Template: Systems Disorder to complete this item to include the following sections:

A. Description of Disorder/Disease Process

B. Laboratory Tests

C. Diagnostic Procedures

D. Medications: Describe four medications and one teaching point for each.

APPLICATION EXERCISES KEY

1. A. INCORRECT: Sensory changes are not associated with ALS, but are findings in MS.

    B. INCORRECT: Fluctuations in blood pressure are not findings in a client who has ALS.

    C. **CORRECT:** Incontinence due to muscle weakness is a finding in a client who has ALS.

    D. **CORRECT:** Ineffective cough due to progressive muscle weakness is a finding in a client who has ALS.

    E. INCORRECT: Cognitive changes do not occur in a client who has ALS.

    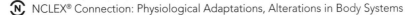 NCLEX® Connection: Physiological Adaptations, Alterations in Body Systems

2. A. INCORRECT: Riluzole should be taken on an empty stomach every 12 hr, either 1 hr before or 2 hr after meals.

    B. INCORRECT: Riluzole should be taken on an empty stomach every 12 hr, either 1 hr before or 2 hr after meals.

    C. **CORRECT:** Riluzole is hepatotoxic, so alcoholic beverages should be avoided to decrease the risk of liver damage.

    D. INCORRECT: Riluzole does not affect blood pressure.

    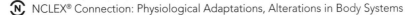 NCLEX® Connection: Pharmacological and Parenteral Therapies, Medication Administration

3. A. **CORRECT:** Lubricating eye drops reduce corneal dryness and irritation caused by weakness of the eyelids.

    B. INCORRECT: Wearing sunglasses does not prevent corneal dryness and irritation.

    C. INCORRECT: Providing head support does not correct drooping eyelids caused by muscle weakness.

    D. **CORRECT:** Taping the eyes closed at night prevents corneal dryness and irritation.

    E. INCORRECT: Promoting rest does not reduce eyelid drooping in the client who has MG.

    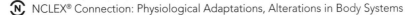 NCLEX® Connection: Physiological Adaptations, Illness Management

4. A. INCORRECT: The client who has MG is instructed to take cholinesterase inhibitors 45 min prior to meals.

    B. INCORRECT: Dysphagia occurs in a client who has MG, and suction equipment should be available in case of choking.

    C. **CORRECT:** Hot temperatures and hot water can cause a client who has MG to have an exacerbation.

    D. INCORRECT: A medical alert bracelet identifies the client who has MG.

    Ⓝ NCLEX® Connection: Physiological Adaptations, Illness Management

5. A. **CORRECT:** Areas of loss of skin sensation are a clinical finding in a client who has MS.

    B. **CORRECT:** Nystagmus is a clinical finding in a client who has MS.

    C. INCORRECT: Hair loss is not a clinical finding in a client who has MS.

    D. INCORRECT: Dysphagia, swallowing difficulty, is a clinical finding in a client who has MS.

    E. **CORRECT:** Ataxia occurs in the client who has MS as muscle weakness develops and there is loss of coordination.

    Ⓝ NCLEX® Connection: Physiological Adaptations, Pathophysiology

6. *Using the ATI Active Learning Template: Systems Disorder*

    A. Description of Disorder/Disease Process: MS is an autoimmune disorder characterized by the development of plaque in the white matter of the central nervous system. Plaque damages the myelin sheath and interferes with impulse transmission between the CNS and the body.

    B. Laboratory Tests: Cerebrospinal fluid analysis.

    C. Diagnostic Procedures: MRI of the brain and spine

    D. Medications

    • Immunosuppressive agents such as azathioprine (Imuran) and cyclosporine (Sandimmune) – Long-term effects include increased risk for infection, hypertension, and kidney dysfunction.

    • Corticosteroids such as prednisone – Increased risk for infection, hypervolemia, hypernatremia, hypokalemia, GI bleeding, and personality changes.

    • Antispasmodics such as dantrolene (Dantrium), tizanidine (Zanaflex), baclofen (Lioresal) and diazepam (Valium) are used to treat muscle spasticity. Report increased weakness and jaundice to provider. Avoid stopping baclofen abruptly.

    • Immunomodulators such as interferon beta (Betaseron) are used to prevent and treat relapses.

    • Anticonvulsants such as carbamazepine (Tegretol) are used for paresthesia.

    • Stool softeners such as docusate sodium (Colace) are used for constipation.

    • Anticholinergics such as propantheline are used for bladder dysfunction.

    • Beta-blockers such as primidone (Mysoline) and clonazepam (Klonopin) are used for tremors.

    Ⓝ NCLEX® Connection: Physiological Adaptations, Alterations in Body Systems

chapter 11

Overview

- Headaches may be acute or chronic, temporary or life-threatening.
- Headaches are a common occurrence and affect individuals of all ages; headaches are associated with other conditions such as colds, allergies, and stress or muscle tension.
- Primary headaches have no organic cause that can be identified. They include migraine headaches, tensionlike, and cluster headaches. They can be managed in the primary care setting.
- Secondary headaches are associated with an organic cause, such as a brain tumor or aneurysm, and warrant further investigation and medical management.
- This chapter includes migraine headaches and cluster headaches.

Health Promotion and Disease Prevention

- Promote stress management strategies and recognition of triggers of the onset of a headache.
- Promote hand hygiene to prevent the spread of viruses that produce coldlike symptoms.
- Review pain management to include over-the-counter medications and herbal remedies.
- Review risk factors (triggers) for both migraine and cluster headaches.
  - Alcohol or environmental allergies
  - Intense odors, bright lights, overuse of certain medications
  - Fatigue, sleep deprivation, depression, emotional or physical stress, anxiety
  - Menstrual cycles and oral contraceptive use
  - Foods containing tyramine, monosodium glutamate (MSG), nitrites, or milk products

---

MIGRAINE HEADACHES

Assessment

- Subjective Data
  - Photophobia and phonophobia (sensitivity to sounds)
  - Nausea and vomiting
  - Stress and anxiety
  - Unilateral pain, often behind one eye or ear
- Objective Data
  - Health history and family history for headache patterns
  - Alterations in ADLs for 4 to 72 hr

- Clinical manifestations that are similar with each headache
- Classified by categories and stages
  - With aura
    - Prodromal stage: includes awareness of findings for hours to days before onset: irritability, depression, food cravings, diarrhea/constipation, and frequent urination.
    - Aura stage: develops over minutes to an hour to include neurologic findings: numbness and tingling of mouth, lips, face, or hands; visual disturbances (light flashes, bright spots).
    - Second stage: severe, incapacitating, throbbing headache that intensifies over several hours and is accompanied by nausea, vomiting, drowsiness, and vertigo.
    - Third stage (4 to 72 hr): headache is dull. Older adults may continue with aura, and pain subsides (visual migraine).
    - Recovery with pain and aura subsiding. Muscle aches and contraction of head and neck muscles are common. Physical activity worsens pain, and client may sleep.
  - Without aura
    - Pain is aggravated by physical activity.
    - Unilateral, pulsating pain.
    - One or more of these manifestations present: photophobia, phonophobia, nausea, and/or vomiting.
    - Persists for 4 to 72 hr; often occurs in early morning, during periods of stress, or with premenstrual tension or fluid retention.
  - Atypical
    - Headache lasts longer than 72 hr.
    - Neurologic manifestations persist for 7 days.
    - Ischemic infarct may be found on neuroimaging.
    - Does not fit other criteria.
- Diagnostic Procedures: neuroimaging if neurologic findings present or client is older with a new onset of headaches.

Patient-Centered Care

- Nursing care (during headache)
  - Maintain a cool, dark, quiet environment.
  - Elevate the head of the bed to 30°.
  - Administer medications as prescribed.
- Medications
  - Abortive therapy to alleviate pain during aura or soon after start of headache.
    - For mild migraines: NSAIDs (ibuprofen, naproxen), acetaminophen, and over-the-counter anti-inflammatory medications in formulations for migraines (Advil Migraine Capsules).
    - Antiemetics (metoclopramide [Reglan]) to relieve nausea and vomiting.

- Severe migraines
  - □ Triptan preparations (zolmitriptan [Zomig], sumatriptan [Imitrex], eletriptan [Relpax]) to produce a vasoconstrictive effect.
  - □ Ergotamine preparations with caffeine (Cafergot, dihydroergotamine [Migranal]) to narrow blood vessels and reduce inflammation.
  - □ Isometheptene in combination formulations (Midrin) when other medications do not work.
- ○ Preventive therapy for frequent headaches or when other therapies are ineffective.
  - NSAIDs with beta-blocker (propranolol [Inderal]), calcium channel blocker, beta-adrenergic blocker or antiepileptic medications (divalproex [Depakote], topiramate [Topamax]).
  - Client is instructed to check pulse when taking beta-adrenergic blockers and calcium channel blockers.
- Client Education
  - ○ Review "Three R" approach with client (www.headaches.org).
    - Recognize migraine manifestations.
    - Respond and seek provider.
    - Relieve pain and manifestations.
  - ○ Remain in a cool, dark, quiet environment.
  - ○ Elevate the head of the bed as desired.
  - ○ Educate women over age 50 about risk factors for cardiovascular disease and stroke.

  - ○ Review trigger avoidance and management.
    - Educate about foods with tyramine (such as pickles, caffeine, beer, wine, aged cheese, artificial sweeteners) and foods with MSG or preservatives.
    - Review current medications for those known to induce migraines: ranitidine, estrogen, nitroglycerin, and nifedipine.
    - Discuss anger issues and handling conflict.
    - Reinforce the need for adequate rest and sleep.
    - Review travel involving a change in altitude.
    - Reinforce the need to avoid light glare or flickering lights.
    - Review client's menstrual cycle pattern and hormone fluctuations.
    - Discuss avoiding intense environmental odors, perfumes, and tobacco smoke.
  - ○ Educate client about use of complementary and alternative therapies.
    - Provide referral to community centers offering yoga, meditation, tai chi, exercise, and massage for relaxation and to alleviate muscle tension.
    - Provide referral to acupuncture and acupressure therapy, which may be helpful for pain management.
    - Herbal remedies and nutrition supplements should be reviewed with the provider because there is insufficient evidence to support their use in management of migraines.

CLUSTER HEADACHES

Assessment

- Subjective
  - Brief episode of intense, unilateral, nonthrobbing pain lasting 30 min to 2 hr that can radiate to forehead, temple, or cheek
    - Occurring daily at about the same time for 4 to 12 weeks
    - Followed by period of remission for up to 9 to 12 months
  - More frequent during spring and fall
  - No warning signs
  - Less common than migraines
- Objective
  - Men between 20 to 50 years of age
  - Tearing of the eye with runny nose and nasal congestion
  - Facial sweating
  - Drooping eyelid and eyelid edema
  - Miosis
  - Facial pallor
  - Nausea and vomiting
  - Pacing, walking, or sitting and rocking activities

Patient-Centered Care

- Medications (see medications for Migraine Headaches)
  - Triptans
  - Ergotamine preparations
  - Antiepileptic medications
  - Calcium channel blockers
  - Corticosteroids
  - Over-the-counter capsaicin
  - Melatonin
  - Glucosamine
- Home oxygen therapy at 7 to 10 L/min for 15 to 30 min may be helpful at onset of headache.
- Client education
  - Remain in a cool, dark, quiet environment with head elevated.

○ Remain in sitting position when using oxygen, and maintain safety precautions when using oxygen in the home.

○ Review prevention strategies.

- Wear sunglasses to reduce light and glare.

- Obtain adequate rest and sleep, exercise, and relaxation.

- Avoid foods containing tyramine, MSG, and nitrites (preservatives).

- Review of risk factors (triggers) for headaches.

  □ Anger outburst

  □ Anxiety and prolonged anticipation, or periods of stress

  □ Excessive physical activity, fatigue

  □ Altered sleep-wake cycles

APPLICATION EXERCISES

1. A nurse in a clinic is caring for a client who has frequent migraine headaches. The client asks about foods that may cause headaches. The nurse should recommend that the client avoid which of the following foods?

    A. Baked salmon

    B. Salted cashews

    C. Frozen strawberries

    D. Fresh asparagus

2. A nurse in a clinic is teaching a client who has a history of migraine headaches about a new prescription for zolmitriptan (Zomig). Which of the following statements by the client indicates understanding of the teaching?

    A. "This medication will relieve my symptoms by causing my blood vessesls to dilate."

    B. "This medication should prevent the headache from occurring."

    C. "I should take this medication as soon as I notice symptoms developing."

    D. "I should take this medication to lower my sensitivity to food triggers."

3. A nurse in a provider's office is obtaining a nursing history from a client who has cluster headaches. Which of the following are expected findings? (Select all that apply.)

    _____ A. Pain is bilateral across the posterior occipital area.

    _____ B. Client is experiencing altered sleep-wake cycle.

    _____ C. Headache occurs at approximately the same time of the day.

    _____ D. Client describes headache pain as dull and throbbing.

    _____ E. Nasal congestion and drainage occur.

4. A nurse is reviewing discharge instructions with a client who has a new diagnosis of migraine headaches. Which of the following instructions should the nurse include?

    A. Use music therapy for relaxation with the onset of the headache.

    B. Increase physical activity when a headache is present.

    C. Drink sugar-free beverages to prevent headaches.

    D. Apply a cool cloth to the face during a headache.

5. A nurse is obtaining a health history from a client who is being evaluated for the cause of frequent headaches. Which of the following questions should the nurse ask to identify the clinical findings of migraine headaches?

    A. Do the headaches occur at the same time each day?

    B. Is your headache accompanied by profuse facial sweating?

    C. Do you have seasonal headaches?

    D. Is there a pattern of headaches among family members?

6. A nurse in a clinic is caring for a client who has migraine headaches and is reviewing a new prescription for sumatriptan (Imitrex) nasal spray 5 mg. Using the ATI Active Learning Template: Medication and the ATI Pharmacology Review Module, complete this item to include the following: expected pharmacological action, and at least one statement under each of the subsequent sections of the template.

APPLICATION EXERCISES KEY

1. A. INCORRECT: Fish that is smoked contains tyramine and should be avoided. Baked salmon does not contain tyramine and is not a trigger for migraine headaches.

    B. **CORRECT:** Nuts contain tyramine, which may trigger migraine headaches.

    C. INCORRECT: Fruits are not a source of tyramine, which may trigger migraine headaches.

    D. INCORRECT: Vegetables are not a source of tyramine, which may trigger migraine headaches.

    Ⓝ NCLEX® Connection: Basic Care and Comfort, Nutrition and Oral Hydration

2. A. INCORRECT: Zolmitriptan causes cranial arteries, the basilar arteries, and blood vessels in the dura mater to constrict.

    B. INCORRECT: Zolmitriptan is used for abortive therapy in treating migraine headaches. It is not used for headache prevention.

    C. **CORRECT:** Zolmitriptan is a medication used to treat migraine headaches.

    D. INCORRECT: Zolmitriptan is used as a component of abortive therapy for treatment of migraine headaches and does not affect a client's sensitivity to food triggers.

    Ⓝ NCLEX® Connection: Pharmacological and Parenteral Therapies, Medication Administration

3. A. INCORRECT: Cluster headaches typically cause pain on one side of the head and radiate to the forehead, temple, or cheek.

    B. **CORRECT:** Cluster headaches may be caused by a lack of continuity in the sleep-wake cycle.

    C. **CORRECT:** Cluster headaches occur at about the same time of day for 4 to 12 weeks.

    D. INCORRECT: Cluster headaches are typically described as unilateral, intense, and nonthrobbing.

    E. **CORRECT:** A client may have a runny nose and nasal congestion with a cluster headache.

    Ⓝ NCLEX® Connection: Physiological Adaptations, Pathophysiology

4. A. INCORRECT: A quiet environment should be maintained during a migraine headache.

    B. INCORRECT: Increasing physical activity during a migraine headache may worsen the pain.

    C. INCORRECT: Sugar-free beverages contain tyramine, which can trigger a migraine headache.

    D. **CORRECT:** A cool cloth is an appropriate action that promotes comfort and may relieve pain.

    Ⓝ NCLEX® Connection: Basic Care and Comfort, Non-Pharmacological Comfort Interventions

5.   A. INCORRECT: Cluster headaches typically occur at the same time each day.

     B. INCORRECT: Profuse facial sweating is typical in the presence of cluster headaches.

     C. INCORRECT: A seasonal pattern is seen with cluster headaches.

     D. **CORRECT:** A familial pattern of headaches is a common finding with migraines.

     (N) NCLEX® Connection: Health Promotion and Maintenance, Health Promotion/Disease Prevention

6.   *Using the ATI Active Learning Template: Medication*
     - Expected Pharmacological Action
       ○ Vasoconstriction of cranial carotid arteries.
     - Therapeutic Uses
       ○ Abortive treatment of acute migraine attacks with or without aura and cluster headaches.
     - Side/Adverse Effects
       ○ Chest pressure and tightness; mild vertigo, malaise, fatigue and tingling sensations; coronary vasospasm (rare.)
     - Nursing Interventions/Client Education
       ○ Report chest pressure and tightness to provider if does not resolve quickly; do not take medication during pregnancy or if trying to become pregnant as medication may have teratogenic effects.
     - Medication/Food Interactions
       ○ Do not use concurrent with ergot alkaloids, monoamine oxidase inhibitors or selective serotonin reuptake inhibitors (SSRIs) and serotonin/norepinephrine reuptake inhibitors (SNRIs).
     - Nursing Interventions/Client Education
       ○ Avoid use of St. John's wort when on this medication.
     - Nursing Administration
       ○ Administer one unit-dose nasal spray in one nostril. May be repeated in 2 hr if headache remains but not to exceed 40 mg in 24 hr.
     - Evaluation of Medication Effectiveness
       ○ Relief of headache pain should be noted within 15 min after administration, with complete relief anticipated within 2 hr; relief of photophobia, phonophobia, nausea and vomiting associated with migraine attack.

     (N) NCLEX® Connection: Pharmacological and Parenteral Therapies, Medication Administration

chapter **12**

Overview

- Disorders of the eye can be caused by injury, disease process, and the aging process.

- Disorders of the eye that nurses should be knowledgeable about include the following:
  - Macular degeneration
  - Cataracts
  - Glaucoma

MACULAR DEGENERATION

Overview

- Macular degeneration, often called age-related macular degeneration (AMD), is the central loss of vision that affects the macula of the eye.

- There is no cure for macular degeneration.

- AMD is the No. 1 cause of vision loss in people over the age of 60.

- Two types of macular degeneration
  - Dry macular degeneration is the most common and is caused by a gradual blockage in retinal capillary arteries, which results in the macula becoming ischemic and necrotic due to the lack of retinal cells.
  - Wet macular degeneration is a less common form and is caused by the new growth of blood vessels that have thin walls and allow blood and fluid to leak from them.

Assessment

- Risk Factors
  - Dry macular degeneration
    - Smokers
    - Hypertension
    - Female
    - Short body stature
    - Family history
    - Diet lacking carotene and vitamin A
  - Wet macular degeneration can occur at any age
- Subjective Data
  - Lack of depth perception
  - Objects appear distorted
  - Blurred vision
- Objective Data
  - Loss of central vision
  - Blindness
  - Diagnostic Procedures
    - Ophthalmoscopy
      - An ophthalmoscope is used to examine the back part of the eyeball (fundus), including the retina, optic disc, macula, and blood vessels.
    - Visual acuity tests
      - Visual acuity tests include the Snellen and Rosenbaum eye charts.
- Client Education
  - Encourage clients to consume foods high in antioxidants, carotene, vitamin E, and B_{12}. The provider may prescribe a daily supplement high in carotene and vitamin E.
  - Monthly eye exams are essential in managing this disease.
  - As loss of vision progresses, clients will be challenged with the ability to eat, drive, write, and read, as well as other activities of daily living.
  - Refer clients to community organizations that can assist with transportation, reading devices, and large-print books.

CATARACTS

Overview

- A cataract is an opacity in the lens of an eye that impairs vision.
- There are three types of cataracts:
  - A subcapsular cataract begins at the back of the lens.
  - A nuclear cataract forms in the center (nucleus) of the lens.
  - A cortical cataract forms in the lens cortex and extends from the outside of the lens to the center.

 View Image: Cataracts

Health Promotion and Disease Prevention

- Teach clients to wear sunglasses while outside.
- Educate clients to wear protective eyewear while performing hazardous activities, such as welding and yard work.
- Encourage annual eye examinations and good eye health, especially in adults over the age of 40.

Assessment

- Risk Factors
  - Advanced age
  - Diabetes
  - Heredity
  - Smoking
  - Eye trauma
  - Excessive exposure to the sun
  - Chronic corticosteroid use
- Subjective Data
  - Decreased visual acuity (prescription changes, reduced night vision)
  - Blurred vision
  - Diplopia – double vision
  - Glare and light sensitivity – photo sensitivity
  - Halo around lights

- Objective Data
  - Physical Assessment Findings
    - Progressive and painless loss of vision
    - Visible opacity
    - Absent red reflex
  - Diagnostic Procedures
    - Cataracts can be determined upon examination of the lens using an ophthalmoscope.

Patient-Centered Care

- Nursing Care
  - Check the client's visual acuity using the Snellen chart.
  - Examine the external and internal eye structures using an ophthalmoscope.
  - Determine the client's functional capacity due to decreased vision.
  - Increase the amount of light in a room.
  - Provide the client with adaptive devices that accommodate for reduced vision.
    - Magnifying lens and large print books/newspapers
    - Talking devices, such as clocks
- Medications
  - Cycloplegic mydriatic (Atropine 1% ophthalmic solution)
    - This medication prevents pupil constriction for prolonged periods of time and relaxes muscles in the eye. It is used to dilate the eye preoperatively and for visualization of the eye's internal structures.
    - Nursing Considerations
      - The medication has a long duration, but a fast onset.
    - Client Education
      - Remind the client that the effects of the medication can last 7 to 14 days.
      - The medication may cause photosensitivity, so remind the client to wear sunglasses to protect the eyes.
- Teamwork and Collaboration
  - An ophthalmologist (eye surgeon) should be consulted for cataract surgery.

- Surgical Interventions
  - Surgical removal of the lens
    - A small incision is made, and the lens is either removed in one piece, or in several pieces, after being broken up using sound waves. The posterior capsule is retained. A replacement or intraocular lens is inserted. Replacement lenses can correct refractive errors, resulting in improved vision.
    - Nursing Actions
      - Postoperative care should focus on:
        - ▸ Preventing infection
        - ▸ Administering ophthalmic medications
        - ▸ Providing pain relief
        - ▸ Teaching the client about self-care at home and fall prevention
    - Client Education
      - Wear sunglasses while outside or in brightly lit areas.
      - Report signs of infection, such as yellow or green drainage.
      - Avoid activities that increase IOP.
        - ▸ Bending over at the waist
        - ▸ Sneezing
        - ▸ Coughing
        - ▸ Straining
        - ▸ Head hyperflexion
        - ▸ Restrictive clothing, such as tight shirt collars
        - ▸ Sexual intercourse
      - Limit activities.
        - ▸ Avoid tilting the head back to wash hair.
        - ▸ Limit cooking and housekeeping.
        - ▸ Avoid rapid, jerky movements, such as vacuuming.
        - ▸ Avoid driving and operating machinery.
        - ▸ Avoid sports.
      - Report pain with nausea/vomiting – indications of increased IOP or hemorrhage.
      - Best vision is not expected until 4 to 6 weeks following the surgery.
      - The client should report if any changes occur, such as lid swelling, decreased vision, bleeding or discharge, a sharp, sudden pain in the eye, and/or flashes of light or floating shapes.

Complications

- Infection
  - ○ Infection can occur after surgery.
  - ○ Client Education
    - ■ Signs of infection that the client should report include yellow or green drainage, increased redness or pain, reduction in visual acuity, increased tear production, and photophobia.
- Bleeding
  - ○ Bleeding is a potential risk several days following surgery.
  - ○ Client Education
    - ■ Clients should immediately report any sudden change in visual acuity or an increase in pain.

GLAUCOMA

Overview

- Glaucoma is a disturbance of the functional or structural integrity of the optic nerve. Decreased fluid drainage or increased fluid secretion increases intraocular pressure (IOP) and can cause atrophic changes of the optic nerve and visual defects. An expected reference range for IOP is between 10 and 21 mm/Hg.
- There are two primary types of glaucoma:
  - ○ Open-angle glaucoma – most common form of glaucoma. Open-angle refers to the angle between the iris and sclera. The aqueous humor outflow is decreased due to blockages in the eye's drainage system (Canal of Schlemm and trabecular meshwork), causing a rise in IOP.
  - ○ Angle-closure glaucoma – less common form of glaucoma. IOP rises suddenly. With angle-closure glaucoma, the angle between the iris and the sclera suddenly closes, causing a corresponding increase in IOP.
- Glaucoma is a leading cause of blindness. Early diagnosis and treatment is essential in preventing vision loss from glaucoma.

Health Promotion and Disease Prevention

- Encourage annual eye examinations and good eye health, especially adults over the age of 40.
- Educate clients about the disease process and early indications of glaucoma, such as reduced vision and mild eye pain.

Assessment

- Risk Factors
  - Age
  - Infection
  - Tumors
  - Diabetes mellitus
  - Genetic predisposition
  - Hypertension
- Subjective and Objective Data
  - Open-angle glaucoma
    - Headache
    - Mild eye pain
    - Loss of peripheral vision
    - Decreased accommodation
    - Elevated IOP (greater than 21 mm Hg)
  - Angle-closure glaucoma
    - Rapid onset of elevated IOP
    - Decreased or blurred vision
    - Seeing halos around lights
    - Pupils are nonreactive to light
    - Severe pain and nausea
    - Photophobia
  - Diagnostic Procedures
    - Visual assessments
      - Decrease in visual acuity and peripheral vision
    - Tonometry
      - Tonometry is used to measure IOP. IOP (expected reference range is 10 to 21 mm Hg) is elevated with glaucoma, especially angle-closure.
    - Gonioscopy
      - Gonioscopy is used to determine the drainage angle of the anterior chamber of the eyes.

Patient-Centered Care

- Nursing Care
  - Monitor clients for increased IOP (greater than 21 mm Hg).
  - Monitor clients for decreased vision and light sensitivity.
  - Assess clients for aching or discomfort around the eye.

- ○ Explain the disease process to clients and allow them to express their feelings.
- ○ Treat severe pain and nausea that accompanies angle-closure glaucoma with analgesics and antiemetics.
- Medications
  - ○ The priority intervention for treating glaucoma is drug therapy.
  - ○ Client teaching should include the following:
    - Prescribed eye medication is beneficial if used every 12 hr.
    - Instill one drop in each eye twice daily.
    - Wait 10 to 15 min in between eye drops if more than one is prescribed by the provider.
    - Avoid touching the tip of the application bottle to the eye.
    - Always wash hands before and after use.
    - Once eyedrop is instilled, apply pressure using the punctal occlusion technique (placing pressure on the inner corner of the eye).
  - ○ Pilocarpine (Isopto Carpine – ophthalmic solution)
    - Pilocarpine is a miotic, which constricts the pupil and allows for better circulation of the aqueous humor. Miotics can cause blurred vision.
  - ○ Timolol (Timoptic – ophthalmic solution) and acetazolamide (Diamox – oral medication)
    - Beta-blockers (timolol) and carbonic anhydrase inhibitors (acetazolamide) decrease IOP by reducing aqueous humor production.
  - ○ IV mannitol (Osmitrol)
    - IV mannitol is an osmotic diuretic used in the emergency treatment for angle-closure glaucoma to quickly decrease IOP.
  - ○ Prednisolone acetate (Pred Forte – ophthalmic solution)
    - Prednisolone acetate is an ocular steroid used to decrease inflammation.
  - ○ Acetazolamide (Diamox – oral medication)
    - Acetazolamide is administered preoperatively to reduce IOP, to dilate pupils, and to create eye paralysis to prevent lens movement.
    - Nursing Considerations
      - □ Always ask clients whether they are allergic to sulfa. Acetazolamide is a sulfa-based medication.
- Teamwork and Collaboration
  - ○ Referral to an ophthalmologist (eye surgeon) may be indicated if surgery is necessary.
- Surgical Interventions
  - ○ Glaucoma surgery
    - Laser trabeculectomy, iridotomy, or the placement of a shunt are procedures used to improve the flow of the aqueous humor by opening a channel out of the anterior chamber of the eye.
    - Nursing Actions
      - □ IOP is checked 1 to 2 hr postoperatively by the surgeon.
      - □ Educate clients about the disease and importance of adhering to the medication schedule to treat IOP.

- Client Education
  - □ Wear sunglasses while outside or in brightly lit areas.
  - □ Report signs of infection, such as yellow or green drainage.
  - □ Avoid activities that increase IOP.
    - ▶ Bending over at the waist
    - ▶ Sneezing
    - ▶ Coughing
    - ▶ Straining
    - ▶ Head hyperflexion
    - ▶ Restrictive clothing, such as tight shirt collars
    - ▶ Sexual intercourse
  - □ Clients should not lie on the operative side and should report severe pain or nausea (possible hemorrhage).
  - □ Clients should report if any changes occur, such as lid swelling, decreased vision, bleeding or discharge, a sharp, sudden pain in the eye and/or flashes of light or floating shapes.
  - □ Limit activities.
    - ▶ Avoid tilting head back to wash hair.
    - ▶ Limit cooking and housekeeping.
    - ▶ Avoid rapid, jerky movements, such as vacuuming.
    - ▶ Avoid driving and operating machinery.
    - ▶ Avoid sports.
  - □ Report pain with nausea/vomiting – indications of increased IOP or hemorrhage.
  - □ Final best vision is not expected until 4 to 6 weeks after surgery.
- Care after Discharge
  - ○ Set up services such as community outreach programs, meals on wheels, and services for the blind.

Complications

- Blindness
  - ○ Blindness is a potential consequence of undiagnosed and untreated glaucoma.
  - ○ Client Education
    - Encourage adults 40 or older to have an annual examination, including a measurement of IOP.

APPLICATION EXERCISES

1. A nurse is caring for a an older adult client who has diabetes mellitus. The client reports loss of peripheral vision. For which of the following is the client at risk?

    A. Cataracts

    B. Open-angle glaucoma

    C. Macular degeneration

    D. Angle-closure glaucoma

2. A nurse is caring for a client following a trabeculectomy. Which of the following statements should the nurse include in the teaching?

    A. "You may resume playing golf."

    B. "You need to tilt your head back when washing your hair."

    C. "You may continue driving to and from work."

    D. "You need to limit your housekeeping activities."

3. A nurse is caring for a male older adult client who has a new diagnosis of glaucoma. Which of the following should the nurse recognize as risk factors associated with this disease? (Select all that apply.)

    _____ A. Gender

    _____ B. Genetic predisposition

    _____ C. Hypertension

    _____ D. Age

    _____ E. Diabetes mellitus

4. A nurse is caring for a client who has a new diagnosis of cataracts. Which of the following clinical manifestations should the nurse expect to find? (Select all that apply.)

    _____ A. Eye pain

    _____ B. Floating spots

    _____ C. Blurred vision

    _____ D. White pupils

    _____ E. Bilateral red reflexes

5. A nurse is assessing a client following cataract surgery. The client reports nausea and severe eye pain. Which of the following actions should the nurse take?

    A. Notify the provider.

    B. Administer an analgesic.

    C. Administer an antiemetic.

    D. Turn the client onto the operative side.

6. A nurse is reviewing the discharge instructions for a client who has a new diagnosis of primary open-angle glaucoma and a new prescription for timolol (Timpotic) 0.25%. Use the ATI Active Learning Template: Medication and the ATI Pharmacology Review Module to complete this item. Include Adverse Effects: List at least three that should be included in the teaching.

APPLICATION EXERCISES KEY

1. A. INCORRECT: A client who has cataracts experiences a decrease in vision and sensitivity to lights.

    B. **CORRECT:** The nurse should anticipate that the client is experiencing open-angle glaucoma. Loss of peripheral vision is a clinical manifestation associated with this diagnosis.

    C. INCORRECT: A client who has macular degeneration experiences a loss of central vision.

    D. INCORRECT: A client who has angle-closure glaucoma experiences nausea and severe pain.

    Ⓝ NCLEX® Connection: Health Promotion and Maintenance, Health Screening

2. A. INCORRECT: The nurse should not instruct the client to resume playing golf. This could cause the client's intraocular pressure (IOP) to rise or possible injury to the eye.

    B. INCORRECT: The nurse should not instruct the client to tilt his head back when washing his hair. This could cause the client's intraocular pressure (IOP) to rise or possible injury to the eye.

    C. INCORRECT: Driving should be avoided until the client's vision is evaluated following surgery and the provider instructs the client about resuming driving.

    D. **CORRECT:** The nurse should instruct the client to limit housekeeping activities following cataract surgery. This activity could elevate the client's intraocular pressure (IOP) or result in injury to the eye.

    Ⓝ NCLEX® Connection: Physiological Adaptations, Illness Management

3. A. INCORRECT: Gender is not a risk factor associated with glaucoma.

    B. **CORRECT:** Genetic predisposition is a risk factor associated with glaucoma.

    C. **CORRECT:** Hypertension is a risk factor associated with glaucoma.

    D. **CORRECT:** Age is a risk factor associated with glaucoma.

    E. **CORRECT:** Diabetes mellitus is a risk factor associated with glaucoma.

    Ⓝ NCLEX® Connection: Health Promotion and Maintenance, Health Promotion/Disease Prevention

4. A. INCORRECT: Eye pain is not a clinical manifestation associated with cataracts.

    B. INCORRECT: Floating spots are a clinical manifestation associated with retinal detachment.

    C. **CORRECT:** Blurred vision is a clinical manifestation associated with cataracts.

    D. **CORRECT:** White pupils are a clinical manifestation associated with cataracts.

    E. INCORRECT: Bliateral red reflexes are absent in a client who has cataracts.

    Ⓝ NCLEX® Connection: Basic Care and Comfort, Personal Hygiene

5. A. **CORRECT:** Following cataract surgery, the provider should be notified if the client is experiencing nausea and severe pain.

    B. INCORRECT: Analgesic medication should not be administered until the client is evaluated by the provider.

    C. INCORRECT: Antiemetic medication should not be administered until the client is evaluated by the provider.

    D. INCORRECT: Turning the client on hcr operative side could result in increased eye pain and worsen the nausea.

    Ⓝ NCLEX® Connection: Basic Care and Comfort, Rest and Sleep

6. *Using ATI Active Learning Template: Medication and the ATI Pharmacology Review Module*
    - Adverse Effects
      - CNS: lethargy, fatigue, weakness, anxiety, headache, somnolence, confusion, depression, psychotic dissociation
      - CV: bradycardia, palpitations, syncope, hypotension, AV conduction disturbances, aggravation of peripheral vascular insufficiency, CHF
      - Special senses: superficial punctate keratopathy, eye irritation including conjunctivitis, keratitis, blepharitis
      - Skin: urticaria, rash, GI nausea, anorexia, dyspepsia
      - Respiratory: difficulty breathing, bronchospasm
      - Metabolic: hypokalemia, hypoglycemia
      - Body as whole: fever

    Ⓝ NCLEX® Connection: Pharmacological and Parenteral Therapies, Adverse Effects/Contraindications/Side Effects/Interactions

chapter 13

Overview

- The middle ear consists of the tympanic membrane (eardrum) and three ossicular bones (malleus, incus, and stapes), and connects to the oropharynx via the eustachian tube.

- The inner ear consists of the oval window, cochlea (hearing organ), and vestibular system (organ responsible for balance, which includes the semicircular canals).

- Changes in the middle and inner ear related to aging include thickening of the tympanic membrane (loss of elasticity), loss of sensory "hair" cells in the organ of Corti, and limitations to movement of the ossicles (incus, stapes, malleus).

- Middle and inner ear disorders cause many of the same problems due to their close proximity and adjoining structures.

- Disorders related to function of the middle ear can be caused by injury, disease, and/or the aging process.

- Middle ear infections are called otitis media.

  ○ Infection causes inflammation of ossicles and purulent drainage.

  ○ May be acute, chronic, or serous.

  ○ Treated with antibiotics or surgery. (Refer to the chapter on *Acute Otitis Media* in the *Nursing Care of Children Review Module*.)

- Inner ear problems are characterized by tinnitus (continuous ringing in ear), vertigo (whirling sensation), and dizziness.

- Labyrinthitis and Ménière's disease are inner ear problems.

  ○ Labyrinthitis is an infection of the labyrinth, usually secondary to otitis media.

  ○ Ménière's disease is a vestibular disease characterized by a triad of manifestations: tinnitus, unilateral sensorineural hearing loss, and vertigo.

    ▪ Benign paroxysmal vertigo (BPV) occurs in response to a change in position. It is thought to be due to a disturbance of crystals in the semicircular canals, initiating vertigo that lasts from days to months.

- Visual, vestibular, and proprioceptive systems provide the brain with input regarding balance. Problems within any of these systems pose a risk for loss of balance.

- Nurses should be knowledgeable about the types of middle- and inner-ear disorders, including infection, tumors, and issues with balance and coordination.

Assessment

- Risk Factors
  - Middle ear disorders
    - Recurrent colds and otitis media
    - Enlarged adenoids
    - Trauma
    - Changes in air pressure (scuba diving, flying)
  - Inner ear disorders
    - Viral or bacterial infection
    - Damage due to ototoxic medications
- Subjective Data
  - Middle ear disorders
    - Hearing loss
    - Feeling of fullness and/or pain in the ear
  - Inner ear disorders
    - Hearing loss
    - Tinnitus
    - Dizziness or vertigo
- Objective Data
  - Middle ear disorders
    - Red, inflamed ear canal and tympanic membrane (TM)
    - Bulging TM
    - Fluid and/or bubbles behind TM
  - Inner ear disorders
    - Vomiting
    - Nystagmus
    - Alterations in balance
  - Diagnostic Procedures
    - Tympanogram measures the mobility of the TM and middle ear structures relative to sound (effective in diagnosing middle ear disease).
    - Otoscopy
      - An otoscope is used to examine the external auditory canal, the TM, and malleus bone visible through the TM.

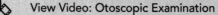
M View Video: Otoscopic Examination

- ▫ Nursing Actions
  - ▸ Otoscopic examination is done if audiometry results indicate a possible impairment or if a client is reporting ear pain.
  - ▸ After selection of a properly sized speculum, an otoscope is introduced into the external ear.
  - ▸ If the ear canal curves, pull up and back on the auricle of adults, and down and back on the auricle of children, to straighten out the canal and enhance visualization.
  - ▸ The TM should be a pearly gray color and intact. It should provide complete structural separation of the outer and middle ear structures.
  - ▸ The light reflex should be visible from the center of the TM anteriorly (5 o'clock right ear; 7 o'clock left ear).

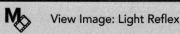 View Image: Light Reflex

  - ▸ In the presence of fluid or infection in the middle ear, the TM becomes inflamed and may bulge from the pressure of the exudate. This also displaces the light reflex, a significant diagnostic finding.
  - ▸ Avoid touching the lining of the ear canal, which causes pain due to sensitivity.
- ▫ Client Education
  - ▸ Warn the client that to see the TM clearly, the auricle may need to be firmly pulled.
- ■ Electronystagmography (ENG) determines the type of nystagmus elicited by the stimulation of the acoustic nerve.
  - ▫ Electrodes are placed around the eyes and movements of the eyes are recorded when the ear canal is stimulated with cold water instillation or injection of air. Recording of eye movements can be interpreted by a specialist as either normal or abnormal.
  - ▫ Nursing Actions
    - ▸ Intraprocedure, the nurse should ask simple questions (name recall, math problems) to ensure the client remains alert.
    - ▸ The client should be maintained on bed rest and NPO postprocedure until vertigo subsides.
  - ▫ Client Education
    - ▸ The client's preparation includes fasting immediately before the procedure, and restricting caffeine, alcohol, sedatives, and antihistamines 24 hr prior to the test.
    - ▸ This test is not performed on clients who have a pacemaker. (Pacemaker signals inhibit sensitivity of ENG.)
- ■ Caloric testing
  - ▫ Water (warmer or cooler than body temperature) is instilled in the ear in an effort to induce nystagmus.
  - ▫ The eyes' response to the instillation of cold and warm water is diagnostic of vestibular disorders.
  - ▫ This can be done concurrently with ENG.
  - ▫ Nursing Actions – The client should follow the same restrictions as those for an ENG.
  - ▫ Client Education – Inform the client of the above restrictions.

Patient-Centered Care

- Nursing Care
  - Monitor the client's functional ability and balance. Take fall risk precautions as necessary.
  - Evaluate the client's home situation. Collaborate with home health to assess home safety and falls risks, as needed.
  - Encourage client who has balance or functional limitations to rise slowly and use assistance and assistive devices as needed.
  - Check the hearing of clients receiving ototoxic medications for more than 5 days. Reduced renal function that occurs with aging increases the risk for ototoxicity. Ototoxic medications include:
    - Multiple antibiotics – gentamicin, amikacin, or metronidazole (Flagyl)
    - Diuretics – furosemide (Lasix)
    - NSAIDs – aspirin or ibuprofen (Advil)
    - Chemotherapeutic agents – cisplatin
  - Assist with ENG and/or caloric testing as needed.
  - Administer antivertigo and antiemetic medications as needed.
- Medications
  - Meclizine (Antivert)
    - Meclizine has antihistamine and anticholinergic effects and is used to treat the vertigo that accompanies inner ear problems.
    - Nursing Considerations
      - Restrict use in clients who have closed-angle glaucoma.
      - Observe the client for sedation and take appropriate precautions to ensure safe ambulation.
    - Client Education – Warn the client about the sedative effects of meclizine (avoid driving, operating heavy machinery).
  - Antiemetics
    - Droperidol (Inapsine) is one of several antiemetics used to treat nausea and vomiting associated with vertigo.
    - Nursing Considerations
      - Observe the client for postural hypotension and tachycardia.
      - Tell the client to avoid abrupt changes in position.
    - Client Education – Warn the client about the hypotensive effects of droperidol.
  - Diphenhydramine and dimenhydrinate
    - Antihistamines are effective in the treatment of vertigo and nausea that accompany inner ear problems.
    - Nursing Considerations
      - Observe the client for urinary retention.
      - Observe the client for sedation, and take appropriate precautions to ensure safe ambulation.
    - Client Education
      - Warn the client about the sedative effects (avoid driving, operating heavy machinery).
      - Inform the client that dry mouth is to be expected.

- ○ Scopolamine (Transderm Scop)
  - ■ Anticholinergics, such as scopolamine, are effective in the treatment of nausea that accompanies inner ear problems.
  - ■ Nursing Considerations
    - □ Observe the client for urinary retention.
    - □ Observe the client for sedation and take appropriate precautions to ensure safe ambulation.
    - □ Clients who have open-angle glaucoma should be monitored for increasing eye pressure; contraindicated in clients who have angle-closure glaucoma.
  - ■ Client Education
    - □ Warn the client about the sedative effects antihistamines (avoid driving, heavy machinery).
    - □ Inform client that dry mouth is to be expected.
- ○ Diazepam (Valium)
  - ■ Diazepam is a benzodiazepine that has antivertigo effects.
  - ■ Nursing Considerations
    - □ Observe for sedation and take appropriate precautions to ensure safe ambulation.
    - □ Restrict use in clients who have closed-angle glaucoma.
    - □ For the older adult client, use the smallest effective dose (prevent oversedation, ataxia).
  - ■ Client Education
    - □ Warn the client about the sedative effects of diazepam (avoid driving, operating heavy machinery).
    - □ Inform the client of diazepam's addictive properties and appropriate use of the medication.
- • Teamwork and Collaboration
  - ○ Vestibular rehabilitation is an option for clients who experience frequent episodes of vertigo and/or are incapacitated due to the vertigo. A team of health care providers treats the cause and teaches the client exercises that can help him adapt to and minimize the effects of vertigo. A combination of biofeedback, physical therapy, and stress management may be used. Postural education can teach the client positions to avoid as well as positional exercises that can terminate an attack of vertigo.
- • Therapeutic Procedures
  - ○ Vertigo-reducing activities
    - ■ Client Education
      - □ The client should be taught how to prevent stimulation/exacerbation of vertigo.
      - □ Have the client avoid caffeine and alcohol.
      - □ Encourage the client to rest in a quiet, darkened environment when vertigo is severe.
      - □ Have the client use assistive devices (cane, walker) as needed for safe ambulation to assist with balance.
      - □ Encourage the client to maintain a safe environment that is free of clutter.
      - □ Instruct the client to take a diuretic, if prescribed, to decrease the amount of fluid in semicircular canals.
      - □ Tell the client to space intake of fluids evenly throughout the day.
      - □ Teach the client to decrease intake of salt and sodium-containing foods (processed meats, MSG).
      - □ Remind the client to resume these precautions if vertigo returns.

- Surgical Interventions
  - Stapedectomy
    - A stapedectomy is a surgical procedure of the middle ear in which the stapes is removed and replaced with a prosthesis.
      - The procedure is done through the external ear canal and TM.
      - The TM is repaired, and sterile ear packing is placed postoperatively.
    - The procedure is done when otosclerosis has developed and the bones of the middle ear fuse together.
    - Otosclerosis is one of the causes of conductive hearing loss in older adults.
    - Nursing Actions
      - Assess the client for facial nerve damage.
      - Intervene for vertigo, nausea, and vomiting (common findings following the procedure).
    - Client Education
      - Hearing is initially worse, but will improve as healing occurs.
      - Avoid straining, coughing, sneezing with mouth closed, air travel, and rapid head movements.
      - Hair can be washed if the ear is covered with a dressing. No water should enter the ear.
  - Cochlear implant – sensorineural hearing loss
    - Cochlear implants consist of a microphone that picks up sound, a speech processor, a transmitter and receiver that converts sounds into electric impulses, and electrodes that are attached to the auditory nerve.
    - The implant's transmitter is located outside the head behind the ear and connects via a magnet to the receiver located immediately below it, under the skin.
    - Young children and adults who lost their hearing after speech development adapt to cochlear implants more quickly than those who were totally deaf at birth. Intensive and prolonged language training is necessary for individuals who did not develop speech.
    - Nursing Actions – follow pre-, intra- and postoperative outpatient surgery guidelines
    - Client Education
      - Inform the client that immediately after surgery, the unit is not turned on.
      - Two to six weeks after surgery, the external unit is applied and the speech processor is programmed.
      - Instruct the client on precautions to prevent infection.
      - Instruct the client that MRIs must be avoided.
  - Labyrinthectomy
    - A labyrinthectomy is a surgical treatment for vertigo that involves removal of the labyrinthine portion of the inner ear.
    - Nursing Actions
      - Client will have severe nausea and vertigo postoperatively. Take appropriate safety precautions and give antiemetics as needed.
    - Client Education
      - Inform the client that hearing loss is to be expected in the affected ear.

APPLICATION EXERCISES

1. A nurse is performing an otoscopic examination of a client. Which of the following is an unexpected finding?

    A. Pearly, gray tympanic membrane (TM)

    B. Malleus visible behind the TM

    C. Flaky skin in the external canal near the TM

    D. Black cerumen partially occluding the TM

2. A nurse in a clinic is caring for a client who has been experiencing mild to moderate vertigo due to benign paroxysmal vertigo for several weeks. Which of the following actions should the nurse recommend to help control the vertigo? (Select all that apply.)

    _____ A. Reduce exposure to bright lighting.

    _____ B. Move head slowly when changing positions.

    _____ C. Avoid fruits high in potassium.

    _____ D. Plan evenly spaced daily fluid intake.

    _____ E. Avoid smoking.

3. A nurse is caring for a client who has suspected Ménière's disease. Which of the following is an expected finding?

    A. Presence of a purulent lesion in the external ear canal

    B. Recent history of plane travel

    C. Bulging, red bilateral tympanic membranes

    D. Unilateral hearing loss

4. A nurse is reviewing the health record of a client who has a middle ear disorder. Which of the following are expected findings? (Select all that apply.)

    _____ A. Enlarged adenoids

    _____ B. Report of recent colds

    _____ C. Discontinued prescription for furosemide 6 months ago

    _____ D. Light reflexes visible on otoscopic exam at 5 and 7 o'clock

    _____ E. Report of frequent ingestion of ibuprofen

5. A nurse is completing discharge teaching to a client following a stapedectomy. Which of the following statements by the client indicates understanding of the teaching?

    A. "I am glad I'll be able to return to my position as an airplane pilot right away."

    B. "I will cover my ear when washing my hair."

    C. "I will remove the dressing behind my ear in 7 days."

    D. "I can expect my hearing to return in 24 hours."

6. A nurse in a clinic is completing preoperative teaching for an adult client who will receive a cochlear implant. What should be included in the teaching? Use the ATI Active Learning Template: Therapeutic Procedure to complete this item to include the following sections:

    A. Description of Procedure: Describe a cochlear implant.

    B. Indications: Describe the indication for a cochlear implant.

    C. Nursing Interventions: List at least four.

APPLICATION EXERCISES KEY

1. A. INCORRECT: A pearly, gray TM is an expected finding during an otoscopic examination.

    B. INCORRECT: Visualization of the malleus behind the TM is an expected finding during an otoscopic examination.

    C. INCORRECT: Flaking skin in the external ear canal is an expected finding during an otoscopic examination.

    D. **CORRECT:** Cerumen varies from light to dark yellowish-brown in color. Black cerumen may indicate the presence of blood and is an unexpected finding during an otoscopic examination.

    Ⓝ NCLEX® Connection: Psychosocial Integrity, Chemical and Other Dependencies/ Substance Use Disorder

2. A. **CORRECT:** Remaining in a darkened, quiet environment can reduce vertigo, particularly when it is severe.

    B. **CORRECT:** Moving slowly when standing or changing positions can reduce vertigo.

    C. INCORRECT: The client who has vertigo should be instructed to avoid foods containing high levels of sodium to reduce fluid retention, which can cause vertigo.

    D. **CORRECT:** Fluid intake should be planned so that it is evenly spaced throughout the day to prevent excess fluid accumulation in the semicircular canals.

    E. INCORRECT: Smoking has no effect on vertigo.

    Ⓝ NCLEX® Connection: Physiological Adaptations, Alterations in Body Systems

3. A. INCORRECT: Ménière's disease is an inner ear disorder. A purulent lesion in the external ear canal is not an expected clinical finding.

    B. INCORRECT: Ménière's disease is an inner ear disorder. Changes in air pressure due to plane travel affect the middle ear.

    C. INCORRECT: Ménière's disease is an inner ear disorder. Bulging, red bilateral tympanic membranes is a finding associated with a middle ear infection.

    D. **CORRECT:** Unilateral sensorineural hearing loss is a clinical finding in Ménière's disease.

    Ⓝ NCLEX® Connection: Physiological Adaptations, Alterations in Body Systems

4.   A. **CORRECT:** Enlarged tonsils are a clinical finding associated with a middle ear infection.

B. **CORRECT:** Frequent colds and otitis media are clinical findings associated with a middle ear disorder.

C. INCORRECT: Furosemide (Lasix) is an ototoxic medication and can cause a middle ear disorder, but the effects would not be present 6 months after discontinuing the prescription.

D. INCORRECT: Light reflexes would be absent or in altered positions in a client who has a middle ear disorder.

E. **CORRECT:** Ibuprofen is an ototoxic medication and can cause a middle ear disorder.

Ⓝ NCLEX® Connection: Physiological Adaptations, Pathophysiology

5.   A. INCORRECT: Airplane travel is limited, as prescribed by the provider, following a stapedectomy.

B. **CORRECT:** Water should be prevented from entering the ear canal until the incision is healed following a stapedectomy.

C. INCORRECT: A stapedectomy is performed through the tympanic membrane, and the client will have sterile ear packing within the ear canal. There is no external excision.

D. INCORRECT: Hearing is usually worse following a stapedectomy and will gradually improve as healing occurs.

Ⓝ NCLEX® Connection: Physiological Adaptations, Alterations in Body Systems

6.   *Using the ATI Active Learning Template: Therapeutic Procedure*

A. Description of Procedure: A cochlear implant consists of a microphone to pick up sound, a speech processor, a transmitter and receiver to convert sounds into electrical impulses, and electrodes that are attached to the auditory nerve. The implant's transmitter is placed outside the head, behind the ear, via a magnet that attaches to the receiver located under the skin below it.

B. Indications: A cochlear implant is performed for sensorineural hearing loss.

C. Nursing Interventions
   • Pre- and postoperative teaching is completed.
   • Intraoperative care is provided in an outpatient setting.
   • Client education includes:
   • The unit is not turned on immediately after surgery
   • Two to 6 weeks after surgery, the external unit is applied and the speech processor is programmed.
   • The client is instructed to prevent infection.
   • MRIs should be avoided by clients who have a cochlear implant.

Ⓝ NCLEX® Connection: Psychosocial Integrity, Chemical and Other Dependencies/ Substance Use Disorder

UNIT 2 **NURSING CARE OF CLIENTS WITH NEUROSENSORY DISORDERS**
SECTION: NEUROLOGIC EMERGENCIES

CHAPTER 14   Head Injury

Overview

- Head injuries are classified as open or penetrating trauma (skull integrity compromised) or closed or blunt trauma (skull integrity maintained). Head injuries are also classified as mild, moderate, or severe, depending upon Glasgow Coma Scale (GCS) ratings and the length of time the client was unconscious.

- Open-head injuries pose a high risk for infection.

- Skull fractures are often accompanied by brain injury. Damage to the brain tissue may be the result of decreased oxygen supply, or the direct impact from the skull fracture, which caused the trauma. The glucose levels in the brain are negatively affected, resulting in an alteration in neurological synaptic ability.

- Head injuries may be associated with hemorrhage (epidural, subdural, and intracerebral) or cerebrospinal fluid leakage. Any collection of fluid or foreign objects that occupies the space within the skull poses a risk for cerebral edema, cerebral hypoxia, and brain herniation.

- A cervical spine injury should always be suspected when a head injury occurs. A cervical spine injury must be ruled out prior to removing any devices used to stabilize the cervical spine.

Health Promotion and Disease Prevention

- Wear helmets when skateboarding, riding a bike or motorcycle, skiing, and playing football or any other sport that could cause a head injury. Depending on the activity or sport, instruct the client to wear a helmet.

- Wear seat belts when driving or riding in a car.

- Avoid dangerous activities (speeding, driving under the influence of alcohol or drugs).

Assessment

- Risk Factors
  - Males under 25 years of age
  - Motor vehicle or motorcycle crashes
  - Age 65 to 75 years old (second highest incidence)
  - Drug and alcohol use
  - Sports injuries
  - Assault
  - Gunshot wounds
  - Falls

- Subjective and Objective Data
  - Presence of alcohol or illicit drugs at time of injury.
  - Amnesia (loss of memory) before or after the injury.
  - Loss of consciousness – Length of time the client is unconscious is significant.
  - Manifestations of increased intracranial pressure include:
    - Severe headache.
    - Deteriorating level of consciousness, restlessness, irritability.
    - Dilated, pinpoint, or asymmetric pupils, slow to react or nonreactive.
    - Alteration in breathing pattern (Cheyne-Stokes respirations, central neurogenic hyperventilation, apnea).
    - Deterioration in motor function, abnormal posturing (decerebrate, decorticate, or flaccidity).
    - Cushing reflex, which is a late finding characterized by severe hypertension with a widening pulse pressure (systolic – diastolic) and bradycardia.
    - Cerebrospinal fluid leakage from the nose and ears ("halo" sign – yellow stain surrounded by blood on a paper towel; fluid tests positive for glucose).
    - Seizures.
  - Laboratory Tests
    - ABGs
    - Blood alcohol and toxicology screen
    - CBC with differential and BUN
      - BUN is used to determine the client's renal status. This information is needed prior to administration of radiology contrast media.
  - Diagnostic Procedures
    - Cervical spine films are used to diagnose a cervical spine injury.
    - Computerized tomography (CT) and/or a magnetic resonance imaging (MRI) of the head and/or neck (with and without contrast if indicated).

Patient-Centered Care

- Nursing Care
  - There is a 1 hr "golden window" for treatment of head injuries. Emergency treatment provided during this time frame decreases the morbidity and mortality rates associated with these conditions, especially for epidural hematomas.

  - Educate the client's family on effective ways to communicate with the client (touch, talk, and assist with care as appropriate).
  - Assess/monitor the client at regularly scheduled intervals:
    - Respiratory status – the priority assessment
      - The brain is dependent upon oxygen to maintain function and has little reserve available if oxygen is deprived. Brain function begins to diminish after 3 min of oxygen deprivation.
    - Changes in level of consciousness, using the GCS, which provides the earliest indication of neurological deterioration.
    - Cranial nerve function (eye blink response, gag reflex, tongue and shoulder movement)
    - Pupillary changes (PERRLA)

- Findings of infection (nuchal rigidity occurs with meningitis)
- Bilateral sensory and motor responses
- Intracranial pressure (ICP)
  - Four methods are used to monitor.
    - Use a thin tube inserted into the lateral ventricle (intraventricular).
    - Use a bolt or screw placed in the subarachnoid area (subarachnoid).
    - Place a sensor in the epidural space (epidural).
    - Place a fiberoptic transducer-tipped catheter into the subdural or subarachnoid space, ventricle, or brain tissue.
  - Expected reference range for ICP level is 10 to 15 mm Hg.
  - ICP may be increased by
    - Hypercarbia, which leads to cerebral vasodilation
    - Endotracheal or oral tracheal suctioning
    - Coughing
    - Blowing the nose forcefully
    - Extreme neck or hip flexion/extension
    - Maintaining the head of the bed at an angle less than 30°
    - Increasing intra-abdominal pressure (restrictive clothing, Valsalva maneuver).
  - Implement actions that will decrease ICP.
    - Elevate head at least 30° to reduce ICP and to promote venous drainage.
    - Avoid extreme flexion, extension, or rotation of the head, and maintain the body in a midline neutral position.
    - Maintain a patent airway. Provide mechanical ventilation as indicated.
    - Administer oxygen as indicated to maintain an oxygen saturation level of greater than 92%.
    - Hyperventilate clients on mechanical ventilation to keep the $PaCO_2$ between 35 to 38 mm Hg. This reduces cerebral blood flow.
    - Maintain cervical spine stability until cleared by an x-ray.
    - Report presence of cerebrospinal fluid (CSF) from nose or ears to the provider.
    - Provide a calm, restful environment (limit visitors, minimize noise).
    - Implement measures to prevent complications of immobility (turn every 2 hr, footboard, and splints). Specialty beds can be used.
    - Monitor fluid and electrolyte values and osmolarity to detect changes in sodium regulation, the onset of diabetes insipidus, or severe hypovolemia.
    - Provide adequate fluids to maintain cerebral perfusion and to minimize cerebral edema. When a large amount of IV fluids are prescribed, monitor for excess fluid volume which could increase ICP.
    - Maintain safety and seizure precautions (side rails up, padded side rails, call light within the client's reach).
    - Even if the level of consciousness is decreased, explain to the client the actions being taken and why.
      - Hearing is the last sense affected by a head injury

- Secondary brain injury results from client condition following trauma.
  - Causes include hypotension, hypoxia, hyperglycemia, hypoglycemia, acidosis, and hypercapnia.
  - Nursing Actions
    - Monitor vital signs, blood glucose, oxygen saturation, and ABGs.
    - Collaborate with provider and respiratory therapy to correct imbalances and prevent further injury.
- Medications
  - Mannitol (Osmitrol) is an osmotic diuretic used to treat cerebral edema.
    - Nursing Considerations
      - Administer IV to treat acute cerebral edema.
      - Insert indwelling urinary catheter to monitor fluid and renal status. Monitor urine osmolality daily.
      - Monitor serum electrolytes and osmolality every 6 hr.
  - Pentobarbital (Nembutal Sodium) is used to induce a barbiturate coma to decrease cerebral metabolic demands.
    - This treatment is performed when the ICP is refractory to treatment and has exceeded 25 mm Hg for 30 min, 30 mm Hg for 15 min, or 40 mm Hg for 1 min.
    - A barbiturate coma is a treatment of last resort and aims to decrease elevated ICP by inducing vasoconstriction and decreasing cerebral metabolic demands.
    - Nursing Considerations
      - Medication is administered in bursts to decrease cerebral activity. Dosages are controversial outside of the manufacturer's guidelines.
        - ▸ Protocols vary, but can begin with 10 mg/kg over 30 min, then 5 mg/kg every hour for three doses, with a maintenance dose of 1 mg/kg per hour.
      - Treatment continues until the ICP remains below 20 mm Hg for 48 hr.
      - Medication is then slowly withdrawn
      - Nursing care during this treatment requires full physiological support for the client's body functions.
      - If treatment is not successful, a re-evaluation is completed if the client expressed a desire to donate his organs.
  - Phenytoin (Dilantin) is used prophylactically to prevent or treat seizures.
    - Nursing Considerations
      - Dosing for this medication is client-specific and based on therapeutic blood levels.
      - Check for medication interactions.
  - Morphine sulfate or fentanyl (Sublimaze) are analgesics used to control pain and restlessness.
    - Nursing Considerations
      - Calm and reassure clients, clarifying misconceptions (brain surgery can be an extremely fearful procedure).
      - Avoid opioid use with clients who are not mechanically ventilated due to CNS depressant effects.
        - ▸ Prevents accurate assessment of neurological system.
        - ▸ May cause respiratory depression.

□ Monitor blood pressure cautiously with clients who are mechanically ventilated. Opioid use coupled with hypotension may cause increased ICP.

□ Resume preoperative monitoring of vital signs, ICP, and oxygenation as prescribed.

- Teamwork and Collaboration

  ○ Care should include professionals from other disciplines as indicated. This may include physical, occupational, recreational, and/or speech therapists due to neurological deficits that may occur secondary to the area of the brain damaged.

  ○ Social services should be contacted to provide links to social service agencies and schools.

  ○ Rehabilitation facilities are frequently used to compress the time required to recover from a head injury and support re-emergence into society.

- Surgical Interventions

  ○ Craniotomy

    ▪ A craniotomy is the removal of nonviable brain tissue that allows for expansion and/or removal of epidural or subdural hematomas. It involves drilling a burr hole or creating a bone flap to permit access to the affected area. Treatment of intracranial hemorrhages requires surgical evacuation.

    ▪ This is a life-saving procedure, and is associated with many potential complications, such as:

      □ Severe neurological impairment, infection, persistent seizures, neurological deficiencies, and/or death.

    ▪ Nursing Actions

      □ Postoperative treatment will depend upon the neurological status of the client after surgery.

      □ Initially, care will surround the prevention of complications, maximizing cerebral function, and supporting other physiological systems.

      □ For supratentorial surgery, maintain HOB at least 30° with body positioning to prevent increased ICP.

      □ For infratentorial craniotomy, keep client flat and on either side for 24 to 48 hr to prevent pressure on neck incision site.

      □ Hyperventilate the mechanically ventilated client for 24 to 48 hr as prescribed to maintain $PaCO_2$ around 35 mm Hg.

      □ Monitor wound dressing and mark drainage every 1 to 2 hr. Monitor and maintain wound drain, documenting output every 8 hr.

Complications

- Brain herniation

  ○ A brain herniation is the downward shift of brain tissue due to cerebral edema.

  ○ The brain consists of brain matter, cerebrospinal fluid, and intravascular blood.

  ○ The Monro-Kellie doctrine states that any alteration in the volume of one of these results in a compromise in the other components.

  ○ When trauma creates a shift in these components, and the other components are unable to accommodate, the brain shifts from the cranial vault, or herniates.

M ◇ View Image: Brain Herniation

- ○ This can result in brain tissue moving downward, through the foramen magnum.
- ○ Clinical findings include fixed dilated pupils, deteriorating level of consciousness, Cheyne-Stokes respirations, hemodynamic instability, and abnormal posturing.
- ○ Recovery after this occurrence is rare, and urgent medical mannitol (Osmitrol) and/or surgical (debulking) treatment is indicated.
- ○ With treatment, severe neurological impairment usually persists.
- ○ Nursing Actions
  - ▪ This situation should be prevented before treatment is needed.
  - ▪ Close monitoring of the client's vital signs and neurological status will allow early reporting of changes in the GCS score, an increase in the blood pressure, and an alteration in respiratory pattern and effort.
- ○ Client Education
  - ▪ Family members should be frequently updated on the health status of the client member. Frequent updates and repeating medical information is often necessary to ensure comprehension among family members.
  - ▪ The decision to surgically treat brain herniation is made in the presence of a critical situation.
  - ▪ Social service workers and/or pastoral personnel can be helpful to support the family, while reinforcing the medical situation.
- • Hematoma and intracranial hemorrhage
  - ○ Monitor for severe headache, rapid decline in level of consciousness, worsening neurological function and herniation, and changes in ICP.
  - ○ Surgery is required to remove subdural and epidural hematoma.
  - ○ Intracranial hemorrhage is treated with osmotic diuretics.
- • Neurogenic pulmonary edema
  - ○ Findings mimic acute pulmonary edema without cardiac involvement.
  - ○ This is a life-threatening emergency. Immediate, aggressive treatment is used. Survival is rare.
- • Diabetes insipidus or syndrome of inappropriate antidiuretic hormone (SIADH)
- • Cerebral salt wasting (CSW)
  - ○ CSW is caused by effects of atrial natriuretic factor (ANF) located in the hypothalamus.
  - ○ Increased ANF production decreases sodium retention in the kidneys. ANF also may prevent renin and aldosterone release.
  - ○ CSW causes decreased serum osmolality and hyponatremia. CSW is the primary cause of hyponatremia following neurosurgery.
  - ○ CSW causes hypovolemia, compared with increased extracellular fluid in clients with SIADH.
  - ○ Nursing Interventions
    - ▪ Monitor serum electrolytes and osmolality daily.
    - ▪ Document strict intake and output.
    - ▪ Weigh client daily.
    - ▪ Treat electrolyte and fluid imbalance, as prescribed. Monitor for dehydration or fluid overload during treatment.

APPLICATION EXERCISES

1. A nurse is caring for a client who was recently admitted to the emergency department following a head-on motor vehicle crash. The client is unresponsive, has spontaneous respirations of 22/min, and a laceration on his forehead that is bleeding. Which of the following is the priority nursing action at this time?

    A. Keep neck stabilized.

    B. Insert nasogastric tube.

    C. Monitor pulse and blood pressure frequently.

    D. Establish IV access and start fluid replacement.

2. A nurse is caring for a client who has just been admitted following surgical evacuation of a subdural hematoma. Which of the following is the priority assessment?

    A. Glasgow Coma Scale

    B. Cranial nerve function

    C. Oxygen saturation

    D. Pupillary response

3. A nursing is caring for a client who has a closed-head injury with ICP readings range from 16 to 22 mm Hg. Which of the following actions should the nurse take to decrease the potential for raising the client's ICP? (Select all that apply.)

    _____ A. Suction the endotracheal tube.

    _____ B. Hyperventilate the client.

    _____ C. Elevate the client's head on two pillows.

    _____ D. Administer a stool softener.

    _____ E. Keep the client well hydrated.

4. A nurse in the critical care unit is completing an admission assessment of a client who has a gunshot wound to the head. Which of the following assessment findings are indicative of increased ICP? (Select all that apply.)

_____ A. Headache

_____ B. Dilated pupils

_____ C. Tachycardia

_____ D. Decorticate posturing

_____ E. Hypotension

5. A nurse is caring for a client who has increased ICP and a new prescription for mannitol (Osmitrol). For which of the following adverse effects should the nurse monitor?

A. Hyperglycemia

B. Hyponatremia

C. Hypervolemia

D. Oliguria

6. A nurse is reviewing the plan of care for a client who has a head injury. What should be included in the plan of care? Use the ATI Active Learning Template: Systems Disorder to complete this item to include the following:

A. Nursing Care:
- Identify the priority nursing assessment and describe why this is important.
- Identify the nursing assessment that will provide the earliest indication of neurological deterioration.
- Describe two activities the nurse should instruct the client to avoid that will increase ICP.
- Describe three additional nursing actions.

APPLICATION EXERCISES KEY

1. A. **CORRECT:** The greatest risk to the client is permanent damage to the spinal cord if a cervical injury does exist. The priority nursing intervention is to keep the neck immobile until damage to the cervical spine can be ruled out.

   B. INCORRECT: Insertion of a nasogastric tube is not the priority nursing action at this time.

   C. INCORRECT: Frequent monitoring of pulse and blood pressure is important but not the priority nursing action at this time.

   D. INCORRECT: Establishing IV access for fluid replacement is important but not the priority nursing action at this time.

   Ⓝ NCLEX® Connection: Reduction of Risk Potential, Potential for Complications of Diagnostic Tests/ Treatments/Procedures

2. A. INCORRECT: The Glasgow Coma Scale is important but not the priority assessment at this time.

   B. INCORRECT: Assessment of cranial nerve function is important but not the priority assessment at this time.

   C. **CORRECT:** Using the airway, breathing, and circulation (ABC) priority-setting framework, assessment of oxygen saturation is the priority action. Brain tissue can only survive for 3 min before permanent damage occurs.

   D. INCORRECT: Assessment of pupillary response is important but not the priority assessment at this time.

   Ⓝ NCLEX® Connection: Physiological Adaptations, Unexpected Response to Therapies

3. A. INCORRECT: Suctioning increases ICP and should be done only when indicated.

   B. **CORRECT:** Hyperventilation of the client will prevent hypercarbia, which can cause vasodilation with a secondary increase in ICP.

   C. INCORRECT: Hyperflexion of the client's neck with pillows carries the risk of increasing ICP and should be avoided.

   D. **CORRECT:** Administration of a stool softener will decrease the need to bear down (Valsalva maneuver) during bowel movements, which can increase ICP.

   E. INCORRECT: Overhydration carries the risk of increasing ICP and should be avoided.

   Ⓝ NCLEX® Connection: Reduction of Risk Potential, Diagnostic Tests

4. A. **CORRECT:** Headache is a finding associated with increased ICP.

    B. **CORRECT:** Dilated pupils is a finding associated with increased ICP.

    C. INCORRECT: Bradycardia, not tachycardia, is a finding associated with increased ICP.

    D. **CORRECT:** Decorticate or decerebrate posturing is a finding associated with increased ICP.

    E. INCORRECT: Hypertension, not hypotension, is a finding associated with increased ICP.

    (N) NCLEX® Connection: Physiological Adaptations, Alterations in Body Systems

5. A. INCORRECT: Hyperglycemia is not an adverse effect of mannitol.

    B. **CORRECT:** Mannitol is a powerful osmotic diuretic, and adverse effects include electrolyte imbalances such as hyponatremia.

    C. INCORRECT: Hypovolemia is an adverse effect of mannitol, an osmotic diuretic, and should be monitored.

    D. INCORRECT: Polyuria is an adverse of mannitol, an osmotic diuretic, and should be monitored.

    (N) NCLEX® Connection: Physiological Adaptations, Fluid and Electrolyte Imbalances

6. *Using the ATI Active Learning Template: Systems Disorder*

    A. Nursing Care

    • Priority Nursing Assessment: Respiratory status. The brain is dependent on oxygen to maintain function and has minimal reserve if oxygen is not available. Brain function begins to diminish after 3 minutes of oxygen deprivation.

    • Assessment indication of early neurological deterioration: Changes in level of consciousness.

    • Client Activities: Coughing and blowing the nose forcefully.

    • Nursing Actions

      ○ Elevate the head to at least 30°.

      ○ Maintain patent airway.

      ○ Administer oxygen to keep oxygen saturation greater than 92%.

      ○ Maintain cervical spin stability until cleared by x-ray.

      ○ Report presence of cerebrospinal fluid from nose or ears to the provider.

      ○ Provide a calm, restful environment (limit visitors, minimize noise).

      ○ Implement measures to prevent complications of immobility (turn every 2 hr, use footboard and splints); provide a specialty bed.

      ○ Monitor fluid and electrolyte values and osmolarity.

      ○ Provide adequate fluids; monitor IV fluids.

      ○ Maintain safety and seizure precautions (side rails up, padded side rails, call light within client's reach).

      ○ Explain all nursing actions to client and family.

    (N) NCLEX® Connection: Physiological Adaptations, Pathophysiology

UNIT 2   NURSING CARE OF CLIENTS WITH NEUROSENSORY DISORDERS
SECTION: NEUROLOGIC EMERGENCIES

CHAPTER 15   Stroke

Overview

- Strokes, also known as cerebrovascular accidents (CVAs) or brain attacks, involve a disruption in the cerebral blood flow secondary to ischemia, hemorrhage, brain attack, or embolism.

- There are three causes of strokes:

  - Hemorrhagic – These occur secondary to a ruptured artery or aneurysm. The prognosis for a client who has experienced a hemorrhagic stroke is poor due to the amount of ischemia and increased ICP caused by the expanding collection of blood. A stroke, if caught early and evacuation of the clot can be done with cessation of the active bleed, the prognosis of a hemorrhagic stroke improves significantly.

  - Thrombotic – These occur secondary to the development of a blood clot on an atherosclerotic plaque in a cerebral artery that gradually shuts off the artery and causes ischemia distal to the occlusion. Symptoms of a thrombotic stroke evolve over a period of several hours to days.

  - Embolic – These occur secondary to an embolus traveling from another part of the body to a cerebral artery. Blood to the brain distal to the occlusion is immediately shut off causing neurologic deficits or a loss of consciousness to instantly occur. An embolic stroke may be reversed with a thrombolytic enzyme, such as recombinant tissue plasminogen activator (rtPA [Retavase]), if given within 4.5 hours of the initial symptoms.

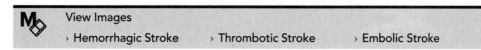

M   **View Images**

     › Hemorrhagic Stroke   › Thrombotic Stroke   › Embolic Stroke

Health Promotion

Q EBP

- Health Promotion and Disease Prevention

  - Hypertension, diabetes mellitus, smoking, and other related disorders can increase a client's risk for a stroke.

  - Early treatment of hypertension, maintenance of blood glucose within expected range, and refraining from smoking will decrease these risk factors.

  - Maintaining a healthy weight and getting regular exercise can also decrease the risk of a stroke.

Assessment

- Risk Factors
  - Cerebral aneurysm
  - Arteriovenous malformation (AV)
  - Diabetes mellitus
  - Obesity
  - Hypertension
  - Atherosclerosis
  - Hyperlipidemia
  - Hypercoagulability
  - Atrial fibrillation
  - Use of oral contraceptives
  - Smoking
  - Cocaine use
- Subjective Data
  - Some clients report transient symptoms, such as visual disturbances, dizziness, slurred speech, and a weak extremity.
  - These symptoms may indicate a transient ischemic attack (TIA), which can be a warning of an impending stroke.
  - Antithrombotic medication and/or surgical removal of atherosclerotic plaques in the carotid artery can prevent the subsequent occurrence of a stroke.
- Objective Data
  - Physical Assessment Findings
    - Symptoms will vary based on the area of the brain that is deprived of oxygenated blood.
      - □ The left cerebral hemisphere is responsible for language, mathematics skills, and analytic thinking.
      - □ Symptoms consistent with a left-hemispheric stroke include the following:
        - ▸ Expressive and receptive aphasia (inability to speak and understand language respectively)
        - ▸ Agnosia (unable to recognize familiar objects)
        - ▸ Alexia (reading difficulty)
        - ▸ Agraphia (writing difficulty)
        - ▸ Right extremity hemiplegia (paralysis) or hemiparesis (weakness)
        - ▸ Slow, cautious behavior
        - ▸ Depression, anger, and quick to become frustrated
        - ▸ Visual changes, such as hemianopsia (loss of visual field in one or both eyes)

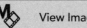 View Image: Hemianopsia

- The right cerebral hemisphere is responsible for visual and spatial awareness and proprioception.

  ▸ Altered perception of deficits (overestimation of abilities)

  ▸ One-sided neglect syndrome (ignore left side of the body – cannot see, feel, or move affected side, so client unaware of its existence). Can occur with left-hemispheric strokes, but is more common with right-hemispheric strokes.

  ▸ Loss of depth perception

  ▸ Poor impulse control and judgment

  ▸ Left hemiplegia or hemiparesis

  ▸ Visual changes, such as hemianopsia

- Diagnostic Procedures

  ▪ A magnetic resonance imaging (MRI), computed tomography (CT) imaging, and/or a computed axial tomography (CAT) scan may be used to identify edema, ischemia, and necrosis.

  ▪ A magnetic resonance angiography (MRA) or a cerebral angiography are used to identify the presence of a cerebral hemorrhage, abnormal vessel structures (AV malformation, aneurysms), vessel ruptures, and regional perfusion of blood flow in the carotid arteries and brain.

  ▪ A lumbar puncture is used to assess for the presence of blood in the cerebrospinal fluid (CSF). A positive finding is consistent with a cerebral hemorrhage or ruptured aneurysm.

  ▪ The Glasgow Coma Scale score is used when the client has a decreased level of consciousness or orientation. The risk for increased ICP exists related to the swelling of the brain that can occur secondary to ischemic insult.

Patient-Centered Care

- Nursing Care

  - Monitor the client's vital signs every 1 to 2 hr. Notify the provider immediately if the client's blood pressure exceeds a systolic greater than 180 mm Hg or a diastolic greater than 110 mm Hg. This can indicate the client is experiencing an ischemic stroke.

  - Monitor the client's temperature. A fever can cause an increase in intracranial pressure.

  - Provide oxygen therapy to maintain the client's oxygen saturation level greater than 92%, or if the client's level of consciousness is decreased.

  - Place the client on a cardiac monitor to detect arrhythmias.

  - Conduct a cardiac assessment, and auscultate the client's apical heart rate to detect murmurs or irregularity.

  - Monitor for changes in the client's level of consciousness (increased ICP sign).

  - Monitor vital signs, electrocardiogram.

  - Elevate the client's head of the bed approximately 30° to reduce ICP and to promote venous drainage. Avoid extreme flexion or extension of the neck, and maintain the client's head in the midline neutral position.

  - Institute seizure precautions.

○ Assist with the client's communication skills if his speech is impaired.

  ▪ Assess the ability to understand speech by asking the client to follow simple commands.

  ▪ Observe for consistently affirmative answers when the client actually does not comprehend what is being said.

  ▪ Assess accuracy of yes/no responses in relation to closed-ended questions.

  ▪ Supply the client with a picture board of commonly requested items/needs.

○ Assist with safe feeding.

  ▪ Assess swallowing and gag reflexes before feeding. Speech therapy may request a swallowing study that can involve swallowing a barium substrate and radiography of the peristaltic activity of the esophagus.

  ▪ If a swallowing deficit is identified, the client's liquids may need to be thickened with a commercial thickener to avoid aspiration.

  ▪ Have the client eat in an upright position and swallow with the head and neck flexed slightly forward.

  ▪ Place food in the back of the mouth on the unaffected side.

  ▪ Have suction on standby.

  ▪ Maintain a distraction-free environment during meals.

○ Prevent complications of immobility, such as atelectasis, pneumonia, pressure sores, and DVTs. While clients who have experienced strokes are ambulated as soon as possible to prevent complications, during periods of inactivity, preventive measures related to complications of immobility should be implemented.

○ Maintain skin integrity.

  ▪ Reposition the client frequently and use padding.

  ▪ Monitor bony prominences, paying particular attention to the affected extremities.

  ▪ If the client has one-sided neglect, teach him to protect and care for the affected extremity to avoid injuring it in the wheel of the wheelchair or hitting/smashing it against a doorway.

○ Encourage passive range of motion every 2 hr to the affected extremities and active range of motion every 2 hr to the unaffected extremities. Teach the client how to use the unaffected side to exercise the affected side of the body.

○ Elevate the affected extremities to promote venous return and reduce swelling. An elastic glove can be placed on the affected hand if swelling is severe. Teach the client to massage the affected hand by stroking it in a distal to proximal manner, encouraging fluid in the hand to move back into the wrist and arm.

○ Maintain a safe environment to reduce the risk of falls. Assistive devices should be used during transfers, such as transfer belts and sliding boards. Sit-to-stand lifts can also facilitate transfers and reduce strain on the care provider's body.

○ If the client has homonomous hemianopsia (loss of the same visual field in both eyes), instruct him to use a scanning technique (turning head from the direction of the unaffected side to the affected side) when eating and ambulating.

○ To prevent deep vein thrombosis (DVT) from developing, provide preventive measures, such as sequential compression stockings, frequent position changes, and mobilization.

- Provide assistance with ADLs as needed. Instruct the client to dress the affected side first and sit in a supportive chair that aids in balance. Have occupational therapy assess the client for adaptive aids, such as a plate guard, utensils with built-up handles, a reaching tool to pick things up, and shirts and shoes that have hook and loop fasteners/tape instead of buttons and ties.

- Clients who have experienced strokes have decreased endurance and impaired balance due to paralysis on one side of the body. Frequent rest periods from sitting in the wheelchair should be provided by returning the client to bed after therapies and meals. When sitting the client up in bed or in the wheelchair, leaning to the affected side typically occurs and should be countered with some manner of support.

- Shoulder subluxation can occur if the affected arm is not supported. The weight of the arm is such that it can actually cause a painful dislocation of the shoulder from its socket. Supporting the arm while in bed, the wheelchair, or during ambulation should be accomplished with an arm sling or strategically placed pillows.

- Support the client during periods of emotional lability and depression.

- Medications
  - Anticoagulants (heparin sodium, enoxaparin [Lovenox], warfarin [Coumadin])
    - Use of anticoagulants is controversial and not recommended due to the high risk of intracerebral bleeding.
  - Antiplatelets (aspirin)
    - Low-dose aspirin is given within 24 to 48 hr following a stroke to prevent further clot formation.
    - Other antiplatelets, such as clopidogrel (Plavix), are not recommended.
  - Thrombolytic medications reteplase recombinant (rtPA [Retavase])
    - Give within 4.5 hours of the initial symptoms.
  - Antiepileptic medications (phenytoin [Dilantin], gabapentin [Neurontin])
    - These medications are not commonly given following a stroke unless the client develops seizures.
    - Gabapentin can be given for paresthetic pain in an affected extremity.

- Teamwork and Collaboration
  - Speech and language therapists can be consulted for language therapy and swallowing exercises.
  - Physical therapy can be consulted for assistance with reestablishment of ambulation with or without assistive devices (single or quad cane, walker) or wheelchair support. Wheelchair adaptations, such as an extended brake handle on the client's affected side of the wheelchair, may be necessary. Safety features, such as placing the brakes on when preparing to transfer and the use of a cushion on the seat, may also be integrated by physical therapy into the client's plan of care.
  - Occupational therapy can be consulted for assistance with reestablishment of partial or full function of the affected hand and arm. If function does not return to the extremity, measures, such as massage and elastic gloves will be prescribed by occupational therapy to prevent swelling of the extremity.
  - Social services can be consulted to make arrangements for rehabilitation services and temporary placement on a skilled rehabilitation unit or extended-care facility during provision of these services. Prior to discharge, the social worker may make a home visit with selected therapists and nurses to evaluate the need for environmental alterations in the home and adaptive equipment needed for ADLs.

- Therapeutic Procedures
  - Systemic or catheter-directed thrombolytic therapy restores cerebral blood flow. It must be administered within 6 hr of the onset of symptoms. It is contraindicated for treatment of a hemorrhagic stroke and for clients with an increased risk of bleeding due to anticoagulant therapy or other bleeding anomaly. Possibility of a hemorrhagic stroke is ruled out with an MRI prior to the initiation of thrombolytic therapy
- Surgical Interventions
  - Carotid artery angioplasty with stenting (CAS) involves inserting a catheter in the femoral artery and placing a distal/embolic protection device to catch clot debris during the procedure while a stent is being placed in the carotid artery to open a blockage. CAS is less invasive, blood loss is decreased, and length of hospitalization is shorter. Postoperative care is the same as carotid endarterectomy.
  - Carotid endarterectomy is performed to open the artery by removing atherosclerotic plaque. This procedure is performed when the carotid artery is blocked or when the client is experiencing TIAs.
  - Assess for increased headache, neck swelling, and hoarseness of the throat.

Complications

- Dysphagia and aspiration
  - Dysphagia can result from neurological involvement of the cranial nerves that innervate the face, tongue, soft palate, and throat. As a result, the client's risk of aspiration is great.
  - Not all clients who have experienced a stroke have dysphagia, but all should be evaluated prior to reestablishing oral nutrition and hydration.
  - Nursing Actions
    - Assess the client's gag reflex.
    - If the gag reflex is present, give the client a small sip of water to determine if choking occurs.
    - If the client exhibits some difficulty managing food or fluids, a swallowing evaluation should be done by a speech therapist.
    - Begin the client with a prescribed diet and observe closely for choking. Have the suction equipment available. Initial feedings should be done by an RN, so appropriate interventions can be taken if choking occurs.
    - Thicker liquids are usually tolerated better than thin liquids; therefore, thickener may need to be added to oral fluids. Use the appropriate amount of thickener to obtain the prescribed consistency.
  - Client Education
    - Teach the client's family how to thicken liquids to the proper consistency.
    - Instruct the client to flex his head forward when swallowing to decrease the risk of choking.

- Unilateral neglect
  - Unilateral neglect is the loss of awareness of the side affected by the stroke. The client cannot see, feel, or move the affected side of his body; therefore, he forgets that it exists.
  - This lack of awareness poses a great risk for injury to the neglected extremities and creates a self-care deficit.
  - Nursing Actions
    - Observe the client's affected extremities for injury (bruises and abrasions of the affected hand and arm, hyperflexion of the foot from it falling off of the wheelchair during transport).
    - Apply an arm sling if the client is unable to remember to care for the affected extremity.
    - Ensure the foot rest is on the wheelchair and an ankle brace is on the affected foot.
  - Client Education
    - Instruct the client to dress the affected side first.
    - Teach the client how to care for the affected side.
    - Use the unaffected hand to pull the affected extremity to midline and out of danger from the wheel of the wheelchair or from hitting or smashing it against a doorway.
    - Teach the client to look over the affected side periodically.

APPLICATION EXERCISES

1. A nurse is caring for a client who has experienced a right-hemispheric stroke. Which of the following are expected findings? (Select all that apply.)

___X___ A. Impulse control difficulty

___X___ B. Left hemiplegia

___X___ C. Loss of depth perception

_____ D. Aphasia

___X___ E. Lack of awareness

2. A nurse is caring for a client who has left homonymous hemianopsia. Which of the following is an appropriate nursing intervention?

A. Teach the client to scan to the right to see objects on the right side of her body.

(B.) Place the client's bedside table on the right side of the bed.

C. Orient the client to the food on her plate using the clock method.

D. Place the client's wheelchair on her left side.

3. A nurse is planning care for a client who has dysphagia and has a new dietary prescription. Which of the following should the nurse include in the plan of care? (Select all that apply.)

___X___ A. Have suction equipment available for use.

___X___ B. Use thickened liquids.

___X___ C. Place food on the client's unaffected side of her mouth.

_____ D. Assign an assistive personnel to feed the client slowly.

___X___ E. Teach the client to swallow with her neck flexed.

4. A nurse is caring for a client who has global aphasia (both receptive and expressive). Which of the following should the nurse include in the client's plan of care? (Select all that apply.)

___X___ A. Speak to the client at a slower rate.

___X___ B. Look directly at the client when speaking.

___X___ C. Allow extra time for the client to answer.

_____ D. Complete sentences that the client cannot finish.

___X___ E. Give instructions one step at a time.

5. A nurse is assessing a client who has experienced a left-hemispheric stroke. Which of the following is an expected finding?

     A. Impulse control difficulty

     B. Poor judgment

     C. Inability to recognize familiar objects

     D. Loss of depth perception

6. A nurse is caring for a client who has dysphagia. Using the ATI Active Learning Template: Nursing Skill, list three nursing actions the nurse should include while caring for this client.

APPLICATION EXERCISES KEY

1.　A. **CORRECT:** A client who has experienced a right-hemispheric stroke will exhibit impulse control difficulty, such as the urgency to use the restroom.

　　B. **CORRECT:** A client who has experienced a right-hemispheric stroke will exhibit left-sided hemiplegia.

　　C. **CORRECT:** A client who has experienced a right-hemispheric stroke will experience a loss in depth perception.

　　D. INCORRECT: A client who has experienced a left-hemispheric stroke will experience aphasia.

　　E. **CORRECT:** A client who has experienced a right-hemispheric stroke will demonstrate a lack of awareness of surroundings.

　　Ⓝ NCLEX® Connection: Physiological Adaptations, Pathophysiology

2.　A. INCORRECT: A client who has left homonymous hemianopsia has lost the left visual field of both eyes. Scanning to the right will decrease the client's field of vision.

　　B. **CORRECT:** The client is unable to visualize to the left midline of her body. Placing the client's bedside table on the right side of her bed will permit visualization of items on the table.

　　C. INCORRECT: Using the clock method of food placement will be ineffective because only half of the plate can be seen.

　　D. INCORRECT: The client's wheelchair should be placed to the client's right or unaffected side.

　　Ⓝ NCLEX® Connection: Physiological Adaptations, Illness Management

3.　A. **CORRECT:** Have suction equipment available for use is correct. Suction equipment should be available in case of choking and aspiration.

　　B. **CORRECT:** The client should be given thickened liquids, which are easier to swallow.

　　C. **CORRECT:** Placing food on the unaffected side of the client's mouth will allow her to have better control of the food and reduce the risk of aspiration.

　　D. INCORRECT: Due to the risk of aspiration, an assistive personnel should not be assigned to feed the client because the client's swallowing ability should be assessed, and suctioning may be needed if choking occurs.

　　E. **CORRECT:** The client should be taught to flex her neck, tucking the chin down and under, to close the epiglottis during swallowing.

　　Ⓝ NCLEX® Connection: Reduction of Risk Potential, Potential for Alterations in Body Systems

4. A. **CORRECT:** Clients who have global aphasia will have difficulty with both speaking and understanding speech. One strategy that can enhance client understanding is speaking to the client at a slower rate.

    B. **CORRECT:** One strategy that can enhance understanding while speaking is looking directly at the client.

    C. **CORRECT:** One strategy that can enhance understanding is allowing the client extra time to answer.

    D. INCORRECT: The nurse should allow the client adequate time to finish sentences and not complete the sentences for him.

    E. **CORRECT:** One strategy that can enhance understanding is giving instructions one step at a time.

    Ⓝ NCLEX® Connection: Reduction of Risk Potential, System Specific Assessments

5. A. INCORRECT: A client who has experienced a right-hemispheric stroke will experience difficulty with impulse control.

    B. INCORRECT: A client who has experienced a right-hemispheric stroke will experience poor judgment.

    C. **CORRECT:** A client who experienced a left-hemispheric stroke will demonstrate the inability to recognize familiar objects. This is also known as agnosia.

    D. INCORRECT: A client who experienced a right-hemispheric stroke will experience a loss of depth perception.

    Ⓝ NCLEX® Connection: Physiological Adaptations, Pathophysiology

6. *Using the ATI Active Learning Template: Nursing Skill*
    - Nursing Actions include the following:
        ○ Assess the client's gag reflex.
        ○ If the gag reflex is present, give the client a small sip of water to determine if choking occurs.
        ○ If the client exhibits some difficulty managing food or fluids, a swallowing evaluation should be done by a speech therapist.
        ○ Begin the client with a prescribed diet and observe closely for choking. Have suction equipment available. Initial feedings should be done by an RN, so appropriate interventions can be taken if choking occurs.
        ○ Thicker liquids are usually tolerated better than thin liquids. Therefore, thickener may need to be added to oral fluids. Use the appropriate amount of thickener to obtain the prescribed consistency.

    Ⓝ NCLEX® Connection: Physiological Adaptations, Illness Management

chapter 16

Overview

- Spinal cord injuries (SCIs) involve the loss of motor function, sensory function, reflexes, and control of elimination. Injuries in the cervical region result in quadriplegia – paralysis/paresis of all four extremities and trunk. Injuries below T1 result in paraplegia – paralysis/paresis of the lower extremities. Truncal instability also results if the lesion is in the upper thoracic region.

- The level of cord involved dictates the consequences of spinal cord injury. For example, an injury at C4 or above poses a great risk for impaired spontaneous ventilation because of the involvement of the phrenic nerve.

> **M**   View Image: Spinal Cord and Cauda Equina

- Not all fractures of the vertebrae cause SCIs. Direct injury to the spinal cord secondary to the trauma or bone fragments in the spinal canal must occur for the spinal cord itself to become damaged.

- SCIs range from contusions or incomplete lesions of the spinal cord to complete lesions caused by a lesion that extends across the entire diameter of the cord, or an actual transection of the spinal cord. Complete lesions result in the loss of all voluntary movement and sensation below the level of the injury. Incomplete lesions result in varying losses of voluntary movement and sensation below the level of the injury.

Health Promotion and Disease Prevention

- Most SCIs are caused by trauma, such as motor vehicle crashes, diving accidents, and gunshot wounds.

- Hyperflexion injuries are caused by acceleration injuries that cause sharp forward flexion of the spine (head-on collision, fall, or diving). Hyperextension injuries are caused by a backward snap of the spine (rear-end collision or a downward fall onto the chin).

Assessment

- Risk Factors

  - Males age 16 to 30
  - High-risk activities (extreme sports or high-speed driving)
  - Active in impact sports (football or diving)
  - Acts of violence (gunshot and knife wounds)
  - Alcohol and/or drug use
  - Disease (metastatic cancer or arthritis of the spine)
  - Falls, especially in older adults

- Subjective Data
  - ○ Report of lack of sensation of dermatomes below the level of the lesion
  - ○ Report of neck or back pain
- Objective Data
  - ○ Physical Assessment Findings
    - ▪ Inability to feel light touch when touched by a cotton ball, inability to discriminate between sharp and dull when touched with a safety pin or other sharp objects, and an inability to discriminate between hot and cold when touched with containers of hot and cold water.
    - ▪ Absent deep tendon reflexes.
    - ▪ Flaccidity of muscles.
    - ▪ Hypotension that is more severe when the client is in sitting in an upright position.
    - ▪ Shallow respirations.
    - ▪ Dependent edema.
    - ▪ Neurogenic shock, which accompanies spinal trauma, causes a total loss of all reflexive and autonomic function below the level of the injury for a period of several days to weeks.
    - ▪ Loss of temperature regulation: hyperthermia or hypothermia.
  - ○ Laboratory Tests
    - ▪ Urinalysis, hemoglobin, ABGs, CBCs (for evaluation of platelets and WBCs)
      - ▫ Used to monitor for undiagnosed internal bleeding (the client may not feel pain from internal injuries) and impaired respiratory exchange (due to phrenic nerve involvement and/or inability to voluntarily increase depth and rate of respirations).
  - ○ Diagnostic Procedures
    - ▪ X-rays, magnetic resonance imaging (MRI), and computed tomography (CT) imaging/computed axial tomography (CAT) scan can be used to assess the extent of the damage and the location of blood and bone fragments.

Patient-Centered Care

- Nursing Care
  - ○ Respiratory status
    - ▪ Monitoring the client's respiratory status is the first priority. Involuntary respirations can be affected due to a lesion at or above the phrenic nerve or swelling from a lesion immediately below C4. Lesions in the cervical or upper thoracic area will also impair voluntary movement of muscles used in respiration (increase in depth or rate).
    - ▪ Provide the client with oxygen and suction as needed.
    - ▪ Assist with intubation and mechanical ventilation if necessary.
    - ▪ Assist the client to cough by applying abdominal pressure when attempting to cough.
    - ▪ Teach client about use of incentive spirometer, and encourage client to perform coughing and deep breathing regularly.

○ Tissue perfusion – Neurogenic shock occurs after a SCI and can cause total loss of voluntary and autonomic function for several days to weeks. Hypotension, dependent edema, and loss of temperature regulation are common symptoms.

   ▪ When in an upright position, clients who are in neurogenic shock will experience postural hypotension. Transferring the client to a wheelchair should occur in stages.

   ▪ Raise the client's head of the bed and be ready to lower the angle if the client reports dizziness.

   ▪ Transfer the client into a reclining wheelchair with the back of the wheelchair reclined.

   ▪ Be ready to lock and lean the wheelchair back onto the knee to a fully reclined position if the client reports dizziness after the transfer. Do not attempt to return the client to the bed.

   ▪ Monitor the client for signs of thrombophlebitis (swelling of extremity, absent/decreased pulses, and areas of warmth and/or tenderness). The client may be on anticoagulants to prevent development of lower extremity thrombi.

○ Intake and output – The client may be NPO for several days. Regulation of fluid balance and nutritional support is necessary. Maintain an adequate fluid intake for the client; fluid will aid in preventing urinary calculi and bladder infections, and maintain soft stools.

○ Neurological status – After determining the baseline, monitor for an increasing loss of neurological function.

○ Muscle strength and tone – After determining the baseline, monitor for an increasing loss of muscle strength in the affected extremities.

   ▪ Clients who have upper motor neuron injuries (above L1 and L2) will convert to a spastic muscle tone after neurogenic shock.

   ▪ Paraplegics who have lower motor neuron injuries (below L1 and L2) will convert to a flaccid type of paralysis.

   ▪ Because most lower motor neuron lesions involve the cauda equina, the motor and sensory deficits can be patchy, with some areas of innervation and others without.

   ▪ Encourage active range-of-motion (ROM) exercises when possible and assist with passive ROM if the client lacks all motor function.

○ Mobility – Clients who have complete injuries will not regain mobility. Clients who have incomplete injuries can regain some function that will allow mobility with various types of braces. However, functional mobility can still be best attained through the use of a wheelchair.

○ Sensation – Varying degrees of loss of sensation will be experienced depending on whether the lesion is complete or incomplete. Care must be taken to prevent skin breakdown both in the bed and wheelchair. Various types of foam and air mattresses are available for beds and wheelchairs.

○ Bowel and bladder function

   ▪ Spastic neurogenic bladder – Clients who have upper motor neuron injuries will develop a spastic bladder after the neurogenic shock resolves. Bladder management options for male clients include condom catheters and stimulation of the micturition reflex by tugging on the pubic hair. Female clients will need to use an indwelling urinary catheter due to the unpredictably of the release of urine.

   ▪ Flaccid neurogenic bladder – Clients who have lower motor neuron injuries will develop a flaccid bladder. Bladder management options for males and females include intermittent catheterization and Credé's method (downward pressure placed on the bladder to manually express the urine).

- Neurogenic bowel functioning does not differ a lot between upper and lower motor neuron injuries. Daily use of stool softeners or bulk-forming laxatives is recommended to keep the stool soft. A bowel movement can be stimulated daily or every other day by administration of a bisacodyl (Dulcolax) suppository or digital stimulation (stimulation of the rectal sphincter with a gloved and lubricated finger) only if requested by the provider. Digital stimulation should be used cautiously to avoid provoking a vagal response, which can result in bradycardia and syncope.
- Development of a schedule as part of bladder and bowel training is critical in preventing complications related to immobility and promoting adequate nutrition and fluid balance.

- ○ Gastrointestinal function – An ileus can develop immediately after injury. Monitor for bowel sounds.
- ○ Skin Integrity – Changing the client's position every 2 hr is critical (every 1 hr when in a wheelchair). Clients who have a SCI can neither move nor feel pain from prolonged pressure. Pressure-relief devices in both the bed and the wheelchair must be consistently used.
- ○ Sexual Function – Teach the client about alterations in sexual function and possible adaptive strategies. Quadriplegics and other clients who have upper motor neuron lesions are usually capable of reflexogenic erections (erections secondary to manual manipulation). Ejaculation coordinated with emission may or may not occur. Clients who have lower motor neuron injuries are less able to have reflexogenic erections, but clients who have incomplete injuries may be able to have a combination of reflexogenic and psychogenic erections (erections stimulated by sexual thoughts and images). Administer medications as prescribed.

- Medications
  - ○ Glucocorticoids
    - Adrenocortical steroids such as methylprednisolone (Solu-Medrol) aid in decreasing edema of the spinal cord, which can cause spinal cord compression and areas of ischemia.
  - ○ Vasopressors
    - Norepinephrine and dopamine are given to treat hypotension, particularly during neurogenic shock.
  - ○ Antimuscarinic
    - Atropine sulfate may be used to treat bradycardia.
  - ○ Plasma expanders
    - Dextran, a volume expander, is used to treat hypotension secondary to spinal shock.
    - Nursing Considerations
      - □ Observe the client for symptoms of fluid overload.
  - ○ Muscle relaxants
    - Baclofen (Lioresal) and dantrolene sodium (Dantrium) – Given to clients who have severe muscle spasticity. Spasticity can be so severe that clients develop pressure ulcers, which can make sitting in a wheelchair very difficult.
    - Monitor for drowsiness, muscle weakness.
    - Baclofen may be given intrathecally to reduce the sedative effects.

- ○ Cholinergics
  - ▪ Bethanechol (Urecholine) – Decreases spasticity of the bladder, allowing for easier bladder training and fewer accidents.
  - ▪ Nursing Considerations
    - ▫ Observe the client for urinary retention. Measure residual periodically.
- ○ Analgesics
  - ▪ Opioids, nonopioids, and NSAIDs are given for pain. Clients may or may not be able to feel pain from spinal cord injury. Clients who do have muscle spasticity may report feeling discomfort from the muscle spasms.
- ○ Anticoagulants
  - ▪ Heparin or low-molecular-weight heparins are used for deep-vein thrombosis prophylaxis.
  - ▪ Nursing Considerations
    - ▫ Monitor INR, PT, and aPTT for therapeutic levels of anticoagulation.
    - ▫ Observe for signs of gastrointestinal bleeding or bleeding secondary to unrecognized injury.
- ○ Stool softeners and bulk-forming laxatives
  - ▪ Docusate sodium (Colace) or polycarbophil (Fibercon) prevent constipation and keep the stool soft.
- ○ Vasodilators
  - ▪ Hydralazine (Apresoline) and nitroglycerin (Nitrostat) – Use PRN to treat episodes of hypertension during automatic dysreflexia.
  - ▪ Nursing Considerations
    - ▫ Monitor blood pressure frequently.
- • Teamwork and Collaboration
  - ○ The client will need intensive occupational and physical therapy to learn how to perform ADLs and reestablish mobility using either a manual or electric wheelchair or braces and crutches. The client also will be fitted for splints to prevent contractures and provide wrist support for eating and manipulating joy stick on electric wheelchair.
  - ○ Social services will need to determine the client's financial resources, home care needs, and adaptations needed in the home prior to discharge.
  - ○ Referral of the client to an SCI support group can aid in emotionally adapting to changes in body image and role.
- • Therapeutic Procedures
  - ○ Application of immobilization devices and traction
    - ▪ Clients who have cervical fractures may be placed in a halo fixation device or cervical tongs. The purpose is to provide traction and/or immobilize the spinal column.

M⬧ View Image: Halo Traction

- Nursing Actions
  - Maintain body alignment and ensure cervical tong weights hang freely.
  - Monitor skin integrity by providing pin care and assessing the skin under the halo fixation vest as appropriate.
  - Do not use the halo device to turn or move a client.
- Client Education
  - If the client goes home with a halo fixation device on, provide instruction on pin and vest care.
  - Teach the client signs of infection and skin breakdown.

- Surgical Interventions
  - Spinal Surgery
    - Spinal fusion is commonly done when a spinal fracture creates an area of instability of the spine.
    - Spinal fusions done in the cervical area usually are done using an anterior approach through the front of the neck.
    - Spinal fusions in the thoracic or lumbar areas are done using a posterior approach and can be combined with a decompressive laminectomy.
    - A decompressive laminectomy is done by removing a section of lamina, accessing the spinal canal, and removing bone fragments, foreign bodies, or hematomas that may be placing pressure on the spinal cord.

 M View Image: Laminectomy

    - Donor bone often is obtained from the iliac crest and used to fuse together the vertebrae that are unstable.
    - Application of paravertebral rods can be used to mechanically immobilize several vertebral levels.
    - Nursing Actions
      - In clients who have undergone an anterior cervical fusion, monitor for possible airway compromise from swelling or hemorrhage. Observe for deviation of the trachea.
      - Assess neuro status and vital signs every hour for the first 4 hr following spinal fusion.
    - Client Education
      - Inform the client that an area of decreased range-of-motion will always exist in the area of fusion or paravertebral rods.
      - Rods are usually not removed unless they cause pain. Removal can be done after the spine has restabilized.

- Care After Discharge
  - Clients who have experienced SCI with subsequent loss of function will need varying levels of support upon discharge.
  - Clients who have quadriplegia will require a lengthy and extensive rehabilitative experience, which can occur on an outpatient or in-home basis.

○ Family members will need to be instructed on all aspects of clients' personal needs.

○ Referrals will need to be made, with the assistance of social services, for a home health nurse, home health aide, and in-home physical and occupational therapists.

○ Many adaptations may also need to be made to the home to make it wheelchair accessible.

○ Although clients who have paraplegia will require less intensive therapy, all of the referrals and accommodations necessary for clients with quadriplegia also will be needed for clients with paraplegia.

○ Client Education

  ▪ Clients and family members will need to be taught all aspects of clients' care (ADLs, transfers, and medication regimen).

Complications

- Orthostatic hypotension

  ○ Occurs when clients change position due to the interruption in functioning of the automatic nervous system and pooling of blood in lower extremities when in an upright position.

  ○ Nursing Actions

    ▪ Change the client's positioning slowly and place the client in a wheelchair that reclines.

    ▪ Use thigh-high elastic hose or elastic wraps to increase venous return. Elastic wraps may need to extend all the way up the client's legs and include the client's abdomen.

- Neurogenic shock

  ○ Neurogenic shock is a common response of the spinal cord following an injury.

  ○ Symptoms of bradycardia, hypotension, flaccid paralysis, loss of reflex activity below level of injury, and paralytic ileus accompany neurogenic shock due to the loss of autonomic function.

  ○ Nursing Actions

    ▪ Monitor vital signs for hypotension and bradycardia.

    ▪ Treat symptoms with appropriate medications (vasopressors or atropine).

- Autonomic dysreflexia

  ○ Occurs secondary to the stimulation of the sympathetic nervous system and inadequate compensatory response by the parasympathetic nervous system. Clients who have lesions below T6 do not experience dysreflexia because the parasympathetic nervous system is able to neutralize the sympathetic response.

  ○ Sympathetic stimulation is usually caused by a triggering stimulus in the lower part of the body (refer to list under Nursing Actions).

  ○ Stimulation of the sympathetic nervous system causes extreme hypertension, sudden severe headache, pallor below the level of the spinal cord's lesion dermatome, blurred vision, diaphoresis, restlessness, nausea, and piloerection (goose bumps).

  ○ Stimulation of the parasympathetic nervous system causes bradycardia, flushing above the corresponding dermatome to the spinal cord lesion (flushed face and neck), and nasal stuffiness.

○ Nursing Actions

  ▪ Determine and treat the cause.

    ▫ Sit the client up (to decrease blood pressure secondary to postural hypotension).

    ▫ Notify the provider.

    ▫ Determine the cause.

      ▸ Distended bladder – most common cause (kinked or blocked urinary catheter, urinary retention, or urinary calculi)

      ▸ Fecal impaction

      ▸ Cold stress or drafts on lower part of the body

      ▸ Tight clothing

      ▸ Undiagnosed injury or illness (kidney infection or stone, lower extremity fracture)

    ▫ Treat the cause.

      ▸ Relieve the kink in the catheter or irrigate to remove blockage.

      ▸ Catheterize the client (use anesthetic ointment on the tip of the catheter).

      ▸ Remove the impaction (use anesthetic ointment prior to removal).

      ▸ Adjust the room temperature and block drafts.

      ▸ Remove tight clothing.

      ▸ Assess for injury, such as lower extremity fracture or kidney/bladder infection.

  ▪ Monitor vital signs for severe hypertension and bradycardia.

  ▪ Administer antihypertensives (nitrates or hydralazine).

○ Client Education

  ▪ Provide client education regarding potential causes of dysreflexia.

  ▪ Instruct the client to space out fluid intake and increase frequency of intermittent catheterizations if fluid intake is temporarily increased.

  ▪ Provide a list of possible actions to pursue if an episode of dysreflexia does occur.

APPLICATION EXERCISES

1. A nurse is planning care for a client who suffered a spinal cord injury (SCI) involving a T12 fracture 1 week ago. The client has no muscle control of the lower limbs, bowel, or bladder. Which of the following should be the nurse's highest priority?

    A. Prevention of further damage to the spinal cord

    B. Prevention of contractures of the lower extremities

    C. Prevention of skin breakdown of areas that lack sensation

    D. Prevention of postural hypotension when placing the client in a wheelchair

2. A nurse is caring for a client with a spinal cord injury who reports a severe headache and is sweating profusely. Vital signs include BP of 220/110 mm Hg, with an apical heart rate of 54/min. Which of the following actions should the nurse take first?

    A. Notify the provider.

    B. Sit the client upright in bed.

    C. Check the client's urinary catheter for blockage.

    D. Administer antihypertensive medication.

3. A nurse is caring for a client who has a C4 spinal cord injury. Which of the following should the nurse recognize the client as being at the greatest risk for?

    A. Neurogenic shock

    B. Paralytic ileus

    C. Stress ulcer

    D. Respiratory compromise

4. A nurse is caring for a client who experienced a cervical spine injury 24 hr ago. Which of the following types of prescribed medications should the nurse clarify with the provider?

    A. Glucocorticoids

    B. Plasma expanders

    C. H2 antagonists

    D. Muscle relaxants

5. A nurse is caring for a client who experienced a cervical spine injury 3 months ago. Which of the following types of bladder management methods should the nurse use for this client?

    A. Condom catheter

    B. Intermittent urinary catheterization

    C. Credé's method

    D. Indwelling urinary catheter

6. A nurse is assessing a client who has suffered a spinal cord injury. Use the ATI Active Learning Template: Systems Disorder. List three physical assessment findings the nurse should look for.

APPLICATION EXERCISES KEY

1. A. **CORRECT:** The greatest risk to the client during the acute phase of a SCI is further damage to the spinal cord. Therefore, when planning care, the priority should be the prevention of further damage to the spinal cord by administration of corticosteroids, minimizing movement of the client until spinal stabilization is accomplished through either traction or surgery, and adequate oxygenation of the client to decrease ischemia of the spinal cord.

   B. INCORRECT: Preventing contractures is important, but it is not the highest priority.

   C. INCORRECT: Preventing skin breakdown is important, but is not the highest priority.

   D. INCORRECT: Preventing postural hypotension is important, but it is not the highest priority.

    NCLEX® Connection: Physiological Adaptations, Pathophysiology

2. A. INCORRECT: Notifying the provider is important, but it is not the priority action for the nurse to take.

   B. **CORRECT:** The greatest risk to the client is experiencing a cerebrovascular accident (stroke) secondary to elevated blood pressure. The first action by the nurse is to elevate the head of the bed until the client is in an upright position. This will lower the blood pressure secondary to postural hypotension.

   C. INCORRECT: Checking the client's catheter for blockage is important, but it is not the priority action the nurse should take.

   D. INCORRECT: Administering an antihypertensive medication may be indicated, but it is not the priority action the nurse should take.

    NCLEX® Connection: Reduction of Risk Potential, Changes/Abnormalities in Vital Signs

3. A. INCORRECT: Neurogenic shock is a complication, but it is not the greatest risk to the client at this time.

   B. INCORRECT: A paralytic ileus is a complication, but it is not the greatest risk to the client at this time.

   C. INCORRECT: A stress ulcer is a complication, but it is not the greatest risk to the client at this time.

   D. **CORRECT:** Using the airway, breathing, and circulation (ABC) priority-setting framework, the greatest risk to the client with an SCI at the level of C4 is respiratory compromise secondary to involvement of the phrenic nerve. Maintenance of an airway and provision of ventilatory support as needed is the priority intervention.

    NCLEX® Connection: Physiological Adaptations, Pathophysiology

4. A. INCORRECT: Glucocorticoids are appropriate medications to administer at this time.

    B. INCORRECT: Plasma expanders are appropriate medications to administer at this time.

    C. INCORRECT: H_2 antagonists are appropriate medications to administer at this time.

    D. **CORRECT:** The client will still be in spinal shock 24 hr following the injury. The client will not experience muscle spasms until after the spinal shock has resolved, making muscle relaxants unnecessary at this time.

     NCLEX® Connection: Pharmacological and Parenteral Therapies, Adverse Effects/Contraindications/ Side Effects/Interactions

5. A. **CORRECT:** A client who has a cervical spinal cord injury will also have an upper motor neuron injury, which is manifested by a spastic bladder. Because the bladder will empty on its own, a condom catheter is an appropriate method and is noninvasive.

    B. INCORRECT: Intermittent urinary catheterization is an appropriate method for a client who has a flaccid bladder.

    C. INCORRECT: Credé's method is appropriate for a client who has a flaccid bladder.

    D. INCORRECT: An indwelling urinary catheter is invasive and another bladder management method should be used.

     NCLEX® Connection: Basic Care and Comfort, Elimination

6. *Using the ATI Active Learning Template: Systems Disorder*
    - Physical Assessment Findings
        ○ Inability to feel light touch when touched by a cotton ball, inability to discriminate between sharp and dull when touched with a safety pin or other sharp objects, and an inability to discriminate between hot and cold when touched with containers of hot and cold water.
        ○ Absent deep tendon reflexes
        ○ Flaccidity of muscles
        ○ Hypotension that is more severe when the client is in sitting in an upright position
        ○ Shallow respirations
        ○ Dependent edema
        ○ Neurogenic shock, which accompanies spinal trauma, causes a total loss of all reflexive and autonomic function below the level of the injury for a period of several days to weeks.
        ○ Loss of temperature regulation – hyperthermia or hypothermia

     NCLEX® Connection: Reduction of Risk Potential, System Specific Assessments

UNIT 3   Nursing Care of Clients with Respiratory Disorders

SECTIONS

› Diagnostic and Therapeutic Procedures
› Respiratory System Disorders
› Respiratory Emergencies

NCLEX® CONNECTIONS

When reviewing the chapters in this unit, keep in mind the relevant sections of the NCLEX® outline, in particular:

Client Needs: Pharmacological and Parenteral Therapies	Client Needs: Reduction of Risk Potential	Client Needs: Physiological Adaptation
› Relevant topics/tasks include: » Adverse Effects/Contraindications/Side Effects/Interactions › Manage the client experiencing side effects and adverse reactions of medication. » Expected Actions/Outcomes › Evaluate the client's use of medications over time. » Medication Administration › Educate the client on medication self-administration procedures.	› Relevant topics/tasks include: » Laboratory Values › Identify laboratory values for ABGs, BUN, cholesterol, glucose, hematocrit, hemoglobin, glycosylated hemoglobin, platelets, potassium, sodium, WBC, creatinine, PT, PTT and APTT, INR. » Potential for Complications of Diagnostic Tests/Treatments/Procedures › Maintain tube patency. » Therapeutic Procedures › Educate the client about home management of care (tracheostomy and ostomy).	› Relevant topics/tasks include: » Alterations in Body Systems › Monitor and care for clients on a ventilator. » Pathophysiology › Understand general principles of pathophysiology. » Medical Emergencies › Apply knowledge of nursing procedures and psychomotor skills when caring for a client experiencing a medical emergency.

chapter 17

Overview

- Respiratory diagnostic procedures are used to evaluate a client's respiratory status by checking indicators such as the oxygenation of the blood, lung functioning, and the integrity of the airway.

- Respiratory diagnostic procedures that nurses should be knowledgeable about include the following:

  ○ Pulmonary function tests (PFTs)

  ○ ABGs

  ○ Bronchoscopy

  ○ Thoracentesis

Pulmonary Function Tests (PFTs)

- Pulmonary function tests determine lung function and breathing difficulties.

  ○ PFTs measure lung volumes and capacities, diffusion capacity, gas exchange, flow rates, airway resistance along with distribution of ventilation.

  ○ Helpful in identifying clients for lung disease.

  ○ Commonly performed for clients who have dyspnea.

  ○ Can be performed before surgical procedures to identify clients with respiratory risks.

  ○ If client is smoker, instruct client not to smoke 6 to 8 hr prior to testing.

  ○ If a client uses inhalers, withhold 4 to 6 hr prior to testing. (This may vary according to facility policy.)

ABGs

- An ABG sample reports the status of oxygenation and acid-base balance of the blood.

  ○ An ABG measures the following:

    ▪ pH – the amount of free hydrogen ions in the arterial blood (H^+).

    ▪ PaO_2 – the partial pressure of oxygen.

    ▪ $PaCO_2$ – the partial pressure of carbon dioxide.

    ▪ HCO_3^- – the concentration of bicarbonate in arterial blood.

    ▪ SaO_2 – percentage of oxygen bound to Hgb as compared with the total amount that can be possibly carried.

  ○ ABGs can be obtained by an arterial puncture or through an arterial line.

- Indications
  - Potential Diagnoses
    - Blood pH levels may be affected by any number of disease processes (respiratory, renal, malnutrition, electrolyte imbalance, endocrine, or neurologic).
    - These assessments are helpful in monitoring the effectiveness of various treatments (such as acidosis interventions), in guiding oxygen therapy, and in evaluating client responses to weaning from mechanical ventilation.
- Interpretation of Findings

ABG MEASURE	NORMAL RANGE		ABG MEASURE	NORMAL RANGE
pH	7.35 to 7.45		HCO_3^-	21 to 28 mEq/L
PaO_2	80 to 100 mm Hg		SaO_2	95 to 100%
$PaCO_2$	35 to 45 mm Hg			

  - Blood pH levels below 7.35 reflect acidosis, and levels above 7.45 reflect alkalosis.
- Arterial Puncture
  - Preprocedure
    - Nursing Actions
      - Obtain a heparinized syringe for the sample collection.
      - Perform an Allen's test prior to arterial puncture to verify patent radial and ulnar circulation. The nurse should compress the ulnar and radial arteries simultaneously while instructing the client to form a fist. Then, have the client relax his hand while releasing pressure on the radial artery. His hand should turn pink quickly, indicating patency of the radial artery. Repeat this process for the ulnar artery.

> **M** View Image: Allen's Test

    - Client Education
      - Explain and reinforce the procedure with the client. Clients often experience pain with repeated ABG level checks and are often unaware of the purpose of the puncture.
  - Intraprocedure
    - Nursing Actions
      - Perform an arterial puncture using surgical aseptic technique, and collect a specimen into a heparinized syringe.
      - Place the collected and capped specimen into a basin of ice and water to preserve pH levels and oxygen pressure. The specimen should be transported to the laboratory immediately.

      - Accessing the radial artery for sampling may be more difficult with older adult clients because of impaired peripheral vasculature.

- ○ Postprocedure
  - ▪ Nursing Actions
    - □ Immediately after an arterial puncture, hold direct pressure over the site for at least 5 min. Pressure must be maintained for at least 20 min if the client is receiving anticoagulant therapy. Ensure that bleeding has stopped prior to removing direct pressure.
    - □ Monitor the ABG sampling site for bleeding, loss of pulse, swelling, and changes in temperature and color.
    - □ Document all interventions and client response.
    - □ Report results to the provider as soon as they are available.
    - □ Administer oxygen as prescribed. Change ventilator settings as ordered or notify a respiratory therapist.
  - ▪ Note: Arterial puncture is frequently done by a respiratory therapist in hospital settings.
- • Arterial Line
  - ○ Preprocedure
    - ▪ Nursing Actions
      - □ Verify that the arterial line may be used for specimen collection.
      - □ Obtain a heparinized syringe for the sample collection and a standard syringe for waste.
    - ▪ Client Education
      - □ Explain and reinforce the procedure with the client.
  - ○ Intraprocedure
    - ▪ Nursing Actions
      - □ Follow specific facility protocols for collection procedures.
      - □ Collect waste and specimen. Place both on ice for transport to the laboratory immediately.
      - □ Flush the arterial line with the preconnected flushing system.
  - ○ Postprocedure
    - ▪ Nursing Actions
      - □ Assess the arterial waveform upon completion.
      - □ Document all interventions and the client's response.
      - □ Report results to the provider as soon as they are available.
      - □ Administer oxygen to the client as prescribed. Change the ventilator settings as ordered, or notify a respiratory therapist.

- Complications
  - Hematoma, arterial occlusion
    - A hematoma occurs when blood accumulates under the skin at the IV site.
    - Nursing Actions
      - Observe the client for changes in temperature, swelling, color, loss of pulse, or pain.
      - Notify the provider immediately if symptoms persist.
      - Apply pressure to the hematoma site.

  - Air embolism
    - Air enters the arterial system during catheter insertion.
    - Nursing Actions
      - Place the client on his left side in the Trendelenburg position.
      - Monitor the client for a sudden onset of shortness of breath, decrease in SaO_2 levels, chest pain, anxiety, and air hunger.
      - Notify the provider immediately if symptoms occur, administer oxygen therapy, and obtain ABGs. Continue to assess the client's respiratory status for any deterioration.

Bronchoscopy

- Bronchoscopy permits visualization of the larynx, trachea, and bronchi through either a flexible fiberoptic bronchoscope or a rigid bronchoscope.
  - Bronchoscopy can be performed as an outpatient procedure, in a surgical suite under general anesthesia, or at the bedside under local anesthesia and moderate (conscious) sedation.
  - Bronchoscopy also can be performed on clients who are receiving mechanical ventilation by inserting the scope through the client's endotracheal tube.
- Indications
  - Potential Diagnoses
    - Visualization of abnormalities such as tumors, inflammation, and strictures
    - Biopsy of suspicious tissue (lung cancer)
      - Clients undergoing a bronchoscopy with biopsy have additional risks for bleeding and/or perforation.
    - Aspiration of deep sputum or lung abscesses for culture and sensitivity and/or cytology (pneumonia)
  - Note: Bronchoscopy is also performed for therapeutic reasons, such as removal of foreign bodies and secretions from the tracheobronchial tree, treating postoperative atelectasis, and to destroy and excise lesions.

- Preprocedure
  - Nursing Actions
    - Assess the client for allergies to anesthetic agents or routine use of anticoagulants.
    - Ensure that a consent form is signed by the client prior to the procedure.
    - Remove the client's dentures, if applicable, prior to the procedure.
    - Maintain the client on NPO status prior to the procedure as ordered, usually 8 to 12 hr, to reduce the risk of aspiration when the cough reflex is blocked by anesthesia.
    - Administer preprocedure medications as prescribed, such as viscous lidocaine or local anesthetic throat sprays.
- Intraprocedure
  - Nursing Actions
    - Position the client in a sitting position.
    - Administer medications as prescribed, such as sedatives, antianxiety agents, and/or atropine to reduce oral secretions.
    - Assist in collecting and labeling specimens. Ensure prompt delivery to the laboratory.
    - Monitor the client's vital signs, respiratory pattern, and oxygenation status throughout the procedure.
    - Sedation given to older adult clients who have respiratory insufficiency may precipitate respiratory arrest.
- Postprocedure
  - Nursing Actions
    - Continuously monitor the client's respirations, blood pressure, pulse oximetry, heart rate, and level of consciousness during the recovery period.
      - □ Assess the client's level of consciousness while recognizing that older adult clients may develop confusion or lethargy due to the effects of medications given during the bronchoscopy.
    - Assess the client's level of consciousness, presence of gag reflex, and ability to swallow prior to resuming oral intake (usually takes about 2 hr).
      - □ Allow adequate time for the cough and gag reflex to return prior to resuming oral intake. The cough reflex may be slower to return in older adult clients receiving local anesthesia due to impaired laryngeal reflex.
      - □ Once the cough reflex returns, the nurse may offer ice chips to the client and eventually fluids.
    - Monitor the client for development of significant fever (mild fever for less than 24 hr is not uncommon), productive cough, significant hemoptysis indicative of hemorrhage (a small amount of blood-tinged sputum is expected), hypoxemia.
    - Be prepared to intervene for unexpected responses and/or aspiration, laryngospasm.
    - Provide oral hygiene to the client.
    - Evaluate and document the client's response to the procedure (stable vital signs, return of gag reflex).

- For older adult clients, encourage coughing and deep breathing every 2 hr. There is an increased risk of respiratory infection and pneumonia in older adult clients due to decreased cough effectiveness and decreased secretion clearance. Respiratory infections may be more severe and last longer in older adult clients.

- The client is not discharged from the recovery room until adequate cough reflex and respiratory effort are present.

  ○ Client Education

    - Instruct clients that gargling with salt water or using throat lozenges may provide comfort for soreness of the throat.

- Complications

  ○ Laryngospasm

    - Laryngospasm is uncontrolled muscle contractions of the laryngeal cords (vocal cords) that impede the client's ability to inhale.

    - Nursing Actions

      □ Continuously monitor the client for signs of respiratory distress.

      □ Maintain a patent airway by repositioning the client or inserting an oral or nasopharyngeal airway as appropriate.

      □ Administer oxygen therapy to the client as prescribed. Humidification can decrease the likelihood of laryngeal edema.

  ○ Pneumothorax

    - Pneumothorax can occur following a rigid bronchoscopy.

    - Assess client's breath sounds and oxygen saturation, and obtain a follow-up chest x-ray.

  ○ Aspiration

    - Aspiration can occur if the client chokes on oral or gastric secretions.

    - Nursing Actions

      □ Prevent aspiration in the client by withholding oral fluids or food until the gag reflex returns (usually 2 hr).

      □ Perform suctioning as needed.

Thoracentesis

- Thoracentesis is the surgical perforation of the chest wall and pleural space with a large-bore needle. It is performed to obtain specimens for diagnostic evaluation, instill medication into the pleural space, and remove fluid (effusion) or air from the pleural space for therapeutic relief of pleural pressure.

  ○ Thoracentesis is performed under local anesthesia by a provider at the client's bedside, in a procedure room, or in a provider's office.

  ○ Use of an ultrasound for guidance decreases the risk of complications.

- Indications
  - Potential Diagnoses
    - Transudates (heart failure, cirrhosis, nephritic syndrome)
    - Exudates (inflammatory, infectious, neoplastic conditions)
    - Empyema
    - Pneumonia
    - Blunt, crushing, or penetrating chest injuries/trauma, or invasive thoracic procedures, such as lung and/or cardiac surgery
  - Client Presentation
    - Large amounts of fluid in the pleural space compress lung tissue and can cause pain, shortness of breath, cough, and other symptoms of pleural pressure.
    - Assessment of the effusion area may reveal decreased breath sounds, dull percussion sounds, and decreased chest wall expansion. Pain may occur due to inflammatory process.
- Interpretation of Findings
  - Aspirated fluid is analyzed for general appearance, cell counts, protein and glucose content, the presence of enzymes such as lactate dehydrogenase (LDH) and amylase, abnormal cells, and culture.
- Preprocedure
  - Percussion, auscultation, radiography, or sonography is used to locate the effusion and needle insertion site.

  - Changes in fat deposition in many older adult clients may make it difficult for the provider to identify the landmarks for insertion of the thoracentesis needle.
  - Nursing Actions
    - Ensure that the client has signed the informed consent form.
    - Gather all needed supplies.
    - Obtain preprocedure x-ray as prescribed to locate pleural effusion and to determine needle insertion site.
    - Position the client sitting upright with his arms and shoulders raised and supported on pillows and/or on an overbed table and with his feet and legs well-supported.
  - Client Education
    - Instruct the client to remain absolutely still (risk of accidental needle damage) during the procedure and not to cough or talk unless instructed by the primary care provider.
- Intraprocedure
  - Nursing Actions
    - Assist the provider with the procedure (strict surgical aseptic technique). *sterile*
    - Prepare the client for a feeling of pressure with needle insertion and fluid removal.
    - Monitor the client's vital signs, skin color, and oxygen saturation throughout the procedure.
    - Measure and record the amount of fluid removed from the client's chest.
    - Label specimens at the bedside, and promptly send them to the laboratory.
  - Note: The amount of fluid removed is limited to 1 L at a time to prevent cardiovascular collapse.

- Postprocedure
  - Nursing Actions
    - Apply a dressing over the puncture site, and assess dressing for bleeding or drainage.
    - Monitor the client's vital signs and respiratory status (respiratory rate and rhythm, breath sounds, oxygenation status) hourly for the first several hours after the thoracentesis.
    - Auscultate lungs for reduced breath sounds on side of thoracentesis.
    - Encourage the client to deep breathe to assist with lung expansion.
    - Obtain a postprocedure chest x-ray (check resolution of effusions, rule out pneumothorax).
- Complications
  - Mediastinal shift
    - Shift of thoracic structures to one side of the body.
      - Monitor client's vital signs.
      - Auscultate client's lungs for a decrease in or absence of breath sounds.
  - Pneumothorax
    - Pneumothorax is a collapsed lung. It can occur due to injury to the lung during the procedure.
    - Nursing Actions
      - Monitor the client for signs and symptoms of pneumothorax, such as diminished breath sounds.
      - Monitor postprocedure chest x-ray results.
      - Educate the client on indications of a pneumothorax, which can develop during the first 24 hr following a thoracentesis. Indications include deviated trachea, pain on the affected side that worsens upon exhalation, affected side does not move in and out upon inhalation and exhalation, increased heart rate, rapid shallow respirations, "nagging" cough, or feeling of air hunger.
  - Bleeding
    - Bleeding can occur if the client is moved during the procedure or is at an increased risk for bleeding.
    - Nursing Actions
      - Monitor the client for coughing and/or hemoptysis.
      - Monitor the client's vital signs and laboratory results for evidence of bleeding (hypotension, reduced Hgb level).
      - Assess thoracentesis site for bleeding.
  - Infection
    - Infection can occur due to the introduction of bacteria with the needle puncture.
    - Nursing Actions
      - Ensure that sterile technique is maintained.
      - Monitor the client's temperature following the procedure.

APPLICATION EXERCISES

1. A nurse is caring for a client who is scheduled for a thoracentesis. Prior to the procedure, which of the following actions should the nurse take?

    A. Position the client in an upright position, leaning over the bedside table.

    B. Explain the procedure to the client.

    C. Obtain ABGs from the client.

    D. Administer benzocaine spray to the client.

2. A nurse is assessing a client who is in respiratory distress. The nurse should recognize that which of the following can cause a low pulse oximetry reading? (Select all that apply.)

    _____ A. Nail polish

    _____ B. Inadequate peripheral circulation

    _____ C. Hyperthermia

    _____ D. Increased Hgb level

    _____ E. Edema

3. A nurse is assessing a client following a bronchoscopy. Which of the following findings should the nurse report to the provider?

    A. Blood-tinged sputum

    B. Dry, nonproductive cough

    C. Sore throat

    D. Bronchospasms

4. A nurse is caring for a client who is scheduled for a thoracentesis. Which of the following supplies should the nurse ensure is in the client's room? (Select all that apply.)

    _____ A. Oxygen equipment

    _____ B. Incentive spirometer

    _____ C. Pulse oximeter

    _____ D. Sterile dressing

    _____ E. Suture removal kit

5. A nurse is caring for a client following a thoracentesis. Which of the following clinical manifestations should the nurse recognize as risks for complications? (Select all that apply.)

_____ A. Dyspnea

_____ B. Localized bloody drainage on the dressing

_____ C. Fever

_____ D. Hypotension

_____ E. Report of pain at the puncture site

6. A nurse is assessing a client following an arterial line placement. Use the ATI Active Learning Template: Therapeutic Procedure. List three postprocedure nursing actions the nurse should take while caring for this client.

APPLICATION EXERCISES KEY

1. A. **CORRECT:** Positioning the client in an upright position and bent over the bedside table widens the pleural space for the provider to access the pleural fluid.

    B. INCORRECT: It is not the role of the nurse to explain the procedure to the client. This is the responsibility of the provider.

    C. INCORRECT: It is not indicated that the client needs ABGs drawn.

    D. INCORRECT: Benzocaine spray is not administered with a thoracentesis. It is used for a bronchoscopy.

     NCLEX® Connection: Reduction of Risk Potential, Diagnostic Tests

2. A. **CORRECT:** Nail polish can affect the accuracy of pulse oximetry and result in an incorrect pulse oximetry level.

    B. **CORRECT:** Inadequate peripheral circulation can result in a low reading while obtaining a client's pulse oximetry level.

    C. INCORRECT: Hypothermia can result in a low reading while obtaining a client's pulse oximetry level.

    D. INCORRECT: A decreased Hgb level can result in a low reading while obtaining a client's pulse oximetry level.

    E. **CORRECT:** Edema can result in a low reading while obtaining a client's pulse oximetry level.

     NCLEX® Connection: Reduction of Risk Potential, Diagnostic Tests

3. A. INCORRECT: Blood-tinged sputum is an expecting finding following a bronchoscopy.

    B. INCORRECT: A dry, nonproductive cough is an expected finding following a bronchoscopy.

    C. INCORRECT: A sore throat is an expected finding following a bronchoscopy.

    D. **CORRECT:** Bronchospams can indicate the client is having difficulty maintaining a patent airway. The nurse should notify the provider immediately.

     NCLEX® Connection: Reduction of Risk Potential, Diagnostic Tests

4. A. **CORRECT:** Oxygen equipment is necessary to have in the client's room if the client becomes short of breath following the procedure.

    B. INCORRECT: An incentive spirometer is indicated for a client following thoracic surgery to promote improved oxygenation and pulmonary function.

    C. **CORRECT:** Pulse oximetry is necessary to monitor the client's oxygen saturation level during the procedure.

    D. **CORRECT:** A sterile dressing is necessary to apply to the puncture site following the procedure.

    E. INCORRECT: A suture removal kit is needed to remove sutures following surgery.

    (N) NCLEX® Connection: Reduction of Risk Potential, Diagnostic Tests

5. A. **CORRECT:** Dyspnea can indicate a pneumothorax or a reaccumulation of fluid. The nurse should notify the provider immediately.

    B. INCORRECT: Localized bloody drainage contained on a dressing is an expected finding following a thoracentesis.

    C. **CORRECT:** Fever can indicate an infection. The nurse should notify the provider immediately.

    D. **CORRECT:** Hypotension can indicate intrathoracic bleeding. The nurse should notify the provider immediately.

    E. INCORRECT: The client's report of pain at the puncture site is an expected finding following a thoracentesis.

    (N) NCLEX® Connection: Reduction of Risk Potential, Potential for Complications of Diagnostic Tests/Treatments/Procedures

6. *Using the ATI Active Learning Template: Therapeutic Procedure*
    - Postprocedure Nursing Actions
      - Assess the arterial waveform upon completion.
      - Document all interventions and the client's response.
      - Report results to the provider as soon as they are available.
      - Administer oxygen to the client as prescribed. Change the ventilator settings as ordered, or notify a respiratory therapist.

    (N) NCLEX® Connection: Reduction of Risk Potential, Diagnostic Tests

chapter **18**

Overview

- Chest tubes are inserted into the pleural space to drain fluid, blood, or air; reestablish a negative pressure; facilitate lung expansion; and restore normal intrapleural pressure.

- Chest tubes can be inserted in the emergency department, at the client's bedside, or in the operating room through a thoracotomy incision.

- Chest tubes are removed when the lungs have reexpanded and/or there is no more fluid drainage.

Chest Tube Systems

- A disposable three-chamber drainage system is most often used.

  - First chamber: drainage collection

  - Second chamber: water seal

  - Third chamber: suction control

 View Image: Chest Tube Drainage System

- Water seals are created by adding sterile fluid to a chamber up to the 2 cm line. The water seal allows air to exit from the pleural space on exhalation and stops air from entering with inhalation.

  - To maintain the water seal, the chamber must be kept upright and below the chest tube insertion site at all times. The nurse should routinely monitor the water level due to the possibility of evaporation. The nurse should add fluid as needed to maintain the 2 cm water seal level.

  - The height of the sterile fluid in the suction control chamber determines the amount of suction transmitted to the pleural space. A suction pressure of -20 cm H_2O is common. The application of suction results in continuous bubbling in the suction chamber. The nurse should monitor the fluid level and add fluid as needed to maintain the prescribed level of suctioning.

  - Tidaling (movement of the fluid level with respiration) is expected in the water seal chamber. With spontaneous respirations, the fluid level will rise with inspiration (increase in negative pressure in lung) and will fall with expiration. With positive-pressure mechanical ventilation, the fluid level will rise with expiration and fall with inspiration.

  - Cessation of tidaling in the water seal chamber signals lung reexpansion or an obstruction within the system.

Chest Tube Insertion

- Indications
  - Diagnoses
    - Pneumothorax (collapsed lung)
    - Hemothorax (blood in lung)
    - Postoperative chest drainage (thoracotomy or open-heart surgery)
    - Pleural effusion (fluid in lung)
    - Lung abscess (necrotic lung tissue)
  - Client Presentation
    - Dyspnea
    - Distended neck veins
    - Poor circulation
    - Cough
    - Absent or reduced breath sounds
- Preprocedure
  - Nursing Actions
    - Verify that the consent form is signed.
    - Reinforce client teaching. Breathing will improve when the chest tube is in place.
    - Assess for allergies to local anesthetics.
    - Assist the client into the desired position (supine or semi-Fowler's).
    - Prepare the chest drainage system prior to the chest tube insertion per the facility's protocol (fill the water seal chamber).
    - Administer pain and sedation medications as prescribed.
    - Prep the insertion site with povidone-iodine.
- Intraprocedure
  - Nursing Actions
    - Assist the provider with insertion of the chest tube, application of a dressing to the insertion site, and set-up of the drainage system.
      - □ The chest tube tip is positioned up toward the shoulder (pneumothorax) or down toward the posterior (hemothorax or pleural effusion).
      - □ The chest tube is then sutured to the chest wall, and an airtight dressing is placed over the puncture wound.
      - □ The chest tube is then attached to drainage tubing that leads to a drainage system.
      - □ Place the chest tube drainage system below the client's chest level with the tubing coiled on the bed. Ensure that the tubing from the bed to the drainage system is straight to promote drainage via gravity.
    - The nurse should continually monitor the client's vital signs and response to the procedure.

 View Image: Chest Tube

- Postprocedure
  - Nursing Actions
    - Assess the client's vital signs, breath sounds, SaO$_2$, color, and respiratory effort as indicated by the status of the client and at least every 4 hr.
    - Encourage coughing and deep breathing every 2 hr.
    - Keep the drainage system below the client's chest level, including during ambulation.
    - Monitor the chest tube's placement and function.
      - □ Check the water seal level every 2 hr, and add fluid as needed. The fluid level should fluctuate with respiratory effort.
      - □ Document the amount and color of drainage hourly for the first 24 hr and then at least every 8 hr. Mark the date, hour, and drainage level on the container at the end of each shift. Report excessive drainage (greater than 70 mL/hr) or drainage that is cloudy or red to the provider. Drainage will often increase with position changes or coughing.
      - □ Monitor the fluid in the suction control chamber, and maintain the fluid level prescribed by the provider.
      - □ Check for expected findings of tidaling in the water seal chamber and continuous bubbling only in the suction chamber.
    - Routinely monitor tubing for kinks, occlusions, or loose connections.
    - Monitor the chest tube insertion site for redness, pain, infection, and crepitus (air leakage in subcutaneous tissue).
    - Position the client in the semi-Fowler's to high-Fowler's position to promote optimal lung expansion and drainage of the fluid from the lungs.

    - Administer pain medications as prescribed.
    - Obtain a chest x-ray to verify the chest tube's placement.
    - Keep two enclosed hemostats, sterile water, and an occlusive dressing located at the bedside at all times.
    - Due to the risk of causing a tension pneumothorax, chest tubes are clamped only when ordered by the provider in specific circumstances, such as in the case of an air leak, during drainage system change, accidental disconnection of tubing, or damage to the drainage system.
    - Do not strip or milk tubing; only perform this action when prescribed by the provider. Stripping creates a high negative pressure and can damage the client's lung tissue.
- Complications
  - Air leaks
    - Air leaks can result if a connection is not taped securely.
    - Nursing Actions
      - □ Monitor the water seal chamber for continuous bubbling (air leak finding). If observed, locate the source of the air leak, and intervene accordingly (tighten the connection, replace drainage system).
        - ▸ Check all of the connections.
        - ▸ Notify provider if an air leak is noted, and if prescribed, gently apply a padded clamp to determine the location of the air leak. Remove the clamp immediately following assessment.

- ○ Accidental disconnection, system breakage, or removal
  - ▪ These complications can occur at any time.
  - ▪ Nursing Actions
    - ▫ If the tubing separates, the client is instructed to exhale as much as possible and to cough to remove as much air as possible from the pleural space. The nurse cleanses the tips and reconnects the tubing.
    - ▫ If the chest tube drainage system is compromised, the nurse immerses the end of the tube in sterile water to restore the water seal.
    - ▫ If a chest tube is accidentally removed, an occlusive dressing taped on only three sides should be immediately placed over the insertion site. This allows air to escape and reduces risk for development of a tension pneumothorax.
- ○ Tension pneumothorax
  - ▪ Sucking chest wounds, prolonged clamping of the tubing, kinks in the tubing, or obstruction may cause a tension pneumothorax.
  - ▪ Assessment findings include tracheal deviation, absent breath sounds on one side, distended neck veins, respiratory distress, asymmetry of the chest, and cyanosis.

Chest Tube Removal

- Provide pain medication 30 min before removing chest tubes.
- Assist the provider with sutures and chest tube removal.
- Instruct the client to take a deep breath, exhale, and bear down (Valsalva maneuver) or to take a deep breath and hold it (increases intrathoracic pressure and reduces risk of air emboli) during chest tube removal.
- Apply airtight sterile petroleum jelly gauze dressing. Secure in place with a heavyweight stretch tape.
- Obtain chest x-rays as prescribed. This is performed to verify continued resolution of the pneumothorax, hemothorax, or pleural effusion.
- Monitor the client for excessive wound drainage, signs of infection, or recurrent pneumothorax.

APPLICATION EXERCISES

1. A nurse is preparing to care for a client following chest tube placement. Which of the following items should be available in the client's room? (Select all that apply.)

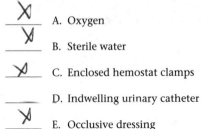

_____ A. Oxygen

_____ B. Sterile water

_____ C. Enclosed hemostat clamps

_____ D. Indwelling urinary catheter

_____ E. Occlusive dressing

2. A nurse is caring for a client who has a chest tube and drainage system in place. The nurse observes that the client's chest tube was accidentally removed. Which of the following actions should the nurse take first?

A. Place the tubing in sterile water to restore the water seal.

B. Apply sterile gauze to the insertion site.

C. Place tape around the insertion site.

D. Assess the client's respiratory status.

3. A nurse is assessing a client who has a chest tube and drainage system in place. Which of the following are expected findings? (Select all that apply.)

_____ A. Continuous bubbling in the water seal chamber

_____ B. Gentle constant bubbling in the suction control chamber

_____ C. Rise and fall in the level of water in the water seal chamber with inspiration and expiration

_____ D. Exposed sutures without dressing

_____ E. Drainage system upright at chest level

4. A nurse is assisting a provider with the removal of a chest tube. Which of the following should the nurse instruct the client to do?

A. Lie on his left side.

B. Use the incentive spirometer.

C. Cough at regular intervals.

D. Perform the Valsalva maneuver. *bare down*

5. A nurse is planning care for a client following the insertion of a chest tube and drainage system. Which of the following should be included in the plan of care? (Select all that apply.)

_____ A. Encourage the client to cough every 2 hr.

_____ B. Check for continuous bubbling in the suction chamber.

_____ C. Strip the drainage tubing every 4 hr.

_____ D. Clamp the tube once a day.

_____ E. Obtain a chest x-ray.

6. A nurse is caring for a client who is scheduled for a chest tube placement. Use the ATI Active Learning Template: Therapeutic Procedure to complete this item. Include three preprocedure nursing actions.

APPLICATION EXERCISES KEY

1. A. **CORRECT:** Oxygen should be readily available in case the client develops respiratory distress following chest tube placement. The nurse should monitor the client's respiration, oxygen saturation, and lung sounds.

    B. **CORRECT:** If the chest tubing becomes disconnected, the end of the tubing should be placed in sterile water to restore the water seal.

    C. **CORRECT:** Hemostat clamps should be available for the nurse to use to check for air leaks.

    D. INCORRECT: An indwelling urinary catheter is not indicated for a client who has a chest tube.

    E. **CORRECT:** If the chest tubing becomes disconnected, the nurse should immediately place an occlusive dressing over the chest tube insertion site. This allows air to escape and reduces the risk for development of a tension pneumothorax.

     NCLEX® Connection: Reduction of Risk Potential, Therapeutic Procedures

2. A. INCORRECT: Placing the tubing in sterile water to restore the water seal is an appropriate action, but it is not the first action.

    B. **CORRECT:** Using the airway, breathing, and circulation (ABC) priority-setting framework, the application of a sterile gauze to the site should be the first action for the nurse to take. This allows air to escape and reduces the risk for development of a tension pneumothorax.

    C. INCORRECT: Placing tape around the insertion site ensures that the sterile gauze remains intact and is an appropriate action, but it is not the first action.

    D. INCORRECT: Assessing the client's respiratory status is an appropriate action, but it is not the first action.

     NCLEX® Connection: Reduction of Risk Potential, Potential for Complications of Diagnostic Tests/ Treatments/Procedures

3. A. INCORRECT: Continuous bubbling in the water seal chamber indicates an air leak.

    B. **CORRECT:** Gentle bubbling in the suction control chamber is an expected finding as air is being removed.

    C. **CORRECT:** A rise and fall of the fluid level in the water seal chamber upon inspiration and expiration indicates that the drainage system is functioning properly.

    D. INCORRECT: The nurse should cover the sutures at the insertion site with an airtight dressing.

    E. INCORRECT: The drainage system should be maintained in an upright position below the level of the client's chest.

     NCLEX® Connection: Reduction of Risk Potential, Potential for Complications of Diagnostic Tests/ Treatments/Procedures

4.   A. INCORRECT: Incorrect: The position the client should assume during removal of a chest tube will depend upon the location of the insertion site.

     B. INCORRECT: The use of an incentive spirometer is not indicated during chest tube removal.

     C. INCORRECT: The client is instructed to breathe normally and remain calm during the procedure.

     D. **CORRECT:** The client should be instructed to take a deep breath, exhale, and bear down (Valsalva maneuver) as the chest tube is being removed. This increases intrathoracic pressure and reduces the risk of an air embolism.

      NCLEX® Connection: Reduction of Risk Potential, Potential for Complications of Diagnostic Tests/Treatments/Procedures

5.   A. **CORRECT:** The nurse should instruct the client to cough every 2 hr. This promotes oxygenation and lung reexpansion.

     B. **CORRECT:** The nurse should check for continuous bubbling in the suction chamber to verify that suction is being maintained at an appropriate level.

     C. INCORRECT: The nurse should not milk or strip the drainage tubing to check for kinks. This action is only to be done when prescribed by the provider. Stripping creates negative high pressure and can damage the client's lung tissue.

     D. INCORRECT: The nurse should not clamp the tubing unless indicated by the provider. This is done to verify for the presence of an air leak or if the tubing accidentally has been disconnected. Clamping may cause a tension pneumothorax.

     E. **CORRECT:** A chest x-ray is obtained following the procedure to verify chest tube placement.

      NCLEX® Connection: Reduction of Risk Potential, Therapeutic Procedures

6.   *Using the ATI Active Learning Template: Therapeutic Procedure*
     - Preprocedure nursing actions
       - Verify that the consent form is signed.
       - Reinforce client teaching. Breathing will improve when the chest tube is in place.
       - Assess for allergies to local anesthetics.
       - Assist the client into the desired position (supine or semi-Fowler's).
       - Prepare the chest drainage system per the facility's protocol (fill the water seal chamber).
       - Administer pain and sedation medications as prescribed.
       - Prep the insertion site with povidone-iodine.

      NCLEX® Connection: Reduction of Risk Potential, Therapeutic Procedures

CHAPTER 19   Respiratory Management and Mechanical Ventilation

Overview

- Oxygen is a tasteless and colorless gas that accounts for 21% of atmospheric air.

- Oxygen is used to maintain adequate cellular oxygenation. It is used in the treatment of many acute and chronic respiratory problems.

- Oxygen is administered in an attempt to maintain an SaO_2 of at least 95% to 100% by using the lowest amount of oxygen without putting the client at risk for complications.

- Clients who cannot spontaneously breathe on their own require mechanical ventilation. This can include clients who need respiratory assistance due to severe respiratory disease, general anesthesia, trauma or other illnesses.

Oxygen Delivery Devices

- Supplemental oxygen can be delivered by a variety of methods based on the client's particular circumstances. The percentage of oxygen delivered to the client is expressed as the fraction of inspired oxygen (FiO_2).

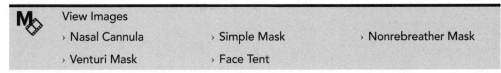

View Images		
› Nasal Cannula	› Simple Mask	› Nonrebreather Mask
› Venturi Mask	› Face Tent	

- Low-flow oxygen delivery systems deliver varying amounts of oxygen based on the method and the client's breathing pattern.

  ○ Nasal cannula – A length of tubing with two small prongs for insertion into the nares

    ▪ FiO_2 – 24 to 44% at flow rates of 1 to 6 L/min

    ▪ Advantages

      □ Safe, easy to apply, comfortable, and well tolerated.

      □ The client is able to eat, talk, and ambulate.

    ▪ Disadvantages

      □ The FiO_2 varies with the flow rate and the client's rate and depth of breathing.

      □ Extended use can lead to skin breakdown and drying of the mucous membranes.

      □ Tubing is easily dislodged.

- Nursing Actions
  - Assess the patency of the nares.
  - Ensure that the prongs fit in the nares properly. *prongs facing down*
  - Use water-soluble gel to prevent dry nares.
  - Provide humidification for flow rates of 4 L/min and above.
- Simple face mask (covers the client's nose and mouth)
  - FiO_2 – 40% to 60% at flow rates of 1 to 6 L/min (the minimum flow rate is 5 L/min to ensure flushing of CO_2 from the mask).
  - Advantages
    - A face mask is easy to apply and may be more comfortable than a nasal cannula.
  - Disadvantages
    - Flow rates of 5 L/min or lower can result in rebreathing of CO_2.
    - Device is poorly tolerated by clients who have anxiety or claustrophobia.
    - Eating, drinking, and talking are impaired.
    - Use caution with clients who have a high risk of aspiration or airway obstruction.
  - Nursing Actions
    - Assess proper fit to ensure a secure seal over the nose and mouth.
    - Ensure that the client wears a nasal cannula during meals.
- Partial rebreather mask (covers the client's nose and mouth)
  - FiO_2 – 60% to 75% at flow rates of 6 to 11 L/min
  - Advantages
    - The mask has a reservoir bag attached with no valve, which allows the client to rebreathe up to one third of exhaled air together with room air.
  - Disadvantages
    - Complete deflation of the reservoir bag during inspiration causes CO_2 buildup.
    - The FiO_2 varies with the client's breathing pattern.
    - Mask is poorly tolerated by clients who have anxiety or claustrophobia.
    - Eating, drinking, and talking are impaired.
    - Use with caution for clients who have a high risk of aspiration or airway obstruction.
  - Nursing Actions
    - Keep the reservoir bag from deflating by adjusting the oxygen flow rate to keep it inflated.
    - Assess proper fit to ensure a secure seal over the nose and mouth.
    - Ensure that the client uses a nasal cannula during meals.

- ○ Nonrebreather mask (covers the client's nose and mouth)
  - ▪ FiO_2 – 80% to 95% at flow rates of 10 to 15 L/min to keep the reservoir bag two-thirds full during inspiration and expiration.
  - ▪ Advantages
    - □ Delivers the highest O_2 concentration possible (except for intubation).
    - □ A one-way valve situated between the mask and reservoir allows the client to inhale maximum O_2 from the reservoir bag. The two exhalation ports have flaps covering them that prevent room air from entering the mask.
  - ▪ Disadvantages
    - □ The valve and flap on the mask must be intact and functional during each breath.
    - □ Poorly tolerated by clients who have anxiety or claustrophobia.
    - □ Eating, drinking, and talking are impaired.
    - □ Use with caution for clients who have a high risk of aspiration or airway obstruction.
  - ▪ Nursing Actions
    - □ Perform an hourly assessment of the valve and flap.
    - □ Assess proper fit to ensure a secure seal over the nose and mouth.
    - □ Ensure that the client uses a nasal cannula during meals.
- • High-flow oxygen delivery systems deliver precise amounts of oxygen when properly fitted.
  - ○ Venturi mask (covers the client's nose and mouth)
    - ▪ FiO_2 – 24% to 55% at flow rates of 2 to 10 L/min via different sizes of adaptors
    - ▪ Advantages
      - □ Delivers the most precise oxygen concentration.
      - □ Humidification is not required.
      - □ Best suited for clients who have chronic lung disease.
    - ▪ Disadvantages
      - □ The use of a Venturi mask is expensive.
    - ▪ Nursing Actions
      - □ Assess frequently to ensure an accurate flow rate.
      - □ Make sure the tubing is free of kinks.
  - ○ Aerosol mask, face tent (fits loosely around the face and neck), and tracheostomy collar (a small mask that covers a surgically created opening in the trachea)
    - ▪ FiO_2 – 24% to 100% at flow rates of at least 10 L/min (provide high humidification with oxygen delivery)
    - ▪ Advantages
      - □ Good for clients who do not tolerate masks well.
      - □ Useful for clients who have facial trauma, burns, and/or thick secretions.

- Disadvantages
  - High humidification requires frequent monitoring.
- Nursing Actions
  - Empty condensation from the tubing often.
  - Ensure that there is adequate water in the humidification canister.
  - Ensure that the aerosol mist leaves from the vents during inspiration and expiration.
  - Make sure the tubing does not pull on the tracheostomy.
- T-piece
  - FiO$_2$ – 24% to 100% at flow rates of at least 10 L/min
  - Advantages
    - This device can be used for clients who have tracheostomies, laryngectomies, or endotracheal tubes (ET).
  - Disadvantages
    - High humidification requires frequent monitoring.
  - Nursing Actions
    - Ensure that the exhalation port is open and uncovered.
    - Make sure that the T-piece does not pull on the tracheostomy or ET tube.
    - Ensure that the mist is evident during inspiration and expiration.

Oxygen Therapy

- Indications
  - Diagnoses
    - Hypoxemia and hypoxia
      - Hypoxemia is an inadequate level of oxygen in the blood. Hypovolemia, hypoventilation, and interruption of arterial flow can lead to hypoxemia.
  - Client Presentation

EARLY FINDINGS	LATE FINDINGS
› Tachypnea	› Confusion and stupor
› Tachycardia	› Cyanotic skin and mucous membranes
› Restlessness	› Bradypnea
› Pale skin and mucous membranes	› Bradycardia
› Elevated blood pressure	› Hypotension
› Symptoms of respiratory distress (use of accessory muscles, nasal flaring, tracheal tugging, and adventitious lung sounds)	› Cardiac dysrhythmias

- Nursing Actions
  - Preparation of the client
    - Explain all procedures to the client.
    - Place the client in semi-Fowler's or Fowler's position to facilitate breathing and promote chest expansion.
    - Ensure that all equipment is working properly.
  - Ongoing care
    - Provide oxygen therapy at the lowest flow that will correct hypoxemia.
    - Assess/monitor respiratory rate, rhythm and effort, and lung sounds to determine the client's need for supplemental oxygen
      - Signs and symptoms of hypoxemia are shortness of breath, anxiety, tachypnea, tachycardia, restlessness, pallor, or cyanosis of the skin and/or mucous membranes, adventitious breath sounds, and confusion.
      - Signs and symptoms of hypercarbia (elevated levels of CO_2) are restlessness, hypertension, and headache.
    - Assess/monitor oxygenation status with pulse oximetry and ABGs.
    - Apply the oxygen delivery device as prescribed. Assess the fit of the mask to ensure a secure seal over the client's nose and mouth.
    - Promote good oral hygiene, and provide as needed.
    - Promote turning, coughing, deep breathing, use of incentive spirometer, and suctioning.
    - Promote rest, and decrease environmental stimuli.

    - Provide emotional support for clients who appear anxious.
    - Assess nutritional status; provide supplements as prescribed.
    - Assess/monitor the client's skin integrity; provide moisture and pressure-relief devices as indicated.
    - Assess/monitor and document the client's response to oxygen therapy.
    - Titrate oxygen to maintain prescribed oxygen saturation.
    - Discontinue supplemental oxygen gradually.
  - Interventions
    - Monitor for signs and symptoms of respiratory depression such as decreased respiratory rate and decreased level of consciousness; notify the provider if these findings are present.
    - Respiratory Distress
      - Position the client for maximum ventilation (Fowler's or semi-Fowler's position).
      - Complete a focused respiratory assessment.
      - Promote deep breathing, and use supplemental oxygen as prescribed.
      - Stay with the client, and provide emotional support to decrease anxiety.
      - Promote airway clearance by encouraging coughing and oral/oropharyngeal suctioning if necessary.

- Complications
  - Oxygen toxicity
    - Oxygen toxicity can result from high concentrations of oxygen (typically above 50%), long durations of oxygen therapy (typically more than 24 to 48 hr), and the client's degree of lung disease.
    - Signs and symptoms include a nonproductive cough, substernal pain, nasal stuffiness, nausea, vomiting, fatigue, headache, sore throat, and hypoventilation.
    - Nursing Actions
      - Use the lowest level of oxygen necessary to maintain an adequate SaO_2.
      - Monitor the ABGs, and notify the provider if SaO_2 levels are outside of the expected reference range.
      - Use an oxygen mask with continuous positive airway pressure (CPAP), bilevel positive airway pressure (BiPAP), or positive end expiratory pressure (PEEP) as prescribed while the client is on a mechanical ventilator to help decrease the amount of needed oxygen.
  - Oxygen-induced hypoventilation
    - Oxygen-induced hypoventilation can develop in clients who have COPD and chronic hypoxemia and hypercarbia. Clients who have COPD rely on low levels of arterial oxygen as their primary drive for breathing. Providing supplemental oxygen at high levels can decrease or eliminate their respiratory drive.
    - Nursing Actions
      - Monitor the client's respiratory rate and pattern, level of consciousness, and SaO_2.
      - Provide oxygen therapy at the lowest flow that corrects hypoxemia.
      - If the client tolerates it, use a Venturi mask to deliver precise oxygen levels.
      - Notify the provider of impending respiratory depression, such as a decreased respiratory rate and a decreased level of consciousness.
  - Combustion
    - Oxygen is combustible.
    - Nursing Actions
      - Post "No Smoking" or "Oxygen in Use" signs to alert others of a fire hazard.
      - Know where the closest fire extinguisher is located.
      - Educate the client and others about the fire hazard of smoking during oxygen use.
      - Have the client wear a cotton gown because synthetic or wool fabrics can generate static electricity.
      - Ensure that all electric devices (razors, hearing aids, radios) are working well.
      - Ensure electric machinery (monitors, suction machines) are well-grounded.
      - Do not use volatile, flammable materials (alcohol or acetone) near clients who are receiving oxygen.

Endotracheal (ET) Tube and Endotracheal Intubation

- Indications
  - A tube is inserted through the client's nose or mouth into the trachea. This allows for emergency airway management of the client.
  - Mouth intubation is the easiest and quickest form of intubation and is often performed in the emergency department.
  - Nasal intubation is performed when the client has facial or oral trauma.
    - This route is not used if the client has a clotting problem.
- Placement:
  - Intubation is typically performed by a nurse anesthetist, anesthesiologist, or pulmonologist.
  - A chest x-ray verifies correct placement of the ET tube.
  - ET tubes may be cuffed or uncuffed. The cuff on the tracheal end of an ET tube is inflated to ensure proper placement and the formation of a seal between the cuff and the tracheal wall. This prevents air from leaking around the ET tube.
  - The seal ensures that an adequate amount of tidal volume is delivered by the mechanical ventilator when attached to the external end of the ET tube.
- The client is unable to talk when the cuff is inflated.
- Nursing Actions
  - Have resuscitation equipment to include a manual resuscitation bag with a face mask at the bedside at all times.
  - Monitor the client's vital signs and check tube placement.

Mechanical Ventilation

- Mechanical ventilation provides breathing support until lung function is restored, delivering warm (body temperature 37° C [98.6° F]), 100% humidified oxygen at FiO2 levels between 21% to 100%.

 View Video: Mechanical Ventilation

  - Positive-pressure ventilators deliver air to the lungs under pressure throughout inspiration and/or expiration to keep the alveoli open during inspiration and to prevent alveolar collapse during expiration. The benefits include the following:
    - Forced/enhanced lung expansion
    - Improved gas exchange (oxygenation)
    - Decreased work of breathing
  - Mechanical ventilation can be delivered via:
    - An ET tube
    - A tracheostomy tube
    - A nasal or face mask (non-invasive modes such as CPAP, BiPAP)

○ Mechanical ventilators can be cycled based on pressure, volume, time, and/or flow.

COMMON MODES OF VENTILATION

Assist-control (AC)	› Preset rate and tidal volume. Client initiates breath and ventilator takes over. › Hyperventilation can result in respiratory alkalosis. › Client may require sedation to decrease respiratory rate.
Synchronized intermittent mandatory ventilation (SIMV)	› Preset rate and tidal volume. › Client initiates breath and tidal volume will depend upon client's effort. › Ventilator initiated breaths are synchronized to reduce competition between ventilator and client. › Used as a regular mode of ventilation or a weaning mode (rate decreased to allow more spontaneous ventilation). › Can increase work of breathing, causing respiratory muscle fatigue.
Pressure support ventilation (PSV)	› Often used with IMV mode. › Augments spontaneous breathing by adding pressure as inspiration occurs. › Lessens endotracheal tube resistance and reduces work of breathing. › Amount of pressure support is reduced as weaning progresses. › Too much pressure support can result in tachypnea.
Positive end expiratory pressure (PEEP)	› Works to keep the alveoli from collapsing during expiration. › Allows for greater oxygenation and makes the work of breathing easier. › Allows for lower levels of FiO_2 to be used. › Can be used with IMV or AC modes to treat or prevent atelectasis. › Settings 5 to 20 cm H_2O (greater than 20 cm H_2O can cause lung damage).
Volume assured pressure support ventilation (VAPSV)	› Similar to PSV with minimal set tidal volume per breath. › Optimizes inspiratory flow, reduces work of breathing, decreases volutrauma and ensures minimal minute ventilation. › Used for clients with severe respiratory disease or those who have difficulty wearning.
Independent lung ventilation (ILV)	› Double lumen ET tube allows ventilation of each lung separately. › Used for clients who have unilateral lung disease. › Requires two ventilators, sedation and/or use of neuromuscular blocking agents.
High-frequency ventilation	› Delivers small amount of gas at rates of 60 to 3,000 cycles/min. › High frequency ventilation often used in children. › Client must be sedated and/or receiving neuromuscular blocking agents. › Breath sounds difficult to assess.
Inverse ratio ventilation (IRV)	› Lengthens inspiratory phase to maximize oxygenation. › Used for hypoxemia refractory to PEEP. › Uncomfortable for clients and requires sedation and/or neuromuscular blocking agents. › High risk of volutrauma and decreased cardiac output due to air trapping.

COMMON MODES OF VENTILATION	
Continuous positive airway pressure (CPAP)	› Positive pressure supplied during spontaneous breathing. No ventilator breaths delivered unless in conjunction with SIMV. › Risks include volutrauma, decreased cardiac output and ICP. › Can be invasive or noninvasive. › Often used for obstructive sleep apnea.
Bilevel positive airway pressure (BiPAP)	› Positive pressure delivered during spontaneous breaths. › Different pressures delivered for inspiration and expiration. › No spontaneous breaths delivered. › Often used to wean client from ventilator. › Used with a nasal or face mask and is noninvasive.

- Indications are to maintain a patent airway and adequate oxygen saturation of 95% or greater.
  - Diagnoses
    - Hypoxemia, hypoventilation with respiratory acidosis
      - Airway trauma
      - Exacerbation of COPD
      - Acute pulmonary edema due to myocardial infarction or heart failure
      - Asthma attack
      - Head injuries, cerebrovascular accident, or coma
      - Neurological disorders (multiple sclerosis, myasthenia gravis, Guillain-Barré)
      - Obstructive sleep apnea
    - Respiratory support following surgery (decrease workload)
    - Respiratory support while under general anesthesia or heavy sedation
- Nursing Actions
  - Preparation of the Client
    - Explain the procedure to the client.
    - Establish a method for client to communicate, such as asking yes/no questions, providing writing materials, using a dry-erase board and/or a picture communication board, or lip reading.
  - Ongoing Care
    - Maintain a patent airway.
      - Assess the position and placement of tube.
      - Document tube placement in centimeters at the client's teeth or lips.
      - Use two staff members for repositioning and resecuring the tube.
      - Apply protective barriers (soft wrist restraints) according to hospital protocol to prevent self-extubation.
      - Use caution when moving the client.

- Suction oral and tracheal secretions to maintain tube patency.

- Support ventilator tubing to prevent mucosal erosion and displacement.

- Have a resuscitation bag with a face mask available at the bedside at all times in case of ventilator malfunction or accidental extubation.

■ Assess respiratory status every 1 to 2 hr: breath sounds equal bilaterally, presence of reduced or absent breath sounds, respiratory effort, or spontaneous breaths.

■ Suction the client's tracheal tube to clear secretions from the airway.

■ Monitor and document ventilator settings hourly.

- Rate, FiO_2, and tidal volume

- Mode of ventilation

- Use of adjuncts (PEEP, CPAP)

- Plateau or peak inspiratory pressure (PIP)

- Alarm settings

■ Monitor the ventilator alarms, which signal if the client is not receiving the correct ventilation.

- Never turn off the ventilator alarms.

- There are three types of ventilator alarms: volume, pressure, and apnea alarms.

  ▸ Volume (low pressure) alarms indicate a low exhaled volume due to a disconnection, cuff leak, and/or tube displacement.

  ▸ Pressure (high pressure) alarms indicate excess secretions, client biting the tubing, kinks in the tubing, client coughing, pulmonary edema, bronchospasm, and/or pneumothorax.

  ▸ Apnea alarms indicate that the ventilator does not detect spontaneous respiration in a preset time period.

■ Maintain adequate (but not excessive) volume in the cuff of the endotracheal tube.

- Assess the cuff pressure at least every 8 hr. Maintain the cuff pressure below 20 mm Hg to reduce the risk of tracheal necrosis.

- Assess for an air leak around the cuff (client speaking, air hissing, or decreasing SaO_2). Inadequate cuff pressure can result in inadequate oxygenation and/or accidental extubation.

■ Administer medications as prescribed.

- Analgesics – morphine and fentanyl (Sublimaze)

- Sedatives – propofol (Diprivan), diazepam (Valium), lorazepam (Ativan), midazolam (Versed), and haloperidol (Haldol)

  ▸ Clients receiving mechanical ventilation may require sedation or paralytic agents to prevent competition between extrinsic and intrinsic breathing and the resulting effects of hyperventilation.

- Neuromuscular blocking agents – pancuronium bromide (Pavulon), atracurium (Tracrium), and vecuronium (Norcuron)

  ▸ Neuromuscular blocking agents paralyze muscles, but do not sedate or relieve pain. The use of a sedative or analgesic agent in conjunction with a neuromuscular blocking agent is typically prescribed by the provider.

- □ Ulcer-preventing agents – famotidine (Pepcid) or lansoprazole (Prevacid)
- □ Antibiotics for established infections
- Reposition the oral endotracheal tube every 24 hr or according to protocol. Assess for skin breakdown.
  - □ Older adult clients have fragile skin and are more prone to skin and mucous membrane breakdown. Older adult clients have decreased oral secretions. They require frequent, gentle skin and oral care.
- Provide adequate nutrition.
  - □ Assess gastrointestinal functioning every 8 hr.
  - □ Monitor bowel habits.
  - □ Administer enteral or parenteral feedings as prescribed.
- Continually monitor the client during the weaning process and watch for signs of weaning intolerance.
  - □ Respiratory rate greater than 30/min or less than 8/min
  - □ Blood pressure or heart rate changes more than 20% of baseline
  - □ SaO_2 less than 90%
  - □ Dysrhythmias, elevated ST segment
  - □ Significant decrease in tidal volume
  - □ Labored respirations, increased use of accessory muscles, and diaphoresis
  - □ Restlessness, anxiety, and decreased level of consciousness
- Have a manual resuscitation bag with a face mask and oxygen readily available at the client's bedside.
- Have reintubation equipment at bedside.
- Suction the client's oropharynx and trachea.
- Deflate the cuff on the endotrachial tube and remove the tube during peak inspiration.
- Following extubation, monitor the client for signs of respiratory distress or airway obstruction, such as ineffective cough, dyspnea, and stridor.
- Monitor client's SpO_2 and vital signs every 5 min.
- Encourage coughing, deep breathing, and use of the incentive spirometer.
- Reposition the client to promote mobility of secretions.
- Older adult clients have decreased respiratory muscle strength and chest wall compliance, which makes them more susceptible to aspiration, atelectasis, and pulmonary infections. The older adult client will require more frequent position changes to promote mobility of secretions.

- Complications
  - Trauma
    - Barotramua (damage to the lungs by positive pressure)
      - Can occur due to a pneumothorax, subcutaneous emphysema or pneumomediastinum.
    - Volutrauma (damage to the lungs by volume delivered from one lung to the other)
  - Fluid retention
    - Fluid retention in clients who are receiving mechanical ventilation is due to decreased cardiac output, activation of renin-angiotensin-aldosterone system, and/or ventilator humidification.
    - Nursing Actions
      - Monitor the client's intake and output, weight, breath sounds, and endotracheal secretions.
  - Oxygen toxicity
    - Oxygen toxicity can result from high concentrations of oxygen (typically above 50%), long durations of oxygen therapy (typically more than 24 to 48 hr), and/or the client's degree of lung disease.
    - Nursing Actions
      - Monitor for fatigue, restlessness, severe dyspnea, tachycardia, tachypnea, crackles, and cyanosis.
  - Hemodynamic compromise
    - Mechanical ventilation has a risk of increased thoracic pressure (positive pressure), which can result in decreased venous return.
    - Nursing Actions
      - Monitor for tachycardia, hypotension, urine output less than or equal to 30 mL/hr, cool, clammy extremities, decreased peripheral pulses, and a decreased level of consciousness.
  - Aspiration
    - Keep the head of the bed elevated 30° at all times to decrease the risk of aspiration.
    - Nursing Actions
      - Check residuals every 4 hr if the client is receiving enteral feedings to decrease the risk of aspiration.
  - Gastrointestinal ulceration (stress ulcer)
    - Gastric ulcers can be evident in clients receiving mechanical ventilation.
    - Nursing Actions
      - Monitor gastrointestinal drainage and stools for occult blood.
      - Administer ulcer prevention medications (sucralfate and histamine$_2$ blockers) as prescribed.

APPLICATION EXERCISES

1. A nurse is orienting a newly licensed nurse who is caring for a client that is receiving mechanical ventilation, which has been placed on pressure support ventilation (PSV) mode. Which of the following statements by the newly licensed nurse demonstates an understanding of PSV?

    A. "It keeps the alveoli open and prevents atelectasis."

    B. "It permits spontaneous ventilation to decrease the work of breathing."

    C. "It is used with clients who have difficulty weaning from the ventilator."

    D. "It delivers a preset ventilatory rate and tidal volume to the client."

2. A nurse is caring for a client who is experiencing respiratory distress. Which of the following are early clinical manifestations of hypoxemia? (Select all that apply.)

    _____ A. Confusion

    _____ B. Pale skin

    _____ C. Bradycardia

    _____ D. Hypotension

    _____ E. Elevated blood pressure

3. A nurse is orienting a newly licensed nurse on performing routine assessment of a client who is receiving mechanical ventilation via an endotracheal tube. Which of the following should the nurse include in the teaching?

    A. Apply a vest restraint if self-extubation is attempted.

    B. Monitor ventilator settings every 8 hr.

    C. Document tube placement in centimeters at the angle of jaw.

    D. Assess breath sounds every 1 to 2 hr.

4. A nurse is caring for a client who has dyspnea and is to receive oxygen continuously. Which of the following oxygen devices should the nurse use to deliver a precise amount of oxygen to the client?

    A. Nonrebreather mask

    B. Venturi mask

    C. Nasal cannula

    D. Simple face mask

5. A nurse is planning care for a client who is receiving mechanical ventilation. Which mode of ventilation increases the effort of the client's respiratory muscles? (Select all that apply.)

_____ A. Assist-control

_____ B. Synchronized intermittent mandatory ventilation

_____ C. Continous positive aiway pressure

_____ D. Pressure support ventilation

_____ E. Independent lung ventilation

6. A nurse is planning care for a client who is receiving mechanical ventilation. What nursing actions should be included to maintain the client's airway? Use the ATI Active Learning Template: Therapeutic Procedure to describe three nursing actions to maintain the client's airway.

APPLICATION EXERCISES KEY

1. A. INCORRECT: PSV does not maintain pressure in the lungs to keep alveoli open or prevent atelectasis.

   B. **CORRECT:** PSV maintains a preset amount of pressure during spontaneous ventilation to decrease the work of breathing.

   C. INCORRECT: Volume assured pressure support ventilation (VAPSV) mode is used with clients who have difficulty weaning from the ventilator

   D. INCORRECT: Assist-control (AC) mode delivers a preset ventilatory rate and tidal volume to the client.

   Ⓝ NCLEX® Connection: Physiological Adaptations, Alterations in Body Systems

2. A. INCORRECT: Confusion is a late clinical manifestation of hypoxemia.

   B. **CORRECT:** Pale skin is an early clinical manifestation of hypoxemia.

   C. INCORRECT: Bradycardia is a late clinical manifestation of hypoxemia.

   D. INCORRECT: Hypotension is a late clinical manifestation of hypoxemia.

   E. **CORRECT:** Elevated blood pressure is an early clinical manifestation of hypoxemia.

   Ⓝ NCLEX® Connection: Physiological Adaptations, Illness Management

3. A. INCORRECT: Soft wrist restraints should be applied to prevent self-extubation.

   B. INCORRECT: Ventilator settings should be monitored hourly.

   C. INCORRECT: The nurse documents tube placement in centimeters at the client's teeth or lips.

   D. **CORRECT:** The nurse should assess the breath sounds of a client on mechanical ventilation every 1 to 2 hr.

   Ⓝ NCLEX® Connection: Physiological Adaptations, Alterations in Body Systems

4.   A. INCORRECT: A nonrebreather mask delivers an approximated amount of oxygen to the client.

   B. **CORRECT:** A venturi mask incorporates an adapter that allows a precise amount of oxygen to be delivered to the client.

   C. INCORRECT: A nasal cannula delivers an approximated amount of oxygen to the client.

   D. INCORRECT: A simple face mask delivers an approximated amount of oxygen to the client.

   Ⓝ NCLEX® Connection: Physiological Adaptations, Illness Management

5.   A. INCORRECT: Assist-control mode takes over the work of the client's breathing.

   B. **CORRECT:** Sychronized intermittent mandatory ventilation requires that the client generate force to take spontaneous breaths.

   C. **CORRECT:** Continous positive airway pressure requires that the client generate force to take spontaneous breaths.

   D. **CORRECT:** Pressure support ventilation requires that the client generate force to take spontaneous breaths.

   E. INCORRECT: Independent lung ventilation mode is used for unilateral lung disease to ventilate the lung individually.

   Ⓝ NCLEX® Connection: Physiological Adaptations, Alterations in Body Systems

6.   *Using ATI Active Learning Template: Therapeutic Procedure*
   - Nursing Actions
     - Maintain a patent airway.
     - Assess the position and placement of tube.
     - Document the tube placement in centimeters at the client's teeth or lips.
     - Use two staff members for repositioning and resecuring the tube.
     - Apply protective barriers (soft wrist restraints) according to hospital protocol to prevent self-extubation.
     - Use caution when moving the client.
     - Suction oral and tracheal secretions to maintain tube patency.
     - Support ventilator tubing to prevent mucosal erosion and displacement.
     - Have a resuscitation bag with a face mask available at the bedside at all times in case of ventilator malfunction or accidental extubation.

   Ⓝ NCLEX® Connection: Physiological Adaptations, Alterations in Body Systems

chapter 20

Overview

- The airway structures permit air to enter and provide for adequate oxygenation and tissue perfusion.

- Common acute and chronic disorders affect these airway structures.

- A nursing priority for clients who have acute respiratory disorders is to maintain a patent airway to promote oxygenation.

- Acute respiratory disorders include rhinitis, sinusitis, influenza, and pneumonia.

- Pneumonia is an inflammatory process in the lungs that produces excess fluid. Pneumonia is triggered by infectious organisms or by the aspiration of an irritant, such as fluid or a foreign object.

- The inflammatory process in the lung parenchyma results in edema and exudate that fills the alveoli.

Ⓖ - Pneumonia can be a primary disease or a complication of another disease or condition. It affects people of all ages, but the young, older adult clients, and clients who are immunocompromised are more susceptible. Immobility is a contributing factor in the development of pneumonia.

- There are two types of pneumonia. Community-acquired pneumonia (CAP) is the most common type and often occurs as a complication of influenza. Health care-associated pneumonia (HAP) has a higher mortality rate and is more likely to be resistant to antibiotics. It usually takes 24 to 48 hr from the time the client is exposed to acquire HAP.

Ⓖ - Older adult clients are more susceptible to infections and have decreased pulmonary reserves due to normal lung changes, including decreased lung elasticity and thickening alveoli.

Health Promotion and Disease Prevention

- Perform hand hygiene to prevent the spread of infection by bacteria and viruses.

Ⓖ - Encourage immunizations that prevent respiratory disorders, especially immunizations for influenza and pneumonia to younger children and older adults, and those who have chronic illnesses or who are immunocompromised.

- Limit exposure to airborne allergens, which trigger a hypersensitivity reaction.

- Promote smoking cessation.

- Review risk factors for these disorders.

Ⓖ   ○ Extremely young and advanced age

   ○ Recent exposure to viral, bacterial, or influenza infections

   ○ Lack of current immunization status (pneumonia, influenza)

   ○ Exposure to plant pollen, molds, animal dander, foods, medications, and environmental contaminants

- ○ Tobacco smoke

- ○ Substance use (alcohol, cocaine)

- ○ Chronic lung disease (asthma, emphysema)

- ○ Immunocompromised status

- ○ Presence of a foreign body

- ○ Conditions that increase the risk of aspiration (dysphagia)

- ○ Impaired ability to mobilize secretions (decreased level of consciousness, immobility, recent abdominal or thoracic surgery)

- ○ Inactivity and immobility

- ○ Mechanical ventilation (ventilator-acquired pneumonia)

RHINITIS

Overview

- Rhinitis is an inflammation of the nasal mucosa and often the mucosa in the sinuses that can be caused by infection (viral or bacterial) or allergens.

- The common cold (coryza) is caused by viruses spread from person to person in droplets from sneezing and coughing, or by direct contact.

- This disorder often coexists with other disorders, such as asthma and allergies, and may be acute or chronic, nonallergic or allergic (seasonal or perennial).

- The presence of an allergen causes histamine release and other mediators from WBCs in the nasal mucosa. The mediators bind to blood vessel receptors causing capillary leakage, which leads to local edema and swelling.

Assessment

- Subjective Data

  - ○ Excessive nasal drainage, runny nose (rhinorrhea) and nasal congestion

  - ○ Purulent nasal discharge

  - ○ Sneezing and pruritus of the nose, throat and ears

  - ○ Itchy, watery eyes

  - ○ Sore, dry throat

- Objective Data

  - ○ Red, inflamed, swollen nasal mucosa

  - ○ Low-grade fever

- Diagnostic testing may include allergy tests to identify possible allergens.

Patient-Centered Care

- Nursing Care

  - Encourage rest (8 to 10 hr/day) and increased fluid intake (at least 2,000 mL/day).

  - Encourage the use of a home humidifier or breathing steamy air after running hot shower water.

  - Promote proper disposal of tissues and use of cough etiquette (sneeze or cough into tissue, elbow or shoulder and not the hands).

- Medications

  - Antihistamines, such as brompheniramine/pseudoephedrine (Dimetapp); leukotriene inhibitors, such as montelukast (Singulair); and mast cell stabilizers, such as cromolyn (Nasalcrom), are used to block the release of chemicals from WBCs that bind with receptors in nasal tissues, which prevent edema and itching.

    - Nursing Considerations

      - Older adults should be aware of adverse effects such as vertigo, hypertension, and urinary retention.

  - Decongestants, such as phenylephrine (Neo-Synephrine), constrict blood vessels and decrease edema.

    - Nursing Considerations

      - Encourage clients to use as prescribed for 3 to 4 days to avoid rebound nasal congestion.

  - Intranasal glucocorticoid sprays (Flonase) are the most effective for prevention and treatment of seasonal and perennial rhinitis.

  - Antipyretics are used if fever is present.

  - Antibiotics are given if a bacterial infection can be identified.

- Client Education

  - Hand hygiene is reviewed as a measure to prevent transmission.

  - Complementary therapies such as echinacea, large doses of vitamin C, and zinc preparations (lozenges and nasal sprays) may be useful in promoting improved immune response.

  - Limiting exposure to others will prevent and reduce transmission. This is especially important for vulnerable populations such as the very young, older adults and people who are immunosuppressed.

SINUSITIS

Overview

- Sinusitis is an inflammation of the mucous membranes of one or more of the sinuses, usually the maxillary or frontal sinus. Swelling of the mucosa can block the drainage of secretions, which may cause a sinus infection.

- Sinusitis often occurs after rhinitis and may be associated with a deviated nasal septum, nasal polyps, inhaled air pollutants or cocaine, facial trauma, dental infections, or loss of immune function.

- The infection is commonly caused by *Streptococcus pneumoniae*, *Haemophilus influenzae*, diplococcus and bacteroides.

Assessment

- Subjective Data
  - Nasal congestion
  - Headache
  - Facial pressure or pain (worse when head is tilted forward)
  - Cough
  - Bloody or purulent nasal drainage
- Objective Data
  - Tenderness to palpation of forehead, orbital and facial areas
  - Low-grade fever
  - Diagnostic Procedures
    - CT scan or sinus x-rays
      - These procedures confirm the diagnosis, which is typically based upon clinical findings and physical assessment.
    - Endoscopic sinus cavity lavage or surgery to relieve the obstruction and promote drainage of secretions may be done as a diagnostic procedure.

Patient-Centered Care

- Nursing Care
  - Encourage the use of steam humidification, sinus irrigation, saline nasal sprays, and hot and wet packs to relieve sinus congestion and pain.
  - Teach the client to increase fluid intake and rest.
  - Discourage air travel, swimming, and diving.
  - Encourage cessation of tobacco use in any form.
  - Instruct the client on correct technique for sinus irrigation and self-administration of nasal sprays.
- Medications
  - Nasal decongestants, such as phenylephrine (Neo-Synephrine), are used to reduce swelling of the mucosa.
    - Nursing Considerations
      - Clients should be encouraged to begin over-the-counter decongestant use at the first manifestation of sinusitis.
      - Signs of rebound nasal congestion may occur if decongestants are used for more than 3 to 4 days.
  - Broad-spectrum antibiotics, such as amoxicillin (Amoxil), are used on a limited basis for a confirmed causative bacterial pathogen.
  - Pain relief medications include NSAIDs, acetaminophen (Tylenol), and aspirin.

- Client Education
  - Sinus irrigation and saline nasal sprays are an effective alternative to antibiotics for relieving nasal congestion.
  - Contact the provider for manifestations of a severe headache, neck stiffness (nuchal rigidity), and high fever, which may indicate possible complications.

Complications

- Meningitis and encephalitis can occur if pathogens enter the bloodstream from the sinus cavity.

INFLUENZA

Overview

- Seasonal influenza or "flu" occurs as an epidemic, usually in the fall and winter months.
  - It is a highly contagious acute viral infection that occurs in children and adults of all ages.
  - Influenza may be caused by one of several virus families, and this can vary yearly. Adults are contagious from 24 hr before manifestations develop and up to 5 days after they begin.
- Pandemic influenza refers to a viral infection among animals or birds that has mutated and is becoming highly infectious to humans. The resulting viral infection has the potential to spread globally, such as H1N1 ("swine flu") and H5N1 ("avian flu").

Assessment

- Subjective Data
  - Severe headache and muscle aches
  - Chills
  - Fatigue, weakness
  - Severe diarrhea and cough (avian flu)
- Objective Data
  - Fever
  - Hypoxia (avian flu)
  - Diagnostic Procedures
    - AVantage A/H5N1 Flu Test

Patient-Centered Care

- Nursing Care (hospitalized clients)
  - Maintain airborne and contact precautions for hospitalized clients with pandemic influenza.
  - Provide saline gargles.
  - Monitor hydration status, intake and output.
  - Administer fluid therapy as prescribed by the provider.
  - Monitor respiratory status.

- Medications
  - Antivirals
    - Amantadine (Symmetrel), rimantadine (Flumadine), and ribavarin (Virazole) may be prescribed for treatment and prevention of influenza.
    - Duration of the influenza infection may be shortened by antivirals such as the oral inhalant zanamivir (Relenza) and the oral tablet oseltamivir (Tamiflu). In cases of pandemic influenza, these medications may be distributed widely among the population.
    - Client Education
      - Encourage clients to begin antiviral medications within 24 to 48 hr after the onset of manifestations.
  - Influenza vaccines
    - Trivalent vaccines are prepared yearly depending upon the suspected strain of influenza expected to appear. They include an IM injection of Fluvirin or Fluzone and a live attenuated influenza vaccine (LAIV) by intranasal spray (FluMist).
      - Vaccination is encouraged for everyone over 6 months of age.
      - Clients who have a history of pneumonia, chronic medical conditions, and those over age 65, pregnant women, and health care providers are at higher risk and require vaccination.
    - H1N1 vaccine is available for the general population.
    - H5N1 vaccine is stockpiled for distribution if a pandemic occurs.
- Teamwork and Collaboration
  - Respiratory services should be consulted for respiratory support.
  - Community health officials are notified of influenza outbreaks.
  - State and federal public health officials are consulted for containment and prevention directives during pandemic influenza.
- Client Education
  - Encourage annual influenza vaccination when vaccines become available.
  - Reduce the risk for spreading viruses by thoroughly washing hands and following cough etiquette.
  - Avoid places where people gather; avoid close personal contact (handshaking, kissing and hugging).
  - If flu manifestations develop, increase fluid intake, rest and stay home from work or school.
  - Avoid travel to areas where pandemic influenza is identified.
  - Be aware of public health announcements and activation of the early warning system by public health officials in case of pandemic influenza.

Complications

- Pneumonia is a complication of influenza and affects older adults and clients who are debilitated or immunocompromised.

PNEUMONIA

- Subjective Data
  - Anxiety
  - Fatigue
  - Weakness
  - Chest discomfort due to coughing
  - Confusion from hypoxia is the most common manifestation of pneumonia in older adult clients.
- Objective Data
  - Physical Assessment Findings
    - Fever
    - Chills
    - Flushed face
    - Diaphoresis
    - Shortness of breath or difficulty breathing
    - Tachypnea
    - Pleuritic chest pain (sharp)
    - Sputum production (yellow-tinged)
    - Crackles and wheezes
    - Coughing
    - Dull chest percussion over areas of consolidation
    - Decreased oxygen saturation levels (expected reference range is 95 to 100%)
    - Purulent, blood-tinged or rust-colored sputum, which may not always be present
  - Laboratory Tests
    - Sputum culture and sensitivity
      - Obtain specimen before starting antibiotic therapy.
      - Obtain specimen by suctioning if the client is unable to cough.
      - The responsible organism is identified about 50% of the time.
      - Older adult clients have a weak cough reflex and decreased muscle strength. Therefore, older adult clients have trouble expectorating, which can lead to difficulty in breathing and make specimen retrieval more difficult.
    - CBC – Elevated WBC count (may not be present in older adult clients)
    - ABGs – Hypoxemia (decreased PaO_2 less than 80 mm Hg)
    - Blood culture – To rule out organisms in the blood
    - Serum electrolytes – To identify causes of dehydration

- ○ Diagnostic Procedures
  - ▪ Chest x-ray
    - ▫ A chest x-ray will show consolidation (solidification, density) of lung tissue.
    - ▫ Chest x-ray may not indicate pneumonia for a few days after manifestations.
    - ▫ A chest x-ray is an important diagnostic tool because the early manifestations of pneumonia are often vague in older adult clients.

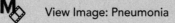
M View Image: Pneumonia

  - ▪ Pulse Oximetry – Clients who have pneumonia usually have oximetry levels less than the expected reference range of 95% to 100%.

Patient-Centered Care

- • Nursing Care
  - ○ Position the client to maximize ventilation (high-Fowler's = 90%) unless contraindicated.
  - ○ Encourage coughing or suction to remove secretions.
  - ○ Administer breathing treatments and medications as prescribed.
  - ○ Administer oxygen therapy as prescribed.
  - ○ Monitor for skin breakdown around the nose and mouth from the oxygen device.
  - ○ Encourage deep breathing with an incentive spirometer to prevent alveolar collapse.
  - ○ Determine the client's physical limitations and structure activity to include periods of rest.
  - ○ Promote adequate nutrition and fluid intake.
    - ▪ The increased work of breathing requires additional calories.
    - ▪ Proper nutrition aids in the prevention of secondary respiratory infections.
    - ▪ Encourage fluid intake of 2 to 3 L/day to promote hydration and thinning of secretions, unless contraindicated due to another condition.
  - ○ Provide rest periods for clients who have dyspnea.
  - ○ Reassure the client who is experiencing respiratory distress.
- • Medications
  - ○ Antibiotics
    - ▪ Antibiotics are given to destroy infectious pathogens; commonly used antibiotics include penicillins and cephalosporins.
    - ▪ Antibiotics are often initially given via IV and then switched to an oral form as the client's condition improves.
    - ▪ It is important to obtain any culture specimens prior to giving the first dose of an antibiotic. Once the specimen has been obtained, the antibiotics can be given while waiting for the results of the prescribed culture.

- Nursing Considerations
  - Observe clients taking cephalosporins for frequent stools.
  - Monitor client's kidney function, especially older adults who are taking penicillins and cephalosporins.
- Client Education
  - Encourage clients to take penicillins and cephalosporins with food. Some penicillins should be taken 1 hr before meals or 2 hr after.

- Bronchodilators
  - Bronchodilators are given to reduce bronchospasms and reduce irritation.
    - Short-acting beta$_2$ agonists, such as albuterol, provide rapid relief.
    - Cholinergic antagonists (anticholinergic medications), such as ipratropium (Atrovent), block the parasympathetic nervous system, allowing for increased bronchodilation and decreased pulmonary secretions.
    - Methylxanthines, such as theophylline (Theo-24), require close monitoring of serum medication levels due to the narrow therapeutic range.
  - Nursing Considerations
    - Monitor serum medication levels for toxicity for clients taking theophylline. Adverse effects will include tachycardia, nausea, and diarrhea.
    - Watch for tremors and tachycardia for clients taking albuterol.
    - Observe for dry mouth in clients taking ipratropium, and monitor heart rate. Adverse effects can include headache, blurred vision, and palpitations, which may indicate toxicity.
  - Client Education
    - Encourage clients to suck on hard candies to help moisten dry mouth while taking ipratropium.
    - Encourage increased fluid intake unless contraindicated.

- Anti-inflammatories decrease airway inflammation.
  - Glucocorticosteroids, such as fluticasone (Flovent) and prednisone (Deltasone), are prescribed to reduce inflammation. Monitor for immunosuppression, fluid retention, hyperglycemia, hypokalemia, and poor wound healing.
  - Nursing Considerations
    - Monitor for decreased immunity function.
    - Monitor for hyperglycemia.
    - Advise the client to report black, tarry stools.
    - Observe for fluid retention and weight gain. This can be common.
    - Monitor the client's throat and mouth for aphthous lesions (canker sores).
  - Client Education
    - Encourage the client to drink plenty of fluids to promote hydration.
    - Encourage the client to take glucocorticosteroids with food.
    - Encourage the client to avoid discontinuing glucocorticosteroids without consulting provider.

- Teamwork and Collaboration
  - ○ Respiratory services should be consulted for inhalers, breathing treatments, and suctioning for airway management.
  - ○ Nutritional services can be contacted for weight loss or gain related to medications or diagnosis.
  - ○ Rehabilitation care can be consulted if the client has prolonged weakness and needs assistance with increasing level of activity.
- Care after Discharge
  - ○ Client Education
    - ▪ Educate the client on the importance of continuing medications for treatment of pneumonia.
    - ▪ Encourage rest periods as needed.
    - ▪ Encourage the client to maintain hand hygiene to prevent infection.
    - ▪ Encourage the client to avoid crowded areas to reduce the risk of infection.
    - ▪ Remind the client that treatment and recovery from pneumonia can take time.
    - ▪ Encourage immunizations for influenza and pneumonia.
    - ▪ Promote smoking cessation if the client is a smoker.

Complications

- Atelectasis
  - ○ Airway inflammation and edema lead to alveolar collapse and increase the risk of hypoxemia.
  - ○ The client reports shortness of breath and exhibits findings of hypoxemia.
  - ○ The client has diminished or absent breath sounds over the affected area.
  - ○ A chest x-ray shows an area of density.
- Bacteremia (sepsis)
  - ○ This occurs if pathogens enter the bloodstream from the infection in the lungs.
- Acute Respiratory Distress Syndrome (ARDS)
  - ○ Hypoxemia persists despite oxygen therapy.
  - ○ The client's dyspnea worsens as bilateral pulmonary edema develops that is noncardiac related.
  - ○ A chest x-ray shows an area of density with a "ground glass" appearance.
  - ○ Blood gas findings demonstrate high arterial blood levels of carbon dioxide (hypercarbia) even though pulse oximetry shows decreased saturation.

APPLICATION EXERCISES

1. Which of the following clients have an increased risk for developing pneumonia? (Select all that apply.)

_____X_____ A. Client who has dysphagia

_____X_____ B. Client who has AIDS

_____ C. Client who was vaccinated for pneumococcus and influenza 6 months ago

_____ D. Client who is postoperative and has received local anesthesia

_____X_____ E. Client who has a closed head injury and is receiving ventilation

_____X_____ F. Client who has myasthenia gravis

2. A nurse in a clinic is caring for a client who was brought to the clinic by her partner. The partner states the client woke up this morning, did not recognize him, and did not know where she was. The client reports chills and chest pain that is worse upon inspiration. Which of the following is the priority nursing action?

A. Obtain baseline vital signs and oxygen saturation.

B. Obtain a sputum culture.

C. Obtain a complete history from the client.

D. Provide a pneumococcal vaccination.

3. A nurse is caring for a client who has pneumonia. Assessment findings include temperature 37.8° C (100° F), respirations 30/min, BP 130/76, heart rate 100/min, and SaO_2 91% on room air. Using a scale of 1 to 4, with 1 being the highest priority, prioritize the following nursing interventions.

_____ A. Administer antibiotics as prescribed.

_____ B. Administer oxygen therapy.

_____ C. Perform a sputum culture.

_____ D. Administer an antipyretic medication to promote client comfort.

4. A nurse in a clinic is caring for a client who has sinusitis. Which of the following techniques should the nurse use to identify clinical manifestations of this disorder?

A. Percussion of posterior lobes of lungs

B. Auscultation of the trachea

C. Inspection of the conjunctiva

D. Palpation of the orbital areas

5. A nurse is teaching a group of clients about influenza. Which of the following statements by a client requires clarification?

    A. "I should wash my hands after blowing my nose to prevent spreading the virus."

    B. "I need to avoid drinking fluids if I develop symptoms."

    C. "I need a flu shot every year because of the different flu strains."

    D. "I should sneeze into my elbow rather than my hands."

6. A nurse in a clinic is discussing health promotion and disease management with a client who has rhinitis. What should the nurse include in this discussion? Use the ATI Active Learning Template: Systems Disorder to complete this item. Include the following:

    A. Risk Factors: Identify three risk factors for rhinitis.

    B. Objective and Subjective: Describe two for each type of data.

    C. Management of Client Care: Describe two client self-care activities.

    D. Medications: Identify two over-the-counter medications the client can use.

APPLICATION EXERCISES KEY

1. A. **CORRECT:** The client who has difficulty swallowing is at increased risk for pneumonia due to aspiration.

    B. **CORRECT:** The client who has AIDS is immunocompromised, which increases the risk of opportunistic infections, such as pneumonia.

    C. INCORRECT: The client who has recently been vaccinated in the past few months is least likely to acquire pneumonia.

    D. INCORRECT: A client who is postoperative and has received local anesthesia has not been ventilated and is least likely to acquire pneumonia.

    E. **CORRECT:** Mechanical ventilation is invasive and increases the risk of pneumonia.

    F. **CORRECT:** A client who has myasthenia gravis has generalized weakness and may have difficulty clearing airway secretions, which increases the risk of pneumonia.

     NCLEX® Connection: Health Promotion and Maintenance, Health Promotion/Disease Prevention

2. A. **CORRECT:** Assessment is the first step of the nursing process and is essential in planning patient-centered care.

    B. INCORRECT: Obtaining a sputum culture is an appropriate action by the nurse, but it is not the priority action.

    C. INCORRECT: Obtaining a complete history from the client is an appropriate action by the nurse, but it is not the priority action.

    D. INCORRECT: Providing for a pneumococcal vaccination is an appropriate action by the nurse, but it is not the priority action.

     NCLEX® Connection: Health Promotion and Maintenance, Techniques of Physical Assessment

3. *Correct order*

    B. The client's respiratory and heart rates are elevated, and her oxygen saturation is 91% on room air. Using the ABC priority framework, providing oxygen is the first intervention.

    C. Obtaining a sputum culture is the second nursing intervention. It should be done prior to administering oral medications to obtain an appropriate and adequate specimen.

    A. Administration of antibiotics is the third action the nurse should take. The sputum culture should be obtained prior to antibiotic administration.

    D. Administering an antipyretic medication is the fourth nursing intervention.

     NCLEX® Connection: Physiological Adaptations, Illness Management

4. A. INCORRECT: Lung percussion is not an appropriate technique to identify clinical manifestations of sinusitis; it is appropriate for a client who has pneumonia.

    B. INCORRECT: Auscultation of the trachea is not an appropriate technique to identify clinical manifestations of sinusitis; it is appropriate for a client who has bronchitis.

    C. INCORRECT: Inspection of the conjunctiva is not an appropriate technique to identify clinical manifestations of sinusitis; it is appropriate for a client who has anemia.

    D. **CORRECT:** Palpation of the orbital, frontal, and facial areas will elicit a report of tenderness, which is a clinical manifestation in a client who has sinusitis.

    (N) NCLEX® Connection: Reduction of Risk Potential, System Specific Assessments

5. A. INCORRECT: Handwashing prevents the spread of influenza viruses.

    B. **CORRECT:** Fluid intake should be increased if findings develop.

    C. INCORRECT: Influenza vaccines are prepared yearly.

    D. INCORRECT: Cough etiquette includes sneezing into the shoulder or elbow rather than the hands.

    (N) NCLEX® Connection: Physiological Adaptations, Alterations in Body Systems

6. *Using the ATI Active Learning Template: Systems Disorder*

    A. Risk Factors
    - Recent exposure to viral, bacterial or influenza infections
    - Lack of current immunization status (pneumonia, influenza)
    - Exposure to plant pollen, molds, animal dander, foods, medications, and environmental contaminants
    - Tobacco smoke
    - Substance use (alcohol, cocaine)
    - Presence of a foreign body
    - Inactivity and immobility

    B. Objective and Subjective Data
    - Subjective
      - Excessive nasal drainage, runny nose (rhinorrhea), nasal congestion
      - Purulent nasal drainage
      - Sneezing and pruritus of the nose, throat, and ears
      - Itchy, watery eyes
      - Sore, dry throat
    - Objective
      - Red, inflamed, swollen nasal mucosa
      - Low-grade fever

    C. Management of Client Care
    - Self-care activities
      - Rest (8 to 10 hr/day), increased fluid intake (at least 2,000 mL/day)
      - Use of a home humidifier or breathing steamy air after running hot shower water
      - Proper disposal of tissues and use of cough etiquette

    D. Medications
    - Brompheniramine/pseudoephedrine (Dimetapp), cromolyn sodium (Nasalcrom), phenylephrine (Neo-synephrine), antipyretics (Tylenol)

    (N) NCLEX® Connection: Health Promotion and Maintenance, Health Promotion/Disease Prevention

chapter 21

Overview

- Asthma is a chronic inflammatory disorder of the airways that results in intermittent and reversible airflow obstruction of the bronchioles.

  ○ The obstruction occurs either by inflammation or airway hyperresponsiveness.

  ○ Asthma can occur at any age.

  ○ The cause of asthma is unknown.

- Manifestations of asthma

  ○ Mucosal edema

  ○ Bronchoconstriction

  ○ Excessive mucus production

 View Image: Normal and Asthmatic Lung Changes

- Asthma diagnoses are based on symptoms and classified into one of the following four categories.

  ○ Mild intermittent – Symptoms occur less than twice a week.

  ○ Mild persistent – Symptoms arise more than twice a week but not daily.

  ○ Moderate persistent – Daily symptoms occur in conjunction with exacerbations twice a week.

  ○ Severe persistent – Symptoms occur continually, along with frequent exacerbations that limit the client's physical activity and quality of life.

Health Promotion and Disease Prevention

- If the client smokes, promote smoking cessation.

- Advise the client to use protective equipment (mask) and ensure proper ventilation while working in environments that contain carcinogens or particles in the air.

- Encourage influenza and pneumonia vaccinations for all clients who have asthma and especially for the older adult.

- Instruct the client how to recognize and avoid triggering agents, such as:

  ○ Environmental factors, such as changes in temperature (especially warm to cold) and humidity

  ○ Air pollutants

  ○ Strong odors (perfume)

  ○ Seasonal allergens (grass, tree, and weed pollens) and perennial allergens (mold, feathers, dust, roaches, animal dander, foods treated with sulfites)

- ○ Stress and emotional distress
- ○ Medications (aspirin, NSAIDS, beta-blockers, cholinergics)
- ○ Enzymes, including those in laundry detergents
- ○ Chemicals (household cleaners)
- ○ Sinusitis with postnasal drip
- ○ Viral respiratory tract infection
- Instruct the client how to properly self-administer medications (nebulizers and inhalers).

 View Video: Asthmatic Breathing – Metered-Dose Inhaler

- Educate the client regarding infection prevention techniques.
- Encourage regular exercise as part of asthma therapy.
  - ○ Promotes ventilation and perfusion.
  - ○ Maintains cardiac health.
  - ○ Enhances skeletal muscle strength.
  - ○ Clients may require pre-medication.
- Instruct client to use hot water to eliminate dust mites in bed linens.

Assessment

- Risk Factors
  - ○ Older adult clients have decreased pulmonary reserves due to physiologic lung changes that occur with the aging process.
    - Older adult clients are more susceptible to infections.
    - The sensitivity of beta-adrenergic receptors decreases with age. As the beta receptors age and lose sensitivity, they are less able to respond to agonists, which relax smooth muscle and can result in bronchospasms.
    - Family history of asthma
    - Smoking
    - Secondhand smoke exposure
    - Environmental allergies
    - Exposure to chemical irritants or dust
    - Gastroesophageal reflux disease (GERD)
- Subjective Data
  - ○ Dyspnea
  - ○ Chest tightness
  - ○ Anxiety and/or stress

- Objective Data
  - Physical Assessment Findings
    - Coughing
    - Wheezing
    - Mucus production
    - Use of accessory muscles
    - Prolonged exhalation
    - Poor oxygen saturation (low SaO_2)
    - Barrel chest or increased chest diameter
  - Obtain the client's history regarding current and previous asthma exacerbations.
    - Onset and duration
    - Precipitating factors (stress, exercise, exposure to irritant)
    - Changes in medication regimen
    - Medications that relieve symptoms
    - Other medications taken
    - Self-care methods used to relieve symptoms

> **M** View Animation: Metered-Dose Inhaler

  - Laboratory Tests
    - ABGs
      - Hypoxemia (decreased PaO_2 less than 80 mm Hg)
      - Hypocarbia (decreased $PaCO_2$ less than 35 mm Hg – early in attack)
      - Hypercarbia (increased $PaCO_2$ greater than 45 mm Hg – later in attack)
    - Sputum cultures
      - Bacteria can indicate infection.
  - Diagnostic Procedures
    - Pulmonary function tests (PFTs) are the most accurate tests for diagnosing asthma and its severity.
      - Forced vital capacity (FVC) is the volume of air exhaled from full inhalation to full exhalation.
      - Forced expiratory volume in the first second (FEV1) is the volume of air blown out as hard and fast as possible during the first second of the most forceful exhalation after the greatest full inhalation.
      - Peak expiratory flow is the fastest airflow rate reached during exhalation.
      - A decrease in FEV1 by 15% to 20% below the expected value is common in clients who have asthma. An increase in these values by 12% following the administration of bronchodilators is diagnostic for asthma.
    - A chest x-ray is used to diagnose changes in the client's chest structure over time.

Patient-Centered Care

- Nursing Care

  ○ Position the client to maximize ventilation (high-Fowler's = 90°).

  ○ Administer oxygen therapy as prescribed.

  ○ Monitor cardiac rate and rhythm for changes during an acute attack (can be irregular, tachycardic, or with PVCs).

  ○ Initiate and maintain IV access.

  ○ Maintain a calm and reassuring demeanor.

  ○ Provide rest periods for older adult clients who have dyspnea. Design room and walkways with opportunities for rest. Incorporate rest into ADLs.

  ○ Encourage prompt medical attention for infections and appropriate vaccinations.

  ○ Administer medications as prescribed.

- Medications

  ○ Bronchodilators (inhalers)

    ▪ Short-acting beta$_2$ agonists, such as albuterol (Proventil, Ventolin), provide rapid relief of acute symptoms and prevent exercise-induced asthma.

    ▪ Anticholinergic medications, such as ipratropium (Atrovent), block the parasympathetic nervous system. This allows for the sympathetic nervous system effects of increased bronchodilation and decreased pulmonary secretions. These medications are long-acting and used to prevent bronchospasms.

    ▪ Methylxanthines, such as theophylline (Theo-24), require close monitoring of serum medication levels due to a narrow therapeutic range. Use only when other treatments are ineffective.

    ▪ Long-acting beta$_2$ agonists, such as salmeterol (Serevent), primarily are used for asthma attack prevention.

    ▪ Nursing Considerations

      □ Theophylline – Monitor the client's serum levels for toxicity. Side effects will include tachycardia, nausea, and diarrhea.

      □ Albuterol – Watch the client for tremors and tachycardia.

      □ Ipratropium – Observe the client for dry mouth.

    ▪ Client Education

      □ Ipratropium – Advise the client to suck on hard candies to help relieve dry mouth; increase fluid intake; and report headache, blurred vision, or palpitations, which may indicate toxicity of ipratropium. Monitor the client's heart rate.

      □ Salmeterol – Advise client to use to prevent an asthma attack and not at the onset of an attack.

  ○ Anti-inflammatory agents

    ▪ These are used to decrease airway inflammation, and they include:

      □ Corticosteroids, such as fluticasone (Flovent) and prednisone (Deltasone)

      □ Leukotriene antagonists, such as montelukast (Singulair), mast cell stabilizers, such as cromolyn sodium (Intal), and monoclonal antibodies, such as omalizumab (Xolair)

- Nursing Considerations
  - Watch the client for decreased immunity function.
  - Monitor for hyperglycemia.
  - Advise the client to report black, tarry stools.
  - Observe the client for fluid retention and weight gain. This can be common.
  - Monitor the client's throat and mouth for aphthous lesions (canker sores).
  - Omalizumab can cause anaphylaxis.
- Client Education
  - Encourage the client to drink plenty of fluids to promote hydration.
  - Encourage the client to take prednisone with food.
  - Advise client to use this medication to prevent asthma, not for the onset of an attack.
  - Encourage client to avoid persons with respiratory infections.
  - Use good mouth care.
  - Do not stop the use of this type of medication suddenly.
- Combination agents (bronchodilator and anti-inflammatory)
  - Ipratropium and albuterol (Combivent)
  - Fluticasone and salmeterol (Advair)
  - If prescribed separately for inhalation administration at the same time, administer the bronchodilator first in order to increase the absorption of the anti-inflammatory agent.
- Teamwork and Collaboration
  - Respiratory services should be consulted for inhalers and breathing treatments for airway management.
  - Nutritional services can be contacted for weight loss or gain related to medications or diagnosis.
  - Rehabilitation care can be consulted if the client has prolonged weakness and needs assistance with increasing level of activity.

Complications

- Respiratory failure
  - Persistent hypoxemia related to asthma can lead to respiratory failure.
  - Nursing Actions
    - Monitor oxygenation levels and acid-base balance.
    - Prepare for intubation and mechanical ventilation as indicated.
- Status asthmaticus
  - This is a life-threatening episode of airway obstruction that is often unresponsive to common treatment. It involves extreme wheezing, labored breathing, use of accessory muscles, distended neck veins, and creates a risk for cardiac and/or respiratory arrest.
  - Nursing Actions
    - Prepare for emergency intubation.
    - As prescribed, administer oxygen, bronchodilators, epinephrine, and initiate systemic steroid therapy.

APPLICATION EXERCISES

1. A nurse in the emergency department is caring for a client who was admitted with an acute asthma attack. Which of the following indicates the client's respiratory status is declining? (Select all that apply.)

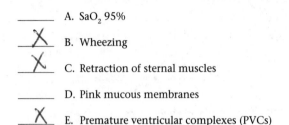

_____ A. SaO$_2$ 95%

___X___ B. Wheezing

___X___ C. Retraction of sternal muscles

_____ D. Pink mucous membranes

___X___ E. Premature ventricular complexes (PVCs)

2. A nurse working on a medical-surgical unit admits a client. Two hours after admission, the client's SaO$_2$ is 91% and he is exhibiting audible wheezes and use of his accessory muscles. Which of the following medications should the nurse expect to administer?

A. Antibiotic

B. Beta-blocker

C. Antiviral

D. Beta$_2$ agonist

3. A nurse is completing discharge teaching with a client who has a new prescription for prednisone (Deltasone) for asthma. Which of the following client statements indicates a need for further teaching?

A. "I will drink plenty of fluids while taking this medication."

B. "I will tell the doctor if I have black, tarry stools."

C. "I will take my medication on an empty stomach."

D. "I will monitor my mouth for canker sores."

4. A nurse is assessing a client with asthma. Which of the following is a risk factor associated with this disease?

A. Gender

B. Environmental allergies

C. Alcohol use

D. Race

5. A nurse is reinforcing teaching with a client on the purpose of taking a bronchodilator. Which of the following statements by the client indicates the teaching was effective?

    A. "This medication can decrease my immune response."

    B. "I take this medication to prevent asthma attacks."

    C. "I need to take this medication with food."

    D. "This medication has a slow onset to treat my symptoms."

6. A nurse is caring for a client with asthma and has a prescription for prednisone (Deltasone). Use the ATI Active Learning Template: Medication to complete this item to include at least three nursing interventions.

APPLICATION EXERCISES KEY

1. A. INCORRECT: An oxygen saturation of 95% is an expected finding within the respiratory system and exhibits no signs of distress.

    B. **CORRECT:** Wheezing is a clinical manifestation indicating that the client's respiratory status is declining.

    C. **CORRECT:** Retraction of sternal muscles is a clinical manifestation that the client's respiratory status is declining.

    D. INCORRECT: Pink mucous membranes is an expected finding within the respiratory system and exhibits no signs of distress.

    E. **CORRECT:** Premature ventricular complexes (PVCs) are a clinical manifestation that the client's respiratory status is declining.

     NCLEX® Connection: Reduction of Risk Potential, Potential for Complications from Surgical Procedures and Health Alterations

2. A. INCORRECT: An antibiotic is not indicated for these symptoms. An antibiotic typically is given for a bacterial infection.

    B. INCORRECT: A beta-blocker is not indicated for these symptoms. A beta blocker typically is given for dysrhythmias, heart disease, or hypertension.

    C. INCORRECT: An antiviral is not indicated for these symptoms. An antiviral typically is given for a virus.

    D. **CORRECT:** A beta$_2$ agonist should be given to relief the client's symptoms.

    NCLEX® Connection: Pharmacological and Parenteral Therapies, Medication Administration

3. A. INCORRECT: The client should drink plenty of fluids while taking this prednisone. This medication can cause the client to have a dry mouth or to become thirsty.

    B. INCORRECT: The client should inform the provider if the client experiences black, tarry stools. This medication can increase the client's bleeding tendency. Black stools can be an indication of blood in the stool.

    C. **CORRECT:** This statement by the client indicates a need for further teaching. The client should take this medication with food. Taking prednisone on an empty stomach can cause gastrointestinal distress.

    D. INCORRECT: The client should monitor their mouth for canker sores. This medication can cause bleeding of the gums and soreness in the mouth. It also decreases the client's immunity function.

    NCLEX® Connection: Pharmacological and Parenteral Therapies, Adverse Effects/Contraindications/Side Effects/Interactions

4. A. INCORRECT: Gender is not a risk factor associated with asthma.

    B. **CORRECT:** Environmental allergies are a risk factor associated with asthma. A client with environmental allergies typically has other allergic problems such as rhinitis or a skin rash.

    C. INCORRECT: Alcohol use is not a risk factor associated with asthma.

    D. INCORRECT: Race is not a risk factor associate with asthma.

    (N) NCLEX® Connection: Health Promotion and Maintenance, Health Promotion/Disease Prevention

5. A. INCORRECT: A bronchodilator does not decrease the body's immune response. An anti-inflammatory medication can cause this effect.

    B. **CORRECT:** A bronchodilator prevents asthma attacks from occurring.

    C. INCORRECT: A bronchodilator does not need to be given with food. An anti-inflammatory medication can cause gastrointestinal distress and needs to be to be given with food.

    D. INCORRECT: A bronchodilator has a fast onset to relieve asthma attack symptoms.

    (N) NCLEX® Connection: Pharmacological and Parenteral Therapies, Medication Administration

6. *Use the ATI Active Learning Template: Medication*
    - Nursing Interventions/Client Education
      ○ Watch the client for decreased immune function.
      ○ Monitor for hyperglycemia.
      ○ Advise the client to report black, tarry stools.
      ○ Observe the client for fluid retention and weight gain. This can be common.
      ○ Monitor the client's throat and mouth for aphthous lesions (cold sores).
      ○ Omalizumab can cause anaphylaxis.

    (N) NCLEX® Connection: Pharmacological and Parenteral Therapies, Medication Administration

chapter 22

Overview

- Chronic obstructive pulmonary disease (COPD) encompasses two diseases: emphysema and chronic bronchitis. Most clients who have emphysema also have chronic bronchitis. COPD is irreversible.

- Emphysema is characterized by the loss of lung elasticity and hyperinflation of lung tissue. Emphysema causes destruction of the alveoli, leading to a decreased surface area for gas exchange, carbon dioxide retention, and respiratory acidosis.

- Chronic bronchitis is an inflammation of the bronchi and bronchioles due to chronic exposure to irritants.

- COPD typically affects middle age to older adults.

Health Promotion and Disease Prevention

- Promote smoking cessation.

- Avoid exposure to secondhand smoke.

- Use protective equipment, such as a mask, and ensure proper ventilation while working in environments that contain carcinogens or particles in the air.

- Influenza and pneumonia vaccinations are important for all clients who have COPD, but especially for the older adult client.

Assessment

- Risk Factors
    - Advanced age – Older adult clients have a decreased pulmonary reserve due to normal lung changes.
    - Cigarette smoking is the primary risk factor for the development of COPD.
    - Alpha$_1$-antitrypsin (AAT) deficiency
    - Exposure to air pollution
- Subjective Data
    - Chronic dyspnea

- Objective Data
  - Physical Assessment Findings
    - Dyspnea upon exertion
    - Productive cough that is most severe upon rising in the morning
    - Hypoxemia
    - Crackles and wheezes
    - Rapid and shallow respirations
    - Use of accessory muscles
    - Barrel chest or increased chest diameter (with emphysema)

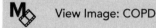 View Image: COPD

    - Hyperresonance on percussion due to "trapped air" (with emphysema)
    - Irregular breathing pattern
    - Thin extremities and enlarged neck muscles
    - Dependent edema secondary to right-sided heart failure
    - Clubbing of fingers and toes
    - Pallor and cyanosis of nail beds and mucous membranes (late stages of the disease)
    - Decreased oxygen saturation levels (expected reference range is 95% to 100%)
    - In clients who have dark-colored skin or in older adults, oxygen saturation levels can be slightly lower.
  - Laboratory Tests
    - An increased hematocrit level is due to low oxygenation levels.
    - Use sputum cultures and WBC counts to diagnose acute respiratory infections.
    - Arterial blood gases (ABGs).
      - Hypoxemia (decreased PaO_2 less than 80 mm Hg)
      - Hypercarbia (increased $PaCO_2$ greater than 45 mm Hg)
      - Respiratory acidosis, metabolic alkalosis compensation
    - Serum electrolytes.
  - Diagnostic Procedures
    - Pulmonary function tests
      - These tests are used for diagnosis, as well as determining the effectiveness of therapy.
      - Comparisons of forced expiratory volume (FEV) to forced vital capacity (FVC) are used to classify COPD as mild to very severe.
      - As COPD advances, the FEV to FVC ratio decreases. The expected reference range is 100%. For mild COPD, the FEV/FVC ratio is decreased to less than 70%. As the disease progresses to moderate and severe, the ratio decreases to less than 50%.

- Chest x-ray
  - □ Reveals hyperinflation of alveoli and flattened diaphragm in the late stages of emphysema.
  - □ It is often not useful for the diagnosis of early or moderate disease.

 M View Image: X-ray of Lungs with Emphysema

- Pulse oximetry
  - □ Clients who have COPD usually have oxygen levels less than the expected reference range of 95% to 100%
- AAT (alpha$_1$ antitrypsin) levels used to assess for AAT deficiency
  - □ A deficiency in a special enzyme produced by the liver that helps regulate other enzymes (that help breakdown pollutants) from attacking lung tissue.

Patient-Centered Care

- Nursing Care
  - ○ Position the client to maximize ventilation (high-Fowler's is 90°).
  - ○ Encourage effective coughing, or suction to remove secretions.
  - ○ Encourage deep breathing and use of an incentive spirometer.
  - ○ Administer breathing treatments and medications as prescribed.
  - ○ Administer oxygen as prescribed.
  - ○ Monitor for skin breakdown around the nose and mouth from the oxygen device.
  - ○ Promote adequate nutrition.
    - Increased work of breathing increases caloric demands.
    - Proper nutrition aids in the prevention of infection.
    - Encourage fluids to promote adequate hydration.
    - Dyspnea decreases energy available for eating, so soft, high-calorie foods should be encouraged.
  - ○ Monitor current weight and note any changes.
  - ○ Instruct the client to practice breathing techniques to control dyspneic episodes.
    - For diaphragmatic, or abdominal, breathing, instruct the client to:
      - □ Take breaths deep from the diaphragm.
      - □ Lie on back with knees bent.
      - □ Rest hand over abdomen to create resistance.
      - □ If the client's hand rises and lowers upon inhalation and exhalation, the breathing is being performed correctly.
    - For pursed lip breathing, instruct the client to:
      - □ Form the mouth as if preparing to whistle.
      - □ Take a breath in through the nose and out through the lips/mouth.
      - □ Do not puff the cheeks.
      - □ Take breaths deep and slow.

○ Incentive spirometry

- This is used to monitor optimal lung expansion.

- Nursing Actions

  □ Show the client how to use the incentive spirometry machine.

- Client Education

  □ Instruct the client to keep a tight mouth seal around mouthpiece and to inhale and hold breath for 3 to 5 seconds. As the client inhales, the needle of the spirometry machine will rise. This promotes lung expansion.

○ Clients who have COPD may need 2 to 4 L/min of oxygen via nasal cannula or up to 40% via Venturi mask.

- Clients who have chronically increased $PaCO_2$ levels usually require 1 to 2 L/min of oxygen via nasal cannula.

- It is important to recognize in COPD that low arterial levels of oxygen serve as the primary drive for breathing.

- Positive Expiratory Pressure Device

  □ Assists client to remove airway secretions.

  □ Client inhales deeply and exhales through device.

  □ While exhaling, a ball moves (that is inside the device), causing a vibration that results in loosening the client's secretions.

- Exercise Conditioning

  □ Includes improving the client's pulmonary status by strengthening the condition of the lungs by exercise.

  □ The client walks daily at a self-paced rate until symptoms of dyspnea occur allowing rest periods and then resuming walking.

  □ The client walks 20 min daily 2 to 3 times weekly.

  □ Determine the client's physical limitations, and structure activity to include periods of rest.

  □ Provide rest periods for older adult clients who have dyspnea. Design the room and walkways with opportunities for relaxation.

○ Provide support to the client and family.

- Talk about disease and lifestyle changes, including home care services such as portable oxygen.

○ Encourage verbalization of feelings.

○ Increase fluid intake.

- Encourage the client to drink 2 to 3 L/day to liquify mucus.

- Medications
  - Bronchodilators (inhalers)
    - Short-acting beta$_2$ agonists, such as albuterol (Proventil, Ventolin) provide rapid relief.
    - Cholinergic antagonists (anticholinergic medications), such as ipratropium (Atrovent), block the parasympathetic nervous system. This allows for the sympathetic nervous system effects of increased bronchodilation and decreased pulmonary secretions. These medications are long acting and are used to prevent bronchospasms.
    - Methylxanthines, such as theophylline (Theo-24), relax smooth muscles of the bronchi. These medications require close monitoring of serum medication levels due to narrow therapeutic ranges. Use only when other treatments are ineffective.
    - Nursing Considerations
      - Monitor the client's serum levels for toxicity when taking theophylline. Side effects will include tachycardia, nausea, and diarrhea.
      - Watch the client for tremors and tachycardia when taking albuterol.
      - Observe the client for dry mouth when taking ipratropium.
    - Client Education
      - Encourage the client to suck on hard candies to help moisten dry mouth while taking ipratropium.
      - Encourage client to increase fluid intake, report headaches, or blurred vision.
      - Monitor heart rate. Palpitations can occur, which may indicate toxicity of ipratropium.
  - Anti-inflammatory agents
    - These medications decrease airway inflammation.
    - If corticosteroids, such as fluticasone (Flovent) and prednisone (Deltasone), are given systemically, monitor for serious side effects (immunosuppression, fluid retention, hyperglycemia, hypokalemia, poor wound healing).
    - Leukotriene antagonists, such as montelukast (Singulair); mast cell stabilizers, such as cromolyn sodium (Intal); and monoclonal antibodies, such as omalizumab (Xolair), can be used.
    - Nursing Considerations
      - Watch the client for a decrease in immunity function.
      - Monitor the client for hyperglycemia.
      - Advise the client to report black, tarry stools.
      - Observe the client for fluid retention and weight gain. This is common.
      - Check the client's throat and mouth for aphthous lesions (cold sores).
      - Omalizumab (Xolair) can cause anaphylaxis.

- Client Education
  - Encourage the client to drink plenty of fluids to promote hydration.
  - Encourage the client to take glucocorticoids (prednisone) with food.
  - Advise client to use medication to prevent and control bronchospasms.
  - Advise client to avoid people who have respiratory infections.
  - Use good mouth care.
  - Use medication as a prophylactic prevention of COPD symptoms.
  - Instruct the client not to stop use of medication suddenly.
- Mucolytic Agents
  - These agents help thin secretions making it easier for the client to expel.
  - Nebulizer treatments include acetylcysteine (Mucomyst), or dornase alfa (Pulmozyme).
  - An oral agent that can be taken is guaifenesin (Mucinex, Robitussin).
  - A combination of guaifenesin and dextrommorphan (Mucinex DM) also can be taken orally to loosen secretions.

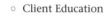

- Interprofessional Care
  - Respiratory services should be consulted for inhalers, breathing treatments, and suctioning for airway management.
  - Nutritional services should be contacted for weight loss or gain related to medications or diagnosis.
  - Rehabilitative care can be consulted if the client has prolonged weakness and needs assistance with increasing level of activity.
- Therapeutic Procedures
  - Chest physiotherapy uses percussion and vibration to mobilize secretions.
  - Raising the foot of the bed slightly higher than the head can facilitate optimal drainage and removal of secretions by gravity.
- Care after Discharge
  - COPD is debilitating for older adult clients. Referrals to assistance programs, such as food delivery services, can be indicated.
  - Set-up referral services, including home care services such as portable oxygen.
  - Client Education
    - Encourage the client to eat high-calorie foods to promote energy.
    - Encourage rest periods as needed.
    - Promote hand hygiene to prevent infection.
    - Reinforce the importance of taking medications (inhalers, oral medications) as prescribed.
    - Promote smoking cessation if the client is a smoker.
    - Encourage immunizations, such as influenza and pneumonia, to decrease the risk of infection.
    - Clients should use oxygen as prescribed. Inform other caregivers not to smoke around the oxygen due to flammability.
    - Provide support to the client and family.

Complications

- Respiratory infection
  - Respiratory infections result from increased mucus production and poor oxygenation levels.
  - Nursing Actions
    - Administer oxygen therapy.
    - Monitor oxygenation levels.
    - Administer antibiotics and other medications as prescribed.
    - Advise client to avoid crowds and people who have respiratory infections.
    - Encourage client to obtain pneumonia and influenza immunizations.
- Right-sided heart failure (cor pulmonale)
  - Air trapping, airway collapse, and stiff alveoli lead to increased pulmonary pressures.
  - Blood flow through the lung tissue is difficult. This increased workload leads to enlargement and thickening of the right atrium and ventricle.
  - Manifestations include the following:
    - Low oxygenation levels
    - Cyanotic lips
    - Enlarged and tender liver
    - Distended neck veins
    - Dependent edema
  - Nursing Actions
    - Monitor respiratory status and administer oxygen therapy.
    - Monitor heart rate and rhythm.
    - Administer medications as prescribed.
    - Administer IV fluids and diuretics to maintain fluid balance.

APPLICATION EXERCISES

1. A nurse is providing discharge teaching to a client who has COPD and has a new prescription for albuterol (Proventil). Which of the following statements made by the client indicates an understanding of the teaching?

    A. "This medication can increase my blood sugar levels."

    B. "This medication can decrease my immune response."

    C. "I can have an increase in my heart rate while taking this medication."

    D. "I can have mouth sores while taking this medication."

2. A nurse is preparing to administer a new prescription prednisone (Deltasone) to a client who has COPD. Which of the following should the nurse monitor for? (Select all that apply.)

    _X_ A. Monitor the client or hypokalemia.

    _____ B. Monitor the client for tachycardia.

    _X_ C. Observe the client for fluid retention.

    _____ D. Monitor the client for nausea.

    _X_ E. Advise the client to report black, tarry stools.

3. A nurse is instructing a client on the use of an incentive spirometer. Which of the following statements made by the client indicates an understanding of the teaching?

    A. "I will place the adapter on my finger to read my blood oxygen saturation level."

    B. "I will lie on my back with my knees bent."

    C. "I will rest my hand over my abdomen to create resistance."

    D. "I will take in a deep breath and hold it before exhaling."

4. A nurse is discharging a client who has COPD. Upon discharge, the client is concerned that he will never be able to leave his house now that he is on continuous oxygen. Which of the following is an appropriate response by the nurse?

    A. "There are portable oxygen delivery systems that you can take with you."

    B. "When you go out, you can remove the oxygen and then reapply it when you get home."

    C. "You probably will not be able to go out as much as you used to."

    D. "Home health services will come to you so you will not need to get out."

5. A nurse is planning to instruct a client on how to perform pursed-lip breathing. Which of the following should the nurse include in the plan of care?

    A. Take quick breaths upon inhalation.

    B. Place your hand over your stomach.

    C. Take a deep breath in through your nose.

    D. Puff your checks upon exhalation.

6. A nurse is reviewing the discharge instructions for a client who has a new prescription for ipratropium (Atrovent). Use the ATI Active Learning Template: Medication to complete this item to include the following section: Nursing Interventions/Client Education. List at least three interventions the nurse should include.

APPLICATION EXERCISES KEY

1. A. INCORRECT: Anti-inflammatory agents such as corticosteroids can cause hyperglycemia.

    B. INCORRECT: Anti-inflammatory agents such as corticosteroids can decrease the immune response.

    C. **CORRECT:** Bronchodilators such as albuterol can cause tachycardia.

    D. INCORRECT: Anti-inflammatory agents such as corticosteroids can cause mouth sores.

    Ⓝ NCLEX® Connection: Pharmacological and Parenteral Therapies, Medication Administration

2. A. **CORRECT:** The nurse should observe the client for a hypokalemia. This is a adverse effect while taking prednisone.

    B. INCORRECT: Tachycardia is an adverse effect of a bronchodilator.

    C. **CORRECT:** The nurse should observe the client for fluid retention. This is an adverse effect while taking prednisone.

    D. INCORRECT: Nausea is an adverse effect of a bronchodilator.

    E. **CORRECT:** The nurse should monitor the client for black, tarry stools. This is an adverse effect while taking prednisone.

    Ⓝ NCLEX® Connection: Pharmacological and Parenteral Therapies, Adverse Effects/Contraindications/ Side Effects/Interactions

3. A. INCORRECT: The client should place an adapter on her finger to read the level of blood oxygen saturation while performing a pulse oximetry reading.

    B. INCORRECT: The client should lie on her back with knees bent while practicing diaphragmatic or abdominal breathing.

    C. INCORRECT: The client should rest her hand over her abdomen while practicing diaphragmatic or abdominal breathing.

    D. **CORRECT:** The client should take in a deep breath and hold it for 3 to 5 seconds before exhaling. As the client exhales, the needle of the spirometer rises. This promotes lung expansion.

    Ⓝ NCLEX® Connection: Physiological Adaptations, Alterations in Body Systems

4. A. **CORRECT:** The client should be informed that there are portable oxygen systems that he can use to leave the house. This should alleviate his anxiety.

    B. INCORRECT: This is not an appropriate statement for the nurse to make. The client should be on oxygen at all times.

    C. INCORRECT: This is not an appropriate statement for the nurse to make. The client should be encouraged to return to his daily routine.

    D. INCORRECT: This is not an appropriate statement for the nurse to make. The client should be encouraged to return to his daily routine. Home health services are to promote a client's independence.

    Ⓝ NCLEX® Connection: Reduction of Risk Potential, Therapeutic Procedures

5. A. INCORRECT: The client should take a slow deep breath upon inhalation. This improves the client's breathing and allows oxygen into lungs.

    B. INCORRECT: The client should place her hand on her stomach while performing diaphragmatic or abdominal breathing. This allows resistance to be met and serves as a guide to the client that she is inhaling and exhaling correctly.

    C. **CORRECT:** The client should take a deep breath in through her nose while performing pursed-lip breathing. This controls the client's breathing.

    D. INCORRECT: The client should not puff her cheeks upon exhalation. This does not allow the client to optimally exhale the carbon dioxide for the her lungs.

    Ⓝ NCLEX® Connection: Reduction of Risk Potential, Therapeutic Procedures

6. *Using ATI Active Learning Template: Medication*
    - Nursing Interventions/Client Education
        - Observe the client for dry mouth when taking this medication.
        - Encourage the client to suck on hard candies to help moisten dry mouth while taking ipratropium.
        - Encourage the client to increase fluid intake, and to report headaches or blurred vision.
        - Monitor the client's heart rate. Palpitations can occur, which may indicate toxicity of ipratropium.

    Ⓝ NCLEX® Connection: Pharmacological and Parenteral Therapies, Medication Administration

chapter 23

Overview

- Tuberculosis (TB) is an infectious disease caused by *Mycobacterium tuberculosis.*

- TB is transmitted through aerosolization (airborne route).

- Once inside the lung, the body encases the TB bacillus with collagen and other cells. This may appear as a Ghon tubercle on a chest x-ray.

- Only a small percentage of people infected with TB actually develop an active form of the infection. The TB bacillus may lie dormant for many years before producing the disease.

- TB primarily affects the lungs but can spread to any organ in the blood.

- The risk of transmission decreases after 2 to 3 weeks of antituberculin therapy.

- A client will have a positive intradermal TB test within 2 to 10 weeks of exposure to the infection.

- Early detection and treatment are vital. TB has a slow onset, and the client may not be aware until the symptoms and disease are advanced. TB diagnosis should be considered for any client who has a persistent cough lasting longer than 3 weeks, chest pain, weakness, weight loss, anorexia, hemoptysis, dyspnea, fever, night sweats, or chills.

- Increasing the percentage of clients who complete treatment for TB should be a goal.

- Individuals who have been exposed to TB but have not developed the disease may have latent TB. This means that *Mycobacterium tuberculosis* is in the body, but the body has been able to fight off the infection. If not treated, it can lie dormant for several years and then become active as the individual becomes older or immunocompromised.

Health Promotion and Disease Prevention

- Clients who live in high-risk areas for tuberculosis should be screened on a yearly basis.

- Family members of clients diagnosed with tuberculosis should be screened.

Assessment

- Risk Factors
  - Frequent and close contact with an untreated individual
  - Lower socioeconomic status and homelessness
  - Immunocompromised status (HIV, chemotherapy, kidney disease, diabetes, Crohn's disease)
  - Poorly ventilated, crowded environments (prisons, long-term care facilities)
  - Advanced age

- ○ Recent travel outside of the United States to areas where TB is endemic
- ○ Substance use
- ○ Health care occupation that involves performance of high-risk activities (respiratory treatments, suctioning, coughing procedures)
- • Subjective Data
  - ○ Persistent cough lasting longer than 3 weeks
  - ○ Purulent sputum, possibly blood-streaked
  - ○ Fatigue and lethargy
  - ○ Weight loss and anorexia
  - ○ Night sweats and low-grade fever in the afternoon
- • Objective Data
  - ○ Physical Assessment Findings
    - ▪ Older adult clients often present with atypical symptoms of the disease (altered mentation or unusual behavior, fever, anorexia, weight loss).
  - ○ Laboratory Tests
    - ▪ QuantiFERON-TB Gold
      - ▫ Blood test that detects release of interferon-gamma (IFN-g) in fresh heparinized whole blood from sensitized people
      - ▫ Diagnostic for infection, whether it is active or latent
  - ○ Diagnostic Procedures
    - ▪ Mantoux test (should be read in 48 to 72 hr)

M◇ View Image: Positive Mantoux Test

- ▫ An intradermal injection of an extract of the tubercle bacillus is made.
- ▫ An induration (palpable, raised, hardened area) of 10 mm or greater in diameter indicates a positive skin test.
- ▫ An induration of 5 mm is considered a positive test for immunocompromised clients.
- ▫ A positive Mantoux test indicates that the client has developed an immune response to TB. It does not confirm that active disease is present. Clients who have been treated for TB may retain a positive reaction.
- ▫ Individuals who have latent TB may have a positive Mantoux test and may receive treatment to prevent development of an active form of the disease.
- ▫ Clients who have received a Bacillus Calmette-Guerin (BCG) vaccine within the past 10 years may have a false-positive Mantoux test. These clients will need a chest x-ray to evaluate the presence of active TB infection.
- ▫ Clients who are immunocompromised (such as those who have HIV) and the elderly should be tested for TB.
- ▫ Client Education
  - ▶ Reinforce to the client the importance of returning for a reading of the injection site by a health care personnel within 48 to 72 hr.

- A chest x-ray may be ordered to detect active lesions in the lungs.
- Acid-fast bacilli smear and culture
  - A positive acid-fast test suggests an active infection.
  - The diagnosis is confirmed by a positive culture for *Mycobacterium tuberculosis*.
  - Nursing Actions
    - Obtain three early-morning sputum samples.
    - Wear personal protective equipment when obtaining specimens.
    - Samples should also be obtained in a negative airflow room.

Patient-Centered Care

- Nursing Care
  - Administer heated and humidified oxygen therapy as prescribed.
  - Prevent infection transmission.
    - Wear an N95 or HEPA respirator when caring for clients who are hospitalized with TB.
    - Place the client in a negative airflow room, and implement airborne precautions.
    - Use barrier protection when the risk of hand or clothing contamination exists.
    - Have the client wear an N95 or HEPA respirator if transportation to another department is necessary. The client should be transported using the shortest and least busy route.
    - Teach the client to cough and expectorate sputum into tissues that are disposed of by the client into provided sacks.
  - Administer medications as prescribed.
  - Promote adequate nutrition.
    - Encourage fluid intake and a well-balanced diet for adequate caloric intake.
    - Encourage foods that are rich in protein, iron, and vitamin C.
  - Provide emotional support.
- Medications
  - Due to the resistance that is developing against the antituberculin medications, combination therapy of up to four medications at a time is presently recommended.
  - Because these medications must be taken for 6 to 12 months, medication noncompliance is a significant contributing factor in the development of resistant strains of TB.
  - The current four-medication regimen includes isoniazid (Nydrazid), rifampin (Rifadin), pyrazinamide, and ethambutol hydrochloride (Myambutol).
  - Client Education
    - Instruct the client to complete a series of medication prescribed by the provider.

- ○ Isoniazid (Nydrazid)
  - ▪ Isoniazid, commonly referred to as INH, is bactericidal and inhibits growth of mycobacteria by preventing synthesis of mycolic acid in the cell wall.
  - ▪ Nursing Considerations
    - □ This medication should be taken on an empty stomach.
    - □ Monitor for hepatotoxicity and neurotoxicity, such as tingling of the hands and feet.
    - □ Vitamin B_6 (pyridoxine) is used to prevent neurotoxicity from isoniazid.
  - ▪ Client Education
    - □ Advise the client not to drink alcohol while taking isoniazid because it may increase the risk for hepatotoxicity.
- ○ Rifampin (Rifadin)
  - ▪ Rifampin, commonly referred to as RIF, is a bacteriostatic and bactericidal antibiotic that inhibits DNA-dependent RNA polymerase activity in susceptible cells.
  - ▪ Nursing Considerations
    - □ Observe for hepatotoxicity.
  - ▪ Client Education
    - □ Inform the client that urine and other secretions will be orange.
    - □ Advise the client to report yellowing of the skin, pain or swelling of joints, loss of appetite, or malaise immediately.
    - □ Inform the client this medication may interfere with the efficacy of oral contraceptives.
- ○ Pyrazinamide
  - ▪ Pyrazinamide, commonly referred to as PZA, is a bacteriostatic and bactericidal, and its exact mechanism of action is unknown.
  - ▪ Nursing Considerations
    - □ Observe for hepatotoxicity.
  - ▪ Client Education
    - □ Instruct the client to drink a glass of water with each dose and increase fluids during the day.
    - □ Advise the client to report yellowing of the skin, pain or swelling of joints, loss of appetite, or malaise immediately.
    - □ Advise the client to avoid using alcohol while taking pyrazinamide.
- ○ Ethambutol (Myambutol)
  - ▪ Ethambutol, commonly referred to as EMB, is a bacteriostatic and works by suppressing RNA synthesis, subsequently inhibiting protein synthesis.
  - ▪ Nursing Considerations
    - □ Obtain baseline visual acuity tests.
    - □ Determine color discrimination ability.
    - □ This medication should not be given to children younger than 13 years of age.
  - ▪ Client Education
    - □ Instruct the client to report changes in vision immediately.

- ○ Streptomycin sulfate (Streptomycin)
  - ▪ Streptomycin sulfate is an aminoglycoside antibiotic. It potentiates the efficacy of macrophages during phagocytosis.
  - ▪ Nursing Considerations
    - ▫ Due to its high level of toxicity, this medication should be used only in clients who have multidrug-resistant TB (MDR-TB).
    - ▫ It can cause ototoxicity, so monitor hearing function and tolerance often.
    - ▫ Report significant changes in urine output and renal function studies.
  - ▪ Client Education
    - ▫ Advise the client to drink at least 2 to 3 L of fluid daily.
    - ▫ Advise the client to notify the provider if hearing declines.
- • Teamwork and Collaboration
  - ○ Contact social services if the client will need assistance in obtaining prescribed medications.
  - ○ Refer the client to a community clinic as necessary for follow-up appointments to monitor medication regimen and status of disease.
  - ○ Client Education
    - ▪ Provide the client and family education because TB is often treated in the home setting.
      - ▫ Exposed family members should be tested for TB.
      - ▫ Educate the client and family to continue medication therapy for its full duration of 6 to 12 months. Emphasize that failure to take the medications may lead to a resistant strain of TB.
      - ▫ Instruct the client to continue with follow-up care for 1 full year.
      - ▫ Inform the client that sputum samples are needed every 2 to 4 weeks to monitor therapy effectiveness. Clients are no longer considered infectious after three negative sputum cultures.
      - ▫ Encourage proper hand hygiene.
      - ▫ Instruct the client to cover mouth and nose when coughing or sneezing.
      - ▫ Inform the client that contaminated tissues should be disposed of in plastic bags.
      - ▫ Advise clients who have active TB to wear an N95 or HEPA respirator when in public places.

Complications

- • Miliary TB
  - ○ The organism invades the bloodstream and can spread to multiple body organs with complications including the following:
    - ▪ Headaches, neck stiffness, and drowsiness (can be life-threatening)
    - ▪ Pericarditis
      - ▫ Dyspnea, swollen neck veins, pleuritic pain, and hypotension due to an accumulation of fluid in pericardial sac that inhibits the heart's ability to pump effectively
  - ○ Nursing Actions
    - ▪ Treatment is the same as for pulmonary TB.

APPLICATION EXERCISES

1. A home health nurse is teaching a client who has active tuberculosis. The provider has prescribed the following medication regimen: isoniazid (Nydrazid) 250 mg PO daily, rifampin (Rifadin) 500 mg PO daily, pyrazinamide 750 mg PO daily, and ethambutol (Myambutol) 1 mg PO daily. Which of the following client statements indicate understanding of the teaching? (Select all that apply.)

_____ A. "I can substitute one medication for another if I run out because they all fight infection."

_____ B. "I will wash my hands each time I cough."

_____ C. "I will wear a mask when I am in a public area."

_____ D. "I am glad I don't have to have any more sputum specimens."

_____ E. "I don't need to worry where I go once I start taking my medications."

2. A nurse is teaching a client who has tuberculosis. Which of the following statements should the nurse include in the teaching?

A. "You will need continue to take the multimedication regimen for 4 months."

B. "You will need to provide sputum samples every 4 weeks to monitor the effectiveness of the medication."

C. "You will need to remain hospitalized for treatment."

D. "You will need to wear a mask at all times."

3. A nurse is caring for a client who has a new diagnosis of tuberculosis and has been placed on a multimedication regimen. Which of the following instructions should the nurse give the client related to the medication ethambutol (Myambutol)?

A. "Your urine may turn a dark orange."

B. "Watch for a change in the sclera of your eyes."

C. "Watch for any changes in vision."

D. "Take vitamin B$_6$ daily."

4. A nurse is preparing to administer a new prescription for isoniazid (INH) to a client who has tuberculosis. Which of the following is an appropriate statement by the nurse about this medication?

    A. "You may notice yellowing of your skin."

    B. "You may experience pain in your joints."

    C. "You may notice tingling of your hands."

    D. "You may experience a loss of appetite."

5. A nurse is providing information to a group of clients at a local community center about tuberculosis. Which of the following clinical manifestations should be included in the teaching? (Select all that apply.)

    _____ A. Persistent cough

    _____ B. Weight gain

    _____ C. Fatigue

    _____ D. Night sweats

    _____ E. Purulent sputum

6. A nurse is caring for a client who has tuberculosis. Use the ATI Active Learning Template: System Disorder to complete this item to include the following:

    A. Description of Disorder/Disease Process

    B. Patient-Centered Care: Include three nursing care interventions.

    C. Complications: Identify one potential complication.

APPLICATION EXERCISES KEY

1. A. INCORRECT: Medications should not be replaced for one another. It is important that the client adhere to the multimedication regimen prescribed by the provider to treat tuberculosis.

    B. **CORRECT:** The client should wash her hands each time she coughs to prevent spreading the infection.

    C. **CORRECT:** The client should wear a mask while in public areas to prevent spreading the infection. The client has active TB, and this is transmitted through the airborne route.

    D. INCORRECT: The client will still need to collect sputum cultures every 2 to 4 weeks until three sputum cultures have come back negative.

    E. INCORRECT: The client will still need to avoid crowded areas if possible and take preventative measures, such as wearing a mask when going out.

     NCLEX® Connection: Safety and Infection Control, Standard Precautions/Transmission-Based Precautions/Surgical Asepsis

2. A. INCORRECT: A client who has tuberculosis needs to continue taking the multimedication regimen for 6 to 12 months.

    B. **CORRECT:** A client who has tuberculosis needs to provide sputum samples every 2 to 4 weeks to monitor the effectiveness of the medication.

    C. INCORRECT: A client who has tuberculosis is often treated in the home setting.

    D. INCORRECT: A client who has tuberculosis needs to wear a mask when in public areas.

     NCLEX® Connection: Reduction of Risk Potential, Therapeutic Procedures

3. A. INCORRECT: Clients receiving rifampin should expect to see their urine turn a dark orange.

    B. INCORRECT: Ethambutol does not affect the sclera of the eyes.

    C. **CORRECT:** Clients receiving ethambutol will need to watch for changes in their vision due to optic neuritis, which can result from taking this medication.

    D. INCORRECT: Clients receiving isoniazid should take vitamin B_6 daily and observe for signs of hepatotoxicity.

     NCLEX® Connection: Pharmacological and Parenteral Therapies, Medication Administration

4. A. INCORRECT: Yellowing of the skin is an adverse effect of rifampin or pyrazinamide.

    B. INCORRECT: Experiencing pain in the joints is an adverse effect of rifampin.

    C. **CORRECT:** Tingling of the hands is an adverse effect of isoniazid.

    D. INCORRECT: Loss of appetite is an adverse effect of rifampin.

     NCLEX® Connection: Pharmacological and Parenteral Therapies, Adverse Effects/Contraindications/ Side Effects/Interactions

5. A. **CORRECT:** Persistent cough is a clinical manifestation of tuberculosis.

    B. INCORRECT: Weight loss is a clinical manifestation of tuberculosis.

    C. **CORRECT:** Fatigue is a clinical manifestation of tuberculosis.

    D. **CORRECT:** Night sweats is a clinical manifestation of tuberculosis.

    E. **CORRECT:** Purulent sputum is a clinical manifestation of tuberculosis.

    (N) NCLEX® Connection: Physiological Adaptations, Pathophysiology

6. *Using the ATI Active Learning Template: System Disorder*
    A. Description of Disorder/Disease Process
      • Tuberculosis (TB) is an infectious disease caused by *Mycobacterium tuberculosis*. TB is transmitted through aerosolization (airborne route). Once inside the lung, the body encases the TB bacillus with collagen and other cells. This may appear as a Ghon tubercle on a chest x-ray. Only a small percentage of people infected with TB actually develop an active form of the infection. The TB bacillus may lie dormant for many years before producing the disease. TB primarily affects the lungs but can spread to any organ in the blood.

    B. Patient-Centered Care
      • Nursing Care Interventions
        ○ Administer heated and humidified oxygen therapy as prescribed.
        ○ Prevent infection transmission.
        ○ Wear an N95 or HEPA respirator when caring for clients who are hospitalized with TB.
        ○ Place the client in a negative airflow room, and implement airborne precautions.
        ○ Use barrier protection when the risk of hand or clothing contamination exists.
        ○ Have the client wear an N95 or HEPA respirator mask if transportation to another department is necessary.
        ○ The client should be transported using the shortest and least busy route.
        ○ Teach the client to cough and expectorate sputum into tissues that are disposed of by the client into provided sacks.
        ○ Administer medications as prescribed.
        ○ Promote adequate nutrition.
        ○ Encourage fluid intake and a well-balanced diet for adequate caloric intake.

    C. Complications
      • Miliary TB
        ○ The organism invades the bloodstream and can spread to multiple body organs with complications including the following:
          ▪ Headaches, neck stiffness, and drowsiness (can be life-threatening)
          ▪ Pericarditis – dyspnea, swollen neck veins, pleuritic pain, and hypotension due to an accumulation of fluid in the pericardial sac that inhibits the heart's ability to pump effectively
        ○ Nursing Actions
          ▪ Treatment is the same as for pulmonary TB.

    (N) NCLEX® Connection: Physiological Adaptations, Alterations in Body Systems

chapter 24

Overview

- A pulmonary embolism (PE) occurs when a substance (solid, gaseous, or liquid) enters venous circulation and forms a blockage in the pulmonary vasculature.

- Emboli originating from deep-vein thrombosis (DVT) are the most common cause. Tumors, bone marrow, amniotic fluid, and foreign matter also can become emboli.

 View Image: Pulmonary Embolism

- Increased hypoxia to pulmonary tissue and impaired blood flow can result from a large embolus. A PE is a medical emergency.

- Prevention, rapid recognition, and treatment of a PE are essential for a positive outcome.

Health Promotion and Disease Prevention

- Promote smoking cessation.

- Encourage maintenance of appropriate weight for height and body frame.

- Encourage a healthy diet and physical activity.

- Prevent deep-vein thrombosis (DVT) by encouraging clients to do leg exercises, wear compression stockings, and avoid sitting for long periods of time.

Assessment

- Risk Factors
  - Long-term immobility
  - Oral contraceptive use and estrogen therapy
  - Pregnancy
  - Tobacco use
  - Hypercoagulability (elevated platelet count)
  - Obesity
  - Surgery (especially orthopedic surgery of the lower extremities or pelvis)
  - Heart failure or chronic atrial fibrillation
  - Autoimmune hemolytic anemia (sickle cell)
  - Long bone fractures

- ○ Advanced age
  - ▪ Older adult clients have decreased pulmonary reserves due to normal lung changes, including decreased lung elasticity and thickening alveoli. Older adult clients can decompensate more quickly.
  - ▪ Certain pathological conditions and procedures that predispose clients to DVT formation (peripheral vascular disease, hypertension, hip and knee orthoplasty) are more prevalent in older adults.
  - ▪ Many older adult clients experience decreased physical activity levels, thus predisposing them to DVT formation and pulmonary emboli.
- Subjective Data
  - ○ Anxiety
  - ○ Feelings of impending doom
  - ○ Pressure in chest
  - ○ Pain upon inspiration and chest wall tenderness
  - ○ Dyspnea and air hunger
- Objective Data
  - ○ Physical Assessment Findings
    - ▪ Pleurisy
    - ▪ Pleural friction rub
    - ▪ Tachycardia
    - ▪ Hypotension
    - ▪ Tachypnea
    - ▪ Adventitious breath sounds (crackles) and cough
    - ▪ Heart murmur in S_3 and S_4
    - ▪ Diaphoresis
    - ▪ Low-grade fever
    - ▪ Decreased oxygen saturation levels (the expected reference range is 95% to 100%), low SaO_2, cyanosis
    - ▪ Petechiae (red dots under the skin) over chest and axillae
    - ▪ Pleural effusion (fluid in the lungs)
  - ○ Laboratory Tests
    - ▪ ABG analysis
      - □ $PaCO_2$ levels are low (the expected reference range is 35 to 45 mm Hg) due to initial hyperventilation (respiratory alkalosis).
      - □ As hypoxemia progresses, respiratory acidosis occurs.
    - ▪ CBC analysis to monitor hemoglobin and hematocrit
    - ▪ D-dimer
      - □ Elevated above expected reference range in response to clot formation and release of fibrin degradation products (the expected reference range is 0.43 to 2.33 mcg/mL).

○ Diagnostic Procedures

▪ Chest x-ray and computed tomography (CT) scan

□ These provide initial identification of a PE. A CT scan is most commonly used. A chest x-ray can show a large PE.

▪ Ventilation-perfusion (V/Q) scan

□ Images show the circulation of air and blood in the lungs and can detect a PE.

▪ Pulmonary Angiography

□ This is the most thorough test to detect a PE, but it is invasive and costly. A catheter is inserted into the vena cava to visually see a PE.

□ Pulmonary angiography is a higher risk procedure than a V/Q scan.

□ Nursing Actions

▸ Verify that informed consent has been obtained.

▸ Monitor the client's status (vital signs, SaO$_2$, anxiety, bleeding with angiography) during and after the procedure.

Patient-Centered Care

- Nursing Care

  ○ Administer oxygen therapy as prescribed to relieve hypoxemia and dyspnea.

  ▪ Position the client to maximize ventilation (high-Fowler's = 90%).

  ○ Initiate and maintain IV access.

  ○ Administer medications as prescribed.

  ○ Provide emotional support and comfort to control client anxiety.

  ○ Monitor changes in level of consciousness and mental status.

- Medications

  ○ Anticoagulants: enoxaparin (Lovenox), heparin, warfarin (Coumadin)

  ▪ Anticoagulants are used to prevent clots from getting larger or additional clots from forming.

  ▪ Nursing Considerations

  □ Assess for contraindications (active bleeding, peptic ulcer disease, history of stroke, recent trauma).

  □ Monitor bleeding times – Prothrombin time (PT) and international normalized ratio (INR) for warfarin, partial thromboplastin time (a PTT) for heparin, and complete blood count (CBC).

  □ Monitor for side effects of anticoagulants (e.g., thrombocytopenia, anemia, hemorrhage).

  ○ Thrombolytic therapy– alteplase (Activase) and streptokinase (Streptase)

  ▪ Used to dissolve blood clots and restore pulmonary blood flow.

  ▪ Similar side effects and contraindications as anticoagulants.

- Nursing Considerations
  - Assess for contraindications (known bleeding disorders, uncontrolled hypertension, active bleeding, peptic ulcer disease, history of stroke, recent trauma or surgery, pregnancy).
  - Monitor for evidence of bleeding, thrombocytopenia, and anemia.
  - Give streptokinase slowly to prevent hypotension.
    - Monitor blood pressure, heart rate, respirations, and oxygen saturation per facility protocol before, during, and after administration of medication.
- Teamwork and Collaboration
  - Cardiology and pulmonary services should be consulted to manage a PE and treatment.
  - Respiratory services should be consulted for oxygen therapy, breathing treatments, and ABGs.
  - Radiology should be consulted for diagnostic studies to determine PE.
- Surgical Interventions
  - Embolectomy
    - Surgical removal of embolus
    - Nursing Actions
      - Prepare the client for the procedure (NPO status, informed consent).
      - Monitor postoperatively (vital signs, SaO$_2$, incision drainage, pain management).
  - Vena cava filter
    - Insertion of a filter in the vena cava to prevent further emboli from reaching the pulmonary vasculature
    - Nursing Actions
      - Prepare the client for the procedure (NPO status, informed consent).
      - Monitor postoperatively (vital signs, SaO$_2$, incision drainage, pain management).
- Care After Discharge
  - If the client is homebound, set up home care services to perform weekly blood draws.
  - Set up referral services to supply portable oxygen for clients who have severe dyspnea.
  - Client Education

    - Provide education to the client for the treatment and prevention of a PE.
      - Promote smoking cessation if the client smokes.
      - Encourage the client to avoid long periods of immobility.
      - Encourage physical activity such as walking.
      - Encourage the client to wear compression stockings to promote circulation.
      - Encourage the client to avoid crossing his legs.
    - Advise the client to monitor intake of foods high in vitamin K (green, leafy vegetables) if taking warfarin. Vitamin K can reduce the anticoagulant effects of warfarin.
    - Advise the client to adhere to a schedule for monitoring PT and INR, follow instructions regarding medication dosage adjustments (for clients on warfarin), and adhere to weekly blood draws.

- Remind the client of the increased risk for bruising and bleeding.
  - □ Instruct the client to avoid taking aspirin products, unless specified by the provider.
  - □ Encourage the client to check his mouth and skin daily for bleeding and bruising.
  - □ Encourage the client to use electric shavers and soft-bristled toothbrushes.
  - □ Instruct the client to avoid blowing his nose hard, and to gently apply pressure if nose bleeds occur.
- Encourage client who is traveling about measures to prevent PE.
- Instruct client to arise from sitting position for 5 min out of every hour.
- Advise client to wear support stockings.
- Inform client to remain hydrated by drinking plenty of water.
- Instruct client to perform active ROM exercises when sitting.

Complications

- Decreased cardiac output – Blood volume is decreased.
  - ○ Nursing Actions
    - Monitor for hypotension, tachycardia, cyanosis, jugular venous distention, and syncope.
    - Assess for the presence of S_3 or S_4 heart sounds.
    - Initiate and maintain IV access.
    - Monitor urinary output (output should be 30 mL/hr or more).
    - Administer IV fluids (crystalloids) to replace vascular volume.
    - Continuously monitor the ECG.
    - Monitor pulmonary pressures. IV fluids can contribute to pulmonary hypertension for clients who have right-sided heart failure (cor pulmonale).
    - Administer inotropic agents (milrinone [Primacor], dobutamine [Dobutrex]), to increase myocardial contractility.
    - Vasodilators may be needed if pulmonary artery pressure is high enough that it interferes with cardiac contractility.
- Hemorrhage – Risk for bleeding increases due to anticoagulant therapy.
  - ○ Nursing Actions
    - Assess for oozing, bleeding, or bruising from injection and surgical sites.
    - Monitor cardiovascular status (blood pressure, heart rate and rhythm).
    - Monitor CBC (hemoglobin, hematocrit, platelets) and bleeding times (PT, aPTT, INR).
    - Administer IV fluids and blood products as required.
    - Test stools, urine, and vomit for occult blood.
    - Monitor for internal bleeding (measure abdominal girth and abdominal or flank pain).

APPLICATION EXERCISES

1. A nurse is caring for several clients. Which of the following clients are at risk for having a pulmonary embolism? (Select all that apply.)

__X__ A. A client who has a BMI of 30

_____ B. A female client who is postmenopausal

__X__ C. A client who has a fractured femur

_____ D. A client who is a marathon runner

__X__ E. A client who has chronic atrial fibrillation

2. A nurse is reviewing prescriptions for a client who has acute dyspnea and diaphoresis. The client states that she is anxious because she feels that she cannot get enough air. Vital signs are: heart rate 117/min, respiratory rate 38/min, temperature 38.4° C (101.2° F), and blood pressure 100/54 mm Hg. Which of the following actions is the priority action at this time?

A. Notify the provider.

B. Administer heparin via IV infusion.

C. Administer oxygen therapy.

D. Obtain a spiral CT scan.

3. A nurse is caring for a client who has a new prescription for heparin therapy. Which of the following statements by the client should indicate an immediate concern for the nurse?

A. "I am allergic to morphine."

B. "I take antacids several times a day."

C. "I had a blood clot in my leg several years ago."

D. "It hurts to take a deep breath."

4. A nurse is assessing a client who has a pulmonary embolism. Which of the clinical manifestations should the nurse expect to find? (Select all that apply.)

_____ A. Bradypnea 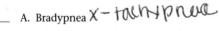 X – tachypnea

__X__ B. Pleural friction rub

_____ C. Hypertension

__X__ D. Petechiae

__X__ E. Tachycardia

5. A nurse is caring for a client who is to receive fibrinolytic thrombolytic therapy. Which of the following should the nurse recognize as a contraindication to the therapy?

A. Hip arthroplasty 2 weeks ago

B. Elevated sedimentation rate

C. Incident of exercise-induced asthma 1 week ago

D. Elevated platelet count

6. A nurse is caring for a client who has a pulmonary embolism. Use the ATI Active Learning Template: Systems Disorder to complete this item to include the following sections:

A. Description of Disorder/Disease Process

B. Patient-Centered Care:
- Describe three nursing interventions.
- Identify two medications.

APPLICATION EXERCISES KEY

1. A. **CORRECT:** A client who has a BMI of 30 is considered obese and is at increased risk for a blood clot.

   B. INCORRECT: A woman who is postmenopausal has decreased estrogen levels and is not at risk for developing a pulmonary embolism.

   C. **CORRECT:** A fractured bone, particularly in a long bone such as the femur, increases the risk of fat emboli.

   D. INCORRECT: A client who is a marathon runner increases the blood flow and circulation of his body, which decreases the risk for developing a pulmonary embolism.

   E. **CORRECT:** A client who has turbulent blood flow in the heart, such as with atrial defibrillation, is also at increased risk of a blood clot.

    NCLEX® Connection: Physiological Adaptations, Unexpected Response to Therapies

2. A. INCORRECT: Notifying the provider about the client's condition is important, but it is not the priority action by the nurse at this time.

   B. INCORRECT: Administration of IV heparin is treatment used to dissolve a blood clot, but it is not the priority action by the nurse at this time.

   C. **CORRECT:** When using the airway, breathing, circulation (ABC) priority approach to care, the nurse determines meeting the client's oxygenation needs by administering oxygen therapy is the priority action.

   D. INCORRECT: Obtaining a spiral CT scan to detect the presence and location of the blood clot is important, but it is not the priority action by the nurse at this time.

    NCLEX® Connection: Physiological Adaptations, Illness Management

3. A. INCORRECT: The nurse should document all allergies. Morphine can be prescribed to manage the client's discomfort due to a blood clot, but is not the immediate concern at this time.

   B. **CORRECT:** The greatest risk to the client is the possibility of bleeding from a peptic ulcer. Further assessment should be completed and the nurse should notify the provider of the finding.

   C. INCORRECT: The client's history of a blood clot is important for the nurse to know, but it is not the immediate concern at this time.

   D. INCORRECT: The client report of pain with breathing is important for the nurse to know, but it is not the immediate concern at this time.

   NCLEX® Connection: Pharmacological and Parenteral Therapies, Adverse Effects/Contraindications/Side Effects/Interactions

4. A. INCORRECT: Tachypnea is a clinical manifestation associated with a pulmonary embolism.

    B. **CORRECT:** A pleural friction rub is a clinical manifestation associated with a pulmonary embolism.

    C. INCORRECT: Hypotension is a clinical manifestation associated with a pulmonary embolism.

    D. **CORRECT:** Petechiae is a clinical manifestation associated with a pulmonary embolism.

    E. **CORRECT:** Tachycardia is a clinical manifestation associated with a pulmonary embolism.

    (N) NCLEX® Connection: Physiological Adaptations, Pathophysiology

5. A. **CORRECT:** Clients who have undergone a major surgical procedure within the last 3 weeks should not receive thrombolytic therapy because of the risk of hemorrhage from the surgical site.

    B. INCORRECT: An elevated sedimentation rate does not place the client at risk for hemorrhage.

    C. INCORRECT: An incident of exercise-induced asthma does not place the client at risk for hemorrhage.

    D. INCORRECT: An elevated platelet count does not place the client at risk for hemorrhage.

    (N) NCLEX® Connection: Pharmacological and Parenteral Therapies, Adverse Effects/Contraindications/ Side Effects/Interactions

6. *Using the Active Learning Template: Systems Disorder*

    A. Description of Disorder/Disease Process

    - A pulmonary embolism (PE) occurs when a substance (solid, gaseous, or liquid) enters venous circulation and forms a blockage in the pulmonary vasculature.
    - Emboli originating from deep-vein thrombosis (DVT) are the most common cause. Tumors, bone marrow, amniotic fluid, and foreign matter can also become emboli.

    B. Patient-Centered Care

    - Nursing Interventions
      - Administer oxygen therapy as prescribed to relieve hypoxemia and dyspnea.
        - Position the client to maximize ventilation (high-Fowler's = 90%).
      - Initiate and maintain IV access.
      - Administer medications as prescribed.
      - Provide emotional support and comfort to control client anxiety.
      - Monitor changes in level of consciousness and mental status.
    - Medications
      - Anticoagulants – enoxaparin (Lovenox), heparin, and warfarin (Coumadin)
      - Thrombolytic therapy – alteplase (Activase) and streptokinase (Streptase)

    (N) NCLEX® Connection: Physiological Adaptations, Unexpected Response to Therapies

chapter 25

Overview

- This chapter will review pneumothorax, hemothorax, and flail chest.

- A pneumothorax is the presence of air or gas in the pleural space that causes lung collapse.

- A tension pneumothorax occurs when air enters the pleural space during inspiration through a one-way valve and is not able to exit upon expiration. The trapped air causes pressure on the heart and the lung. As a result, the increase in pressure compresses blood vessels and limits venous return, leading to a decrease in cardiac output. Death can result if not treated immediately.

  - As a result of a tension pneumothorax, air and pressure continue to rise in the pleural cavity, which causes a mediastinal shift.

- A hemothorax is an accumulation of blood in the pleural space.

- A spontaneous pneumothorax can occur when there has been no trauma. A small bleb on the lung ruptures and air enters the pleural space.

- A flail chest occurs when several ribs, usually on one side of the chest, sustain multiple fractures. Ribs and the fractured segments have minimal attachments, and there is instability of the chest wall. This results in significant limitation in chest wall expansion.

Assessment

- Risk Factors

  - Blunt chest trauma.

  - Penetrating chest wounds.

  - Closed/occluded chest tube.

  - Older adult clients have decreased pulmonary reserves due to normal lung changes, including decreased lung elasticity and thickening alveoli.

  - Older adult clients are more susceptible to infections.

  - Chronic obstructive pulmonary disease (COPD).

- Subjective Data

  - Anxiety

  - Pleuritic pain

- Objective Data
  - ○ Physical Assessment Findings
    - ▪ Signs of respiratory distress (tachypnea, tachycardia, hypoxia, cyanosis, dyspnea, and use of accessory muscles)
    - ▪ Tracheal deviation to the unaffected side (tension pneumothorax)
    - ▪ Reduced or absent breath sounds on the affected side
    - ▪ Asymmetrical chest wall movement
    - ▪ Hyperresonance on percussion due to trapped air (pneumothorax)
    - ▪ Dull percussion (hemothorax)
    - ▪ Subcutaneous emphysema (air accumulating in subcutaneous tissue)
  - ○ Laboratory Tests
    - ▪ ABGs
      - □ Hypoxemia (PaO_2 less than 80 mm Hg)
  - ○ Diagnostic Procedures
    - ▪ Chest x-ray
      - □ Used to confirm pneumothorax or hemothorax

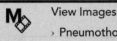

View Images
> Pneumothorax   > Hemothorax

-
  -
    - ▪ Thoracentesis may be used to confirm hemothorax.
      - □ Thoracentesis is the surgical perforation of the chest wall and pleural space with a large-bore needle.
      - □ Nursing Actions
        - ▸ Ensure that informed consent has been obtained.
        - ▸ Make sure the client understands the importance of remaining still during the procedure.
        - ▸ Assist with client positioning and specimen transport. Monitor the client's status (vital signs, SaO_2, injection site). Assist the client to the the edge of the bed and to lean over a bedside table.
        - ▸ Inform the client he will feel discomfort when the local anesthetic solution is injected. When the needle is inserted into the lung, some pressure may be felt, but no pain.

Patient-Centered Care

- Nursing Care
  - ○ Administer oxygen therapy.
  - ○ Auscultate heart and lung sounds and monitor vital signs every 4 hr.
  - ○ Document ventilator settings hourly if the client is receiving ventilation.
  - ○ Check ABGs, SaO_2, CBC, and chest x-ray results.
  - ○ Position the client to maximize ventilation (high-Fowler's = 90%).

Q
EBP

- ○ Provide emotional support to the client and family.
- ○ Monitor chest tube drainage.
- ○ Administer medications as prescribed.
- ○ Encourage prompt medical attention when evidence of infection occurs.
- • Medications
    - ○ Benzodiazepines (sedatives)
        - ▪ Lorazepam (Ativan) or midazolam may be used to decrease anxiety.
        - ▪ Nursing Considerations
            - □ Monitor vital signs. (Benzodiazepines may cause hypotension and respiratory distress.)
            - □ The medications have amnesiac effect.
            - □ Monitor for paradoxical effects (euphoria, rage).
        - ▪ Client Education
            - □ Remind the client that medications will have amnesic effect and cause drowsiness.
    - ○ Opioid agonists (pain medications)
        - ▪ Morphine sulfate and fentanyl (Duragesic) are opioid agents used to treat moderate to severe pain. These medication acts on the mu and kappa receptors that help alleviate pain.
        - ▪ Activation of these receptors produces analgesia (pain relief), respiratory depression, euphoria, sedation, and a decrease in gastrointestinal motility.
        - ▪ Nursing Considerations
            - □ Use cautiously with clients who have asthma or emphysema, due to the risk of respiratory depression.
            - □ Assess pain every 4 hr.
            - □ Remind clients who are receiving a fentanyl patch that the initial patch takes several hours to take effect. A short-acting pain medication will be administered for breakthrough pain.
            - □ Monitor clients, especially older adults, for manifestations of respiratory depression. If respirations are 12/min or less, stop the medication and notify provider immediately.
            - □ Monitor vital signs for hypotension and bradypnea.
            - □ Assess for nausea and vomiting.
            - □ Assess level of sedation (drowsiness, level of consciousness).
            - □ Monitor for constipation.
            - □ Encourage fluid intake and activity related to a decrease in gastric motility.
            - □ Monitor intake and output and fluid retention (common in clients who have an enlarged prostate).
        - ▪ Client Education
            - □ Encourage clients who do not have fluid restrictions due to other conditions to drink plenty of fluids to prevent constipation.
            - □ Teach the client how to use a patient-controlled analgesia (PCA) pump if applicable. The client is the only person who should push the medication administration button. Reassure the client that the safety lockout mechanism on the PCA prevents overdosing of medication.
            - □ If the client is receiving ventilation, the above nursing considerations and client education may vary.

- Teamwork and Collaboration
  - ○ Respiratory services should be consulted for ABGs, breathing treatments, and suctioning for airway management.
  - ○ Pulmonary services may be consulted for chest tube management and pulmonary care.
  - ○ Pain management services may be consulted if pain persists and/or is uncontrolled.
  - ○ Rehabilitation care may be consulted if the client has prolonged weakness and needs assistance with an increasing level of activity.
- Surgical Interventions
  - ○ Chest tube insertion
    - ▪ Chest tubes are inserted in the pleural space to drain fluid, blood, or air; re-establish a negative pressure; facilitate lung expansion; and restore normal intrapleural pressure.
    - ▪ Nursing Actions
      - □ Obtain informed consent, gather supplies, monitor the client's status (vital signs, SaO$_2$, chest tube drainage), report abnormalities to the health care provider, and administer pain medications.
      - □ Continually monitor vital signs and the client's response to the procedure.
      - □ Monitor chest tube placement and function.
- Care After Discharge
  - ○ Set up referral services (home health, respiratory services) to provide portable oxygen if needed.
  - ○ Client Education
    - ▪ Encourage the client to take rest periods as needed.
    - ▪ Remind the client to use proper hand hygiene to prevent infection.
    - ▪ Encourage immunizations for influenza and pneumonia.
    - ▪ Remind the client that recovery from a pneumothorax/hemothorax may be lengthy.
    - ▪ Educate the client and family about the illness, and encourage them to express their feelings.
    - ▪ Encourage smoking cessation if the client currently smokes.
    - ▪ Stress the importance of follow-up care, and instruct the client to report the following to the provider.
      - □ Upper respiratory infection
      - □ Fever
      - □ Cough
      - □ Difficulty breathing
      - □ Sharp chest pain

Complications

- Decreased cardiac output
    - ○ The amount of blood pumped by the heart decreases as intrathoracic pressure rises.
    - ○ Hypotension develops.
    - ○ Nursing Actions
        - ■ Administer IV fluids and blood products as prescribed.
        - ■ Monitor heart rate and rhythm.
        - ■ Monitor intake and output (chest tube drainage).
- Respiratory failure
    - ○ Inadequate gas exchange due to lung collapse
    - ○ Nursing Actions
        - ■ Prepare for mechanical ventilation.
        - ■ Continue respiratory assessment.

FLAIL CHEST

- Flail chest is the inability of the injured side of the chest to expand adequately upon inhalation and contract upon exhalation.
- One side of the chest is typically affected due to multiple rib fractures.

Assessment

- Risk Factors
    - ○ Multiple rib fractures (often caused by motor-vehicle crash or as a result of cardiopulmonary resuscitation on older adults)
- Objective Data
    - ○ Unequal chest expansion (the unaffected side of the chest will expand, while the affected side may appears to diminish in size or remain stationary)
    - ○ Tachycardia
    - ○ Hypotension
    - ○ Dyspnea
    - ○ Cyanosis
- Subjective Data
    - ○ Anxiety
    - ○ Chest pain

- Patient-Centered Care
  - Nursing Care
    - Administer humidified oxygen.
    - Monitor vital signs and SaO_2.
    - Review findings of pulmonary function tests, periodic chest x-rays, and ABGs.
    - Assess lung sounds, color, and capillary refill.
    - Promote lung expansion by encouraging deep breathing and proper positioning.
    - Maintain mechanical ventilation in the event of severe injury to establish adequate gas exchange and stabilize the injury.
    - Suction trachea and endotracheal tube as needed.
    - Administer pain medication as prescribed. Patient-controlled analgesia or an epidural block commonly is used.
    - Administer IV fluids as prescribed.
    - Monitor intake and output.
    - Offer support and reassurance by explaining all procedures.

APPLICATION EXERCISES

1. A nurse is assessing a client who has experienced a gunshot wound. Findings include blood pressure 108/55 mm Hg, heart rate 124/min, respiratory rate 36/min, temperature 38.6° C (101.4° F), and SaO$_2$ 95% on oxygen 15 L/min via nonrebreather mask. The client reports dyspnea and pain. The nurse reassesses the client 30 min later. Which of the following should the nurse report to the provider? (Select all that apply.)

_____ A. Distended neck veins

_____ B. Tracheal deviation

_____ C. Headache

_____ D. Nausea

_____ E. Heart rate 154/min

2. A nurse is reviewing the prescriptions for a client who has a pneumothorax. Which of the following actions should the nurse perform first?

A. Assess the client's pain.

B. Obtain a large-bore IV needle for decompression.

C. Administer lorazepam (Ativan).

D. Prepare for chest tube insertion.

3. A nurse is reviewing discharge instructions for a client who experienced a pneumothorax. Which of the following should be included in the teaching?

A. "Notify your provider if you experience weakness."

B. "You should be able to return to work in 1 week."

C. "You need to wear a mask when in crowded areas."

D. "Notify your provider if you experience a cough."

4. A nurse is preparing to administer morphine 2.5 mg IV bolus to a client who has a pneumothorax. Available is morphine injection 10 mg/mL. How many mL should the nurse administer? (Round the answer to the nearest tenth.)

5. A nurse in the emergency department is assessing a client with a suspected flail chest. Which of the following clinical findings confirm this diagnosis? (Select all that apply.)

_____ A. Bradycardia

_____ B. Cyanosis

_____ C. Hypotension

_____ D. Dyspnea

_____ E. Paradoxic chest movement

6. A nurse is teaching a newly licensed nurse regarding care for a client who has a hemothorax. What should be included in this review? Use the ATI Active Learning Template: System Disorder to complete this item to include the following:

A. Description of Disorder/Disease Process

B. Nursing Interventions: Describe three nursing interventions.

C. Medications: Describe two medications used for hemothorax.

APPLICATION EXERCISES KEY

1. A. **CORRECT:** Distended neck veins indicate that the client's condition is worsening and should be reported to the provider. Distended neck veins are due to impaired gas exchange, which compresses the blood vessels and limits blood return.

    B. **CORRECT:** Tracheal deviation indicates that the client's condition is worsening and should be reported to the provider. Tracheal deviation is due to altered intrathoracic pressure, which moves the trachea toward the unaffected side.

    C. INCORRECT: Headache is not indicated with this client's condition and does not need to be reported to the provider.

    D. INCORRECT: Nausea is not indicated with this client's condition and does not need to be reported to the provider.

    E. **CORRECT:** A heart rate of 154/min indicates that the client's condition is worsening and should be reported to the provider. An increased heart rate is due to impaired cardiac output as a result of trauma.

    Ⓝ NCLEX® Connection: Physiological Adaptations, Unexpected Response to Therapies

2. A. INCORRECT: Assessing the client's pain is important, but this is not the priority action at this time.

    B. **CORRECT:** According to the airway, breathing, circulation (ABC) priority-setting framework, establishing and maintaining the client's respiratory function is the priority. Therefore, obtaining a large-bore IV needle for decompression is the priority action by the nurse.

    C. INCORRECT: The client will likely be anxious, and a benzodiazepine medication can be administered, but this is not the priority action at this time.

    D. INCORRECT: The nurse should gather supplies to prepare for chest tube insertion, but this is not the priority action at this time.

    Ⓝ NCLEX® Connection: Pharmacological and Parenteral Therapies, Dosage Calculation

3. A. INCORRECT: The client does not need to report weakness. This is an expected finding following recovery from a pneumothorax.

    B. INCORRECT: The client should not expect to return to work in 1 week. The client should expect a lengthy recovery following a pneumothorax.

    C. INCORRECT: The client does not need to wear a mask following a pneumothorax. A mask is required for clients who are immunosuppressed.

    D. **CORRECT:** The client should notify the provider of a cough. This may indicate that the client has a respiratory infection and should be treated.

    Ⓝ NCLEX® Connection: Physiological Adaptations, Medical Emergencies

4. **0.3** mL

Using Ratio and Proportion

STEP 1: *What is the unit of measurement to calculate?*
mL

STEP 2: *What is the dose needed?*
Dose needed = Desired
2.5 mg

STEP 3: *What is the dose available? Dose available = Have*
10 mg

STEP 4: *Should the nurse convert the units of measurement?*
No

STEP 5: *What is the quantity of the dose available?*
1 mL

STEP 6: *Set up an equation and solve for X.*

$$\frac{Have}{Quantity} = \frac{Desired}{X}$$

$$\frac{10 \text{ mg}}{1 \text{ mL}} = \frac{2.5 \text{ mg}}{X \text{ mL}}$$

X = 0.25

STEP 7: *Round if necessary.*
0.25 = 0.3

STEP 8: *Reassess to determine whether the amount to give makes sense.*
If there is 10 mg/mL and the prescribed amount is 2.5 mg, it makes sense to give 0.3 mL. The nurse should administer morphine injection 0.3 mL IV bolus.

Using Desired Over Have

STEP 1: *What is the unit of measurement to calculate?*
mL

STEP 2: *What is the dose needed?*
Dose needed = Desired
2.5 mg

STEP 3: *What is the dose available? Dose available = Have*
10 mg

STEP 4: *Should the nurse convert the units of measurement?*
No

STEP 5: *What is the quantity of the dose available?*
1 mL

STEP 6: *Set up an equation and solve for X.*

$$\frac{Desired \times Quantity}{Have} = X$$

$$\frac{2.5 \text{ mg} \times 1 \text{ mL}}{10 \text{ mg}} = X \text{ mL}$$

X = 0.25

STEP 7: *Round if necessary.*
0.25 = 0.3

STEP 8: *Reassess to determine whether the amount to give makes sense.*
If there is 10 mg/mL and the prescribed amount is 2.5 mg, it makes sense to give 0.3 mL. The nurse should administer morphine injection 0.3 mL IV bolus.

Using Dimensional Analysis

STEP 1: *What is the unit of measurement to calculate?*
mL

STEP 2: *What quantity of the dose is available?*
1 mL

STEP 3: *What is the dose available? Dose available = Have*
10 mg

STEP 4: *What is the dose needed?*
Dose needed = Desired
2.5 mg

STEP 5: *Should the nurse convert the units of measurement?*
No

STEP 6: *Set up an equation of factors and solve for X.*

$$X = \frac{Quantity}{Have} \times \frac{Conversion (Have)}{Conversion (Desired)} \times \frac{Desired}{}$$

$$X \text{ mL} = \frac{1 \text{ mL}}{10 \text{ mg}} \times \frac{2.5 \text{ mg}}{}$$

X = 25

STEP 7: *Round if necessary.*
0.25 = 0.3

STEP 8: *Reassess to determine whether the amount to give makes sense.*
If there is 10 mg/mL and the prescribed amount is 2.5 mg, it makes sense to give 0.3 mL. The nurse should administer morphine injection 0.3 mL IV bolus.

(N) NCLEX® Connection: Physiological Adaptations, Illness Management

5. A. INCORRECT: Tachycardia is a clinical manifestation indicative of flail chest due to inadequate oxygenation.

    B. **CORRECT:** Cyanosis is a clinical manifestation indicative of flail chest due to inadequate oxygenation.

    C. **CORRECT:** Hypotension is a clinical manifestation indicative of flail chest.

    D. **CORRECT:** Dyspnea is a clinical manifestation indicative of flail chest. This is due to injury and the client's inability to effectively inhale and exhale.

    E. **CORRECT:** Paradoxic chest movement is a clinical manifestation indicative of flail chest. This is due to injury to the chest and the inability to inhale and exhale.

    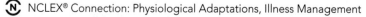 NCLEX® Connection: Physiological Adaptations, Pathophysiology

6. *Using the ATI Active Learning Template: System Disorder*

    A. Description of Disorder/Disease Process
    *   A hemothorax is an accumulation of blood in the pleural space.

    B. Nursing Interventions
    *   Administer oxygen therapy.
    *   Document ventilator settings hourly if the client is receiving ventilation.
    *   Monitor ABGs, SaO_2, CBC, and chest x-ray findings.
    *   Position the client to maximize ventilation (high-Fowler's = 90%).
    *   Provide emotional support to the client and family.
    *   Monitor chest tube drainage.
    *   Administer medications as prescribed.
    *   Encourage prompt medical attention when manifestations of infection occur.
    *   Auscultate heart and lung sounds and monitor vital signs every 4 hr.

    C. Medications
    *   Benzodiazepines (sedatives) – Lorazepam (Ativan) or midazolam may be used to decrease the client's anxiety.
    *   Opioid agonists (pain medications) – Morphine sulfate and fentanyl (Duragesic) are opioid agents used to treat moderate to severe pain. These medication acts on the mu and kappa receptors that help alleviate pain.

    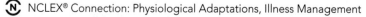 NCLEX® Connection: Physiological Adaptations, Illness Management

chapter 26

Overview

- Acute respiratory failure (ARF)
  - ARF is caused by failure to adequately ventilate and/or oxygenate.
  - Ventilatory failure is due to a mechanical abnormality of the lungs or chest wall, impaired muscle function (the diaphragm), or a malfunction in the respiratory control center of the brain.
  - Oxygenation failure can result from a lack of perfusion to the pulmonary capillary bed (pulmonary embolism) or a condition that alters the gas exchange medium (pulmonary edema, pneumonia).
  - Both inadequate ventilation and oxygenation can occur in individuals with diseased lungs (asthma, emphysema). Diseased lung tissue can cause oxygenation failure and increased work of breathing, eventually resulting in respiratory muscle fatigue and ventilatory failure.
  - Criteria for acute respiratory failure are based on ABG values.
  - ABGs that indicate ARF
    - Room air, PaO_2 less than 60 mm Hg, and SaO_2 less than 90%
    - $PaCO_2$ greater than 50 mm Hg in conjunction with a pH less than 7.30
- Acute respiratory distress syndrome (ARDS)
  - ARDS is a state of acute respiratory failure with a mortality rate of 25% to 40%.
  - Indicators present with ARDS
    - Dyspnea
    - Bilateral noncardiogenic pulmonary edema
    - Reduced lung compliance
    - Diffuse patchy bilateral pulmonary infiltrates
    - Severe hypoxemia despite administration of 100% oxygen
  - A systemic inflammatory response injures the alveolar-capillary membrane. It becomes permeable to large molecules, and the lung space is filled with fluid.
  - A reduction in surfactant weakens the alveoli, which causes collapse or filling of fluid, leading to worsening edema.
- Severe acute respiratory syndrome (SARS)
  - SARS is the result of a viral infection from a mutated strain of the coronaviruses, a group of viruses that also cause the common cold.
  - The virus invades the pulmonary tissue, which leads to an inflammatory response.
  - The virus is spread easily through airborne droplets from sneezing, coughing, or talking.
  - The virus does not spread to the bloodstream because it flourishes at temperatures slightly below normal core body temperature.
- Older adult clients have decreased pulmonary reserves due to normal lung changes, including decreased lung elasticity and thickening alveoli. Older adult clients may decompensate more quickly.

Assessment

- Risk Factors
  - ARF
    - Ventilatory failure
      - COPD
      - Pulmonary embolism
      - Pneumothorax
      - Flail chest
      - ARDS
      - Asthma
      - Pulmonary edema
      - Fibrosis of lung tissue
      - Neuromuscular disorders (multiple sclerosis, Guillain-Barré syndrome), spinal cord injuries, and cerebrovascular accidents that impair the client's rate and depth of respiration
      - Elevated intracranial pressure (closed-head injuries, cerebral edema, hemorrhagic stroke)
    - Oxygenation failure
      - Pneumonia
      - Hypoventilation
      - Hypovolemic shock
      - Pulmonary edema
      - Low hemoglobin
      - Low concentrations of oxygen (carbon monoxide poisoning, high altitude, smoke inhalation)
    - Combined ventilatory and oxygenation failure
      - Decreased gas exchange results in poor diffusion of oxygen into arterial blood with carbon dioxide retention
      - Hypoventilation (poor respiratory movement)
      - Chronic bronchitis
      - Asthma attack
      - Emphysema
      - Cardiac failure
        - Objective Data
          - Dyspnea
          - Orthopnea
        - Subjective Data
          - Cyanosis
          - Pallor
          - Hypoxemia

▷ Tachycardia

▷ Confusion

▷ Restlessness

▷ Hypercarbia (high levels of carbon dioxide in the blood)

▸ Laboratory Tests

▷ ABGs to confirm and monitor combined ventilatroy and oxygenation failure

▷ PaO$_2$ less than 60 mm Hg and oxygen saturation less than 90% on room air (hypoxemia, hypercarbia)

○ ARDS

▪ May result from localized lung damage or from the effects of other systemic problems

▪ Aspiration

▪ Pulmonary emboli (fat, amniotic fluid)

▪ Pneumonia and other pulmonary infections

▪ Sepsis

▪ Near-drowning accident

▪ Trauma

▪ Damage to the central nervous system

▪ Smoke or toxic gas inhalation

▪ Drug ingestion/overdose (heroin, opioids, salicylates)

○ SARS

▪ Exposure to an infected individual

▪ Immunocompromised individuals (chemotherapy, AIDS)

• Subjective Data

○ Shortness of breath

○ Dyspnea with or without exertion

○ Orthopnea (difficulty breathing lying flat)

• Objective Data

○ Physical Assessment Findings

▪ Rapid, shallow breathing

▪ Cyanotic, mottled, dusky skin

▪ Tachycardia

▪ Hypotension

▪ Substernal or suprasternal retractions

▪ Decreased SaO$_2$ (less than 90%)

▪ Adventitious breath sounds (wheezing, rales)

▪ Cardiac arrhythmias

▪ Confusion

▪ Lethargy

- ○ Laboratory Tests
  - ▪ ABGs to confirm and monitor ARF, ARDS, and SARS
    - ▫ PaO$_2$ less 60 mm Hg and oxygen saturation less than 90% on room air (hypoxemia)
    - ▫ PaCO$_2$ greater than 50 mm Hg and pH less than 7.30 (hypoxemia, hypercarbia)
- ○ Diagnostic Procedures
  - ▪ Chest x-ray
    - ▫ Results may include:
      - ▸ Pulmonary edema (ARF, ARDS)
      - ▸ Cardiomegaly (ARF)
      - ▸ Diffuse infiltrates and white-out or ground glass appearance (ARDS)
      - ▸ Infiltrates (SARS)
    - ▫ Nursing Actions
      - ▸ Assist with client positioning before and after the x-ray.
      - ▸ Interpret and communicate the results to the appropriate personnel in a timely manner.
  - ▪ Electrocardiogram (ECG) to rule out cardiac involvement
  - ▪ Hemodynamic monitoring
    - ▫ Pulmonary capillary wedge pressure with ARDS is usually low or within the expected reference range (4 to 12 mm Hg). Continuous hemodynamic monitoring is important for fluid management.
    - ▫ Nursing Actions
      - ▸ Monitor the ECG during placement of central venous pressure catheter and hemodynamic monitor.
      - ▸ Have resuscitation medications and equipment available.
      - ▸ Monitor hemodynamic waveforms and readings.
      - ▸ Confirm catheter placement using a chest x-ray.

Patient-Centered Care

- • Nursing Care
  - ○ Maintain a patent airway and monitor respiratory status every hour and more often as needed.
  - ○ Mechanical ventilation often is required. Positive-end expiratory pressure (PEEP) often is used to prevent alveolar collapse during expiration. Follow facility protocol for monitoring and documenting ventilator settings.
  - ○ Oxygenate before suctioning secretions to prevent further hypoxemia.
  - ○ Suction the client as needed.
  - ○ Assess and document sputum color, amount, and consistency.
  - ○ Assess lung sounds per facility protocol.
  - ○ Monitor for pneumothorax (a high PEEP may cause the lungs to collapse).

- ○ Obtain ABGs as prescribed and following each ventilator setting adjustment.
- ○ Maintain continuous ECG monitoring for changes that may indicate increased hypoxemia, especially when repositioning and applying suction.
- ○ Continually monitor vital signs, including SaO_2. Assess pain level.
- ○ Position the client to facilitate ventilation and perfusion.
- ○ Prevent infection.
  - ▪ Perform frequent hand hygiene.
  - ▪ Use appropriate suctioning technique.
  - ▪ Provide oral care every 2 hr and as needed.
  - ▪ Wear protective clothing (gown, gloves, mask) when appropriate.
- ○ Promote nutrition
  - ▪ Assess bowel sounds.
  - ▪ Monitor elimination patterns.
  - ▪ Obtain daily weights.
  - ▪ Monitor intake and output.
  - ▪ Administer enteral and/or parenteral feedings as prescribed.
  - ▪ Prevent aspiration with enteral feedings (elevate the head of the bed 30° to 45°).
    - □ Confirm nasogastric (NG) tube placement prior to feeding.
- ○ Provide emotional support to the client and family.
  - ▪ Encourage verbalization of feelings.
  - ▪ Provide alternative communication means (dry erase board, pen and paper).

- Medications

PHARMACOLOGIC AGENTS	
BENZODIAZEPINES	
Examples	› Lorazepam (Ativan) › Midazolam
Actions	› Reduces anxiety and resistance to ventilation and decreases oxygen consumption
Nursing Considerations	› Monitor respirations on clients who are not ventilated. › Monitor blood pressure and SaO_2. › Use cautiously in conjunction with opioid narcotics.
GENERAL ANESTHESIA	
Examples	› Propofol (Diprivan)
Actions	› Induces and maintains anesthesia › Sedates clients who are to be placed on mechanical ventilation
Nursing Considerations	› Contraindicated for clients with hyperlipidemia and egg allergies. › Administer only to clients who are intubated and ventilated. › Monitor ECG, blood pressure, and sedation levels. › IV rate must be slowed to assess neurological status. (Follow facility protocol.) › Monitor for hypotension. › Titrate to desired sedation.

PHARMACOLOGIC AGENTS

CORTICOSTEROIDS

Examples	› Methylprednisolone sodium succinate (Solu-Medrol) › Dexamethasone sodium phosphate
Actions	› Reduces WBC migration, decreases inflammation, and helps stabilize the alveolar-capillary membrane during ARDS
Nursing Considerations	› Discontinue medication gradually. › Administer with an antiulcer medication to prevent peptic ulcer formation. › Monitor weight and blood pressure. › Monitor glucose and electrolytes. › Advise the client to take oral doses with food and avoid stopping the medication suddenly.

OPIOID ANALGESICS

Examples	› Morphine sulfate › Fentanyl citrate (Sublimaze)
Actions	› Provides pain management
Nursing Considerations	› Monitor respirations on clients who are not ventilated. › Monitor blood pressure, heart rate, and SaO_2. › Monitor ABGs (hypercapnia can result from depressed respirations). › Use cautiously in conjunction with hypnotic sedatives. › Assess pain level and response to medication. › Have naloxone hydrochloride and resuscitation equipment available for severe respiratory depression in clients who are not receiving ventilation.

NEUROMUSCULAR BLOCKING AGENTS

Examples	› Vecuronium
Actions	› Facilitates ventilation and decreases oxygen consumption › Often used with painful ventilatory modes (inverse ratio ventilation and PEEP)
Nursing Considerations	› Administer only to clients who are intubated and ventilated. › Monitor ECG, blood pressure, and muscle strength. › Give pain medication and sedatives with neuromuscular blocking agents. › Neuromuscular blocking agents do not sedate or relieve pain. (Clients may be awake and frightened.) › Have neostigmine methylsulfate and atropine sulfate (Atropair) available to reverse the effects of the neuromuscular blocking agent. › Have resuscitation equipment available. › Reassure the client that paralysis is medication induced. › Explain all procedures.

PHARMACOLOGIC AGENTS	
ANTIBIOTICS SENSITIVE TO CULTURED ORGANISM(S)	
Examples	› Vancomycin (Vancocin)
Actions	› Treats identified organisms
Nursing Considerations	› Culture sputum prior to administration of first dose. › Monitor for a hypersensitivity reaction. › Give IV doses slowly. › Monitor the IV site for infiltration. › Do not give with other medications. › Monitor coagulopathy and renal function. › Advise client to take oral doses with food and finish the prescribed dose.

- Teamwork and Collaboration
  - Respiratory therapy
    - The respiratory therapist typically manages the ventilator, adjusts the settings, and provides chest physiotherapy to improve ventilation and chest expansion.
    - The respiratory therapist also may suction the endotracheal tube and administer inhalation medications, such as bronchodilators.
  - Physical therapy for extended ventilatory support and rehabilitation
  - Nutritional therapy
    - Enteral or parenteral feeding
    - Nutritional support following extubation
- Therapeutic Procedures
  - Intubation and mechanical ventilation
    - Artificial airway insertion with mechanical ventilation
    - Nursing Actions
      - Monitor ECG, SaO$_2$, lung sounds, and color.
      - Sedate as needed.
      - Provide reassurance to calm the client.
      - Have suction equipment, manual resuscitation bag, and face mask available at all times.
      - Suction secretions as needed.
      - Preintubation
        - Oxygenate with 100% oxygen.
        - Assist ventilation with manual resuscitation bag and face mask.
        - Have emergency resuscitation equipment readily available.

◻ Postintubation

▸ Assess bilateral lung sounds, symmetrical chest movement, and chest x-ray findings to confirm placement of the endotracheal tube.

▸ Secure the endotracheal tube per facility guidelines.

▸ Assess the balloon cuff for air leaks periodically.

◻ PEEP

▸ Positive pressure is applied at the end of expiration to keep the alveoli expanded.

▸ PEEP is added to the ventilator setting to increase oxygenation and improve lung expansion.

▪ Client Education

◻ Explain all procedures to the client.

◻ Reassure and calm the client.

◻ Explain to the client and family that the client will be unable to speak while the endotracheal tube is in place.

○ Kinetic therapy

▪ A special kinetic bed that rotates laterally alters client positioning to reduce atelectasis and improve ventilation.

▪ Nursing Actions

◻ Begin slowly and gradually to increase the degree of rotation as tolerated.

◻ Monitor ECG, SaO_2, breath sounds, and blood pressure.

◻ Stop rotation if the client becomes distressed.

◻ Provide routine skin care to prevent breakdown.

◻ Sedate as needed.

▪ Client Education

◻ Explain all procedures to the client.

Complications

• Endotracheal tube

○ Trauma during intubation or long-term intubation

▪ Can cause damage to trachea and vocal cords

▪ Nursing Actions

◻ Consider a tracheostomy for long-term ventilation.

○ Altered position of endotracheal tube

▪ Nursing Actions

◻ Check tube positioning every 1 to 2 hr and as needed.

◻ Assess lung sounds, SaO_2, and chest movement.

◻ Secure endotracheal tube per facility guidelines to maintain tube placement.

- ○ Aspiration pneumonia
  - ▪ Nursing Actions
    - ▫ Check the cuff on the endotracheal tube for leaks.
    - ▫ Assess suction contents for gastric secretions.
    - ▫ Verify NG tube placement.
- ○ Infection
  - ▪ Nursing Actions
    - ▫ Prevent infection by using proper hand hygiene and suctioning technique.
    - ▫ Assess color, amount, and consistency of secretions.
- ○ Blocked endotracheal tube indicated by high-pressure alarm on ventilator
  - ▪ Nursing Actions
    - ▫ Suction secretions to relieve a mucous plug or insert an oral airway to prevent biting on the tube.

- Mechanical Ventilation
  - ○ Increased intrathoracic pressure
    - ▪ PEEP increases intrathoracic pressure, which can cause a decreased blood return to the heart, decreased cardiac output, and/or hypotension.
    - ▪ Decreased cardiac output can activate the renin-angiotensin-aldosterone system, leading to fluid retention and/or decreased urine output.
    - ▪ Nursing Actions
      - ▫ Monitor input and output, weight, and hydration status.
    - ▪ Client Education
      - ▫ Advise the client to avoid using the Valsalva maneuver (straining with bowel movement), because it can further increase intrathoracic pressure.
  - ○ Barotrauma
    - ▪ Ventilation with positive pressure causes damage to the lungs (pneumothorax, subcutaneous emphysema).
    - ▪ Nursing Actions
      - ▫ Monitor oxygenation status and chest x-ray.
      - ▫ Assess for subcutaneous emphysema (crackles and/or air movement felt under skin).
      - ▫ Document all ventilator changes made.
        - ▸ A high-pressure ventilator alarm may indicate pneumothorax.
  - ○ Immobilization
    - ▪ Can result in muscle atrophy, pneumonia, and pressure sores
    - ▪ Nursing Actions
      - ▫ Reposition and suction every 2 hr and as needed.
      - ▫ Provide routine skin care.
      - ▫ Implement range-of-motion exercises to prevent muscle atrophy.

APPLICATION EXERCISES

1. A nurse in the emergency department is assessing a client who was in a motor vehicle crash. Findings include absent breath sounds in the left lower lobe with dyspnea, blood pressure 118/68 mm Hg, heart rate 124/min, respiratory rate 38/min, temperature 38.6° C (101.4° F), and SaO_2 92% on room air. Which of the following actions should the nurse take first?

    A. Obtain a chest x-ray.

    B. Prepare for chest tube insertion.

    C. Administer oxygen via a high-flow mask.

    D. Initiate IV access.

2. A nurse is orienting a newly licensed nurse on the purpose of administering vecuronium (Norcuron) to a client who has acute respiratory distress syndrome. Which of the following statements by the newly licensed nurse indicates understanding of the teaching?

    A. "This medication is given to treat infection."

    B. "This medication is given to facilitate ventilation."

    C. "This medication is given to decrease inflammation."

    D. "This medication is given to reduce anxiety."

3. A nurse is reviewing the health records of five clients. Which of the following clients are at risk for developing acute respiratory distress syndrome (ARDS)? (Select all that apply.)

    _____ A. A client who experienced a near-drowning incident

    _____ B. A client following coronary artery bypass graft surgery

    _____ C. A client who has a hemoglobin of 15.1 mg/dL

    _____ D. A client who has dysphagia

    _____ E. A client who experienced a drug overdose

4. A nurse is planning care for a client who has severe acute respiratory distress system (SARS). Which of the following should be included in the plan of care for this client? (Select all that apply.)

_____ A. Administration of antibiotics

_____ B. Providing supplemental oxygen

_____ C. Administration of antiviral medications

_____ D. Administration of bronchodilators

_____ E. Maintaining ventilatory support

5. A nurse is caring for a client who is receiving vecuronium (Norcuron) for acute respiratory distress syndrome (ARDS). Which of the following medications should the nurse anticipate administering with this medication? (Select all that apply.)

_____ A. Fentanyl (Duragesic)

_____ B. Furosemide (Lasix)

_____ C. Midazolam (Versed)

_____ D. Famotidine (Pepcid)

_____ E. Dexamethasone (Decadron)

6. A nurse is reviewing the plan of care for a client who has acute respiratory distress syndrome (ARDS). What should be included in the plan of care? Use the ATI Active Learning Template: Systems Disorder to complete this item to include the following sections:

A. Risk Factors: Describe three conditions related to acute respiratory distress syndrome (ARDS).

B. Patient-Centered Care: Describe three nursing care interventions to maintain oxygenation.

C. Complications: Identify two complications of ARDS.

APPLICATION EXERCISES KEY

1. A. INCORRECT: Obtaining a chest x-ray to determine the level of injury to the client's lungs is important, but is not the priority action at this time.

    B. INCORRECT: Preparing the client for chest tube insertion is important to facilitate lung expansion and restore normal intrapleural pressure, but is not the priority action at this time.

    C. **CORRECT:** According to the airway, breathing, and circulation (ABC) priority-setting framework, administering oxygen via high-flow mask is the priority action for the nurse to take.

    D. INCORRECT: Initiating IV access to administer medications as prescribed is important, but is not the priority action at this time.

    ⊗ NCLEX® Connection: Physiological Adaptations, Illness Management

2. A. INCORRECT: Antibiotics are given to treat infection.

    B. **CORRECT:** Vecuronium (Norcuron) is a neuromuscular blocking agent given to facilitate ventilation and decrease oxygen consumption.

    C. INCORRECT: Corticosteroids are given to treat inflammation.

    D. INCORRECT: Benzodiazepines are given to treat anxiety.

    ⊗ NCLEX® Connection: Pharmacological and Parenteral Therapies, Expected Actions/Outcomes

3. A. **CORRECT:** A client who experienced a near-drowning incident is at risk for developing ARDS due to trauma to the lungs and cerebral edema.

    B. **CORRECT:** A client following coronary artery bypass graft surgery is at risk for developing ARDS due to trauma to the chest.

    C. INCORRECT: Hemoglobin of 15.1 mg/dL is within the expected reference range. A client who has a low hemoglobin is at risk for developing ARDS.

    D. **CORRECT:** A client who has dysphagia is at risk for developing ARDS due to difficulty swallowing and risk for aspiration.

    E. **CORRECT:** A client who experienced a drug overdose is at risk for developing ARDS due to damage to the central nervous system.

    ⊗ NCLEX® Connection: Physiological Adaptations, Alterations in Body Systems

4. A. INCORRECT: Antibiotics are given to treat bacterial infections. This would not be indicated for SARS.

    B. **CORRECT:** Providing supplemental oxygen should be included in the plan of care for SARS. Oxygen is administered given to treat severe hypoxemia.

    C. INCORRECT: SARS is caused by the coronavirus. There are no effective antiviral medications to treat this virus.

    D. **CORRECT:** Administration of bronchodilators should be included in the plan of care for SARS. Bronchodilators are used to vasodilate the client's airway.

    E. **CORRECT:** Maintaining ventilatory support should be included in the plan of care for SARS. Intubation may be required to maintain a patent airway.

    Ⓝ NCLEX® Connection: Physiological Adaptations, Illness Management

5. A. **CORRECT:** Fentanyl (Duragesic) is a pain medication used to treat clients who have ARDS when a neuromuscular blocking agent such as vecuronium (Norcuron) is administered.

    B. INCORRECT: Furosemide (Lasix) is a diuretic used to release fluid from the body.

    C. **CORRECT:** Midazolam (Versed) is a sedative medication used to treat clients who have ARDS when a neuromuscular blocking agent such as vecuronium (Norcuron) is administered.

    D. INCORRECT: Famotidine (Pepcid) is a H_2 receptor antagonist given to treat upset stomach and heartburn.

    E. INCORRECT: Dexamethasone (Decadron) is a corticosteroid used to treat inflammation such as arthritis or an immune disorder.

    Ⓝ NCLEX® Connection: Pharmacological and Parenteral Therapies, Medication Administration

6. *Using the ATI Active Learning Template: Systems Disorder*

    A. Risk Factors

    -   May result from localized lung damage or from the effects of other systemic problems
    -   Aspiration
    -   Pulmonary emboli (fat, amniotic fluid)
    -   Pneumonia and other pulmonary infections
    -   Sepsis
    -   Near-drowning accident
    -   Trauma
    -   Damage to the central nervous system
    -   Smoke or toxic gas inhalation
    -   Drug ingestion/overdose (heroin, opioids, salicylates)

    B. Patient-Centered Care

    -   Maintain a patent airway and monitor respiratory status every hour as needed.
    -   Suction the client as needed.
    -   Assess lung sounds.
    -   Assess and document sputum color, amount, and consistency.
    -   Oxygenate before suctioning secretions to prevent further hypoxemia.
    -   Mechanical ventilation often is required. Positive-end expiratory pressure (PEEP) often is used to prevent alveolar collapse during expiration.
    -   Monitor for pneumothorax. (A high PEEP may cause the lungs to collapse.)
    -   Obtain ABGs as prescribed and following each ventilator setting adjustment.
    -   Maintain continuous ECG monitoring for changes that may indicate increased hypoxemia, especially when repositioning and applying suction.
    -   Continually monitor vital signs, including SaO_2.
    -   Position the client to facilitate ventilation and perfusion.

C. Complications

- Endotracheal tube
  - Trauma during intubation or long-term intubation
    - Can cause damage to trachea and vocal cords
    - Nursing Actions
      - Consider a tracheostomy for long-term ventilation.
  - Aspiration pneumonia
    - Nursing Actions
      - Check the cuff on the endotracheal tube for leaks.
      - Assess suction contents for gastric secretions.
      - Verify NG tube placement.
  - Infection
    - Nursing Actions
      - Prevent infection by using proper hand hygiene and suctioning technique.
      - Assess color, amount, and consistency of secretions.
  - Blocked endotracheal tube
    - The high-pressure alarm on the ventilator may indicate a blocked endotracheal tube.
    - Nursing Actions
      - Suction secretions to relieve a mucous plug or insert an oral airway to prevent biting on the tube.
  - Altered position of endotracheal tube
    - Nursing Actions
      - Check tube positioning every 1 to 2 hr and as needed.
      - Assess breath sounds, SaO_2, and chest movement.
      - Secure endotracheal tube per institution's guidelines to maintain tube placement.
- Mechanical Ventilation
  - Increased intrathoracic pressure
    - Positive pressure (PEEP) increases intrathoracic pressure, which can cause a decreased blood return to the heart, decreased cardiac output and/or hypotension.
    - Decreased cardiac output can activate the renin-angiotensin-aldosterone system, leading to fluid retention and/or decreased urine output.
    - Nursing Actions
      - Monitor input and output, weight, and hydration status.
    - Client Education
      - Advise the client to avoid using the Valsalva maneuver (straining with bowel movement), because it can further increase intrathoracic pressure.
  - Barotrauma
    - Ventilation with positive pressure causes damage to the lungs (pneumothorax, subcutaneous emphysema).

Ⓝ NCLEX® Connection: Physiological Adaptations, Pathophysiology

UNIT 4   Nursing Care of Clients with Cardiovascular Disorders

SECTIONS

› Diagnostic and Therapeutic Procedures
› Cardiac Disorders
› Vascular Disorders

NCLEX® CONNECTIONS

When reviewing the chapters in this unit, keep in mind the relevant sections of the NCLEX® outline, in particular:

Client Needs: Pharmacological and Parenteral Therapies	Client Needs: Reduction of Risk Potential	Client Needs: Physiological Adaptation
› Relevant topics/tasks include: » Adverse Effects/ Contraindications/Side Effects/Interactions › Identify a contraindication to the administration of a medication to the client. » Central Venous Access Devices › Provide care for the client with a central venous access device. » Parenteral/Intravenous Therapy › Apply knowledge and concepts of mathematics/ nursing procedures/ psychomotor skills when caring for a client receiving intravenous and parenteral therapy.	› Relevant topics/tasks include: » Diagnostic Tests › Apply knowledge of related nursing procedures and psychomotor skills when caring for clients undergoing diagnostic testing. » Changes/Abnormalities in Vital Signs › Evaluate invasive monitoring data. » System Specific Assessment › Assess the client for abnormal peripheral pulses after a procedure or treatment.	› Relevant topics/tasks include: » Alterations in Body Systems › Assist with invasive procedures. » Hemodynamics › Identify cardiac rhythm strip abnormalities. » Unexpected Responses to Therapies › Assess the client for unexpected adverse responses to therapy.

chapter 27

Overview

- Cardiovascular diagnostic procedures evaluate the functioning of the heart by monitoring for enzymes in the blood; using ultrasound to visualize the heart; determining the heart's response to exercise; and using catheters to determine blood volume, perfusion, fluid status, how the heart is pumping, and degree of artery blockage.

- Cardiovascular diagnostic procedures that nurses should be familiar with include:

  ○ Cardiac enzymes and lipid profile

  ○ Echocardiogram

  ○ Stress testing

  ○ Hemodynamic monitoring

  ○ Angiography

  ○ Vascular Access

Cardiac Enzymes and Lipid Profile

- Cardiac enzymes are released into the bloodstream when the heart muscle suffers ischemia. A lipid profile provides information regarding cholesterol levels and is used for early detection of heart disease.

- Cardiac enzymes are specific markers in diagnosing a myocardial infarction (MI).

- Indications

  ○ Angina

  ○ MI

  ○ Heart disease

  ○ Hyperlipidemia

- Interpretation of Findings

CARDIAC ENZYME	EXPECTED REFERENCE RANGE	ELEVATED LEVELS FIRST DETECTABLE FOLLOWING MYOCARDIAL INJURY	EXPECTED DURATION OF ELEVATED LEVELS
Creatine kinase MB isoenzyme (CK-MB) – more sensitive to myocardium	0% of total CK (30 to 170 units/L)	4 to 6 hr	3 days
Troponin T	Less than 0.2 ng/L	3 to 5 hr	14 to 21 days
Troponin I	Less than 0.03 ng/L	3 hr	7 to 10 days
Myoglobin	Less than 90 mcg/L	2 hr	24 hr

TEST	EXPECTED REFERENCE RANGE	PURPOSE
Cholesterol (total)	› Less than 200 mg/dL	› Screening for heart disease
HDL	› Females – 35 to 80 mg/dL › Males – 35 to 65 mg/dL	› "Good" cholesterol produced by the liver
LDL	› Less than 130 mg/dL	› "Bad" cholesterol can be up to 70% of total cholesterol
Triglycerides	› Males – 40 to 160 mg/dL › Females – 35 to 135 mg/dL › Older adults (over age 65) – 55 to 220 mg/dL	› Evaluating for atherosclerosis

- Preprocedure – Explain the purpose for the test to the client.
- Intraprocedure – A blood specimen is obtained via venipuncture.
- Postprocedure – Lab findings are discussed by the provider, and choice of treatment is determined.

Echocardiogram

- An echocardiogram is an ultrasound of the heart, which is used to diagnose valve disorders and cardiomyopathy.
- Indications
  - Cardiomyopathy
  - Heart failure
  - Angina
  - Myocardial infarction
- Preprocedure – Explain the reason for the test to the client. This is a noninvasive test and takes up to 1 hr.
- Intraprocedure – Instruct the client to lie on left side and remain still.
- Postprocedure – Provider reviews test results and a plan for follow-up care with the client.

Stress Testing

- The cardiac muscle is exercised by the client walking on a treadmill. This provides information regarding the workload of the heart. Once the client's heart rate reaches a certain rate, the test is discontinued.
  - Clients can become too tired, may be disabled or physically challenged, and be unable to finish the test. The provider can prescribe the test to be done as a pharmacological stress test.
- Indications
  - Angina
  - Heart Failure
  - Myocardial Infarction
  - Dysrhythmia

- Preprocedure
  - Nursing Actions
    - Ensure that a signed informed consent form is obtained.
    - Explain to the client that he will be walking on a treadmill, and comfortable shoes and clothing are recommended.
      - □ If a pharmacological stress test is prescribed, a medication such as adenosine (Adenocard) or dobutamine (Dobutrex) is given to stress the heart instead of walking on the treadmill.
    - Instruct the client to fast 2 to 4 hr before the procedure according to facility policy and to avoid tobacco, alcohol, and caffeine before the test.
- Intraprocedure
  - Nursing Actions
    - Apply a 12-lead ECG to monitor the client's heart rate during the test.
- Postprocedure
  - Nursing Actions
    - The client is monitored by 12-lead ECG and his blood pressure is checked frequently until he is stable.
    - The provider reviews findings with client.

Hemodynamic Monitoring

- Hemodynamic monitoring involves special indwelling catheters, which provide information about blood volume and perfusion, fluid status, and how well the heart is pumping.

 View Image: Hemodynamic Monitoring

  - Hemodynamic status is assessed with several parameters.
    - Central venous pressure (CVP)
    - Pulmonary artery pressure (PAP)
    - Pulmonary artery wedge pressure (PAWP)
    - Cardiac output (CO)
    - Intra arterial pressure
  - Mixed venous oxygen saturation (SvO_2) indicates the balance between oxygen supply and demand. It is measured by a pulmonary artery catheter with fiberoptics.
  - A hemodynamic monitoring system is used to display a client's hemodynamic data and includes:
    - Pressure transducer
    - Pressure tubing
    - Monitor
    - Pressure bag and flush device

- Arterial lines are placed in the radial (most common), brachial, or femoral artery.
    - Arterial lines provide continuous information about changes in blood pressure and permit the withdrawal of samples of arterial blood. Intra-arterial pressures can differ from cuff pressures.
    - The integrity of the arterial waveform should be assessed to verify the accuracy of blood pressure readings.
    - Monitor circulation in the limb with the arterial line (capillary refill, temperature, color).
    - Arterial lines are not used for IV fluid administration.
- Pulmonary Artery (PA) Catheters
    - The PA catheter is inserted into a large vein (internal jugular, femoral, subclavian, brachial) and threaded through the right atria and ventricle into a branch of the pulmonary artery.
    - PA catheters have multiple lumens, ports, and components that allow for various hemodynamic measurements, blood sampling, and infusion of IV fluids.
        - Proximal lumen can be used to measure right atrial pressure (CVP), infuse IV fluids, and obtain venous blood samples.
        - Distal lumen can be used to measure pulmonary artery pressures (PA systolic, PA diastolic, mean PA pressure, and PA wedge pressure). This lumen is not used for IV fluid administration.
        - Balloon inflation port is intermittently used for PAWP measurements. When not in use, it should be left deflated and in the "locked" position.
        - Thermistor measures the temperature differences between the right atrium and the pulmonary artery in order to determine cardiac output.
        - Additional infusion ports may be available, depending on the brand.
- Indications
    - Serious or critical illness
    - Heart failure
    - Post coronary artery bypass graft (CABG) clients
    - ARDS
    - Acute kidney injury
    - Burn injury
    - Trauma injury
- Interpretation of Findings

HEMODYNAMIC MONITORING	EXPECTED REFERENCE RANGES
Central venous pressure (CVP)	1 to 8 mm Hg
Pulmonary artery systolic (PAS)	15 to 26 mm Hg
Pulmonary artery diastolic (PAD)	5 to 15 mm Hg
Pulmonary artery wedge pressure (PAWP)	4 to 12 mm Hg
Cardiac output (CO)	4 to 7 L/min
Mixed venous oxygen saturation (SvO_2)	60% to 80%

- The intravascular volume in older adult clients is often reduced. Therefore, the nurse should anticipate lower hemodynamic values, particularly if dehydration is a complication.

- Preprocedure
  - Nursing Actions
    - Line Insertion
      - Ensure the client's understanding of the procedure prior to obtaining signed informed consent form.
      - Assemble the pressure monitoring system. Purge air from system and maintain sterility of connections.
      - Place the client in supine or Trendelenburg position.
      - Administer sedation and pain medications as prescribed.
      - Level transducer with phlebostatic axis (4th intercostal space, midaxillary line), which corresponds with the right atrium.
      - Zero system with atmospheric pressure, because the hemodynamic pressure lines must be calibrated to read zero atmospheric pressure.
      - Obtain initial readings as prescribed. Compare arterial blood pressure to noninvasive cuff pressure (NIBP).
      - Document the client's response.
- Intraprocedure

MONITOR FOR MANIFESTATIONS OF ALTERED HEMODYNAMICS			
PRELOAD		**AFTERLOAD**	
Right heart – CVP Left heart – PAWP		Right heart – pulmonary vascular resistance (PVR) Left heart – systemic vascular resistance (SVR)	
Elevated	Decreased	Elevated	Decreased
› Crackles in lungs › Jugular vein distention › Hepatomegaly › Peripheral edema › Taut skin turgor	› Poor skin turgor › Dry mucous membranes	› Cool extremities › Weak peripheral pulses	› Warm extremities › Bounding peripheral pulses

hypervolemia (handwritten annotation left margin, with *)
hypervolemia (handwritten annotation in table)
hypovolemia (handwritten annotation in table)

- Postprocedure
  - Nursing Actions
    - Obtain chest x-ray to confirm catheter placement.
    - Continually monitor respiratory and cardiac status (vital signs, heart rhythm, SaO_2).
      - Observe respiratory pattern and effort.
      - Compare noninvasive cuff pressure (NIBP) to arterial blood pressure.
    - Maintain line placement and integrity.
      - Observe and document waveforms. Report changes in waveforms to the provider, as this can indicate catheter migration or displacement.
      - Document catheter placement each shift and as needed (after movement for transport).
      - Monitor and secure connections between pressure tubing, transducers, and catheter ports.

- Obtain readings from hemodynamic catheter as prescribed.
  - Place the client in supine position prior to recording hemodynamic values. Head of bed can be elevated 15° to 30°.
  - Level the transducer at the phlebostatic axis before readings and with all position changes.
  - Zero system to atmospheric pressure.
  - Compare hemodynamic findings to physical assessment.
  - Monitor trends in values obtained over time.
- Complications
  - Infection/Sepsis
    - Infection at insertion site can occur if aseptic technique is not used.
    - Nursing Actions
      - Change dressings per facility protocol and as needed.
      - Use surgical aseptic technique with dressing changes (mask, sterile gloves, maintain sterile field).
      - Monitor for evidence of infection (elevated WBC count or temperature).
      - Perform thorough hand hygiene.
      - Collect specimens (blood cultures, catheter tip cultures) and deliver to the laboratory.
      - Administer antibiotic therapy as prescribed.
      - Administer IV fluids for intravascular support.
      - Administer vasopressors (dopamine) for vasodilation secondary to sepsis.
  - Embolism
    - Plaque or a clot can become dislodged during the procedure.
    - Nursing Actions
      - Use 0.9% sodium chloride for flushing system. (Heparin is not used, and heparin-coated catheters are no longer used due to the possibility of heparin-induced thrombocytopenia.)
      - Avoid introduction of air into flushing system to prevent air embolism.
      - Recognize that there is a risk of pneumothorax with insertion of the line.
      - Recognize that there is a risk of dysrhythmias with insertion/movement of the line.

Angiography

- A coronary angiogram, also called a cardiac catheterization, is an invasive diagnostic procedure used to evaluate the presence and degree of coronary artery blockage.
  - Angiography also can be done on the lower extremities to determine blood flow and areas of blockage.
  - Angiography involves the insertion of a catheter into a femoral (sometimes a brachial) vessel and threading it into the right or left side of the heart. Coronary artery narrowings and/or occlusions are identified by the injection of contrast media under fluoroscopy.

View Image: Cardiac Catheter

- Indications
  - Unstable angina and ECG changes (T wave inversion, ST segment elevation, depression)
  - Confirm and determine location and extent of heart disease.
- Preprocedure
  - Nursing Actions
    - Maintain the client on NPO status for at least 8 hr (due to the risk for aspiration when lying flat for the procedure).
    - Ensure that the consent form is signed.
    - Assess that the client and family understand the procedure.
    - Assess for iodine/shellfish allergy (contrast media).
    - Assess renal function prior to introduction of contrast dye.
    - Administer premedications as prescribed (methylprednisone [Solu-Medrol], diphenhydramine [Benadryl]).
  - Client Education
    - Instruct the client that he is awake and sedated during procedure. A local anesthetic is used. A small incision is made, often in the groin to insert the catheter. The client can feel warmth and flushed when the dye is inserted. After the procedure, the client must keep the affected leg straight. Pressure (a sandbag) can be placed on the incision to prevent bleeding.
- Intraprocedure
  - Nursing Actions
    - Administer sedatives and analgesia as prescribed.
    - Continually monitor vital signs and heart rhythm.
    - Be prepared to intervene for dysrhythmias.
    - Have resuscitation equipment and emergency medications readily available.
- Postprocedure
  - Nursing Actions
    - Assess vital signs every 15 min x 4, every 30 min x 2, every hour x 4, and then every 4 hr (follow facility protocol).
    - Assess the groin site at the same intervals for:
      - Bleeding and hematoma formation
      - Thrombosis; document pedal pulse, color, temperature
    - Maintain bed rest in supine position with extremity straight for prescribed time.
      - A vascular closure devise may be used to hasten hemostasis following catheter removal.
      - Older adult clients can have arthritis, which can make lying in bed for 4 to 6 hr after the procedure painful. The provider can be notified for prescribed medication.

- Conduct continuous cardiac monitoring for dysrhythmias (reperfusion following angioplasty can cause dysrhythmias).

- Administer antiplatelet or thrombolytic agents as prescribed to prevent clot formation and restenosis.

  □ Aspirin

  □ Clopidogrel (Plavix), ticlopidine (Ticlid)

  □ Heparin

  □ Low molecular weight heparin (enoxaparin [Lovenox])

  □ GP IIb/IIIa inhibitors, such as eptifibatide (Integrilin)

- Administer anxiolytics (Ativan) and analgesia (morphine) as needed.

- Monitor urine output and administer IV fluids for hydration.

  □ Contrast media acts as an osmotic diuretic.

- Perform/assist with sheath removal from vessel.

  □ Apply pressure to arterial/venous sites for the prescribed period of time (varies depending upon the method used for vessel closure).

  □ Observe for vagal response (hypotension, bradycardia) from compression of nerves.

  □ Apply pressure dressing.

- Client Education

  - Instruct the client to:

    □ Avoid strenuous exercise for the prescribed period of time.

    □ Immediately report bleeding from the insertion site, chest pain, shortness of breath, and changes in the color or temperature of the extremity.

    □ Restrict lifting (less than 10 lb [4.5 kg]) for the prescribed period of time.

  - Clients who have stent placement will receive anticoagulation therapy for 6 to 8 weeks. Instruct the client to:

    □ Take the medication at the same time each day.

    □ Have regular laboratory tests to determine therapeutic levels.

    □ Avoid activities that could cause bleeding (use soft toothbrush, wear shoes when out of bed).

  - Encourage the client to follow lifestyle guidelines (manage weight, consume a low-fat/low-sodium diet, get regular exercise, stop smoking, decrease alcohol intake).

- Complications

  - Cardiac Tamponade

    - Cardiac tamponade can result from fluid accumulation in the pericardial sac.

      □ Manifestations include hypotension, jugular venous distention, muffled heart sounds, and paradoxical pulse (variance of 10 mm Hg or more in systolic blood pressure between expiration and inspiration).

      □ Hemodynamic monitoring reveals intracardiac and pulmonary artery pressures are similar and elevated (plateau pressures).

- Nursing Actions
  - Notify the provider immediately.
  - Administer IV fluids to combat hypotension as prescribed.
  - Obtain a chest x-ray or echocardiogram to confirm diagnosis.
  - Prepare the client for pericardiocentesis (informed consent, gather materials, administer medications as appropriate).
    - ▸ Monitor hemodynamic pressures as they normalize.
    - ▸ Monitor heart rhythm; changes indicate improper positioning of the needle.
    - ▸ Monitor for reoccurrence of signs after the procedure.

- Hematoma Formation
  - Blood clots may form near the insertion site.
  - Nursing Actions
    - Assess the groin at prescribed intervals and as needed.
    - Hold pressure for uncontrolled oozing/bleeding.
    - Monitor peripheral circulation.
    - Notify the provider.

- Restenosis of Treated Vessel
  - Clot reformation in the coronary artery can occur immediately or several weeks after procedure.
  - Nursing Actions
    - Assess ECG patterns and for occurrence of chest pain.
    - Notify the provider immediately.
    - Prepare the client for return to the cardiac catheterization laboratory.

- Retroperitoneal Bleeding
  - Bleeding into retroperitoneal space (abdominal cavity behind the peritoneum) can occur due to femoral artery puncture.
  - Nursing Actions
    - Assess for flank pain and hypotension.
    - Notify the provider immediately.
    - Administer IV fluids and blood products as prescribed.

Vascular Access

- The site and type of vascular access is determined by the characteristics of the prescribed therapy (medication type, pH and osmolality, length of time for therapy). The goal is to minimize the number of catheter insertions and the risk for adverse reactions.
  - ○ Age-related loss of skin turgor and poor vein conditions pose challenges to vascular access. Using veins in the hand is not appropriate for older adult clients.
- Central Catheters
  - ○ Central catheters are appropriate for any fluids due to rapid hemodilution in the superior vena cava (SVC).
  - ○ Ensure x-ray verification of tip placement prior to use.
  - ○ All central catheters are inserted by a provider with the exception of peripherally inserted central catheter (PICC) lines, which may be inserted by a specially trained nurse. Insertion occurs in the OR, the client's room, or in an outpatient facility.
  - ○ Tunneled and implanted catheters require surgical removal.
  - ○ Central catheter types include nontunneled percutaneous central catheter (triple lumen), PICC, tunneled percutaneous central catheter (Hickman, Groshong), and implanted port.
    - Nontunneled percutaneous central catheter
      - □ Description – 15 to 20 cm in length with one to three lumens
      - □ Length of use – short-term use only
      - □ Insertion location – subclavian vein, jugular vein; tip in the distal third of the superior vena cava
      - □ Indications – administration of blood, long-term administration of chemotherapeutic agents, antibiotics, and total parenteral nutrition
    - Peripherally inserted central catheter
      - □ Description – 40 to 65 cm with single or multiple lumens
      - □ Length of use – up to 12 months
      - □ Insertion location – basilic or cephalic vein at least one finger's breadth below or above the antecubital fossa; the catheter should be advanced until the tip is positioned in the lower one-third of the superior vena cava.
      - □ Indications – administration of blood, long-term administration of chemotherapeutic agents, antibiotics, and total parenteral nutrition
      - □ Preprocedure
        - ▸ PICCs may be inserted by specially trained nurses.
        - ▸ Apply local anesthetic at insertion site and insert the catheter using surgical aseptic technique.

- ▫ Postprocedure
  - ▸ Apply an initial dressing of gauze and replace with a transparent dressing within 24 hr.
  - ▸ An initial x-ray should be taken to ensure proper placement.
  - ▸ Care of a PICC line includes:
    - ▹ Assessing the site at least every 8 hr. Note redness, swelling, drainage, tenderness, and condition of the dressing.
    - ▹ Changing the tube and positive pressure cap per facility protocol (usually a minimum of every 3 days for the hospitalized client).
    - ▹ Using 10 mL or larger syringe to flush the line.
    - ▹ Cleaning the insertion port with alcohol for 3 seconds and allowing it to dry completely prior to accessing it.
    - ▹ Performing flush for intermittent medication administration per facility protocol, usually with 10 mL of 0.9% sodium chloride before, between, and after medications.
    - ▹ Obtaining blood samples by withdrawing 10 mL of blood and discarding; taking a second syringe and withdrawing 10 mL of blood for sample; taking a third syringe and flushing with 10 mL of 0.9% sodium chloride (follow facility protocol for specific flushing guidelines).
    - ▹ Using transparent dressing. Follow facility protocol for dressing changes, usually every 7 days and when indicated (wet, loose, soiled).
    - ▹ Advising the client not to immerse his arm in water. To shower, cover dressing site to avoid water exposure.
    - ▹ Educating the client not to have blood pressure taken in arm with PICC line.
- ▪ Tunneled percutaneous central catheter
  - ▫ Description – 48 to 104 cm (19 to 41 in) in length.
  - ▫ For long-term use.
  - ▫ Insertion location – A portion of the catheter lies in a subcutaneous tunnel separating the point where the catheter enters the vein from where it enters the skin with a cuff. Tissue granulates into the cuff to provide a mechanical barrier to organisms and an anchoring for the catheter.
  - ▫ Indications – Frequent and long-term need for vascular access.
  - ▫ No dressing is needed because entrance into skin and vein are separate and tissue granulates into catheter cuff, providing a barrier. Groshong catheters have pressure-sensitive valves to prevent blood reflux and do not require a clamp.

- Implanted port
  - □ Description – Port is comprised of a small reservoir covered by a thick septum.
  - □ Insertion location – Port is surgically implanted into chest wall pocket; the catheter is inserted into the subclavian vein with the tip in the superior vena cava.
  - □ Indications – Long-term (a year or more) need for vascular access; commonly used for chemotherapy.
  - □ Preprocedure
    - ‣ To access an implanted port:
      - ▷ Apply local anesthetic to skin if indicated. Palpate skin to locate the port body septum to ensure proper insertion of the needle.
      - ▷ Clean the skin with alcohol for at least 3 seconds and allow to dry prior to insertion of the needle.
      - ▷ Access with a noncoring (Huber) needle.
  - □ Postprocedure
    - ‣ Flush (with 10 mL 0.9% sodium chloride or per facility protocol) after every use and at least once per month.
- Complications
  - ○ Phlebitis can be chemical (osmolarity or pH is different, veins too small for substance), bacterial, or mechanical irritation (excess IV manipulation).
    - Nursing Actions
      - □ Monitor for findings of:
        - ‣ Erythema at the site (usual initial sign)
        - ‣ Pain or burning at the site and the length of the vein
        - ‣ Discomfort when the skin over the tip is palpated
        - ‣ Warmth over the site
        - ‣ Edema at the site
        - ‣ Vein indurated (hard), red streak, and/or cordlike
        - ‣ Slowing infusion rate
        - ‣ Temperature elevation of 1° F or more
        - ‣ Infection appearing 7 to 10 days after insertion

- Take preventive measures.
  - ▸ Observe the site every 2 hr for infection or infiltration.
  - ▸ Nontunneled catheters require an intact sterile dressing (tunneled catheters do not).
  - ▸ Clean the site with 2% chlorhexidine-based preparation, 70% alcohol, or tincture of iodine per facility protocol with friction. Let preparation air dry before insertion.
  - ▸ Change IV sites every 3 days or per facility protocol.
- Provide treatment.
  - ▸ Discontinue the IV.
  - ▸ Apply warm compresses.
  - ▸ Restart with new tubing/infusate.

○ Occlusion is a blockage in the access device that impedes flow.
- ■ Nursing Actions
  - Flush the line at least every 12 hr (3 mL for peripheral, 10 mL for central lines) to maintain patency.
    - ▸ Studies show that 0.9% sodium chloride is as effective as heparinized flush solutions to maintain catheter patency. Follow facility policy.
  - Flush ports after every use and at least once a month while implanted.
  - Administer urokinase (Abbokinase) to lyse obstructions per facility protocol.

○ Catheter Thrombosis/Emboli – Blood can coagulate and cause an occlusion.
- ■ Nursing Actions
  - Flush the line per facility protocol.
  - Do not force fluid if resistance is encountered (may dislodge thrombosis).
  - Use a 10 mL or larger syringe to avoid excess pressure per square inch (PSI) that could cause catheter fracture/rupture.

○ Infiltration and Extravasation
- ■ Infiltration is fluid leaking into surrounding subcutaneous tissue, and extravasation is unintentional infiltration of a vesicant medication that causes tissue damage.
- ■ Causes
  - Improper IV insertion
  - Improper vein selection (too small, too fragile, poor location)
  - Irritating infusates that weaken and rupture the vein wall
  - Overmanipulation of the IV catheter
  - Improper taping that allows IV catheter movement and vein compromise
  - Tape too tight, becoming a tourniquet
- ■ Nursing Actions
  - Monitor for evidence of:
    - ▸ Swelling around the site and proximal or distal to the IV
    - ▸ Edema "puffiness" in the dependent area of the extremity
    - ▸ Skin taut or rigid with blanching
    - ▸ Sensation of coolness

□ Check the client and the system.

▶ Putting pressure on the vein just beyond the tip of the catheter should stop the IV flow. If flow is not affected, the fluid is probably going into the subcutaneous tissue.

▶ The infusion pump alarm may sound due to occlusion. (Do not rely on the alarm because pressure must be significant to activate.)

▶ "Leaking" at the site after confirming tube connections indicates a problem.

▶ Blood return is not considered a reliable indicator.

□ Take preventive measures.

▶ Do not use arm with midline catheter (MIL) or PICC for blood pressure or phlebotomy.

▶ Do not use hand veins in older adult clients who have minimal subcutaneous tissue.

▶ Do not use hand veins for vesicant medication.

▶ Use an arm board for sites affected by the motion of a joint.

□ Provide treatment.

▶ Remove using direct pressure with gauze sponge until bleeding stops.

▶ Apply cool compresses.

▶ Elevation is optional.

▶ Avoid starting a new IV site in the same extremity.

○ Air Embolism – Vascular access can result in gas bubbles being introduced into the vascular system.

▪ Nursing Actions

□ Leave central lines clamped when not in use.

□ Have the client hold breath while the tubing is changed.

□ If the client has sudden shortness of breath, place in Trendelenburg on left side, give oxygen, and notify the provider (to trap and aspirate air).

○ Mechanical Complications

▪ Mechanical complications include accidental dislodgement, mesh damage on port catheters, and catheter migration.

▪ Nursing Actions

□ To prevent accidental dislodgement:

▶ Cover the extremity site with stretch netting.

▶ Wrap a washcloth folded in thirds around the arm before applying a needed restraint. This prevents the restraint from sliding and dislodging the catheter.

▶ Only tape the catheter hub to minimize manipulation.

▶ When removing the dressing, pull from distal to proximal.

▶ If the skin is oily, "defat" oils with alcohol and air-dry before antiseptic cleansing.

□ Use only a noncoring (Huber) needle to avoid damaging the mesh on port catheters.

□ Note the length to help detect catheter migration. Notify the provider of any changes in length.

APPLICATION EXERCISES

1. A nurse is orienting a newly licensed nurse on the care of a client who is receiving hemodynamic monitoring. Which of the following statements by the newly licensed nurse indicates the teaching was effective?

    A. "Air should be instilled into the monitoring system."

    B. "The client should be in the prone position."

    C. "The transducer should be level with the 2nd intercostal space."

    D. "A chest x-ray is needed to verify placement."

2. A nurse is caring for a client following a coronary artery bypass graft (CABG). Hemodynamic monitoring has been initiated. Which of the following actions by the nurse facilitate correct monitoring readings? (Select all that apply.)

    _____ A. Place the client in high-Fowler's position.

    _____ B. Level transducer to phlebostatic axis.

    _____ C. Zero transducer to room air.

    _____ D. Observe trends in readings.

    _____ E. Compare readings to physical assessment.

3. A nurse is caring for a client who is receiving hemodynamic monitoring and has the following hemodynamic readings: PAS 34 mm Hg, PAD 21 mm Hg, PAWP 16 mm Hg, and CVP 12 mm Hg. For which of the following is the client at risk? (Select all that apply.)

    _____ A. Heart failure

    _____ B. Cor pulmonale

    _____ C. Hypovolemic shock

    _____ D. Pulmonary hypertension

    _____ E. Peripheral edema

4. A nurse is teaching a client the importance of remaining still following angiography. Which of the following is an appropriate statement by the nurse?

    A. "Moving in bed raises your blood pressure."

    B. "Too much activity increases your risk for infection."

    C. "Moving in bed increases your risk of a complication due to anesthesia."

    D. "Too much activity places you at risk for bleeding."

5. A nurse is reviewing a new prescription to administer 0.9% sodium chloride IV at 50 mL/hr to a client who is receiving hemodynamic monitoring and has an indwelling IV catheter in the left hand. Which of the following sites can be used for administering this solution? (Select all that apply.)

_____ A. Peripheral saline lock

_____ B. Port on the arterial line

_____ C. Port on proximal (CVP) lumen of pulmonary artery (PA) catheter

_____ D. Port on distal lumen of PA catheter

_____ E. Balloon inflation port

6. A nurse is reviewing the plan of care with a client who is scheduled for a stress test. What should the nurse include in the review? Use the ATI Active Learning Template: Diagnostic Procedure to complete this item to include the following:

    A. Purpose of the Procedure

    B. Indications: List at least two.

    C. Nursing Actions: Describe at least two preoperative actions.

APPLICATION EXERCISES KEY

1. A. INCORRECT: Air should be purged from, not instilled into, the monitoring system.

    B. INCORRECT: The client should be placed in the supine or Trendelenburg position.

    C. INCORRECT: For hemodynamic monitoring, the transducer should be level with the 4th intercostal space, which is at the base of the right atrium.

    D. **CORRECT:** A chest x-ray is obtained to confirm proper placement of the lines.

     NCLEX® Connection: Reduction of Risk Potential, Potential for Complications of Diagnostic Tests/ Treatments/Procedures

2. A. INCORRECT: The client is placed with the head elevated to 45° during hemodynamic readings.

    B. **CORRECT:** The level of the transducer should be at the phlebostatic axis (right atrium) to ensure an accurate reading is obtained.

    C. **CORRECT:** The transducer is zeroed to room air to ensure an accurate reading is obtained. Hemodynamic pressure lines should be calibrated to read atmospheric pressure as zero.

    D. **CORRECT:** The trend of the client's pressure readings assists in providing appropriate medical treatment.

    E. **CORRECT:** Readings are compared to the client's physical assessment findings to evaluate the client's condition and the appropriate treatment provided.

     NCLEX® Connection: Reduction of Risk Potential, Potential for Complications of Diagnostic Tests/ Treatments/Procedures

3. A. **CORRECT:** Heart failure is associated with left ventricular failure and would be indicated by elevated hemodynamic readings.

    B. **CORRECT:** Cor pulmonale is associated with the right side of the heart, and pulmonary problems would be indicated by elevated hemodynamic readings.

    C. INCORRECT: Hypovolemic shock is associated with fluid loss and would be indicated by low hemodynamic readings.

    D. **CORRECT:** Pulmonary hypertension is associated with high blood pressure in the pulmonary arteries, affects the right side of the heart, and would be indicated by elevated hemodynamic readings.

    E. **CORRECT:** Peripheral edema is associated with left ventricular failure and would be indicated by elevated hemodynamic readings.

    NCLEX® Connection: Physiological Adaptations, Hemodynamics

4. A. INCORRECT: Avoiding an increase in blood pressure is not the purpose the client should remain still.

   B. INCORRECT: Decreasing the risk for infection is not the purpose the client should remain still.

   C. INCORRECT: Anesthesia risk is not the purpose that the client should remain still.

   D. **CORRECT:** Following angiography, it is important that the client lie still due to the increased risk for bleeding at the insertion site.

   Ⓝ NCLEX® Connection: Reduction of Risk Potential, Potential for Complications of Diagnostic Tests/ Treatments/Procedures

5. A. **CORRECT:** IV fluid administration can occur via a lock on a peripheral IV catheter.

   B. INCORRECT: An arterial line is used for hemodynamic monitoring and the collection of blood samples. It should not be used for IV fluid administration.

   C. **CORRECT:** The proximal (CVP) lumen of a PA catheter is used for hemodynamic monitoring and can also be used for IV fluid administration.

   D. INCORRECT: The distal lumen of a PA catheter is used for hemodynamic monitoring and the collection of blood samples. It should not be used for IV fluid administration.

   E. INCORRECT: The balloon inflation port is intermittently used for pulmonary artery wedge pressure (PAWP) measurements. When not in use, the balloon is deflated.

   Ⓝ NCLEX® Connection: Physiological Adaptations, Hemodynamics

6. *Using the ATI Active Learning Template: Diagnostic Procedure*

   A. Purpose of the Procedure
      * The cardiac muscle is exercised by walking on a treadmill. This provides information regarding the workload of the heart.

   B. Indications
      * Angina
      * Heart Failure
      * Myocardial Infarction
      * Dysrhythmia

   C. Nursing Actions
      * Ensure that a signed informed consent form is obtained.
      * Explain to the client that he will be walking on a treadmill. Comfortable shoes and clothing are recommended.
      * Explain that a pharmacological stress test can be prescribed if the client cannot walk on the treadmill and complete the test. A medication such as adenosine (Adenocard) or dobutamine (Dobutrex) is administered to stress the heart instead of walking on the treadmill.
      * The client is instructed to fast 2 to 4 hr before the procedure or according to facility policy and to avoid tobacco, alcohol, and caffeine before the test.

   Ⓝ NCLEX® Connection: Reduction of Risk Potential, Diagnostic Tests

chapter 28

Overview

- Cardiac electrical activity can be monitored by using an ECG. The heart's electrical activity can be monitored by a standard 12-lead ECG (resting ECG), ambulatory ECG (Holter monitoring), continuous cardiac monitoring, or by telemetry.

 View Image: ECG Strip

- Cardiac dysrhythmias are heartbeat disturbances (beat formation, beat conduction, or myocardial response to beat).

- Nurses should be familiar with cardioversion and defibrillation procedures for treating dysrhythmias.

Electrocardiography

- Electrocardiography uses an electrocardiograph to record the electrical activity of the heart over time. The electrocardiograph is connected by wires (leads) to skin electrodes placed on the chest and limbs of a client.

  ○ Continuous cardiac monitoring requires the client to be in close proximity to the monitoring system.

  ○ Telemetry allows the client to ambulate while maintaining proximity to the monitoring system.

- Indications

 View Images
› Premature Atrial Complexes (PACs)   › Premature Ventricular Complexes (PVCs)
› Ventricular Tachycardia   › Atrial Fibrillation

  ○ Dysrhythmias

    ▪ Sinus bradycardia and tachycardia

    ▪ Atrioventricular (AV) blocks

    ▪ Atrial fibrillation

    ▪ Ventricular asystole

    ▪ Premature atrial complexes (PACs) and premature ventricular complexes (PVCs)

    ▪ Supraventricular tachycardia

    ▪ Ventricular tachycardia

    ▪ Ventricular fibrillation

- ○ Client Presentation
  - ▪ Cardiovascular disease
  - ▪ Myocardial infarction (MI)
  - ▪ Hypoxia
  - ▪ Acid-base imbalances
  - ▪ Electrolyte disturbances
  - ▪ Kidney failure, liver, or lung disease
  - ▪ Pericarditis
  - ▪ Drug or alcohol use
  - ▪ Hypovolemia
  - ▪ Shock
- Preprocedure
  - ○ Nursing actions
    - ▪ Prepare the client for a 12-lead ECG, if prescribed.
      - □ Position the client in a supine position with chest exposed.
      - □ Wash the client's skin to remove oils.
      - □ Attach one electrode to each of the client's extremities by applying electrodes to flat surfaces above the wrists and ankles and the other six electrodes to the chest, avoiding chest hair. (Chest hair may need to be shaved on male clients).

 View Image: ECG Lead Placement

- Intraprocedure
  - ○ Nursing actions
    - ▪ Instruct the client to remain still and breathe normally while the 12-lead ECG is performed.
    - ▪ Monitor the client for manifestations of dysrhythmia (chest pain, decreased level of consciousness, and shortness of breath) and hypoxia.
- Postprocedure
  - ○ Nursing actions
    - ▪ Remove leads from client, print ECG report, and notify the provider.
    - ▪ Apply a Holter monitor if the client is on a telemetry unit and/or needs continuous cardiac monitoring.
    - ▪ Continue to monitor the client for dysrhythmia.

Dysrhythmias

- Dysrhythmias are classified by the following:
  - Site of origin – sinoatrial (SA) node, atria, atrioventricular (AV) node, or ventricle
    - Electrophysiological study to determine the area of the heart causing the dysrhythmia. Ablation of the area is possible.
  - Effect on the rate and rhythm of the heart – bradycardia, tachycardia, heart block, premature beat, flutter, fibrillation, or asystole
- Dysrhythmias can be benign or life-threatening.
- The life-threatening effects of dysrhythmias are generally related to decreased cardiac output and ineffective tissue perfusion.
- Cardiac dysrhythmias are a primary cause of death in clients suffering acute MI and other sudden death disorders.
- Rapid recognition and treatment of serious dysrhythmias is essential to preserve life. Treatment is based on the cardiac rhythm, which can require cardioversion, defibrillation or pacemaker insertion, and/or medications.

DYSRHYTHMIA	MEDICATION	ELECTRICAL MANAGEMENT
› Bradycardia (any rhythm less than 60/min) › Treat if the client is symptomatic	› Atropine and isoproterenol	› Pacemaker
› Atrial fibrillation, supraventricular tachycardia (SVT), or ventricular tachycardia with pulse	› Amiodarone, adenosine, and verapamil	› Synchronized cardioversion
› Ventricular tachycardia without pulse or ventricular fibrillation	› Amiodarone, lidocaine, and epinephrine	› Defibrillation

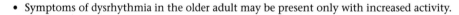

- Symptoms of dysrhythmia in the older adult may be present only with increased activity.
- Risks for heart disease, hypertension, dysrhythmias, and atherosclerosis increase with age.
- Treatment of dysrhythmias follows Advanced Cardiac Life Support (ACLS) evidence-based protocols. See the *Emergency Nursing Principles and Management* chaper for further information.

Cardioversion and Defibrillation

- Cardioversion is the delivery of a direct countershock to the heart synchronized to the QRS complex.
- Defibrillation is the delivery of an unsynchronized, direct countershock to the heart. Defibrillation stops all electrical activity of the heart, allowing the SA node to take over and reestablish a perfusing rhythm.
- Indications
  - Cardioversion – Elective treatment of atrial dysrhythmias, supraventricular tachycardia, and ventricular tachycardia with a pulse. Cardioversion is the treatment of choice for clients who are symptomatic.
  - Defibrillation – Ventricular fibrillation or pulseless ventricular tachycardia.

- Preprocedure
  - Clients who have atrial fibrillation of unknown duration must receive adequate anticoagulation for 4 to 6 weeks prior to cardioversion therapy to prevent dislodgement of thrombi into the bloodstream.
  - Nursing Actions
    - Explain the procedure to the client, and obtain consent.
    - Administer oxygen.
    - Document preprocedure rhythm.
    - Have emergency equipment available.
- Intraprocedure
  - Nursing Actions
    - Administer sedation as prescribed.
    - Administer a prescribed antidysrhythmic agent or other prescribed medications. Digoxin is held for 48 hr prior to elective cardioversion.
    - Ensure proper placement of leads and machine settings, including joules to be delivered.
    - Monitor the client in a lead that provides an upright QRS complex.
    - All staff must stand clear of the client, equipment connected to the client, and the bed when a shock is delivered.
    - Cardioversion requires activation of the synchronizer button in addition to charging the machine. This allows the shock to be in sync with the client's underlying rhythm. Failure to synchronize can lead to development of a lethal dysrhythmia, such as ventricular fibrillation.
    - Perform CPR for cardiac asystole or other pulseless rhythms.
    - Defibrillate the client immediately for ventricular fibrillation.
    - Monitor the client for pulmonary or systemic emboli following cardioversion.
- Postprocedure
  - Nursing Actions
    - After cardioversion or defibrillation, monitor vital signs, assess airway patency, and obtain an ECG.
    - Provide the client/family with reassurance and emotional support.
    - Document
      - Postprocedure rhythm
      - Number of defibrillation or cardioversion attempts, energy settings, time, and response
      - The client's condition and state of consciousness following the procedure
      - Skin condition under the electrodes
  - Client Education
    - Teach the client and family how to assess pulse.
    - Advise the client to report palpitations or irregularities.

- Complications
  - Embolism
    - Cardioversion can dislodge blood clots, potentially causing
      - A pulmonary embolism (evidenced by dyspnea, chest pain, air hunger, and decreasing SaO_2)
      - A cerebrovascular accident (evidenced by decreased level of consciousness, slurred speech, and muscle weakness/paralysis)
      - An MI (evidenced by chest pain and ST segment depression or elevation)
    - Nursing Actions
      - Provide therapeutic anticoagulation for clients who have dysrhythmias.
  - Decreased cardiac output and heart failure
    - Cardioversion may damage heart tissue and impair heart function.
    - Nursing Actions
      - Monitor the client for signs of decreased cardiac output (hypotension, syncope, and increased heart rate) and heart failure (dyspnea, productive cough, edema, and venous distention).
      - Provide medications to increase output (inotropic agents) and to decrease cardiac workload.

APPLICATION EXERCISES

1. A nurse on a cardiac unit is caring for a group of clients. The nurse should recognize which of the following clients as being at risk for the development of a dysrhythmia? (Select all that apply.)

_____ ✗ A. A client who has metabolic alkalosis

_____ B. A client who has a serum potassium level of 4.3 mEq/L

_____ C. A client who has an SaO$_2$ of 96%

_____ ✗ D. A client who has COPD

_____ ✗ E. A client who underwent stent placement in a coronary artery

2. A nurse working on a cardiac unit is admitting a client who is to undergo a cardioversion and is reviewing the health record. Which of the following data requires that the nurse notify the provider to cancel the procedure? (Review the data below for additional client information.)

MAR	VITAL SIGNS	HISTORY AND PHYSICAL
› Ferrous Sulfate (Feosol) 200 mg PO 0800 and 2000 › Diazepam (Valium) 2 mg PO 0800 and 2000 › Isosorbide (Isordil) 2.5 mg PO 4 times a day AC and HS	0800 › T 99° F (37.2° C) › Blood pressure 142/86 mm Hg › Heart rate 88/min and irregular › Respirations 20/min	› Bariatric surgery 10 years ago › Dyspnea with exertion for 3 years › Atrial fibrillation began 3 years ago › Client reports taking the following medications for the past 6 weeks: iron supplement, multivitamin, antilipemic, and nitroglycerin

A. Respiratory history

B. Vital signs

C. Medication history

D. Medications to be administered

3. A nurse is caring for a client who experienced defibrillation. Which of the following should be included in the documentation of this procedure? (Select all that apply.)

_____X_____ A. Follow-up ECG

_____X_____ B. Energy settings used

_____ C. IV fluid intake

_____ D. Urinary output

_____X_____ E. Skin condition under electrodes

4. A nurse on a cardiac unit is caring for a client who is on telemetry. The nurse recognizes the client's heart rate is 46/min and notifies the provider. The nurse should anticipate that which of the following management strategies will be used for this client?

A. Defibrillation

B. Pacemaker insertion

C. Synchronized cardioversion

D. Administration of IV lidocaine

5. A student nurse is observing a cardioversion procedure and hears the team leader call out, "Stand clear." The student should recognize the purpose of this action is to alert personnel that

A. the cardioverter is being charged to the appropriate setting.

B. they should initiate CPR due to pulseless electrical activity.

C. they cannot be in contact with equipment connected to the client.

D. a time-out is being called to verify correct protocols.

6. A nurse educator is reviewing electrocardiography with a group of nurses. What information should be included in this discussion? Use the ATI Active Learning Template: Therapeutic Procedure to complete this item to include the following:

A. Procedure Name: Describe electrocardiography, and describe the difference between continuous cardiac monitoring and telemetry.

B. Indications: List four dysrhythmias that can be identified.

C. Nursing Actions: Identify at least two preprocedure, one intraprocedure, and two postprocedure.

APPLICATION EXERCISES KEY

1. A. **CORRECT:** A client who has an acid-base imbalance such as metabolic alkalosis is at risk for a dysrhythmia.

    B. INCORRECT: A serum potassium of 4.3 mEq/L is within the expected reference range and does not increase the risk of a dysrhythmia.

    C. INCORRECT: SaO_2 of 96% is within the expected reference range and does not increase the risk of a dysrhythmia.

    D. **CORRECT:** A client who has lung disease, such as COPD, is at risk for a dysrhythmia.

    E. **CORRECT:** A client who has cardiac disease and underwent a stent placement is at risk for a dysrhythmia.

     NCLEX® Connection: Physiological Adaptations, Pathophysiology

2. A. INCORRECT: A client who has a dysrhythmia often has a history of lung disease, which can make him a candidate for cardioversion.

    B. INCORRECT: A client who has a dysrhythmia may have an irregular pulse, which can make him a candidate for cardioversion.

    C. **CORRECT:** A client who is to undergo cardioversion needs to be on anticoagulant therapy for 4 to 6 weeks prior to the procedure.

    D. INCORRECT: A client who has a dysthymia often has a history of cardiac disease and angina, which can make him a candidate for cardioversion.

     NCLEX® Connection: Reduction of Risk Potential, Potential for Complications of Diagnostic Tests/ Treatments/Procedures

3. A. **CORRECT:** The client's ECG rhythm is documented following the procedure.

    B. **CORRECT:** Energy settings used during the procedure are documented.

    C. INCORRECT: IV fluid intake is not documented during defibrillation.

    D. INCORRECT: Urinary output is not documented during defibrillation.

    E. **CORRECT:** The condition of the client's skin where electrodes were placed is documented.

     NCLEX® Connection: Reduction of Risk Potential, Therapeutic Procedures

4.   A. INCORRECT: Defibrillation is used when a client has ventricular fibrillation or pulseless ventricular tachycardia.

   B. **CORRECT:** A client who has bradycardia is a candidate for a pacemaker to increase his heart rate.

   C. INCORRECT: Synchronized cardioversion is used when a client has a dysrhythmia such as atrial fibrillation, supraventricular tachycardia (SVT), or ventricular tachycardia with pulse.

   D. INCORRECT: The administration of IV lidocaine is used in clients with a pulseless ventricular dysrhythmia to stimulate cardiac electrical function.

   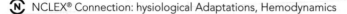 NCLEX® Connection: hysiological Adaptations, Hemodynamics

5.   A. INCORRECT: The cardioverter is charged prior to the delivery of the shock during cardioversion.

   B. INCORRECT: The team leader calls out "Initiate CPR" when members of the team are to begin CPR.

   C. **CORRECT:** A safety concern for personnel performing cardioversion is to "stand clear" of the client and equipment connected to the client when a shock is delivered to prevent them from also receiving a shock.

   D. INCORRECT: A "time-out" is called by personnel during a procedure to verify that proper protocols are being followed.

   NCLEX® Connection: Physiological Adaptations, Medical Emergencies

6. *Using the ATI Active Learning Template: Therapeutic Procedure*

A. Procedure Name

- Electrocardiography is the use of an electrocardiograph to record the electrical activity of the heart over time by connecting wires (leads) to skin electrodes placed on the chest and limbs of the client.

- Continuous monitoring requires the client to be in close proximity to the monitoring system. Telemetry allows the client to ambulate.

B. Indications

- Sinus bradycardia and tachycardia
- Atrioventricular (AV) blocks
- Atrial fibrillation
- Supraventricular tachycardia

- Ventricular fibrillation
- Ventricular asystole
- Premature ventricular complexes (PVCs)
- Premature atrial complexes (PACs)

C. Nursing Actions

- Preprocedure

  ○ Position the client in a supine position with chest exposed.

  ○ Wash the skin to remove oils.

  ○ Attach one electrode to each of the client's extremities by applying electrodes to flat surfaces above the wrists and ankles and the other six electrodes to the chest, avoiding chest hair, which may need to be shaved on male clients.

- Intraprocedure

  ○ Instruct the client to remain still and breathe normally.

  ○ Monitor for manifestations of dysrhythmia (chest pain, decreased level of consciousness, shortness of breath), and hypoxia.

- Postprocedure

  ○ Remove leads, print ECG report, and notify provider.

  ○ Apply Holter monitor if client is on telemetry unit and/or needs continuous monitoring.

  ○ Continue monitoring for manifestations of dysrhythmia and hypoxia.

Ⓝ NCLEX® Connection: Reduction of Risk Potential, Diagnostic Tests

- An arti........aker is a battery-operated device that electrically stimulates the heart when the natural pacemaker of the heart fails to maintain an acceptable rhythm.

M◇   View Image: Pacemaker

- Pacemakers may be temporary or permanent.
- Pacemakers are composed of two parts:
  - The pulse generator houses the energy source (battery) and the control center.
  - The electrodes are wires that attach to the myocardial muscle on one side and connect to the pulse generator on the other.
- Nurses should be familiar with the various types of pacemakers, how they function, and the care involved with their placement/insertion.

- Conduction of electrical impulses through the sinoatrial (SA) node may be slowed with aging, causing bradycardia and conduction defects.

Types of Pacemakers

- Temporary pacemakers (the energy source is provided by an external battery pack)
  - External (transcutaneous)
    - Pacing energy is delivered transcutaneously through the thoracic musculature to the heart via two electrode patches placed on the skin.
    - It requires large amounts of electricity, which can be painful for a client.
    - It is used only in emergency resuscitation of a client who does not have pacing wires inserted.
  - Epicardial
    - Pacemaker leads are attached directly to the heart during open-heart surgery. Wires run externally through the chest incision and may be attached to an external impulse generator if needed.
    - It is commonly used during and immediately following open-heart surgery.
  - Endocardial (transvenous)
    - Pacing wires are threaded through a large central vein (subclavian, jugular, or femoral) and lodged into the wall of the right ventricle (ventricular pacing), right atrium (atrial pacing), or both chambers (dual chamber pacing).

- Permanent pacemakers (contain an internal pacing unit)
  - Indicated for chronic or recurrent dysrhythmias due to sinus or atrioventricular (AV) node malfunction
  - Can be programmed to pace the atrial (A) or ventricular (V) chamber, or both (AV)
  - Pacemaker modes
    - Fixed rate (asynchronous) – Fires at a constant rate without regard for the heart's electrical activity.
    - Demand mode (synchronous) – Detects the heart's electrical impulses and fires at a preset rate only if the heart's intrinsic rate is below a certain level. Pacemaker response modes include the following:
      - Inhibited – Pacemaker activity is inhibited/does not fire.
      - Triggered – Pacemaker activity is triggered/fires when intrinsic activity is sensed.
    - Tachydysrhythmia function – Can overpace a tachydysrhythmia and/or deliver an electrical shock.

FIVE-LETTER SYSTEM TO IDENTIFY PACEMAKER FUNCTION				
Chamber paced	Chamber sensed	Response mode	Programmable functions	Tachydysrhythmic functions
O – None	O – None	O – None	O – None	O – None
A – Atria	A – Atria	T – Triggered	P – Simple	P – Pacing (anti-tachydysrhythmia)
V – Ventricle	V – Ventricle	I – Inhibited	M – Multiple	S – Shock
D – Dual (AV)	D – Dual (AV)	D – Dual (AV)	C – Communicating	D – Dual (P + S)
			R – Rate Modulation	

- Often, the first three letters are used to describe the pacemaker function:
  - Example: VVI mode
    - Function: Ventricular paced, ventricular sensed, inhibited
    - If no QRS detected within desired time, pacemaker fires.
    - If QRS detected, pacemaker does not fire.

Pacemaker Placement

- Indications
  - Diagnoses
    - Symptomatic bradycardia
    - Complete heart block
    - Sick sinus syndrome
    - Sinus arrest
    - Asystole
    - Atrial tachydysrhythmias
    - Ventricular tachydysrhythmias
  - Client presentation
    - Subjective data
      - Dizziness
      - Palpitations (racing heart)
      - Chest pain or pressure

□ Anxiety

□ Fatigue

□ Nausea

□ Breathing difficulties

- Objective data

  □ Bradycardia or tachycardia

  □ Abnormal ECG

  □ Dyspnea, tachypnea

  □ Restlessness

  □ Jugular venous distention

  □ Vomiting

  □ Hypotension

  □ Diaphoresis

  □ Decreased cardiac output

- Preprocedure

  ○ Nursing actions

    - Assess the client's knowledge of the procedure and need for pacemaker (if nonemergent situation).

    - Obtain signed informed consent form from the client.

    - Prepare client's skin (clean with soap and water; trim excess hair). Do not shave, rub, or apply alcohol to the skin.

  ○ Client education

    - Teach the client about the type of pacemaker that is to be inserted and information about the procedure.

      □ Temporary pacemaker

        ▸ Explain that wires and a pacemaker box will be on the client's chest after the procedure.

        ▸ Instruct the client not to touch the dials on the pacemaker box.

        ▸ The wires and box need to be kept dry. The client will not be able to shower.

      □ Permanent pacemaker

        ▸ Explain that a small incision is made using a local anesthetic and IV sedation.

        ▸ The pacemaker may be reprogrammed externally after the procedure.

        ▸ The pacemaker battery will last about 10 years. The pacemaker pulse generator must be replaced when this occurs.

- Intraprocedure

  ○ Nursing actions

    - Monitor the client's status (vital signs, SaO_2, and comfort).

    - Administer medications as prescribed (analgesia, anxiolytics, and antiarrhythmics).

    - Set pacemaker settings as prescribed. Establish a threshold (lowest stimulation that achieves capture).

- Postprocedure
  - ○ Nursing actions
    - ▪ Document the time and date of insertion, model (permanent pacemaker), settings, rhythm strip, presence of adequate pulse and blood pressure, and client response.
    - ▪ Continually monitor heart rate and rhythm. Compare ECG rhythm to prescribed pacemaker settings. Notify provider of any discrepancies.
    - ▪ Obtain chest x-ray as prescribed to assess lead placement and for pneumothorax, hemothorax, or pleural effusion.
    - ▪ Provide analgesia as prescribed.
    - ▪ Minimize shoulder movement initially, and provide a sling (if prescribed) to allow leads to anchor.
    - ▪ Assess the client for hiccups, which may indicate that the generator is pacing the diaphragm.
    - ▪ Maintain the client's safety.
      - □ Ensure that all electrical equipment has grounded connections.
      - □ Remove any electrical equipment that is damaged.
      - □ Make sure all equipment is grounded with a three-pronged plug.
      - □ For a temporary pacemaker
        - ▸ Unattached pacemaker wires can cause cardiac arrhythmias or ventricular fibrillation, even when not attached to pacemaker generator.
        - ▸ Wear gloves when handling pacemaker leads.
        - ▸ Insulate pacemaker terminals and leads with nonconductive material when not in use (rubber gloves).
        - ▸ Keep spare generator, leads, and batteries at the client's bedside.
        - ▸ Secure the pacemaker battery pack. Take care when moving the client, and ensure that there is enough wire slack.
      - □ For a permanent pacemaker
        - ▸ Provide the client with a pacemaker identification card including the manufacturer's name, model number, mode of function, rate parameters, and expected battery life.
  - ○ Client education
    - ▪ Temporary pacemakers are used only in a controlled facility with telemetry for continuous ECG monitoring. If needed, a permanent pacemaker is inserted before discharge to home.
    - ▪ Permanent pacemaker discharge teaching
      - □ Carry a pacemaker identification card at all times.
      - □ Prevent wire dislodgement (wear sling when out of bed, do not raise arm above shoulder for 1 to 2 weeks).
      - □ Take pulse daily at the same time. Notify the provider if heart rate is less than five beats below the pacemaker rate.
      - □ Report signs of dizziness, fainting, fatigue, weakness, chest pain, hiccupping, or palpitations.
      - □ For clients with pacemaker-defibrillators, when the device delivers a shock, anyone touching the client will feel a slight electrical impulse, but the impulse will not harm the person.
      - □ Follow activity restrictions as prescribed, including no contact sports or heavy lifting for 2 months.

- □ Avoid direct blows or injury to the generator site.

- □ Resume sexual activity as desired, avoiding positions that put stress on the incision site.

- □ Never place items that generate a magnetic field directly over the pacemaker generator. These items can affect function and settings. This includes garage door openers, burglar alarms, strong magnets, generators and other power transmitters, and large stereo speakers.

- □ Inform other providers and dentists about the pacemaker. Some tests, such as magnetic resonance imaging and therapeutic diathermy (heat therapy), may be contraindicated.

- □ Pacemakers will set off airport security detectors, and officials should be notified. The airport security device should not affect pacemaker functioning. Airport security personnel should not place wand detection devices directly over the pacemaker.

- Complications
  - ○ Pacemaker insertion complications
    - ▪ Infection or hematoma at insertion site
      - □ Nursing actions
        - ▸ Assess the incision site for redness, pain, drainage, or swelling.
        - ▸ Administer antibiotics as prescribed.
        - ▸ Monitor PT, PTT, and CBC.
    - ▪ Pneumothorax or hemothorax
      - □ Nursing actions
        - ▸ Assess the client's breath sounds and chest movement.
        - ▸ Monitor oxygen saturation.
        - ▸ Obtain a chest x-ray after the procedure.
    - ▪ Arrhythmias related to ventricular irritation from pacemaker electrode
      - □ Nursing actions
        - ▸ Monitor ECG and blood pressure.
        - ▸ Administer antiarrhythmics as prescribed.
        - ▸ Have emergency resuscitation equipment and medications readily available.
  - ○ Pacemaker complications
    - ▪ Pacemaker complications relate to improper sensing or pacing electrical charge being outside the heart.
    - ▪ Causes include insufficient pacemaker settings, lead wire placement and function, battery function, myocardial damage, and electrolyte imbalance.
    - ▪ Complications often are detectable by ECG.
      - □ Monitor ECG to ensure heart rate is within programmed parameters. Pacer spikes should be adequate in number and occur directly before P or QRS complexes.
      - □ Pacer spikes that occur on the T wave can cause life-threatening arrhythmias.
    - ▪ Unintended electrical stimulation of chest muscles results in hiccups and muscle twitching and may lead to cardiac tamponade.
    - ▪ Treatment of complications is related to identifying the cause.
    - ▪ Pacemaker settings should be manipulated only as prescribed by the provider.

APPLICATION EXERCISES

1. A nurse is admitting a client to the coronary care unit following placement of a temporary pacemaker. Which of the following nursing actions should the nurse use to promote client safety? (Select all that apply.)

_____ A. Wear gloves when handling pacemaker leads.

_____ B. Verify the use of three-pronged grounding plugs.

_____ C. Minimize client's shoulder movements.

_____ D. Keep the lead wires taut when turning the client.

_____ E. Additional batteries should be kept at the nurses' station.

2. A nurse is admitting a client who has complete heart block as demonstrated by ECG. The client's pulse rate is 34/min, blood pressure is 83/48 mm Hg, and he is lethargic and unable to complete sentences. Which of the following actions should the nurse perform first?

A. Cleanse the client's skin with soap and water.

B. Prepare the client for insertion of a permanent pacemaker.

C. Obtain signed informed consent form for a pacemaker.

D. Apply transcutaneous pacemaker pads.

3. A nurse is caring for a client following the insertion of a temporary venous pacemaker via the femoral artery that is set as a VVI pacemaker rate of 70/min. Which of the following findings should the nurse report to the provider? (Select all that apply.)

_____ A. Cool and clammy foot with capillary refill of 5 seconds

_____ B. Observed pacing spike followed by a QRS complex

_____ C. Twitching of intercostal muscle

_____ D. Heart rate of 84/min

_____ E. Blood pressure of 104/62 mm Hg

4. A nurse is completing discharge teaching with a client who has a permanent pacemaker. Which of the following statements by the client indicates a need for further teaching?

A. "I will notify the airport screeners about my pacemaker."

B. "I will call my doctor about hiccups."

C. "I will have to disconnect my garage door opener."

D. "I will take my pulse every morning when I awaken."

5. A cardiac nurse educator is reviewing the use of the fixed rate mode pacemaker with a group of newly hired nurses. Which of the following statements by a newly hired nurse indicates understanding of the review?

 A. "This means the pacemaker fires in an asynchronous pattern."

 B. "This means the pacemaker fires only when the heart rate is below a certain rate."

 C. "The pacemaker can automatically adjust to a client's increased activity level."

 D. "The pacemaker activity is triggered by heart muscle activity."

6. A coronary care nurse is orienting a newly hired nurse to the unit and discussing nursing care of a client who has complications related to pacemaker insertion. What should be included in the discussion? Use the ATI Active Learning Template: Therapeutic Procedure to complete this item to include the following sections:

 A. Complications:
 - Describe two.
 - Describe at least two nursing actions for each complication.

APPLICATION EXERCISES KEY

1. A. **CORRECT:** Gloves are worn when handling pacemaker leads.

    B. **CORRECT:** Three-pronged grounding plugs reduce the risk of accidental electrical discharge by equipment being used.

    C. **CORRECT:** The client's shoulder movement should be minimized or the client should wear a sling to promote secure anchoring of the lead wires.

    D. INCORRECT: The lead wires should have some slack in them to prevent dislodging the wires when the client is turned.

    E. INCORRECT: Additional batteries should be kept at the client's bedside for quick access when needed.

     NCLEX® Connection: Physiological Adaptations, Hemodynamics

2. A. **CORRECT:** Before applying transcutaneous pacemaker pads, the client's skin is cleaned with soap and water and dried thoroughly.

    B. INCORRECT: A client in complete heart block should be prepared for the insertion of a permanent pacemaker, but this is not the first action by the nurse.

    C. INCORRECT: Informed consent form is needed before transcutaneous pacing can occur, but this is not the first action by the nurse.

    D. INCORRECT: A client in complete heart block requires external (transcutaneous) pacing prior to the insertion of a permanent pacemaker, but this is not the first action by the nurse.

     NCLEX® Connection: Physiological Adaptations, Hemodynamics

3. A. **CORRECT:** A cool, clammy foot may be an indication of a femoral hematoma secondary to insertion of the lead wires and should be reported.

    B. INCORRECT: A pacing spike followed by a QRS complex is an expected finding.

    C. **CORRECT:** Twitching of the intercostal muscle may indicate lead wire perforation and stimulation of the diaphragm and should be reported.

    D. INCORRECT: A heart rate of 84/min is an expected finding.

    E. INCORRECT: A blood pressure of 104/62 mm Hg is an expected finding.

     NCLEX® Connection: Physiological Adaptations, Unexpected Response to Therapies

4. A. INCORRECT: Clients are instructed to notify airport screening personnel about a pacemaker.

    B. INCORRECT: Hiccups should be reported to the provider because they may indicate improper lead placement.

    C. **CORRECT:** The use of household appliances, such as microwaves and garage door openers, does not affect pacemaker function.

    D. INCORRECT: Discharge teaching includes reminding clients to check their pulse rate on a regular basis.

    Ⓝ NCLEX® Connection: Physiological Adaptations, Hemodynamics

5. A. **CORRECT:** Fixed rate mode is asynchronous, meaning the pacemaker fires without regard for electrical activity in the heart.

    B. INCORRECT: Demand mode detects an electrical impulse, and the pacemaker will then fire only if this impulse remains below a certain level.

    C. INCORRECT: Fixed rate pacemaker mode means the rate does not change in relation to the client's activity level.

    D. INCORRECT: Fixed rate mode means the pacemaker fires without regard for electrical activity in the heart.

    Ⓝ NCLEX® Connection: Physiological Adaptations, Hemodynamics

6. *Using ATI Active Learning Template: Therapeutic Procedure*

    A. Complications and nursing actions for each
    - Infection or hematoma
      ○ Assess incision site for redness, pain, drainage, or swelling.
      ○ Administer antibiotics as prescribed.
      ○ Monitor PT, PTT, and CBC.
    - Pneumothorax or hemothorax
      ○ Monitor breath sounds and chest movement.
      ○ Monitor oxygen saturation.
      ○ Obtain a chest x-ray following the procedure.
    - Arrhythmias
      ○ Monitor ECG and blood pressure.
      ○ Administer antiarrhythmics as prescribed.
      ○ Have emergency resuscitation equipment and medications readily available.

    Ⓝ NCLEX® Connection: Physiological Adaptations, Hemodynamics

chapter 30

Overview

- Cardiovascular procedures reviewed include invasive methods used to improve blood flow for occluded arteries and veins.

- Invasive cardiovascular procedures are indicated after noninvasive interventions have been tried, such as diet, exercise, and medications.

- Invasive cardiovascular procedures that nurses should be knowledgeable about

    ○ Percutaneous coronary intervention (PCI)

    ○ Coronary artery bypass grafts

    ○ Peripheral bypass grafts

Percutaneous Coronary Intervention (PCI)

- PCI is a nonsurgical procedure performed to open coronary arteries through one of the following means:

    ○ Atherectomy – used to break up and remove plaques within cardiac vessels

    ○ Stent – placement of a mesh-wire device to hold an artery open and prevent restenosis

    ○ Percutaneous transluminal coronary angioplasty (PTCA), or angioplasty, involves inflating a balloon to dilate the arterial lumen and the adhering plaque, thus widening the arterial lumen. This can include stent placement.

 View Animation: Stent Placement

- Indications for PCI

    ○ Can be performed on an elective basis to treat coronary artery disease when there is greater than 50% occlusion of one to two coronary arteries. The area of occlusion is confined, not scattered, and easy to access (proximal).

    ○ May reduce ischemia during the occurrence of an acute myocardial infarction (MI), and it is most effective if it is done within 90 min of chest pain.

    ○ May be used as an alternative to coronary artery bypass graft.

    ○ May be used with stent placement to prevent artery reocclusion and to dilate the left main coronary artery, which supplies blood flow to a large area of the heart.

- Client Presentation
  - Subjective Data
    - Chest pain may occur with or without exertion. Pain may radiate to the jaw, left arm, through the back, or to the shoulder. Manifestations may increase in cold weather or with exercise. Other manifestations may include dyspnea, nausea, fatigue, and diaphoresis.
  - Objective Data
    - ECG changes may include ST elevation, depression, or nonspecific ST changes. Other findings may include bradycardia, tachycardia, hypotension, elevated blood pressure, vomiting, and mental disorientation.

- Preprocedure
  - Nursing Actions
    - Ensure that the client signs the consent form.
    - Maintain the client on NPO status for at least 8 hr if possible (risk for aspiration when lying flat for the procedure).
    - Assess that the client and family understand the procedure.
    - Assess the client for an iodine/shellfish allergy. (Contrast dye is used instead of contrast media for consistency.)
    - Assess renal function prior to introduction of contrast dye.
    - Administer premedications as prescribed (antiplatelet medications).
  - Client Education
    - Instruct the client that he may be awake and sedated for the procedure. A local anesthetic may be administered. A small incision is made, often in the groin, to insert the catheter. The client may feel warmth and flushed when the dye is inserted. After the procedure, the client will be asked to keep the affected leg straight. Pressure (a sandbag) may be placed on the incision to prevent bleeding.

- Intraprocedure
  - Nursing Actions
    - Administer sedatives, such as midazolam (Versed), and analgesia, such as fentanyl (Sublimaze), as prescribed.
    - Monitor the client for chest pain.
    - Continually monitor vital signs and heart rhythm.
    - Have resuscitation equipment and emergency medications readily available.
    - Be prepared to intervene for dysrhythmias.

- Postprocedure
  - Nursing Actions
    - Assess the client's vital signs every 15 min x 4, every 30 min x 2, every hour x 4, and then every 4 hr (or per facility protocol).
    - Assess the groin site at the same intervals for bleeding and hematoma formation.
    - Assess for signs of thrombosis. Document pedal pulse, capillary refill, color, and temperature of extremity.

- Maintain bed rest in a supine position with leg straight for prescribed time.
  - □ Older adult clients may have arthritis, which can make lying in bed for 4 to 6 hr after the procedure painful.
- Conduct continuous cardiac monitoring for dysrhythmias. (Reperfusion following angioplasty may cause dysrhythmias.)
- Administer antiplatelet or thrombolytic agents as prescribed to prevent clot formation and restenosis.
  - □ Aspirin
  - □ Clopidogrel (Plavix), tirofiban (Aggrastat)
  - □ Heparin
  - □ Enoxaparin (Lovenox)
  - □ Glycoprotein (GP IIb/IIIa) inhibitors (antiplatelet), such as eptifibatide (Integrilin)
- Administer anxiolytics and analgesics as needed.
- Monitor urine output, and administer IV fluids for hydration.
  - □ Contrast dye acts as an osmotic diuretic.
- Assist with sheath removal from insertion site (artery or vein).
  - □ The catheter sheath is a short hollow tube placed inside the artery or vein at the insertion site. It is used as a guide for the balloon catheter. After angioplasty, the catheter sheath may be left in for access, so that the angioplasty may be repeated, if needed (for restenosis or perforation).
  - □ Apply pressure to arterial/venous sites for prescribed period of time (varies depending upon method used for vessel closure).
  - □ Observe for vagal response (hypotension, bradycardia) from compression of vagus nerve.
  - □ Apply a pressure dressing.
- ○ Client Education
  - Avoid strenuous exercise for prescribed period of time.
  - Immediately report bleeding from insertion site, chest pain, shortness of breath, and changes in color or temperature of extremity.
  - Restrict lifting (less than 10 lb) for prescribed period of time.
  - Client who had a stent placement receives anticoagulation therapy for 6 to 8 weeks. Instruct client to:
    - □ Take medication at the same time each day.
    - □ Have regular laboratory tests to determine therapeutic levels.
    - □ Avoid activities that could cause bleeding (use a soft toothbrush, wear shoes when out of bed, use an electric razor).
  - Encourage client to follow lifestyle guidelines (manage weight, consume a low-fat/low-cholesterol diet, exercise regularly, stop smoking, and decrease alcohol intake).

- Complications
  - Artery dissection
    - Perforation of an artery by the catheter may cause cardiac tamponade or require emergency bypass surgery.
    - Artery dissection findings include severe hypotension and tachycardia, and may require extended occlusion of perforation with a balloon catheter and reversal of anticoagulants.
  - Cardiac tamponade
    - Cardiac tamponade can result from fluid accumulation in the pericardial sac.
      - Findings include hypotension, jugular venous distention, muffled heart sounds, and paradoxical pulse (variance of 10 mm Hg or more in systolic blood pressure between expiration and inspiration).
      - Hemodynamic monitoring reveals that intracardiac and pulmonary artery pressures are similar and elevated (plateau pressures) and that cardiac output is decreased.
    - Nursing Actions
      - Notify the provider immediately.
      - Administer IV fluids to manage hypotension as prescribed.
      - Obtain a chest x-ray or echocardiogram to confirm findings.
      - Prepare the client for pericardiocentesis or return to surgical suite (informed consent, gather materials, administer medications as appropriate).
        - ▸ Monitor hemodynamic pressures and heart rhythm for reoccurrence of findings after the procedure.
  - Hematoma formation near insertion site
    - Nursing Actions
      - Monitor for sensation, color, capillary refill, and peripheral pulses in the extremity distal to the insertion site.
      - Assess groin for development of a hematoma at prescribed intervals and as needed.
      - Hold pressure for uncontrolled oozing/bleeding.
      - Notify the provider.
  - Allergic reaction related to the contrast dye
    - Clinical manifestations can include chills, fever, rash, wheezing, tachycardia, and bradycardia.
    - Nursing Actions
      - Monitor for an allergic reaction.
      - Have resuscitation equipment readily available.
      - Administer diphenhydramine or epinephrine if prescribed.
  - External bleeding at the insertion site
    - Nursing Actions
      - Monitor insertion site for bleeding or swelling.
      - Apply pressure to site.
      - Keep client's leg straight.

- ○ Embolism – plaque or clot can become dislodged
    - ▪ Nursing Actions
        - ▫ Monitor client for chest pain during and after the procedure.
        - ▫ Monitor client's vital signs and SaO_2.
- ○ Retroperitoneal bleeding in the retroperitoneal space (abdominal cavity behind the peritoneum) due to femoral artery puncture
    - ▪ Nursing Actions
        - ▫ Assess for flank pain and hypotension.
        - ▫ Notify the provider immediately.
        - ▫ Administer IV fluids and blood products as prescribed.
    - ▪ Client Education
        - ▫ Advise client that pressure will be applied to insertion site.
        - ▫ Remind client to keep his leg straight.
        - ▫ Advise client to report chest pain, shortness of breath, cardiac manifestations.
- ○ Restenosis of treated vessel – Clot formation in coronary vessel immediately or several days after the procedure.
    - ▪ Nursing Actions
        - ▫ Assess ECG patterns and for report of chest pain.
        - ▫ Notify the provider immediately.
        - ▫ Prepare the client for return to the cardiac catheterization laboratory.
    - ▪ Client Education
        - ▫ Advise the client to notify the provider of cardiac manifestations and to take medications as prescribed.

Coronary Artery Bypass Grafts

- Coronary artery bypass grafting (CABG) is an invasive surgical procedure that aims to restore vascularization of the myocardium.

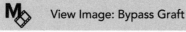

View Image: Bypass Graft

- ○ Performed to bypass an obstruction in one or more of the coronary arteries, CABG does not alter the atherosclerotic process but improves the quality of life for clients restricted by painful coronary artery disease.
- ○ The procedure is most effective when a client has sufficient ventricular function (ejection fraction greater than 40% to 50%).
- ○ Older adult clients are more likely to experience transient neurological changes, toxic effects from cardiac medications, and dysrhythmias.
- Less invasive revascularization procedures have been developed to reduce risk and improve client outcomes (off-pump coronary artery bypass, robotic heart surgery, minimally invasive direct coronary artery bypass). These procedures have characteristics similar to traditional CABG.

- Indications
  - Diagnoses
    - Over 50% blockage of left main coronary artery with anginal episodes (blockage inaccessible to angioplasty and stenting)
    - Significant two-vessel disease with unstable angina
    - Triple-vessel disease with or without angina
    - Persistent ischemia or likely MI following coronary angiography, PCI, or stent placement
    - Heart failure or cardiogenic shock with acute MI or ischemia (may not be reasonable for clients who have poor ejection fractions)
    - Coronary arteries that are unable to be accessed or treated by angioplasty and stent placement (narrow or calcified)
    - Coronary artery disease nonresponsive to medical management
    - Heart valve disease
  - Client Presentation
    - Subjective Data
      - Chest pain may occur with or without exertion. Pain may radiate to jaw, left arm, through the back, or to the shoulder. Effects may increase in cold weather or with exercise. Other findings can include dyspnea, nausea, fatigue, and diaphoresis.
    - Objective Data
      - ECG changes may include ST elevation, depression, or nonspecific ST changes. Other findings may include bradycardia, tachycardia, hypotension, elevated blood pressure, vomiting, and mental disorientation.
- Preprocedure
  - Nursing Actions
    - A CABG may be an elective procedure or done as an emergency. When planned, preparation begins before the client comes to the facility for the procedure.
    - Verify that client has signed the informed consent form.
    - Confirm that recent chest x-ray, ECG, and laboratory reports are available if needed.
    - Administer preoperative medications as prescribed.
      - Anxiolytics, such as lorazepam (Ativan) and diazepam (Valium)
      - Prophylactic antibiotics
      - Anticholinergics, such as scopolamine, to reduce secretions
    - Provide safe transport of the client to the operating suite. Monitor heart rate and rhythm, oxygenation, and other vital indicators.
  - Client Education
    - Provide instruction to the client and family about the procedure and postsurgical environment.
      - Inform the client of the importance of coughing and deep breathing after the procedure to prevent complications.
      - Instruct the client to splint the incision when coughing and deep breathing. Allow the client to provide a return demonstration.

- Instruct the client to report pain to the nursing staff. The majority of pain stems from the harvest site for the vein.
- Inform the client and family to expect the following postoperatively:
  - Endotracheal tube and mechanical ventilator for airway management for several hours following surgery
  - Inability to talk while endotracheal tube is in place
  - Sternal incision and possible leg incision
  - One to two mediastinal chest tubes
  - Indwelling urinary catheter
  - Pacemaker wires
  - Hemodynamic monitoring devices (pulmonary artery catheter, arterial line)
- Instruct client to alter or discontinue regular medications as prescribed by provider.
  - Medications frequently discontinued for CABG
    - ▷ Diuretics 2 to 3 days before surgery
    - ▷ Aspirin and other anticoagulants 1 week before surgery
  - Medications often continued for CABG
    - ▷ Potassium supplements
    - ▷ Scheduled antidysrhythmics, such as amiodarone (Cordarone)
    - ▷ Scheduled antihypertensives, such as metoprolol (Lopressor), a beta-blocker, and diltiazem (Cardizem), a calcium-channel blocker
    - ▷ Insulin (clients who have diabetes mellitus and are insulin-dependent usually receive half the regular insulin dose)
- Assess client and family anxiety levels surrounding the procedure.
  - Encourage the client to verbalize his feelings.
- Intraprocedure
  - An extracardiac vein (saphenous vein), artery (usually the radial or mammary artery), or synthetic graft is used to bypass an obstruction in one or more of the coronary arteries.
  - Most often, a median sternotomy incision is made to visualize the heart and the great vessels.
  - The client is placed on cardiopulmonary bypass, and the client's core temperature may be lowered to decrease the rate of metabolism and demand for oxygen. A normal core temperature may be maintained during cardiopulmonary bypass to improve postoperative myocardial function and reduce postoperative complications.
  - A cardioplegic solution is used to stop the heart. This prevents myocardial ischemia and allows for a motionless operative field.
  - The artery or vein to be used is harvested. When a saphenous vein is used, it is reversed to prevent the valves from interfering with blood flow.
  - The harvested vessel is anastomosed from the aorta to the affected coronary artery distal to the occlusion.
  - Once the bypass is complete, the hypothermic client is rewarmed by heat exchanges on the bypass machine. Grafts are monitored for patency and leakage as the client is weaned from the bypass machine and blood is redirected through coronary vasculature.

- ○ Lastly, pacemaker wires may be sutured into the myocardium, and chest tubes are placed. The incision is closed with wire sutures, and the client is transported to the intensive care unit.
- ○ Nursing Actions
    - ▪ Provide padding to bony prominences to provide comfort and prevent skin breakdown.
    - ▪ Communicate surgical progress to family members, if appropriate.
    - ▪ Assist in monitoring urine output and blood loss.
    - ▪ Document appropriate surgical events.
    - ▪ Assist in arranging intensive care unit placement, and communicate client postoperative needs.
- • Postprocedure
    - ○ Nursing Actions
        - ▪ Maintain patent airway and adequate ventilation.
            - □ Monitor respiratory rate and effort.
            - □ Auscultate breath sounds. Report crackles.
            - □ Monitor SaO_2.
            - □ Document ventilator settings.
            - □ Suction as needed.
            - □ Assist with extubation.
        - ▪ Encourage the client to splint the incision while deep breathing and coughing.
        - ▪ Dangle and turn the client from side to side as tolerated within 2 hr following extubation. Assist the client to a chair within 24 hr. Ambulate the client 25 to 100 ft by first postoperative day.
        - ▪ Consult respiratory services to aid in recovery and client education.
        - ▪ Consult case management services to initiate discharge planning: need for home oxygen therapy, transfer to tertiary care facility.
        - ▪ Continually monitor client's heart rate and rhythm. Treat dysrhythmias per protocol.
        - ▪ Maintain an adequate circulating blood volume.
            - □ Monitor blood pressure.
                - ▸ Hypotension may result in graft collapse.
                - ▸ Hypertension may result in bleeding from grafts and sutures.
                - ▸ Titrate IV drips (dopamine [Intropin], dobutamine [Dobutrex], milrinone [Primacor], sodium nitroprusside [Nipride]) per protocol to control blood pressure and/or increase cardiac output.
            - □ Monitor hemodynamic pressures, and monitor catheter placement. Observe waveforms and markings on catheter.
            - □ Monitor the client's level of consciousness. Assess neurological status every 30 to 60 min until the client awakens from anesthesia, then every 2 to 4 hr, or per facility policy.
            - □ Notify the surgeon of significant changes in values.
        - ▪ Monitor chest tube patency and drainage.
            - □ Measure drainage at least once an hour.
            - □ Volume exceeding 150 mL/hr could be a sign of possible hemorrhage and should be reported to the surgeon.
            - □ Avoid dependent loops in tubing to facilitate drainage.

- Assess and control pain.
  - Determine source of pain (angina, incisional pain).
    - Anginal pain often radiates and is unaffected by breathing.
    - Incisional pain is localized, sharp, aching, burning, and often worsens with deep breathing.
- Administer analgesics as prescribed (morphine, fentanyl).
  - Pain will stimulate sympathetic nervous system, resulting in increased heart rate and systemic vascular resistance.
  - Provide frequent and adequate doses to control pain. Maintain around-the-clock administration.
- Monitor fluid and electrolyte status.
  - Fluid administration is determined by blood pressure, pulmonary artery wedge pressure, right atrial pressure, cardiac output and index, systemic vascular resistance, blood loss, and urine output.
  - Follow provider or unit-specific orders for fluid administration.
  - Monitor the client for electrolyte imbalances, especially for hypokalemia and hyperkalemia.
- Prevent and monitor for infection.
  - Practice proper hand hygiene.
  - Use surgical aseptic technique during procedures such as dressing changes and suctioning.
  - Administer antibiotics.
  - Monitor WBC counts, incisional redness and drainage, and fever.
  - Monitor the client's temperature, and provide warming measures if indicated.
- Client Education
  - Instruct the client to monitor and report manifestations of infection such as fever, incisional drainage, and redness.
  - Instruct the client to treat angina.
    - Maintain a fresh supply of sublingual nitroglycerin.
    - Store nitroglycerin in a light-resistant container.
    - Discontinue activity and rest with onset of pain. Follow directions for treating anginal pain.
    - Instruct the older female client that she may show milder symptoms (dyspnea, indigestion).
  - Instruct the client to adhere to pharmacological regimen.
  - Instruct the client who has diabetes mellitus to closely monitor blood glucose levels.
  - Encourage the client to consume a heart-healthy diet (low fat, low cholesterol, high fiber, low salt).
  - Encourage the client to quit smoking if applicable. Provide resources on smoking cessation.
  - Encourage physical activity. Consult the cardiac rehabilitation program or a physical therapist to devise a specific program.
  - Discuss home environment and social supports. Consult case management to assist with home planning needs.

- Instruct the client to remain home during the first week after surgery and to resume normal activities slowly.
  - ▢ Week 2 – possible return to work part time, increase in social activities
  - ▢ Week 3 – lifting of up to 15 lb, avoidance of heavier lifting for 6 to 8 weeks
- Clients can resume sexual activity based on the advice of the provider.
  - ▢ Walking one block or climbing two flights of stairs symptom-free generally indicates that it is safe for the client to resume normal sexual activity.
- Encourage the client to verbalize his feelings.
- Complications
  - ○ Pulmonary complications include primary complication of atelectasis, as well as pneumonia and pulmonary edema.
    - Nursing Actions
      - ▢ While the client is intubated, suction every 1 to 2 hr and as needed.
      - ▢ Turn the client every 2 hr, and advance him out of bed as soon as possible.
      - ▢ Monitor breath sounds, SaO_2, ABGs, pulmonary artery pressures, cardiac output, and urine output, and obtain a chest x-ray as indicated.
    - Client Education
      - ▢ Encourage coughing, deep breathing, and use of an incentive spirometer. Explain that increasing activity reduces postoperative complications.
  - ○ Hypothermia can cause vasoconstriction, metabolic acidosis, and hypertension.
    - Nursing Actions
      - ▢ Monitor temperature, and provide warming measures, such as warm blankets and heat lamps.
      - ▢ Monitor blood pressure.
      - ▢ Administer vasodilators if prescribed.
    - Client Education
      - ▢ Assure the client that shivering is common following surgery.
  - ○ Decreased cardiac output
    - Decreased cardiac output can result from dysrhythmias, cardiac tamponade, hypovolemia, left ventricular failure, or MI.
      - ▢ Cardiac tamponade results from bleeding while chest tubes are occluded, causing fluid to build up in the pericardium. Increased pericardial fluid compresses heart chambers and inhibits effective pumping.
        - ▸ Indications include a sudden decrease/cessation of chest-tube drainage following heavy drainage, jugular-venous distension with clear lung sounds, and equal pulmonary artery wedge pressure and central venous pressure values.
      - ▢ Hypovolemia may be the result of bleeding, decreased intravascular volume, or vasodilation, and hypotension and decreased urine output are the results.
      - ▢ Left ventricular heart failure may occur with a MI or hypervolemia.

- Nursing Actions

  - □ Monitor ECG, blood pressure, pulmonary artery pressures, cardiac output, urine output, and bleeding through chest tube.

  - □ Administer inotropic medications and fluid and blood products as prescribed.

  - □ Treat dysrhythmias as prescribed.

    - ▸ Use pacemaker wires if heart block is present.

  - □ Treatment of cardiac tamponade involves volume expansion (fluid administration) and an emergency sternotomy with drainage. Pericardiocentesis is avoided because blood may have clotted.

  - ○ Electrolyte Disturbances

    - Potassium and magnesium depletion is common.

    - Nursing Actions

      - □ Always dilute potassium supplements in adequate fluid (40 to 80 mEq in 100 mL of IV solution).

      - □ Administer supplements via infusion pump to control the rate of delivery. Maximum administration rate varies from 10 to 20 mEq/hr.

      - □ Administer supplements through a central catheter.

      - □ Monitor ECG and electrolytes.

  - ○ Neurologic deficits

    - Transient hypertension, hypotension, or a blood clot may cause an intraoperative cerebrovascular accident.

    - Nursing Actions

      - □ Assess neurologic status, including pupils, level of consciousness, and sensory and motor function.

      - □ Maintain client's blood pressure within prescribed parameters.

    - Client Education

      - □ Explain procedures to client.

      - □ Assure the client that memory loss and neurological deficits may be temporary.

Peripheral Bypass Grafts

- Bypass graft surgery aims to restore adequate blood flow to the areas affected by peripheral artery disease.

  - ○ A peripheral bypass graft involves suturing graft material or autogenous saphenous veins proximal and distal to occluded area of an artery. This procedure improves blood supply to the area normally served by the blocked artery.

  - ○ If bypass surgery fails to restore circulation, the client may need to undergo amputation of the limb.

- Indications

  - ○ Acute circulatory compromise in limb

  - ○ Severe pain at rest that interferes with ability to work

- ○ Client Presentation
  - ▪ Subjective Data
    - ▫ Numbness or burning pain to the lower extremity with exercise, and may stop with rest (intermittent claudication)
    - ▫ Numbness or burning pain to the lower extremity at rest, and may wake the client at night; pain may be relieved by lowering the extremity below the level of the heart
  - ▪ Objective Data
    - ▫ Decreased or absent pulses to feet. Dry, hairless, shiny skin on calves. Muscles may atrophy with advanced disease. Skin may be cold and dark colored. Feet and toes may be mottled and dusky, and toenails may be thick. Skin may become reddened (rubor) when extremity is dropped to a dependent position. Ulcers or lesions may be noted on toes (arterial ulcers) or ankles (venous ulcers).
- • Preprocedure
  - ○ Nursing Actions
    - ▪ Assess the client and family's understanding of the procedure.
    - ▪ Verify that the client has signed the informed consent form.
    - ▪ Assess for allergies.
    - ▪ Document baseline vital signs and peripheral pulses.
    - ▪ Administer prophylactic antibiotic therapy as prescribed.
    - ▪ Instruct the client to maintain NPO status for at least 8 hr prior to surgery.
  - ○ Client Education
    - ▪ Include information about postoperative pain management, and teach deep breathing/incentive spirometer exercises.
    - ▪ Advise the client not to cross his legs.
    - ▪ The client may have an arterial line inserted for blood and blood pressure.
    - ▪ Explain that pedal pulses will be checked frequently.
- • Intraprocedure
  - ○ Nursing Actions
    - ▪ Provide padding to bony prominences to provide comfort and to prevent skin breakdown.
    - ▪ Communicate surgical progress to family members, if appropriate.
    - ▪ Assist in monitoring urine output and blood loss.
    - ▪ Document appropriate surgical events.
    - ▪ Communicate client postoperative needs to postanesthesia care unit.
- • Postprocedure
  - ○ Nursing Actions
    - ▪ Assess and monitor vital signs every 15 min for 1 hr and then hourly after the first hour (or per facility policy).
    - ▪ Follow standing orders to maintain blood pressure within the prescribed range. Hypotension may reduce blood flow to graft, and hypertension may cause bleeding.

- Assess and monitor the operative limb every 15 min for 1 hr and then hourly after that, paying particular attention to the following:
    - Incision site for bleeding.
    - Peripheral pulses, capillary refill, and skin color/temperature for signs of bypass graft occlusion. In clients who have dark skin, assess nail beds and soles of feet to detect early cyanosis.
    - Site is marked with an indelible marker.
- Administer IV fluids as prescribed.
- Assess type of pain experienced by the client.
    - Throbbing pain is experienced due to an increase in blood flow to extremity.
    - Ischemic pain is often difficult to relieve with opioid administration.
- Administer analgesics, such as morphine sulfate and fentanyl (Sublimaze).
- Administer antibiotics as prescribed.
- Use surgical aseptic technique for dressing changes.
- Monitor incision sites for evidence of infection, such as erythema, tenderness, and drainage.
- Administer anticoagulant therapy, such as warfarin (Coumadin), heparin, and enoxaparin (Lovenox), to prevent reocclusion.
- Administer antiplatelet therapy, such as clopidogrel (Plavix), tirofiban (Aggrastat), and aspirin.
- Help client turn, cough, and deep breathe every 2 hr.
- Maintain bed rest for 18 to 24 hr. The leg should be kept straight during this time.
- Assist the client to get out of bed and ambulate. Encourage the use of a walker initially.
- Discourage the client from sitting for long periods of time.
- Apply antiembolic stockings to promote venous return.
- Set up a progressive exercise program that includes walking. Consider a physical therapy consult.
- Client Education
    - Advise the client to completely abstain from smoking. Suggest smoking-cessation program.
    - Reinforce activity restrictions.
    - Remind the client to avoid crossing his legs.
    - Advise the client to avoid risk factors for atherosclerosis (smoking, sedentary lifestyle, uncontrolled diabetes mellitus).
    - Teach techniques of foot inspection and care.
        - Keep feet dry and clean.
        - Avoid extreme temperatures.
        - Use lotion.
        - Avoid socks with tight cuffs.
        - Wear clean, white, cotton socks, and always wear shoes.

- Complications
  - Graft occlusion
    - The graft may occlude due to reduced blood flow and clot formation. Occurs primarily in first 24 hr postoperative.
    - Nursing Actions
      - Notify the provider immediately for changes in pedal pulse, extremity color, or temperature.
      - Prepare the client for thrombectomy or thrombolytic therapy.
      - Monitor for bleeding with thrombolytics.
      - Monitor coagulation studies.
      - Monitor for anaphylaxis.
  - Compartment syndrome
    - Pressure from tissue swelling or bleeding within a compartment or a restricted space causes reduced blood flow to the area. Untreated, the affected tissue will become necrotic and die.
    - Nursing Actions
      - Assess for worsening pain, swelling, and tense or taut skin.
      - Report unusual findings to the provider immediately.
      - Prepare the client for a fasciotomy to relieve compartmental pressure.
  - Infection
    - Infection of the surgical site may result in the loss of the graft and increased ischemia.
    - Nursing Actions
      - Assess the wound for increased redness, swelling, and drainage.
      - Monitor WBC count and temperature.
      - Collect specimens (wound or blood cultures).
      - Administer antibiotic therapy.
    - Client Education
      - Advise the client to notify the provider of decreased sensation, increased ischemic pain, redness, or swelling at incisional site or in affected limb.

APPLICATION EXERCISES

1. A nurse is caring for a client who is 4 hr postoperative following coronary artery bypass grafting (CABG) surgery. He is able to inspire 200 mL with the incentive spirometer, then refuses to cough because he is tired and it hurts too much. Which of the following is an appropriate nursing intervention?

    A. Allow the client to rest, and return in 1 hr.

    B. Administer IV bolus analgesic, and return in 15 min.

    C. Document the 200 mL as an appropriate inspired volume.

    D. Tell the client that he must try to cough if he does not want to get pneumonia.

2. A nurse is caring for a client following peripheral bypass graft surgery of the left lower extremity. Which of the following client findings pose an immediate concern? (Select all that apply.)

    _____ A. Trace of bloody drainage on dressing

    _____ B. Capillary refill of affected limb of 6 seconds

    _____ C. Mottled appearance of the limb

    _____ D. Throbbing pain of affected limb that is decreased following IV bolus analgesic

    _____ E. Pulse of 2+ in the affected limb

3. A nurse educator is reviewing the use of cardiopulmonary bypass during surgery for coronary artery bypass grafting with a group of nurses. Which of the following should be included in the discussion? (Select all that apply.)

    _____ A. The client's demand for oxygen is lowered.

    _____ B. Motion of the heart ceases.

    _____ C. Rewarming of the client takes place.

    _____ D. The client's metabolic rate is increased.

    _____ E. Blood flow to the heart is stopped.

4. A nurse is caring for a client following an angioplasty that was inserted through the femoral artery. While turning the client, the nurse discovers blood underneath the client's lower back. The nurse should suspect

    A. retroperitoneal bleeding.

    B. cardiac tamponade.

    C. bleeding from the incisional site.

    D. heart failure.

5. A nurse is completing the admission assessment of a client who will undergo peripheral bypass graft surgery on the left leg. Which of the following is an expected finding?

    A. Rubor of the affected leg when elevated

    B. 3+ dorsal pedal pulse in left foot

    C. Thin, peeling toenails of left foot

    D. Report of intermittent claudication in the affected leg

6. A nurse is developing the plan of care for a client who is returning to the unit following angioplasty. What should be included in the plan of care? Use the ATI Active Learning Template: Therapeutic Procedure to complete this item to include the following sections:

    A. Nursing Actions: Describe five postprocedure nursing actions.

    B. Potential Complications:
- Describe at least two.
- Describe at least two actions related to each of these complications.

APPLICATION EXERCISES KEY

1. A. INCORRECT: Turning, coughing, and deep breathing should be performed every 2 hr to promote oxygenation and circulation.

    B. **CORRECT:** Providing adequate analgesia and returning in 15 min will reduce pain and improve coughing effectiveness.

    C. INCORRECT: This is not an adequate inspired air volume to promote effective oxygenation.

    D. INCORRECT: This intervention is non-therapeutic communication.

    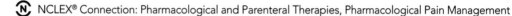 NCLEX® Connection: Pharmacological and Parenteral Therapies, Pharmacological Pain Management

2. A. INCORRECT: A trace of bloody drainage on the dressing is an expected finding and does not require immediate concern.

    B. **CORRECT:** Capillary refill greater than 2 to 4 seconds is outside the expected reference range and should be reported to the provider.

    C. **CORRECT:** Mottled appearance of the affected extremity is an unexpected finding and should be reported to the provider.

    D. INCORRECT: Pain that is decreased following IV bolus analgesia is an expected finding and does not require immediate concern.

    E. INCORRECT: Pulse of 2+ in the affected extremity is an expected finding and does not require immediate concern.

     NCLEX® Connection: Reduction of Risk Potential, Potential for Complications of Diagnostic Tests/ Treatments/Procedures

3. A. **CORRECT:** The use of cardiopulmonary bypass reduces the client's demand for oxygen, which reduces the risk of inadequate oxygenation of vital organs.

    B. **CORRECT:** Motion of the heart ceases during cardiopulmonary bypass to allow for placement of the graft near the affected coronary artery.

    C. **CORRECT:** The core body temperature is lowered for the procedure, and rewarming then occurs through heat exchanges on the cardiopulmonary bypass machine.

    D. INCORRECT: The use of cardiopulmonary bypass decreases the rate of metabolism.

    E. INCORRECT: Blood flow to the heart is maintained by the action of the cardiopulmonary bypass machine.

     NCLEX® Connection: Reduction of Risk Potential, Potential for Complications of Diagnostic Tests/ Treatments/Procedures

4. A. INCORRECT: Retroperitoneal bleeding is internal bleeding.

    B. INCORRECT: Cardiac tamponade includes manifestations of bleeding in the pericardial sac, which is internal.

    C. **CORRECT:** Bleeding is occurring from the incision site and then draining under the client. The nurse should assess the incision for hematoma, apply pressure, monitor the client, and notify the provider.

    D. INCORRECT: Heart failure does not including findings of blood underneath the client's lower back.

    Ⓝ NCLEX® Connection: Reduction of Risk Potential, Therapeutic Procedures

5. A. INCORRECT: Reddening (rubor) of a leg affected by peripheral artery disease occurs when it is placed in a dependent position.

    B. INCORRECT: Pulses are decreased or absent in the feet in cases of peripheral artery disease.

    C. INCORRECT: Toenails are thickened in cases of peripheral artery disease.

    D. **CORRECT:** A client who has peripheral artery disease may report that numbness or burning pain in the extremity ceases with rest (intermittent claudication).

    Ⓝ NCLEX® Connection: Physiological Adaptations, Alterations in Body Systems

6. *Using ATI Active Learning Template: Therapeutic Procedure*

    A. Nursing Actions

    - Assess vital signs every 15 min x 4, every 30 min x 2, every hour x 4, and then every 4 hr (or per facility protocol).
    - Assess the groin site with vital signs.
    - Maintain bed rest in supine position with leg straight for prescribed time.
    - Conduct continuous cardiac monitoring for dysrhythmia.
    - Administer antiplatelet or thrombolytic agents as prescribed.
    - Administer anxiolytics and analgesics as prescribed.
    - Monitor urine output, and administer IV fluids for hydration.
    - Assist with sheath removal from insertion site.

    B. Potential Complications

    - Cardiac tamponade: Notify the provider; administer IV fluids to manage hypotension; obtain chest x-ray or echocardiogram; prepare for pericardiocentesis.
    - Hematoma formation: Monitor sensation, color, capillary refill, and pulse in extremity distal to insertion site; hold pressure for uncontrolled oozing/bleeding; notify the provider.
    - Allergic reaction: Monitor the client; have resuscitation equipment available; administer diphenhydramine or epinephrine as needed.
    - External bleeding: Monitor insertion site for bleeding or swelling; apply pressure to insertion site; keep client's leg straight.
    - Embolism: Monitor for chest pain; monitor vital signs and SaO_2.
    - Retroperitoneal bleeding: Assess for flank pain and hypotension; notify the provider; administer IV fluids and blood products as prescribed.
    - Restenosis of vessel: Assess ECG pattern and for report of chest pain; notify the provider; prepare for return to cardiac catheterization laboratory.

    Ⓝ NCLEX® Connection: Physiological Adaptations, Alterations in Body Systems

UNIT 4   **NURSING CARE OF CLIENTS WITH CARDIOVASCULAR DISORDERS**
          SECTION: CARDIAC DISORDERS

CHAPTER 31   Angina and Myocardial Infarction

Overview

- The continuum from angina to myocardial infarction (MI) is termed acute coronary syndrome. Symptoms of acute coronary syndrome are due to an imbalance between myocardial oxygen supply and demand.

 View Image: Myocardial Infarction

- Angina pectoris is a warning sign of an impending acute MI.

- Women and older adults do not always experience manifestations typically associated with angina or MI.

- The majority of deaths from an MI occur within 1 hr of onset of findings. The average time for a person seeking treatment is 4 hr. Early recognition and treatment of an acute MI is essential to prevent death.

- Research shows improved outcomes following an MI in clients treated with aspirin, beta-blockers, and angiotensin-converting enzyme (ACE) inhibitors.

- When blood flow to the heart is compromised, ischemia causes chest pain. Anginal pain is often described as a tight squeezing, heavy pressure, or constricting feeling in the chest. The pain can radiate to the jaw, neck, or arm.

- There are three types of angina:

  ○ Stable angina (exertional angina) occurs with exercise or emotional stress and is relieved by rest or nitroglycerin (Nitrostat).

  ○ Unstable angina (preinfarction angina) occurs with exercise or emotional stress, but it increases in occurrence, severity, and duration over time.

  ○ Variant angina (Prinzmetal's angina) is due to a coronary artery spasm, often occurring during periods of rest.

- Pain unrelieved by rest or nitroglycerin and lasting for more than 15 min differentiates an MI from angina.

- An abrupt interruption of oxygen to the heart muscle produces myocardial ischemia. Ischemia can lead to tissue necrosis (infarction) if blood supply and oxygen are not restored. Ischemia is reversible. An infarction results in permanent damage.

- When the cardiac muscle suffers ischemic injury, cardiac enzymes are released into the bloodstream, providing specific markers of MI.

- MIs are classified based on the following:

  ○ Affected area of the heart (anterior, anterolateral)

  ○ Depth of involvement (transmural versus nontransmural)

  ○ ECG changes produced (Q wave, non-Q wave); non-Q-wave MIs are more common in older adults, women, and clients who have diabetes mellitus.

ANGINA	MYOCARDIAL INFARCTION
› Precipitated by exertion or stress	› Can occur without cause, often in the morning after rest
› Relieved by rest or nitroglycerin	› Relieved only by opioids
› Symptoms last less than 15 min	› Symptoms last more than 30 min
› Not associated with nausea, epigastric distress, dyspnea, anxiety, diaphoresis	› Associated with nausea, epigastric distress, dyspnea, anxiety, diaphoresis

Health Promotion and Disease Prevention

- Encourage the client to maintain an exercise routine to remain physically active. The client should consult with a provider before starting any exercise regimen.
- The client should have cholesterol level and blood pressure checked regularly.
- The client should consume a diet low in saturated fats and sodium. The client also should consult with a provider regarding diet restrictions.
- If the client is a smoker, promote smoking cessation.

Assessment

- Risk Factors
  - Male gender or postmenopausal women
  - Hypertension
  - Tobacco use
  - Hyperlipidemia
  - Metabolic disorders (diabetes mellitus, hyperthyroidism)
  - Methamphetamine or cocaine use
  - Stress (occupational, physical exercise, sexual activity)
  - An increased risk of coronary artery disease exists for older adult clients who are physically inactive, have one or more chronic diseases (hypertension, heart failure, and diabetes mellitus), or have lifestyle (smoking and diet) habits that contribute to atherosclerosis. Atherosclerotic changes related to aging predispose the heart to poor blood perfusion and oxygen delivery.
  - The incidence of cardiac disease increases with age, especially in the presence of hypertension, diabetes mellitus, hypercholesterolemia, elevated homocysteine, and highly sensitive C-reactive protein (HS-CRP).
- Subjective Data
  - Anxiety, feeling of impending doom
  - Chest pain (substernal or precordial)
    - Pain can radiate down the shoulder or arm, or may present in the form of jaw pain.
    - Pain may be described as a crushing or aching pressure.
  - Nausea
  - Dizziness

- Objective Data
  - Physical Assessment Findings
    - Pallor, and cool, clammy skin
    - Tachycardia and/or heart palpitations
    - Diaphoresis
    - Vomiting
    - Decreased level of consciousness
  - Laboratory Tests
    - Cardiac enzymes released with cardiac muscle injury:
      - Myoglobin – Earliest marker of injury to cardiac or skeletal muscle. Levels no longer evident after 24 hr.
      - Creatine kinase-MB – Peaks around 24 hr after onset of chest pain. Levels no longer evident after 3 days.
      - Troponin I or T – Any positive value indicates damage to cardiac tissue and should be reported.
        - ▸ Troponin I – Levels no longer evident after 7 days.
        - ▸ Troponin T – Levels no longer evident after 14 to 21 days.
  - Diagnostic Procedures (Refer to the chapter on *Cardiovascular Diagnostic and Therapeutic Procedures.*)
    - Electrocardiogram (ECG) – recording of electrical activity of the heart over time
      - Nursing Actions
        - ▸ Assess for changes on serial ECGs.
        - ▸ Client who has angina – ST depression and/or T-wave inversion indicates presence of ischemia.
        - ▸ Client who has MI – T-wave inversion indicates ischemia; ST-segment elevation indicates injury; abnormal Q-wave indicates necrosis.
    - Stress test – Also known as exercise electrocardiography. Client tolerance of activity is tested using a treadmill, bicycle, or medication to evaluate response to increased heart rate.
    - Thallium scan – Assesses for ischemia or necrosis. Radioisotopes cannot reach areas with decreased or absent perfusion, and the areas appear as "cold spots."
      - Nursing Actions
        - ▸ Instruct the client to avoid smoking and consuming caffeinated beverages 4 hr prior to the procedure. These can affect the test.
    - Cardiac catheterization
      - A coronary angiogram, also called a cardiac catheterization, is an invasive diagnostic procedure used to evaluate the presence and degree of coronary artery blockage.
      - Angiography involves the insertion of a catheter into a femoral (sometimes a brachial) vessel and threading it into the right or left side of the heart. Coronary artery narrowing and occlusions are identified by the injection of contrast media under fluoroscopy.
      - Nursing Actions
        - ▸ Ensure the client understands the procedure prior to signing informed consent.
        - ▸ Ensure that the client remains NPO 8 hr prior to procedure.
        - ▸ Assess that the client and family understand the procedure.
        - ▸ Assess for iodine/shellfish allergy (contrast media).

Patient-Centered Care

- Nursing Care
  - Monitor
    - Vital signs every 15 min until stable, then every hour
    - Serial ECG, continuous cardiac monitoring
    - Location, precipitating factors, severity, quality, and duration of pain
    - Hourly urine output – greater than 30 mL/hr indicates renal perfusion
    - Laboratory data (cardiac enzymes, electrolytes, ABGs)
  - Administer oxygen (2 to 4 L/min).
  - Obtain and maintain IV access.
  - Promote energy conservation (cluster nursing interventions).
- Medications
  - Vasodilators
    - Nitroglycerin (Nitrostat) prevents coronary artery vasospasm and reduces preload and afterload, decreasing myocardial oxygen demand.
    - Nursing Considerations
      - □ Used to treat angina and help control blood pressure.
      - □ Used cautiously with other antihypertensive medications.
      - □ Vasodilators can cause orthostatic hypotension.
    - Client Education
      - □ Client education regarding response to chest pain:
        - ▸ Stop activity and rest.
        - ▸ Place nitroglycerin tablet under tongue to dissolve (quick absorption).
        - ▸ If pain is unrelieved in 5 min, the client should call 911 or be driven to an emergency department.
        - ▸ The client can take up to two more doses of nitroglycerin at 5-min intervals.
      - □ Remind the client that a headache is a common side effect of this medication.
      - □ Encourage the client to sit and lie down slowly.
  - Analgesics
    - Morphine sulfate is an opioid analgesic used to treat moderate to severe pain. Analgesics act on the mu and kappa receptors that help alleviate pain.
    - Activation of these receptors produces analgesia (pain relief), respiratory depression, euphoria, sedation, and a decrease in gastrointestinal (GI) motility.
    - Use cautiously with clients who have asthma or emphysema due to the risk of respiratory depression.

- Nursing Considerations
  - For the client having chest pain, assess pain every 5 to 15 min.
  - Watch for manifestations of respiratory depression, especially in older adults. If respirations are 12/min or less, stop medication, and notify the provider immediately.
  - Monitor vital signs for signs of hypotension and decreased respirations.
  - Assess for nausea and vomiting.
- Client Education
  - If nausea and vomiting persist, advise the client to notify a nurse.
  - Teach the client to use the PCA pump, if applicable.
    - The client is the only person who should push the medication administration button. Reassure the client that the safety lockout mechanism on the PCA pump prevents overdosing of the medication.

- Beta-blockers
  - Metoprolol tartrate (Lopressor) has antidysrhythmic and antihypertensive properties that decrease the imbalance between myocardial oxygen supply and demand by reducing afterload and slowing heart rate.
  - In an acute MI, beta-blockers decrease infarct size and improve short- and long-term survival rates.
  - Nursing Considerations
    - Beta-blockers can cause bradycardia and hypotension. Hold the medication if the apical pulse rate is less than 60/min, and notify the provider.
    - Avoid giving to clients who have asthma. Cardioselective beta blockers (affect only beta 1 receptors) are preferred to minimize effects on the respiratory system.
    - Use with caution in clients who have heart failure.
  - Client Education
    - Encourage the client to sit and lie down slowly.
    - Remind the client to notify the provider immediately if shortness of breath, edema, weight gain, or cough occur.
- Thrombolytic agents
  - Streptokinase (Streptase) and alteplase (Activase) are used to break up blood clots.
  - Thrombolytic agents have similar side effects and contraindications as anticoagulants.
  - For best results, give within 6 hr of infarction.
  - Nursing Considerations
    - Assess for contraindications (active bleeding, peptic ulcer disease, history of CVA, recent trauma).
    - Monitor for effects of bleeding (mental status changes, hematuria).
    - Monitor bleeding times – PT, aPTT, INR, fibrinogen levels, and CBC.
    - Monitor for same side effects as anticoagulants (thrombocytopenia, anemia, hemorrhage).
    - Administer streptokinase slowly to prevent hypotension.
  - Client Education
    - Remind the client of the risk for bruising and bleeding while on this medication.

○ Antiplatelet agents

- Aspirin (Ecotrin) and clopidogrel (Plavix) prevent platelets from forming together, which can produce arterial clotting.

- Aspirin prevents vasoconstriction. Due to this and antiplatelet effects, it should be administered with nitroglycerin at the onset of chest pain.

- Nursing Considerations

  □ Antiplatelet agents can cause GI upset.

  □ Use cautiously with clients who have a history of GI ulcers.

  □ Tinnitus, ringing in the ears, can be a sign of aspirin toxicity.

- Client Education

  □ Remind the client of the risk for bruising and bleeding while on this medication.

  □ Encourage the client to use aspirin tablets with enteric coating and to take with food.

  □ Tell the client to report ringing in the ears.

○ Anticoagulants

- Heparin and enoxaparin (Lovenox) are used to prevent clots from becoming larger or other clots from forming.

- Nursing Considerations

  □ Assess for contraindications (active bleeding, peptic ulcer disease, history of CVA, recent trauma).

  □ Monitor bleeding times – PT, aPTT, INR, and CBC.

  □ Monitor for adverse effects of anticoagulants (thrombocytopenia, anemia, hemorrhage).

- Client Education

  □ Remind the client of the risk for bruising and bleeding while on this medication.

○ Glycoprotein IIB/IIIA inhibitors

- Eptifibatide (Integrilin) is used to prevent binding of fibrogen, in turn blocking platelet aggregation. In combination with aspirin therapy, IIB/IIA inhibitors are standard therapy.

- Nursing Considerations

  □ This medication can cause active bleeding.

- Client Education

  □ Instruct the client to report evidence of bleeding during medication therapy.

• Teamwork and Collaboration

○ Pain management services can be consulted if pain persists and/or is uncontrolled.

○ Cardiac rehabilitation care can be consulted if the client has prolonged weakness and needs assistance with increasing level of activity.

○ Nutritional services can be consulted for diet modification to promote low-sodium and low-saturated fat food choices.

• Surgical Interventions

○ Percutaneous transluminal coronary angioplasty (PTCA)

○ Bypass graft (also known as CABG)

- Care after Discharge
  - Cardiac rehabilitation should be consulted for a specific exercise program related to the heart.
  - Nutritional services, such as a dietitian, can be consulted for diet modification or weight management.
  - Client Education
    - Instruct the client to monitor and report signs of infection, such as fever, incisional drainage, and redness.
    - Teach the client to avoid straining, strenuous exercise, or emotional stress when possible.
    - Client education regarding response to chest pain – follow instructions on use of sublingual nitroglycerin.
    - If client is a smoker, encourage smoking cessation.
    - Encourage the client to remain active and to exercise regularly.

Complications

- Acute MI – a complication of angina not relieved by rest or nitroglycerin.
  - Nursing Actions
    - Administer oxygen to the client.
    - Notify the provider immediately.
- Heart failure/cardiogenic shock
  - Injury to the left ventricle can lead to decreased cardiac output and heart failure.
  - Progressive heart failure can lead to cardiogenic shock.
    - This is a serious complication of pump failure, commonly following an MI of 40% blockage.
    - Manifestations include tachycardia; hypotension; inadequate urinary output; altered level of consciousness; respiratory distress (crackles and tachypnea); cool, clammy skin; decreased peripheral pulses; and chest pain.
  - Nursing Actions
    - Administration of oxygen; possible intubation and ventilation may be required.
    - IV administration of morphine, diuretics, and/or nitroglycerin to decrease preload; IV administration of vasopressors and/or positive inotropes to increase cardiac output and to maintain organ perfusion.
    - Maintain continuous hemodynamic monitoring.
- Ischemic mitral regurgitation – evidenced by development of a new cardiac murmur.
  - Nursing Actions
    - Administer oxygen to the client.
    - Notify the provider immediately.

- Ventricular aneurysms/rupture – may be due to necrosis from MI; can present as sudden chest pain, dysrhythmias, and severe hypotension
  - Nursing Actions
    - Administer oxygen to the client.
    - Notify the provider immediately.
- Dysrhythmias
  - An inferior wall MI may lead to an injury to the AV node, resulting in bradycardia and second-degree AV heart block.
  - An anterior wall MI may lead to an injury to the ventricle, resulting in premature ventricular contractions, bundle branch, or complete heart block.
  - Nursing Actions
    - Monitor ECG and vital signs.
    - Administer oxygen.
    - Administer antidysrhythmic medications as indicated.
    - Prepare for cardiac pacemaker if needed.

APPLICATION EXERCISES

1. A nurse is admitting a client who has a suspected myocardial infarction (MI) and a history of angina. Which of the following findings will help the nurse distinguish angina from an MI?

A. Angina can be relieved with rest and nitroglycerin.

B. The pain of an MI resolves in less than 15 min.

C. The type of activity that causes an MI can be identified.

D. Angina can occur for longer than 30 min.

2. A nurse on a cardiac unit is reviewing the laboratory findings of a client who has a diagnosis of myocardial infarction (MI) and reports that his dyspnea began 2 weeks ago. Which of the following cardiac enzymes would confirm the infarction occurred 14 days ago?

A. CK-MB

B. Troponin I

C. Troponin T

D. Myoglobin

3. A nurse is caring for a client in a clinic who asks the nurse why her provider prescribed 1 aspirin per day. Which of the following is an appropriate response by the nurse?

A. "Aspirin reduces the formation of blood clots that could cause a heart attack."

B. "Aspirin relieves the pain due to myocardial ischemia."

C. "Aspirin dissolves clots that are forming in your coronary arteries."

D. "Aspirin relieves headaches that are caused by other medications."

4. A nurse is instructing a client who has angina about a new prescription for metoprolol tartrate (Lopressor). Which of the following statements by the client indicates understanding of the teaching?

A. "I should place the tablet under my tongue."

B. "I should have my clotting time checked weekly."

C. "I will report any ringing in my ears."

D. "I will call my doctor if my pulse rate is less than 60."

5. A nurse is presenting a community education program on recommended lifestyle changes to prevent angina and myocardial infarction. Which of the following changes should the nurse recommend be made first?

    A. Diet modification

    B. Relaxation exercises

    C. Smoking cessation

    D. Taking omega-3 capsules

6. A nurse is teaching a client who has new diagnosis of angina about a new prescription for nitroglycerin (Nitrostat). Which of the following should be included in the teaching? Use the ATI Active Learning Template: Medication and the ATI Pharmacology Review Module to complete this item to include the following sections:

    A. Therapeutic Uses

    B. Side/Adverse Effects:
- Describe two.
- Describe at least one teaching point for each side/adverse effect.

    C. Medication/Food Interactions: Describe two.

    D. Nursing Administration: Describe how the client should be instructed to take the medication in response to chest pain.

APPLICATION EXERCISES KEY

1. A. **CORRECT:** Angina can be relieved by rest and nitroglycerin.

   B. INCORRECT: The pain associated with an MI usually lasts longer than 30 min and requires opioid analgesics for relief.

   C. INCORRECT: There is no specific type of activity that causes an MI. It may occur following rest.

   D. INCORRECT: The pain of angina usually occurs for 15 min or less.

   ⓝ NCLEX® Connection: Physiological Adaptations, Hemodynamics

2. A. INCORRECT: The creatinine kinase MB levels are no longer evident after 3 days.

   B. INCORRECT: Troponin I levels are no longer evident after 7 days.

   C. **CORRECT:** The Troponin T level will still be evident 14 to 21 days following an MI.

   D. INCORRECT: Myoglobin levels are no longer evident after 24 hr.

   ⓝ NCLEX® Connection: Reduction of Risk Potential, Laboratory Values

3. A. **CORRECT:** Aspirin decreases platelet aggregation that can cause a myocardial infarction.

   B. INCORRECT: One aspirin a day is not sufficient to alleviate ischemic pain.

   C. INCORRECT: Aspirin does not dissolve clots.

   D. INCORRECT: Other medications can cause headaches, but one aspirin per day is not administered as an analgesic.

   ⓝ NCLEX® Connection: Pharmacological and Parenteral Therapies, Medication Administration

4. A. INCORRECT: Lopressor is administered orally, not sublingual.

   B. INCORRECT: Lopressor does not affect bleeding or clotting time. A CBC and blood glucose should be monitored periodically.

   C. INCORRECT: Ringing in the ears is not an adverse effect of the medication. Dry mouth and mucous membranes can occur.

   D. **CORRECT:** The client is advised to notify the provider if bradycardia (pulse rate less than 60) occurs.

   ⓝ NCLEX® Connection: Health Promotion and Maintenance, Health Promotion/Disease Prevention

5. A. INCORRECT: Diet modification is an important recommended lifestyle change, but there is another action that is more important.

    B. INCORRECT: The use of relaxation exercises is an important recommended lifestyle change, but there is another action that is more important.

    C. **CORRECT:** According to the airway, breathing, and circulation (ABC) priority-setting framework, adequate oxygenation is the priority. Nicotine causes vasoconstriction, elevates blood pressure, and narrows coronary arteries. Therefore, smoking cessation should be the first recommended lifestyle change.

    D. INCORRECT: Taking omega-3 capsules is an important recommended lifestyle change, but there is another action that is more important.

    (N) NCLEX® Connection: Pharmacological and Parenteral Therapies, Medication Administration

6. *Using the ATI Active Learning Template: Medication*

    A. Therapeutic Uses

    - Treatment of acute angina attack

    B. Side/Adverse Effects

    - Headache

        ○ Take aspirin or acetaminophen to relieve pain.

        ○ Notify the provider if headache persists.

    - Orthostatic hypotension

        ○ Sit or lie down if experiencing dizziness or faintness.

        ○ Avoid sudden position changes, and rise slowly.

    - Reflex tachycardia

        ○ Monitor pulse and BP.

    - Tolerance

        ○ Take lowest dose needed to achieve effect.

    C. Medication/Food Interactions

    - Alcohol can have a hypotensive effect.

    - Other beta-blocker medications, calcium channel blockers, and diuretics can contribute to hypotensive effects.

    - Male clients should not take sildenafil if prescribed nitroglycerin.

    D. Nursing Administration

    - Stop activity and rest. Place tablet under tongue to dissolve. If pain is unrelieved in 5 min, call 911 or ask to be driven to the emergency department. Take two more doses at 5-min intervals.

    (N) NCLEX® Connection: Pharmacological and Parenteral Therapies, Medication Administration

chapter 32

Overview

- Heart failure occurs when the heart muscle is unable to pump effectively, resulting in inadequate cardiac output, myocardial hypertrophy, and pulmonary/systemic congestion. The heart is unable to maintain adequate circulation to meet tissue needs.

- Heart failure is the result of an acute or chronic cardiopulmonary problem, such as systemic hypertension, myocardial infarction (MI), pulmonary hypertension, dysrhythmias, valvular heart disease, pericarditis, and cardiomyopathy.

- Pulmonary edema is a severe, life-threatening accumulation of fluid in the alveoli and interstitial spaces of the lung that can result from severe heart failure.

HEART FAILURE

Overview

- The severity of heart failure is graded on the New York Heart Association's functional classification scale indicating how little, or how much activity it takes to make the client symptomatic (chest pain, or shortness of breath).

  - Class I: Client exhibits no symptoms with activity.

  - Class II: Client has symptoms with ordinary exertion.

  - Class III: Client displays symptoms with minimal exertion.

  - Class IV: Client has symptoms at rest.

- Low-output heart failure can initially occur on either the left or right side of the heart.

  - Left-sided heart (ventricular) failure results in inadequate left ventricle (cardiac) output and consequently in inadequate tissue perfusion. Forms include the following:

    - Systolic heart (ventricular) failure (ejection fraction below 40%, pulmonary and systemic congestion)

    - Diastolic heart (ventricular) failure (inadequate relaxation or "stiffening" prevents ventricular filling)

  - Right-sided heart (ventricular) failure results in inadequate right ventricle output and systemic venous congestion (peripheral edema).

- An uncommon form of heart failure is high-output failure, in which cardiac output is normal or above normal.

Health Promotion and Disease Prevention

- Maintain an exercise routine to remain physically active, and consult with the provider before starting any exercise regimen.
- Consume a diet low in sodium, along with fluid restrictions, and consult with the provider regarding diet specifications.
- Refrain from smoking.
- Follow medication regimen, and follow up with the provider as needed.

Assessment

- Risk Factors
  - Left-sided heart (ventricular) failure
    - Hypertension
    - Coronary artery disease, angina, MI
    - Valvular disease (mitral and aortic)
  - Right-sided heart (ventricular) failure
    - Left-sided heart (ventricular) failure
    - Right ventricular MI
    - Pulmonary problems (COPD, pulmonary fibrosis)
  - High-output heart failure
    - Increased metabolic needs
    - Septicemia (fever)
    - Anemia
    - Hyperthyroidism
  - Cardiomyopathy
    - Coronary artery disease
    - Infection or inflammation of the heart muscle
    - Various cancer treatments
    - Prolonged alcohol use
    - Heredity
  - ⓖ Systolic blood pressure is elevated in older adults, putting them at risk for coronary artery disease and heart failure.
  - Certain medications may increase the risk of heart failure or worsen manifestations in the older adult client.
- Subjective and Objective Data
  - Left-sided failure
    - Dyspnea, orthopnea (shortness of breath while lying down), nocturnal dyspnea
    - Fatigue
    - Displaced apical pulse (hypertrophy)

- S_3 heart sound (gallop)
- Pulmonary congestion (dyspnea, cough, bibasilar crackles)
- Frothy sputum (can be blood-tinged)
- Altered mental status
- Manifestations of organ failure, such as oliguria (decrease in urine output)
○ Right-sided failure
  - Jugular vein distention
  - Ascending dependent edema (legs, ankles, sacrum)
  - Abdominal distention, ascites
  - Fatigue, weakness
  - Nausea and anorexia
  - Polyuria at rest (nocturnal)
  - Liver enlargement (hepatomegaly) and tenderness
  - Weight gain
○ Cardiomyopathy (leading to heart failure)

M ◇ View Image: Cardiomyopathy

- Four types
  □ Dilated (most common)
  □ Hypertrophic
  □ Arrhythmogenic right ventricular
  □ Restrictive
- Blood circulation is impaired to the lungs when the cardiac pump is compromised.
- Manifestations
  □ Fatigue, weakness
  □ Heart failure (left with dilated type, right with restrictive type)
  □ Dysrhythmias (heart block)
  □ S_3 gallop
  □ Cardiomegaly (enlarged heart), more severe with dilated type
  □ Angina (hypertrophic type)
Ⓖ ○ The presence of other chronic illnesses (lung disease, kidney failure) can mask the presence of heart failure in older adult clients.
○ Laboratory Tests
  - Human B-type natriuretic peptides (hBNP): Elevated in heart failure. In clients who have dyspnea, elevated hBNP confirms a diagnosis of heart failure rather than a problem originating in the respiratory system. hBNP levels direct the aggressiveness of treatment interventions.
    □ A level below 100 pg/mL indicates no heart failure.
    □ Levels between 100 to 300 pg/mL suggest heart failure is present.

- □ A level above 300 pg/mL indicates mild heart failure.

- □ A level above 600 pg/mL indicates moderate heart failure.

- □ A level above 900 pg/mL indicates severe heart failure.

- ○ Diagnostic Procedures

  - ▪ Hemodynamic monitoring

    - □ Heart failure generally results in increased central venous pressure (CVP), increased pulmonary wedge pressure (PAWP), increased pulmonary artery pressure (PAP), and decreased cardiac output (CO). See the *Invasive Cardiovascular Procedures* chapter for detailed information related to hemodynamic monitoring.

    - □ Mixed venous oxygen saturation (SvO_2) is directly related to cardiac output. A drop in SvO_2 indicates worsening cardiac function.

  - ▪ Ultrasound

    - □ An ultrasound (also called cardiac ultrasound or echocardiogram), 2-D (two-dimensional) or 3-D (three-dimensional) is used to measure systolic and diastolic function of the heart.

      - ▸ Left ventricular ejection fraction (LVEF): The volume of blood pumped from the left ventricle into the arteries upon each beat. Normal is 55% to 70%.

      - ▸ Right ventricular ejection fraction (RVEF): The volume of blood pumped from the right ventricle to the lungs upon each beat. Normal is 45% to 60%.

  - ▪ Transesophageal echocardiography (TEE) uses a transducer placed in the esophagus behind the heart to obtain a detailed view of cardiac structures. The nurse prepares the client for a TEE in the same manner as for an upper endoscopy.

  - ▪ A chest x-ray can reveal cardiomegaly and pleural effusions.

  - ▪ Electrocardiogram (ECG), cardiac enzymes, electrolytes, and ABGs are used to assess factors contributing to heart failure and/or the impact of heart failure.

Patient-Centered Care

- • Nursing Care

  - ○ Monitor daily weight and I&O.

  - ○ Assess for shortness of breath and dyspnea on exertion.

  - ○ Administer oxygen as prescribed.

  - ○ Monitor vital signs and hemodynamic pressures.

  - ○ Position the client to maximize ventilation (high-Fowler's).

  - ○ Check ABGs, electrolytes (especially potassium if on diuretics), SaO_2, and chest x-ray findings.

  - ○ Assess for signs of medication toxicity (digoxin toxicity).

  - ○ Encourage bed rest until the client is stable.

  - ○ Encourage energy conservation by assisting with care and ADLs.

  - ○ Maintain dietary restrictions as prescribed (restricted fluid intake, restricted sodium intake).

  - ○ Provide emotional support to the client and family.

- Medications

  - Herbal medications can stimulate the cardiovascular system. Obtain a list of herbal supplements the client takes, and advise the client of potential contraindications.

  - Diuretics

    - Diuretics are used to decrease preload.

      - Loop diuretics, such as furosemide (Lasix), bumetanide (Bumex)

      - Thiazide diuretics, such as hydrochlorothiazide (Hydrodiuril)

      - Potassium-sparing diuretics, such as spironolactone (Aldactone)

    - Nursing Considerations

      - Administer furosemide IV no faster than 20 mg/min.

      - Loop and thiazide diuretics can cause hypokalemia, and potassium supplementation may be required.

    - Client Education

      - Teach clients taking loop or thiazide diuretics to ingest foods and drinks that are high in potassium to counter the effects of hypokalemia.

  - Afterload-reducing agents

    - Afterload-reducing agents help the heart pump more easily by altering the resistance to contraction.

      - Angiotensin-converting enzyme (ACE) inhibitors, such as enalapril (Vasotec), captopril (Capoten)

      - Angiotensin receptor II blockers, such as losartan (Cozaar)

      - Calcium channel blockers, such as diltiazem (Cardizem), nifedipine (Procardia)

      - Phosphodiesterase-3 inhibitors, such as milrinone (Primacor)

    - These are contraindicated for clients who have renal deficiency.

    - Nursing Considerations

      - Monitor clients taking ACE inhibitors for hypotension following the initial dose.

        ‣ ACE inhibitors can cause angioedema (swelling of the tongue and throat), a decreased sense of taste, or a skin rash.

        ‣ Monitor for increased levels of potassium.

    - Client Education

      - Inform the client that this medication can cause a dry cough.

      - Notify the provider if the client observes a rash or has a decreased sense of taste.

      - Notify the provider if swelling of the face or extremities occurs.

      - Remind the client that blood pressure needs to be monitored for 2 hr after the initial dose to detect hypotension.

- ○ Inotropic agents
  - ■ Inotropic agents, such as digoxin (Lanoxin), dopamine, dobutamine (Dobutrex), and milrinone (Primacor), are used to increase contractility and thereby improve cardiac output.
  - ■ Nursing Considerations
    - □ For a client taking digoxin, take the apical heart rate for 1 min. Hold the medication if apical pulse is less than 60/min, and notify the provider.
    - □ Observe the client for nausea and vomiting.
    - □ Dopamine, dobutamine, and milrinone are administered via IV. The ECG, blood pressure, and urine output must be closely monitored.
  - ■ Client Education
    - □ Teach clients who are self-administering digoxin to:
      - ▸ Count pulse for 1 min before taking the medication. If the pulse rate is irregular or the pulse rate is outside of the limitations set by the provider (usually less than 60/min or greater than 100/min), instruct the client to hold the dose and contact the provider.
      - ▸ Take the digoxin dose at the same time each day.
      - ▸ Do not take digoxin at the same time as antacids. Separate the two medications by at least 2 hr.
      - ▸ Report signs of toxicity, including fatigue, muscle weakness, confusion, and loss of appetite.
      - ▸ Regularly have digoxin and potassium levels checked.
- ○ Beta-adrenergic blockers (beta-blockers)
  - ■ Medications such as carvedilol (Coreg) and metoprolol (Lopressor) may be used to improve the condition of the client who has sustained increased levels of sympathetic stimulation and catecholamines. This would include clients who have chronic heart failure.
  - ■ Nursing considerations
    - □ Monitor BP, pulse, activity tolerance and orthopnea.
    - □ Check orthostatic blood pressure readings.
  - ■ Client Education
    - □ Instruct the client to weigh daily.
    - □ Advise the client to regularly check BP.
    - □ Tell the client to follow the provider's instructions on increasing medication dosage.
- ○ Vasodilators
  - ■ Nitroglycerine (Nitrostat) and isosorbide mononitrate (Imdur) prevent coronary artery vasospasm and reduce preload and afterload, decreasing myocardial oxygen demand.
  - ■ Nursing Considerations
    - □ Vasodilators are given to treat angina and help control blood pressure.
    - □ Use cautiously with other antihypertensive mediations.
    - □ Vasodilators can cause orthostatic hypotension.
  - ■ Client Education
    - □ Remind the client that a headache is a common side effect of this medication.
    - □ Encourage the client to sit and lie down slowly.

- Human B-type natriuretic peptides (hBNP)
  - hBNPs, such as nesiritide (Natrecor), are used to treat acute heart failure by causing natriuresis (loss of sodium and vasodilation). They are administered IV.
  - Nursing Considerations
    - hBNPs can cause hypotension, as well as a number of cardiac effects, including ventricular tachycardia and bradycardia.
    - BNP levels will increase while on this medication.
    - ECG, blood pressure, and other parameters should be monitored.
  - Client Education
    - The client can be asymptomatic with a low blood pressure.
    - Remind the client to sit and lie down slowly.
- Anticoagulants
  - Anticoagulants, such as warfarin (Coumadin), can be prescribed if the client has a history of thrombus formation.
  - Nursing Considerations
    - Assess for contraindications (active bleeding, peptic ulcer disease, history of cerebrovascular accident, recent trauma).
    - Monitor bleeding times – PT, aPTT, INR, and CBC.
  - Client Education
    - Remind the client of the risk for bruising and bleeding while on this medication.
    - Remind the client to have blood monitored routinely to check bleeding times.
- Teamwork and Collaboration
  - Cardiology and pulmonary services should be consulted to manage heart failure.
  - Respiratory services should be consulted for inhalers, breathing treatments, and suctioning for airway management.
  - Cardiac rehabilitation services can be consulted if the client has prolonged weakness and needs assistance with increasing level of activity.
  - Nutritional services can be consulted for diet modification to promote low-sodium, and low-saturated fat food choices.
- Surgical Interventions
  - Ventricular assist device (VAD)
    - A VAD is a mechanical pump that assists a heart that is too weak to pump blood through the body. A VAD is used in clients who are eligible for heart transplants or who have severe end-stage heart failure and are not candidates for heart transplants. Heart transplantation is the treatment of choice for clients who have severe dilated cardiomyopathy.
    - Nursing Actions
      - Prepare the client for the procedure (NPO status and informed consent).
      - Monitor postoperatively (vital signs, SaO_2, incision drainage, and pain management).

- ○ Heart Transplantation

  - ▪ Heart transplantation is a possible option for clients who have end-stage heart failure. Immunosuppressant therapy is required posttransplantation to prevent rejection.

  - ▪ Eligibility for transplantation depends on several factors, including life expectancy, age, psychosocial status, and absence of drug and alcohol use disorders.

  - ▪ Nursing Actions

    - □ Prepare the client for the procedure (NPO status and informed consent). Laboratory reports and results of diagnostic testing should be available as prescribed.

    - □ Monitor postoperatively (vital signs, SaO_2, incision drainage, and pain management).

    - □ Monitor for complications. Organ transplant recipients are at risk for infection, thrombosis, and rejection. See the *Kidney Transplant* chapter for details related to these complications.

  - ▪ Client Education

    - □ Take medications as prescribed.

    - □ Take diuretics in the early morning and early afternoon.

    - □ Maintain fluid and sodium restriction – a dietary consult can be useful.

    - □ Increase dietary intake of potassium (cantaloupe or bananas) if the client is taking potassium-losing diuretics, such as loop and thiazide diuretics.

    - □ Check weight daily at the same time, and notify the provider for a weight gain of 2 lb in 24 hr or 5 lb in 1 week.

    - □ Schedule regular follow-up visits with the provider.

    - □ Get vaccinations (pneumococcal and yearly influenza vaccines).

PULMONARY EDEMA

Overview

- Cardiogenic factors are the most common cause of pulmonary edema. It is a complication of various heart and lung diseases and usually occurs from increased pulmonary vascular pressure secondary to severe cardiac dysfunction.

- Noncardiac pulmonary edema can occur due to barbiturate or opiate overdose, inhalation of irritating gases, rapid administration of IV fluids, and after a pneumonectomy evacuation of pleural effusion.

- Neurogenic pulmonary edema develops following a head injury.

- ⑤ For older adults, increased risk for pulmonary edema occurs related to decreased cardiac output and heart failure (HF).

- Increased risk for fluid and electrolyte imbalances occurs when the older adult client receives treatment with diuretics.

- For older adults, IV infusions must be administered at a slower rate to prevent circulatory overload.

Health Promotion and Disease Prevention

- Maintain an exercise routine to remain physically active, and consult with the provider before starting any exercise regimen.

- Consume a diet low in sodium along with fluid restrictions, and consult with the provider regarding diet specifications.

- Refrain from smoking.

- Follow medication regimen, and follow up with the provider as needed.

Assessment

- Risk Factors
  - ○ Acute MI
  - ○ Fluid volume overload
  - ○ Hypertension
  - ○ Valvular heart disease
  - ○ Postpneumonectomy
  - ○ Postevacuation of pleural effusion
  - ○ Acute respiratory failure
  - ○ Left-sided heart failure
  - ○ High altitude exposure or deep-sea diving
  - ○ Trauma
  - ○ Sepsis
  - ○ Drug overdose
- Subjective Data
  - ○ Anxiety
  - ○ Inability to sleep
- Objective Data
  - ○ Persistent cough with pink, frothy sputum (cardinal sign)
  - ○ Tachypnea, dyspnea, and orthopnea
  - ○ Hypoxemia (SaO_2 expected reference range greater than 95%)
  - ○ Cyanosis (later stage)
  - ○ Crackles
  - ○ Tachycardia
  - ○ Reduced urine output
  - ○ Confusion, stupor
  - ○ S_3 heart sound (gallop)
  - ○ Increased pulmonary artery occlusion pressure

Patient-Centered Care

- Nursing Care
  - Monitor vital signs every 15 min until stable.
  - Monitor intake and output.
  - Monitor hemodynamic status (pulmonary wedge pressures, cardiac output).
  - Check ABGs, electrolytes (especially potassium if on diuretics), SaO_2, and chest x-ray findings.
  - Maintain a patent airway. Suction as needed.
  - Position the client in high-Fowler's position with feet and legs dependent or sitting on the side of the bed to decrease preload.
  - Administer oxygen using a high-flow rebreather mask. BiPAP or intubation/ventilation can become necessary. Be prepared to intervene quickly.
  - Restrict fluid intake (slow or discontinue infusing IV fluids).
  - Monitor hourly urine output. Watch for intake greater than output or hourly urine less than 30 mL/hr.
- Medications
  - Rapid-acting diuretics, such as furosemide (Lasix) and bumetanide (Bumex), promote fluid excretion.
  - Morphine decreases sympathetic nervous system response and anxiety and promotes mild vasodilation.
  - Vasodilators (nitroglycerin, sodium nitroprusside) decrease preload and afterload.
  - Inotropic agents, such as digoxin (Lanoxin) and dobutamine (Dobutrex), improve cardiac output.
  - Antihypertensives, such as ACE inhibitors and beta-blockers
- Care after Discharge
  - Client Education
    - Provide emotional support for the client and family.
    - Instruct the client on effective breathing techniques.
    - Instruct the client on medications.
    - Stress the importance of continuing to take medications even if the client is feeling better.
    - Teach common side/adverse effects of medications, and reasons to contact the provider.
    - Instruct the client on a low-sodium diet and fluid restriction.
    - The client should measure weight daily at the same time. Notify the provider of a gain of more than 2 lb in 1 day or 5 lb in 1 week.
    - Instruct the client to report swelling of feet or ankles or any shortness of breath or angina.

Complications of Heart Failure

- Acute pulmonary edema
  - Acute pulmonary edema is a life-threatening medical emergency.
  - Nursing Actions
    - Administer prescribed medications to improve cardiac output.
    - Teach the client about measures to improve tolerance to activity, such as alternating periods of activity with periods of rest.

- Findings include anxiety, tachycardia, acute respiratory distress, dyspnea at rest, change in level of consciousness, and an ascending fluid level within the lungs (crackles, cough productive of frothy, blood-tinged sputum).
- Prompt response to this emergency includes the following:
  - Positioning the client in high-Fowler's position.
  - Administration of oxygen, positive airway pressure, and/or intubation and mechanical ventilation.
  - IV morphine (to decrease anxiety, respiratory distress, and decrease venous return).
  - IV administration of rapid-acting loop diuretics, such as furosemide (Lasix).
  - Effective intervention should result in diuresis (carefully monitor output), reduction in respiratory distress, improved lung sounds, and adequate oxygenation.

- Cardiogenic shock
  - This is a serious complication of pump failure that occurs commonly following an MI and injury to greater than 40% of the left ventricle.
  - Findings include tachycardia, hypotension, inadequate urinary output, altered level of consciousness, respiratory distress (crackles, tachypnea), cool, clammy skin, decreased peripheral pulses, and chest pain.
  - Nursing Actions
    - Monitor breath sounds. Assess for crackles or wheezing.
    - Monitor heart sounds.
    - Administration of oxygen; possible intubation and ventilation may be required.
    - IV administration of morphine, diuretics, and/or nitroglycerin to decrease preload; IV administration of vasopressors and/or positive inotropes to increase cardiac output and to maintain organ perfusion.
    - Continuous hemodynamic monitoring.

- Pericardial tamponade
  - Cardiac tamponade can result from fluid accumulation in the pericardial sac.
  - Findings include hypotension, jugular venous distention, muffled heart sounds, and paradoxical pulse (variance of 10 mm Hg or more in systolic blood pressure between expiration and inspiration).
  - Hemodynamic monitoring will reveal intracardiac and pulmonary artery pressures similar and elevated (plateau pressures).
  - Nursing Actions
    - Notify the provider immediately.
    - Administer IV fluids to combat hypotension as prescribed while monitoring for fluid overload.
    - Obtain a chest x-ray or echocardiogram to confirm diagnosis.
    - Prepare the client for pericardiocentesis (informed consent, gather materials, administer medications as appropriate).
    - Monitor hemodynamic pressures as they normalize.
    - Monitor heart rhythm; changes indicate improper positioning of the needle.
    - Monitor for reoccurrence of findings after the procedure.

APPLICATION EXERCISES

1. A nurse is caring for a client who has heart failure and reports increased shortness of breath. The nurse increases the oxygen per protocol. Which of the following actions should the nurse take first?

    A. Obtain the client's weight.

    B. Assist the client into high-Fowler's position.

    C. Auscultate lungs sounds.

    D. Check oxygen saturation with pulse oximeter.

2. A nurse is caring for a client who has heart failure and asks how to limit fluid intake to 2,000 mL/day. Which of the following is an appropriate response by the nurse?

    A. "Pour the amount of fluid you drink into an empty 2 liter bottle to keep track of how much you drink."

    B. "Each glass contains 8 ounces. There are 30 milliliters per ounce, so you can have a total of 8 glasses or cups of fluid each day."

    C. "This is the same as 2 quarts, or about the same as two pots of coffee."

    D. "Take sips of water or ice chips so you will not take in too much fluid."

3. A nurse is teaching a client who has heart failure about the need to limit sodium in the diet to 2,000 mg daily. Which of the following foods should be consumed in limited quantities? (Select all that apply.)

    _X____ A. Cheddar cheese, 2 oz

    _X____ B. Hot dog

    _X____ C. Canned tuna, 3 oz

    _____ D. Roast chicken breast, 3 oz

    _X____ E. Baked ham, 3 oz

4. A nurse is completing discharge teaching to a client who has heart failure and is encouraged to increase potassium in his diet. Which of the following statements by the client indicates understanding of the teaching?

    A. "I will consume more white rice."

    B. "I will eat more baked potatoes."

    C. "I will drink more grape juice."

    D. " I will use more powdered cocoa mixes."

5. A nurse is completing the admission assessment of a client who has suspected pulmonary edema. Which of the following are expected findings? (Select all that apply.)

   __X__ A. Tachypnea

   __X__ B. Persistent cough

   _____ C. Increased urinary output

   _____ D. Thick, yellow sputum

   __X__ E. Orthopnea

6. A nurse in a cardiac rehabilitation program is teaching a class on heart failure to a group of clients. What should be included in this presentation? Use the ATI Active Learning Template: Systems Disorder to include the following:

A. Description of Disorder: Describe the difference between left- and right-sided heart failure.

B. Laboratory Tests: Describe one and its importance.

C. Diagnostic Procedures: Describe two.

D. Medications: Describe two groups of medications and an example of one medication for each group.

APPLICATION EXERCISES KEY

1. A. INCORRECT: Obtaining the client's weight is an appropriate action, but it does not improve the client's oxygenation.

    B. **CORRECT:** Using the airway, breathing, and circulation (ABC) priority-setting framework, the first action is to assist the client into high-Fowler's position. This will decrease venous return to the heart (preload) and help relieve lung congestion.

    C. INCORRECT: Auscultating lung sounds is an appropriate action, but it does not improve the client's oxygenation.

    D. INCORRECT: Checking oxygen saturation is an appropriate action, but it does not improve the client's oxygenation.

    Ⓝ NCLEX® Connection: Physiological Adaptations, Illness Management

2. A. **CORRECT:** Pouring the amount of fluid consumed into an empty 2 L bottle provides a visual guide for the client as to the amount consumed and how to plan daily intake.

    B. INCORRECT: Glasses and cups vary in size and may contain more than 8 oz.

    C. INCORRECT: Offering a vague frame of reference does not assist with accurate fluid measurement.

    D. INCORRECT: Suggesting that the client take sips of water or ice chips does not assist with accurate fluid measurement.

    Ⓝ NCLEX® Connection: Basic Care and Comfort, Nutrition and Oral Hydration

3. A. **CORRECT:** Processed cheese contains 800 mg sodium per 2 oz.

    B. **CORRECT:** A hot dog contains 615 mg sodium.

    C. **CORRECT:** Canned tuna contains 350 mg sodium per 3 oz.

    D. INCORRECT: Lean meats, fish, and poultry contain 30 to 90 mg of sodium per 3 oz.

    E. **CORRECT:** Lean, baked ham contains 1,020 mg sodium per 3 oz.

    Ⓝ NCLEX® Connection: Basic Care and Comfort, Nutrition and Oral Hydration

4. A. INCORRECT: White rice is low in potassium.

    B. **CORRECT:** Baked potatoes are a good source of potassium, containing 854 mg.

    C. INCORRECT: Tomato and orange juices are good sources of potassium.

    D. INCORRECT: Powdered cocoa mixes contain high levels of sodium and minimal potassium.

    Ⓝ NCLEX® Connection: Basic Care and Comfort, Nutrition and Oral Hydration

5. A. **CORRECT:** Tachypnea is an expected finding in a client who has pulmonary edema.

    B. **CORRECT:** A persistent cough with pink, frothy sputum is an expected finding in a client who has pulmonary edema.

    C. INCORRECT: Decreased urinary output is an expected finding in a client who has pulmonary edema.

    D. INCORRECT: Pink, frothy sputum is an expected finding in a client who has pulmonary edema.

    E. **CORRECT:** Orthopnea is an expected finding in a client who has pulmonary edema.

    Ⓝ NCLEX® Connection: Physiological Adaptations, Pathophysiology

6. *Using the ATI Active Learning Template: Systems Disorder*

    A. Description of Disorder: Left-sided heart failure results in inadequate output from the left ventricle, leading to poor tissue perfusion. Systolic failure includes an ejection fraction below 40% with pulmonary and systemic congestion. Diastolic failure includes stiffening or inadequate relaxation of the ventricle. Right-sided heart failure results in inadequate output from the right ventricle, leading to systemic venous congestion and peripheral edema.

    B. Laboratory Tests: Human B-type natriuretic peptides (hBNP) confirms a diagnosis of heart failure, and findings direct the aggressiveness of the treatment.

    C. Diagnostic Procedures
    - Hemodynamic monitoring
    - Ultrasound
    - Chest x-ray
    - Electrocardiogram

    D. Medications
    - Diuretics: furosemide (Lasix), bumetanide (Bumex), hydrochlorothiazide (Hydrodiuril), spironolactone (aldactone)
    - Afterload-reducing agents: enalapril (Vasotec), captopril (Capoten), losartan (Cozaar), diltiazem (Cardizem), nifedipine (Procardia), milrinone (Primacor)

    Ⓝ NCLEX® Connection: Physiological Adaptations, Alterations in Body Systems

chapter 33

Overview

- Valvular heart disease describes an abnormality or dysfunction of any of the heart's four valves: the mitral and aortic valves (left side) and the tricuspid and pulmonic valves (right side).

 View Image: Heart Blood Flow

- Valvular heart disease is classified as:
  - Stenosis – Narrowed opening that impedes blood moving forward.
  - Insufficiency – Improper closure – some blood flows backward (regurgitation).
- Valvular heart disease can have congenital or acquired causes.
  - Congenital valvular heart disease can affect all four valves and cause either stenosis or insufficiency.
  - Acquired valvular heart disease is classified as one of three types:
    - Degenerative disease – Due to damage over time from mechanical stress. The most common cause is hypertension.
    - Rheumatic disease – Gradual fibrotic changes, calcification of valve cusps. The mitral valve is most commonly affected.
    - Infective endocarditis – Infectious organisms destroy the valve. Streptococcal infections are a common cause.

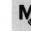 View Image: Heart Valve Comparison

- Valves on the left side are most commonly affected due to higher pressures.
- With age, fibrotic thickening occurs in the mitral and aortic valves. The aorta is stiffer in older adult clients, increasing systolic blood pressure and stress on the mitral valve.

Health Promotion and Disease Prevention

- Early detection and prevention of rheumatic fever helps prevent valvular disease.
- Encourage clients to consume a diet low in sodium and follow fluid restrictions prescribed by the provider to prevent heart failure.

Assessment

- Risk Factors

  - Hypertension

  - Rheumatic fever (mitral stenosis and insufficiency)

  - Infective endocarditis

  - Congenital malformations

  - Marfan syndrome (connective tissue disorder that affects the heart and other areas of the body)

  - In older adult clients, the predominant causes of valvular heart disease are degenerative calcification, papillary muscle dysfunction, and infective endocarditis.

- Subjective and Objective Data

  - Clients who have valvular heart disease are often asymptomatic until late in the progression of the disease.

  - A murmur is heard with turbulent blood flow. The location of the murmur and timing (diastolic versus systolic) help determine the valve involved. Murmurs are graded on a scale of I (very faint) to VI (extremely loud).

  - Left-sided valve damage causes increased pulmonary artery pressure, left ventricular hypertrophy, and decreased cardiac output, resulting in orthopnea, paroxysmal nocturnal dyspnea, and fatigue.

MITRAL STENOSIS	MITRAL INSUFFICIENCY	AORTIC STENOSIS	AORTIC INSUFFICIENCY
› Diastolic murmur	› Systolic murmur	› Systolic murmur	› Diastolic murmur
› Atrial fibrillation	› S_3 and/or S_4 sounds	› S_3 and/or S_4 sounds	› S_3 sounds
› Palpitations	› Atrial fibrillation	› Angina	› Sinus tachycardia
› Jugular venous distention	› Palpitations	› Syncope	› Palpitations
› Pitting edema	› Jugular venous distention	› Decreased SVR	› Angina
› Hemoptysis	› Pitting edema	› Narrowed pulse pressure	› Widened pulse pressure
› Cough	› Crackles in lungs		
› Dysphagia	› Possible diminished lung sounds		
› Hoarseness			

  - Right-sided valve damage results in dyspnea, fatigue, increased right atrial pressure, peripheral edema, jugular vein distention, and hepatomegaly.

TRICUSPID STENOSIS	TRICUSPID INSUFFICIENCY	PULMONIC STENOSIS	PULMONIC INSUFFICIENCY
› Diastolic murmur	› Systolic murmur	› Systolic murmur	› Diastolic murmur
› Atrial dysrhythmias	› Supraventricular tachycardia	› Angina	› Possible split S_2
› Decreased cardiac output	› Conduction delays	› Syncope	
	› "Fluttering" neck vein sensations	› Cyanosis	

○ Diagnostic Procedures

▪ Chest x-ray shows chamber enlargement, pulmonary congestion, and valve calcification.

▪ 12-lead electrocardiogram (ECG) shows chamber hypertrophy.

▪ Echocardiogram shows chamber size, hypertrophy, specific valve dysfunction, ejection function, and amount of regurgitant flow.

▪ Exercise tolerance testing/stress echocardiography is used to assess the impact of the valve problem on cardiac functioning during stress.

▪ Radionuclide studies determine ejection fraction during activity and rest.

▪ Angiography reveals chamber pressures, ejection fraction, regurgitation, and pressure gradients.

Patient-Centered Care

• Nursing Care

○ Monitor current weight, and note recent changes.

○ Assess heart rhythm (can be irregular or bradycardic, assess for murmur).

○ Administer oxygen and medications as prescribed.

○ Assess hemodynamic monitoring.

○ Maintain fluid and sodium restrictions.

○ Assist the client to conserve energy.

• Medications

○ Diuretics

▪ Diuretics are used to decrease preload.

□ Loop diuretics, such as furosemide (Lasix), bumetanide

□ Thiazide diuretics, such as hydrochlorothiazide (Microzide)

□ Potassium-sparing diuretics, such as spironolactone (Aldactone)

▪ Nursing Considerations

□ Administer furosemide IV no faster than 20 mg/min.

□ Loop and thiazide diuretics can cause hypokalemia, and a potassium supplement may be required.

▪ Client Education

□ Teach clients who are taking loop or thiazide diuretics to ingest foods and drinks that are high in potassium to counter hypokalemia effect.

- Afterload-reducing agents
  - Afterload-reducing agents help the heart pump more easily by altering the resistance to contraction.
    - Angiotensin-converting enzyme (ACE) inhibitors, such as enalapril (Vasotec), captopril (Capoten)
    - Beta-blockers, such as atenolol (Tenormin)
    - Calcium-channel blockers, such as amlodipine (Norvasc)
    - Vasodilators, such as hydralazine hydrochloride
  - Nursing Considerations
    - Monitor clients taking ACE inhibitors for initial dose hypotension.
- Inotropic agents
  - Inotropic agents, such as digoxin (Lanoxin), dopamine, dobutamine hydrochloride, and milrinone lactate, are used to increase contractility and thereby improve cardiac output.
  - Client Education
    - Teach clients who are self-administering digoxin to:
      - Count pulse for 1 min before taking the medication. If the pulse rate is irregular or the pulse rate is outside of the limitations set by the provider (usually less than 60/min or greater than 100/min), the client should hold the dose and contact the provider.
      - Take the dose of digoxin at the same time every day.
      - Do not take digoxin at the same time as antacids. Separate the two medications by at least 2 hr.
      - Report signs of toxicity, including fatigue, muscle weakness, confusion, visual changes, and loss of appetite.
- Anticoagulants
  - Anticoagulation therapy is used for clients who have a mechanical valve replacement, atrial fibrillation, or severe left ventricle dysfunction.
- Teamwork and Collaboration
  - Respiratory services should be consulted for inhalers, breathing treatments, and suctioning for airway management.
  - Cardiology can be consulted for cardiac management.
  - Nutritional services can be contacted for weight loss or gain of this client related to medications or diagnosis.
  - Rehabilitative care may need to be consulted if the client has prolonged weakness and needs assistance with increasing level of activity.

- Surgical Interventions
  - ○ Percutaneous balloon valvuloplasty
    - ▪ This procedure can open aortic or mitral valves affected by stenosis. A catheter is inserted through the femoral artery and advanced to the heart. A balloon is inflated at the stenotic lesion to open the fused commissures and improve leaflet mobility.
  - ○ Miscellaneous surgical management
    - ▪ Surgeries used in the treatment of valvular disorders include valve repair, chordae tendineae reconstruction, commissurotomy (relieve stenosis on leaflets), annuloplasty ring insertion (correct dilatation of valve annulus), and prosthetic valve replacement.
      - ▫ Prosthetic valves can be mechanical or tissue. Mechanical valves last longer but require anticoagulation. Tissue valves last 10 to 15 years.
    - ▪ Medical management is appropriate for many older adult clients; surgery is indicated when clinical manifestations interfere with daily activities. The goal of surgery can be to improve the quality of life rather than to prolong life.
    - ▪ Nursing Actions
      - ▫ Postsurgery care is similar to coronary artery bypass surgery (care for sternal incision, activity limited for 6 weeks, report fever).
- Care after Discharge
  - ○ Nutritional services can be contacted for weight loss or weight gain related to medications or diagnosis.
  - ○ Rehabilitative care may need to be consulted if the client has prolonged weakness and needs assistance with increasing level of activity.
  - ○ Client Education
    - ▪ Prophylactic antibiotics are recommended prior to dental work, surgery, or other invasive procedures.
    - ▪ Encourage the client to follow the prescribed exercise program.
    - ▪ Encourage adherence to dietary restrictions; consider nutritional consultation.
    - ▪ Teach the client energy conservation.
    - ▪ Teach symptoms of heart failure; report to provider immediately.

Complications

- Heart Failure
  - ○ Heart failure is the inability of the heart to maintain adequate circulation to meet tissue needs for oxygen and nutrients. Ineffective valves result in heart failure.
  - ○ Nursing Actions
    - ▪ Monitoring a client's heart failure class (I to IV) is often the gauge for surgical intervention for valvular problems.

APPLICATION EXERCISES

1. A nurse is completing discharge teaching with a client who had a surgical placement of a mechanical heart valve. Which of the following statements by the client indicates understanding of the teaching?

 A. "I will be glad to get back to my exercise routine right away."

 B. "I will have my prothrombin time checked on a regular basis."

 C. "I will talk to my dentist about no longer needing antibiotics before dental exams."

 D. "I will continue to limit my intake of foods containing potassium."

2. A nurse is completing the admission physical assessment of client who has a history of mitral valve insufficiency. Which of the following is an expected finding?

 A. Hoarseness

 B. Petechiae

 C. Crackles in lung bases

 D. Splenomegaly

3. A nurse is reviewing the health record of a client who is being evaluated for possible valvular heart disease. The nurse should recognize which of the following data as risk factors for this condition? (Select all that apply.)

 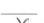 A. Surgical repair of an atrial septal defect at age 2

 _____ B. Measles infection during childhood

 X C. Hypertension for 5 years

 _____ D. Weight gain of 10 lb in past year

  E. Diastolic murmur present

4. A nurse is caring for a 72-year-old client who is to undergo a percutaneous balloon valvuloplasty. The client's daughter asks the nurse to explain the expected outcome of this procedure. Which of the following is an appropriate response by the nurse?

 A. "This will improve blood flow in your mother's coronary arteries."

 B. "This will permit your mother to resume her activities of daily living."

 C. "This will prolong your mother's life."

 D. "This will reverse the effects to the damaged area."

5. A nurse educator is reviewing expected findings in a client who has right-sided valvular heart disease with a group of nurses. Which of the following should be included in the discussion? (Select all that apply.)

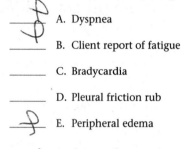

_____ A. Dyspnea

_____ B. Client report of fatigue

_____ C. Bradycardia

_____ D. Pleural friction rub

_____ E. Peripheral edema

6. A nurse educator is preparing a poster on valvular heart disease to be displayed at a health fair. What content should be included on the poster? Use the ATI Active Learning Template: Systems Disorder to complete this item to include the following sections:

A. Description of the Disorder:

- Describe the difference between valve stenosis and insufficiency.
- Describe the difference between acquired and congenital valvular heart disease.
- Describe which valves of the heart are commonly affected and why.

B. Client Education: Describe two actions to prevent valvular disease.

APPLICATION EXERCISES KEY

1. A. INCORRECT: The client will be on activity limitation for 6 weeks following surgery for a heart valve replacement.

    B. **CORRECT:** Anticoagulant therapy with warfarin (Coumadin) is necessary for the client following placement of a mechanical heart valve; the client's prothrombin time will be checked on a regular basis.

    C. INCORRECT: Antibiotic therapy is recommended prior to dental work following placement of a heart valve.

    D. INCORRECT: Dietary recommendations include limiting foods containing sodium.

    Ⓝ NCLEX® Connection: Physiological Adaptations, Alterations in Body Systems

2. A. INCORRECT: Hoarseness is an expected finding in a client who has mitral valve stenosis.

    B. INCORRECT: Petechiae is an expected finding in a client who has infective endocarditis.

    C. **CORRECT:** Crackles in the lung bases is an expected finding in a client who has pulmonary congestion due to mitral valve insufficiency.

    D. INCORRECT: Hepatomegaly, not splenomegaly, is an expected finding in a client who has left-sided heart valve damage.

    Ⓝ NCLEX® Connection: Physiological Adaptations, Pathophysiology

3. A. **CORRECT:** A history of congenital malformations is a risk factor for valvular heart disease.

    B. INCORRECT: Having a streptococcal infection or rheumatic fever during childhood is a risk factor for valvular heart disease.

    C. **CORRECT:** Hypertension places a client at risk for valvular heart disease.

    D. INCORRECT: A sudden weight gain of 10 lb could indicate fluid collection related to left-sided valvular heart disease.

    E. **CORRECT:** A murmur indicates turbulent blood flow, which is often due to valvular heart disease.

    Ⓝ NCLEX® Connection: Health Promotion and Maintenance, Health Promotion/Disease Prevention

4. A. INCORRECT: A valvuloplasty improves blood flow through a heart valve by opening the fused commissures and allowing valve leaflets greater mobility. It does not improve blood flow in the coronary arteries.

    B. **CORRECT:** Surgery is indicated for older adult clients when clinical manifestations interfere with activities of daily living.

    C. INCORRECT: Surgical interventions can improve the client's quality of life, but they will not necessarily prolong life.

    D. INCORRECT: A valvuloplasty improves blood flow through a heart valve by opening the fused commissures and allowing valve leaflets greater mobility. It does not reverse the damage that has already occurred to the valve.

    ⓝ NCLEX® Connection: Reduction of Risk Potential, Therapeutic Procedures

5. A. **CORRECT:** Dyspnea is a clinical manifestation of right-sided valvular heart disease.

    B. **CORRECT:** A client's report of fatigue is a clinical manifestation of right-sided valvular heart disease.

    C. INCORRECT: A normal or rapid pulse and an irregularly irregular rhythm are clinical manifestations of right-sided valvular heart disease.

    D. INCORRECT: A pleural friction rub is a manifestation of pleurisy or pneumonia.

    E. **CORRECT:** Peripheral edema is a clinical manifestation of right-sided valvular heart disease.

    ⓝ NCLEX® Connection: Physiological Adaptations, Pathophysiology

6. *Using ATI Active Learning Template: Systems Disorder*

    A. Description of the Disorder

    - Stenosis is the narrowed opening of a heart valve, which prevents blood from moving forward. Insufficiency is the improper closure of a valve resulting in blood flowing backward (regurgitation) through the valve.

    - Congenital valvular heart disease can affect all four valves and can cause either stenosis or insufficiency. Acquired valvular heart disease occurs due to degenerative changes from mechanical stress over time; rheumatic disease, which causes calcifications, and fibrotic changes, often to the mitral valve; and infective endocarditis, in which infectious organisms destroy the valve.

    - Valves on the left side of the heart are more commonly affected due to higher pressures.

    B. Client Education

    - Prevent and manage hypertension.

    - Early detection and prevention of rheumatic fever.

    - Consume a low-sodium diet.

    ⓝ NCLEX® Connection: Physiological Adaptations, Pathophysiology

chapter 34

Overview

- Inflammation related to the heart is an extended inflammatory response that often leads to the destruction of healthy tissue. This primarily includes the layers of the heart.

- Inflammatory disorders related to the cardiovascular system that nurses should be familiar with include the following:

  ○ Pericarditis

  ○ Myocarditis

  ○ Rheumatic endocarditis

  ○ Infective endocarditis

Health Promotion and Disease Prevention

- Early treatment of streptococcal infections can prevent rheumatic fever.

- Prophylactic treatments (including antibiotics for clients who have cardiac defects) can prevent infective endocarditis.

- Influenza and pneumonia immunizations are important for all clients in order to decrease the incidence of myocarditis, especially in older adults.

Assessment

- Risk Factors

  ○ Congenital heart defect/cardiac anomalies

  ○ Intravenous drug use

  ○ Heart valve replacement

  ○ Immunosuppression

  ○ Rheumatic fever and other infections

  ○ School-age children who have long duration of streptococcus infection

  ○ Malnutrition

  ○ Overcrowding

  ○ Lower socioeconomic status

• Subjective and Objective Data

INFLAMMATORY DISORDER	DESCRIPTION OF DISEASE PROCESS	RELEVANT INFORMATION
Pericarditis	› Inflammation of the pericardium	› Commonly follows a respiratory infection › Can be due to a myocardial infarction › Findings include chest pressure/pain, friction rub auscultated in the lungs, shortness of breath, and pain relieved when sitting and leaning forward
Myocarditis	› Inflammation of the myocardium	› Can be due to a viral, fungal, or bacterial infection, or a systemic inflammatory disease (Crohn's disease) › Findings include tachycardia, murmur, friction rub auscultated in the lungs, cardiomegaly, chest pain, and dysrhythmias
Rheumatic endocarditis	› An infection of the endocardium due to streptococcal bacteria	› Preceded by an upper respiratory infection › Produces lesions in the heart › Occurs with half of the clients who have rheumatic fever › Findings include fever, chest pain, joint pain, tachycardia, shortness of breath, rash on trunk and extremities, friction rub, murmur, and muscle spasms
Infective endocarditis	› Also known as bacterial endocarditis, an infection of the endocardium due to streptococcal or staphylococcal bacteria	› Most common in IV drug users or clients who have cardiac malformations › Findings include fever, flulike symptoms, murmur, petechiae (on the trunk and mucous membranes), positive blood cultures, and splinter hemorrhages (red streaks under the nail beds)

○ Laboratory Tests

▪ Blood cultures to detect a bacterial infection.

▪ An elevated WBC count can be indicative of a bacterial infection.

▪ Cardiac enzymes can be elevated with pericarditis.

▪ Elevated ESR and CRP indicate inflammation in the body.

▪ Throat cultures to detect a streptococcal infection, which can lead to rheumatic fever.

○ Diagnostic Procedures

▪ ECG can detect a murmur or heart block, which is indicative of rheumatic fever.

▪ Echocardiography can reveal inflamed heart layers.

Patient-Centered Care

- Nursing Care
  - Auscultate heart sounds (listen for murmur).
  - Assess breath sounds in all lung fields (listen for friction rub).
  - Review ABGs, SaO_2, and chest x-ray results.
  - Administer oxygen as prescribed.
  - Monitor vital signs (watch for fever).
  - Monitor ECG, and notify the provider of changes.
  - Monitor for cardiac tamponade and heart failure.
  - Obtain throat cultures to identify bacteria to be treated by antibiotic therapy.
  - Administer antibiotics as prescribed.
  - Administer antipyretics as prescribed.
  - Assess onset, quality, duration, and severity of pain.
  - Administer pain medication as prescribed.
  - Encourage bed rest.
  - Provide emotional support to the client and family, and encourage the verbalization of feelings regarding the illness.
- Medications

PENICILLIN	
Type	› Antibiotic
Purpose	› Given to treat infection
Nursing Considerations	› Monitor for skin rash and hives. › Monitor electrolyte and kidney levels.
Client Education	› Instruct clients to report signs of skin rash or hives. › Inform clients that the medication may cause gastrointestinal (GI) distress.
IBUPROFEN (ADVIL)	
Type	› NSAID (nonsteroidal anti-inflammatory drug)
Purpose	› Given to treat fever and inflammation
Nursing Considerations	› Do not use with clients who have peptic ulcer disease. › Watch for signs of GI distress. › Monitor platelets, and liver and kidney levels.
Client Education	› Instruct clients to take the medication with food. › Inform clients that the medication may cause GI distress. › Instruct clients to avoid alcohol consumption while taking the medication.

PREDNISONE (DELTASONE)	
Type	› Glucocorticosteroid
Purpose	› Given to treat inflammation
Nursing Considerations	› Use in low doses. › Monitor blood pressure. › Monitor electrolytes and blood sugar levels. › Clients may heal slowly when taking this medication.
Client Education	› Instruct clients to take the medication with food. › Instruct clients to avoid stopping the medication abruptly. › Instruct clients to report signs of unexpected weight gain.
AMPHOTERICIN B (AMPHOTEC)	
Type	› Antifungal
Purpose	› Given to treat fungus
Nursing Considerations	› Monitor liver and kidney levels.
Client Education	› Inform clients that the medication may cause GI distress.
DIAZEPAM (VALIUM)	
Type	› Benzodiazepine
Purpose	› Given to treat anxiety
Nursing Considerations	› Start in low doses, and monitor for sleepiness and light-headedness. › Monitor liver function.
Client Education	› Instruct clients to take medication as prescribed. › Instruct clients to avoid alcohol consumption while taking the medication. › Instruct clients to avoid stopping the medication abruptly.

- Teamwork and Collaboration
  - Cardiology services may be consulted to manage cardiac dysfunction.
  - Infectious disease services may be consulted to manage infection.
  - Physical therapy may be consulted to increase the client's level of activity once prescribed.
- Surgical Interventions
  - Pericarditis is the insertion of a needle into the pericardium to aspirate pericardial fluid. This can be done in the emergency department or a procedure room.
    - Nursing Actions
      - Pericardial fluid can be sent to the laboratory for culture and sensitivity.
      - Monitor for reoccurrence of cardiac tamponade.
  - Infective Endocarditis
    - Valve debridement, draining of abscess, and repairing congenital shunts are procedures involved with infective endocarditis.
    - Nursing Actions
      - Monitor for signs of bleeding, infection, and alteration in cardiac output.

- Care after Discharge
  - Home health services may be indicated if the client had surgery.
  - Intravenous antibiotic therapy may be given by the home health service.
  - Pharmaceutical services may be indicated for IV supplies and medications.
  - Rehabilitation services may be indicated to help the client increase the level of activity.
  - Client Education
    - Encourage the client to take rest periods as needed.
    - Encourage the client to wash hands to prevent infection.
    - Encourage the client to avoid crowded areas to reduce the risk of infection.
    - Educate the client about the importance of good oral hygiene and the prevention of infection.
    - Educate the client about the importance of taking medications as prescribed.
    - Ask the client to demonstrate the administration of intravenous antibiotics and management before discharge.
    - Encourage the client to participate in smoking cessation (if the client is a smoker).
    - Educate the client and family about the illness, and encourage them to express their feelings.

Complications

- Cardiac Tamponade
  - Pericardial Tamponade
    - Cardiac tamponade can result from fluid accumulation in the pericardial sac.
      - Signs include hypotension, muffled heart sounds, jugular venous distention, and paradoxical pulse (variance of 10 mm Hg or more in systolic blood pressure between expiration and inspiration).
      - Hemodynamic monitoring will reveal intracardiac and pulmonary artery pressures similar and elevated (plateau pressures).
    - Nursing Actions
      - Notify the provider immediately.
      - Administer IV fluids to combat hypotension as ordered.
      - Obtain a chest x-ray or echocardiogram to confirm the diagnosis.
    - Prepare the client for pericardiocentesis (informed consent, gather materials, administer medications as appropriate).
      - Monitor hemodynamic pressures as they normalize.
      - Monitor heart rhythm as changes indicate improper positioning of the needle.
      - Monitor for reoccurrence of signs after the procedure.

APPLICATION EXERCISES

1. A nurse is caring for a client who has pericarditis. Which of the following expected findings should the nurse anticipate?

    A. Petechiae

    B. Murmur

    C. Rash

    D. Friction rub

2. Which of the following clients has the greatest risk of acquiring rheumatic endocarditis?

    A. An older adult who has chronic obstructive pulmonary disease

    B. A child who has an upper respiratory streptococcal infection

    C. A middle-age adult who has lupus erythematosus

    D. A young adult who is at 24 weeks of gestation

3. A nurse in a clinic is caring for a client who has been on long-term NSAID therapy to treat myocarditis. Which of the following laboratory findings should be reported to the provider?

    A. Platelets 100,000/mm^3

    B. Serum glucose 110 mg/dL

    C. Serum creatinine 0.7 mg/dL

    D. Amino alanine transferase (ALT) 30 IU/L

4. A nurse is assessing a client who has splinter hemorrhages in her nail beds and reports a fever. For which of the following conditions is the client at risk?

    A. Infective endocarditis

    B. Pericarditis

    C. Myocarditis

    D. Rheumatic endocarditis

5. A nurse is admitting a client who has suspected rheumatic endocarditis. The nurse should anticipate a prescription from the provider for which of the following laboratory tests to assist in confirmation of this diagnosis?

    A. Arterial blood gases

    B. Serum albumin

    C. Liver enzymes

    D. Throat culture

6. A nurse is reviewing discharge teaching with a client who has myocarditis. What should the nurse include in the teaching? Use the ATI Active Learning Template: Systems Disorder to complete this item to include the following:

    A. Care After Discharge:

      • Identify at least two referral facilities and the services they can provide.

      • Describe at least four actions the client should take when at home.

APPLICATION EXERCISES KEY

1. A. INCORRECT: Petechiae are expected findings in a client who has endocarditis.

    B. INCORRECT: A murmur is an expected finding in a client who has myocarditis and endocarditis.

    C. INCORRECT: Rash is an expected finding in a client who has rheumatic endocarditis.

    D. **CORRECT:** A friction rub can be heard during auscultation of a client who has pericarditis.

    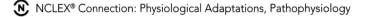 NCLEX® Connection: Physiological Adaptations, Pathophysiology

2. A. INCORRECT: An older adult who has chronic obstructive pulmonary disease is at risk, but this client is not the highest risk.

    B. **CORRECT:** A child who has an upper respiratory due to streptococcal bacteria is at highest risk for developing rheumatic endocarditis. Approximately 50% of clients who have rheumatic fever develop rheumatic endocarditis.

    C. INCORRECT: A middle-age adult who has lupus erythematosus is at risk, but this client is not the highest risk.

    D. INCORRECT: A young adult who is at 24 weeks of gestation is at risk, but this client is not the highest risk.

    NCLEX® Connection: Health Promotion and Maintenance, Health Promotion/Disease Prevention

3. A. **CORRECT:** Long-term NSAID therapy can lower platelets. This finding is outside the expected reference range and should be reported to the provider.

    B. INCORRECT: Serum glucose is not affected by long-term NSAID therapy. This finding is within the expected reference range.

    C. INCORRECT: Kidney function, which is monitored by serum creatinine level, is affected by long-term NSAID therapy. This finding is within the expected reference range.

    D. INCORRECT:Liver function, which is monitored by the ALT level, is affected by long-term NSAID therapy. This finding is within the expected reference range.

    NCLEX® Connection: Physiological Adaptations, Pathophysiology

4. A. **CORRECT:** Splinter hemorrhages in nail beds and a report of fever are findings associated with infective endocarditis.

    B. INCORRECT: A client who has pericarditis would report chest pain.

    C. INCORRECT: A client who has myocarditis would report a rapid heart rate.

    D. INCORRECT: A client who has rheumatic endocarditis would report joint pain.

    Ⓝ NCLEX® Connection: Physiological Adaptations, Illness Management

5. A. INCORRECT: Arterial blood gases are used to monitor the respiratory status of a client who has suspected rheumatic endocarditis, but they do not confirm the diagnosis.

    B. INCORRECT: Serum albumin monitors the nutrition status of a client who has a suspected inflammatory disorder, but it does not confirm the diagnosis.

    C. INCORRECT: Liver enzymes monitor a client's response to antibiotic therapy, which is used to treat rheumatic endocarditis, but they do not confirm the diagnosis.

    D. **CORRECT:** A throat culture can reveal the presence of streptococcus, which is the leading cause of rheumatic endocarditis.

    Ⓝ NCLEX® Connection: Reduction of Risk Potential, Laboratory Values

6. *Using the ATI Active Learning Template: Systems Disorder*

    A. Care After Discharge
    - Referral facilities
        - Home health – postoperative care
        - Pharmaceutical services – intravenous antibiotic therapy, provision of supplies and medications
        - Rehabilitation services – assistance with monitoring and increasing activity level
    - Discharge activities by the client
        - Rest as needed.
        - Wash hands to prevent infection.
        - Avoid crowded areas to reduce the risk of infection.
        - Maintain good oral hygiene to prevent infection.
        - Take medications as prescribed.
        - Administer and manage IV antibiotics.
        - Participate in a smoking cessation program.

    Ⓝ NCLEX® Connection: Physiological Adaptations, Illness Management

chapter 35

Overview

- Peripheral vascular diseases include peripheral arterial disease (PAD) and peripheral venous disorders, both of which interfere with normal blood flow.

- PAD affects the arteries (the blood vessels that carry blood away from the heart), and peripheral venous disease affects the veins (the blood vessels that carry blood toward the heart).

PERIPHERAL ARTERIAL DISEASE (PAD)

Overview

- PAD results from atherosclerosis that usually occurs in the arteries of the lower extremities and is characterized by inadequate flow of blood.

- Atherosclerosis is caused by a gradual thickening of the intima and media of the arteries, ultimately resulting in the progressive narrowing of the vessel lumen. Plaques may form on the walls of the arteries making them rough and fragile.

- Progressive stiffening of the arteries and narrowing of the lumen decreases the blood supply to affected tissues and increases resistance to blood flow.

- Atherosclerosis is actually a type of arteriosclerosis, which means "hardening of the arteries" and alludes to the loss of elasticity of arteries over time due to thickening of their walls.

- PAD is classified as inflow (distal aorta and iliac arteries) or outflow (femoral, popliteal, and tibial arteries) and may range from mild to severe. Tissue damage occurs below the arterial obstruction.

- Buerger's disease, subclavian steal syndrome, thoracic outlet syndrome, Raynaud's disease and Raynaud's phenomenon, and popliteal entrapment are examples of PADs.

Assessment

- Risk Factors
  - Hypertension
  - Hyperlipidemia
  - Diabetes mellitus
  - Cigarette smoking
  - Obesity
  - Sedentary lifestyle

- ○ Familial predisposition
- ○ Age
  - ▪ Older adult clients have a higher incidence of PAD (rate of occurrence is increased in men over 45 and in women who are postmenopausal) and have a higher mortality rate from complications than younger individuals.
- • Subjective Data
  - ○ Burning, cramping, and pain in the legs during exercise (intermittent claudication)
  - ○ Numbness or burning pain primarily in the feet when in bed
  - ○ Pain is relieved by placing legs at rest in a dependent position
- • Objective Data
  - ○ Physical Assessment Findings
    - ▪ Bruit over femoral and aortic arteries

M Listen to Audio: Bruit

- ▪ Decreased capillary refill of toes (greater than 3 seconds)
- ▪ Decreased or nonpalpable pulses
- ▪ Loss of hair on lower calf, ankle, and foot
- ▪ Dry, scaly, mottled skin
- ▪ Thick toenails
- ▪ Cold and cyanotic extremity
- ▪ Pallor of extremity with elevation
- ▪ Dependent rubor

M View Image: Rubor

- ▪ Muscle atrophy
- ▪ Ulcers and possible gangrene of toes
- ○ Diagnostic Procedures
  - ▪ Arteriography
    - ▫ Arteriography of the lower extremities involves arterial injection of contrast medium to visualize areas of decreased arterial flow on an x-ray.
    - ▫ It is usually done only to determine isolated areas of occlusion that can be treated during the procedure with percutaneous transluminal angioplasty and possible stent placement.
    - ▫ Nursing Actions
      - ▸ Observe for bleeding and hemorrhage.
      - ▸ Palpate pedal pulses to identify possible occlusions.

- Exercise tolerance testing

  - □ A stress test is done with or without the use of a treadmill (medications such as dipyridamole [Persantine] and adenosine [Adenocard] may be given to mimic the effects of exercise in clients who cannot tolerate a treadmill) with measurement of pulse volumes and blood pressures prior to and following the onset of symptoms or 5 min of exercise. Delays in return to normal pressures and pulse waveforms indicate arterial disease. It is used to evaluate claudication during exercise.

- Plethysmography

  - □ Plethysmography is used to determine the variations of blood passing through an artery, thus identifying abnormal arterial flow in the affected limb.

  - □ Blood pressure cuffs are attached to the client's upper extremities and a lower extremity and attached to the plethysmograph machine. Variations in peripheral pulses between the upper and lower extremity are recorded.

  - □ A decrease in pulse pressure of the lower extremity indicates a possible blockage in the leg.

- Segmental systolic blood pressure measurements

  - □ A Doppler probe is used to take various blood pressure measurements (thigh, calf, ankle, brachial) for comparison. In the absence of peripheral arterial disease, pressures in the lower extremities are higher than those of the upper extremities.

  - □ With arterial disease, the pressures in the thigh, calf, and ankle are lower.

Patient-Centered Care

- Nursing Care

  - ○ Encourage the client to exercise to build up collateral circulation – Initiate exercise gradually and increase slowly. Instruct the client to walk until the point of pain, stop and rest, and then walk a little farther.

  - ○ Positioning

    - Instruct the client to avoid crossing the legs.

    - Tell the client to refrain from wearing restrictive garments.

    - Tell the client to elevate the legs to reduce swelling, but not to elevate them above the level of the heart because extreme elevation slows arterial blood flow to the feet.

  - ○ Promote vasodilation and avoid vasoconstriction.

    - Provide a warm environment for the client.

    - Have the client wear insulated socks.

    - Tell the client to never apply direct heat to the affected extremity because sensitivity is decreased, and this can cause a burn.

    - Instruct the client to avoid exposure to cold (causes vasoconstriction and decreased arterial flow).

    - Instruct the client to avoid stress, caffeine, and nicotine, which also cause vasoconstriction. Complete abstinence from smoking or chewing tobacco is the most effective method of preventing vasoconstriction. (Vasoconstrictive effects last up to 1 hr after each cigarette smoked.)

- Medications
  - Antiplatelet medications – aspirin (acetylsalicylic acid), clopidogrel (Plavix), pentoxifylline (Trental)
    - Antiplatelet medications reduce blood viscosity by decreasing blood fibrinogen levels, enhancing erythrocyte flexibility, and increasing blood flow in the extremities. Medications, such as aspirin (acetylsalicylic acid) and clopidogrel (Plavix), may be prescribed. Pentoxifylline (Trental), sometimes referred to as a hemorheologic medication, was one of the first to be used and is still used today, but less commonly than the other medications. It may be given to specifically treat intermittent claudication experienced by clients who have PAD.
    - Client Education
      - □ Inform the client that the medication's effects might not be apparent for several weeks.
      - □ Advise the client to monitor for evidence of bleeding such as abdominal pain, coffee-ground emesis, or black, tarry stools.
  - Statins – simvastatin (Zocor), atorvastatin (Lipitor)
    - Can relieve manifestations associated with PAD (intermittent claudication).
- Surgical Interventions
  - Surgical procedures for PAD
    - Percutaneous transluminal angioplasty
      - □ Invasive intra-arterial procedure using a balloon and stent to open and help maintain the patency of the vessel.
      - □ It is used for candidates who are not suitable for surgery or in cases where amputation is inevitable.
    - Laser-assisted angioplasty
      - □ Laser-assisted angioplasty is an invasive procedure in which a laser probe is advanced through a cannula to the site of stenosis.
      - □ The laser is used to vaporize atherosclerotic plaque and open the artery.
    - Nursing Actions
      - □ The priority action is to observe for bleeding at the puncture site.
      - □ Monitor the client's vital signs, peripheral pulses, and capillary refill.
      - □ If prescribed, keep the client on bed rest with his limb straight for 6 to 8 hr before ambulation.
      - □ Anticoagulant therapy is used during the operative procedure, followed by antiplatelet therapy for 1 to 3 months.
    - Arterial revascularization surgery is used with clients who have severe claudication and/or limb pain at rest, or with clients who are at risk for losing a limb due to poor arterial circulation.
      - □ Bypass grafts are used to reroute the circulation around the arterial occlusion.
      - □ Grafts can be harvested from the client (autologous) or made from synthetic materials.
    - Nursing Actions
      - □ The priority action is to maintain adequate circulation in the repaired artery. The location of the pedal or dorsalis pulse should be marked, and its pulsatile strength compared with the contralateral leg on a scheduled basis using a Doppler.
      - □ Color, temperature, sensation, and capillary refill should be compared with the contralateral extremity on a scheduled basis.

- Nursing Actions
  - The priority action is to maintain adequate circulation in the repaired artery. The location of the pedal or dorsalis pulse should be marked, and its pulsatile strength compared with the contralateral leg on a scheduled basis using a Doppler.
  - Color, temperature, sensation, and capillary refill should be compared with the contralateral extremity on a scheduled basis.
  - Assess for warmth, redness, and possibly edema of the affected limb as a result of increased blood flow.
  - Monitor the client for pain. Pain may be severe due to the reestablishment of blood flow to the extremity.
  - Monitor the client's blood pressure. Hypotension may result in an increased risk of clotting or graft collapse, while hypertension increases the risk for bleeding from sutures.
  - Instruct the client to limit bending of the hip and knee to decrease the risk of clot formation.
- Client Education
  - Instruct the client to avoid crossing or raising legs above the level of the heart.
  - Instruct the client to wear loose clothing.
  - Instruct the client on wound care if revascularization surgery was done.
  - Discourage smoking and cold temperatures with the client.
  - Instruct the client about foot care (keep feet clean and dry, wear good-fitting shoes, never go barefoot, cut toenails straight across or have the podiatrist cut nails).

Complications

- Graft Occlusion
  - Graft occlusion is a serious complication of arterial revascularization and often occurs within the first 24 hr following surgery.

  - Nursing Actions
    - Promptly notify the surgeon of manifestations of occlusion, such as absent or reduced pedal pulses, increased pain, change in extremity color, or temperature.
    - Be prepared to assist with treatment, which may include an emergency thrombectomy (removal of a clot), local intra-arterial thrombolytic therapy with an agent such as tissue plasminogen activator, infusion of a platelet inhibitor, or a combination of these. With these treatments, assess the client for manifestations of bleeding.
- Compartment Syndrome
  - Compartment syndrome is considered a medical emergency. Tissue pressure within a confined body space can restrict blood flow and the resulting ischemia can lead to irreversible tissue damage.

> **M** View Image: Compartment Syndrome

- - Nursing Actions

    - Manifestations of compartment syndrome include tingling, numbness, worsening pain, edema, pain on passive movement, and unequal pulses. Immediately report findings to the provider.

    - Loosen dressings.

    - Prepare to assist with fasciotomy (surgical opening into the tissues), which may be necessary to prevent further injury and to save the limb.

PERIPHERAL VENOUS DISORDERS

Overview

- Peripheral venous disorders are problems with the veins that interfere with adequate return of blood flow from the extremities.

- There are superficial and deep veins in the lower extremities that have valves that prevent backflow of blood as it returns to the heart. The action of the skeletal muscles of the lower extremities during walking and other activities also promotes venous return.

- Three peripheral venous disorders that nurses should be familiar with are venous thromboembolism (VTE), venous insufficiency, and varicose veins.

    - A VTE is a blood clot believed to form as a result of venous stasis, endothelial injury, or hypercoagulability. Thrombus formation can lead to a pulmonary embolism, which is a life-threatening complication.

    - Thrombophlebitis refers to a thrombus that is associated with inflammation.

    - Venous insufficiency occurs secondary to incompetent valves in the deeper veins of the lower extremities, which allows pooling of blood and dilation of the veins. The veins' inability to carry fluid and wastes from the lower extremities precipitates the development of swelling, venous stasis ulcers, and in advanced cases, cellulitis.

    - Varicose veins are enlarged, twisted and superficial veins that may occur in any part of the body; however, they are commonly observed in the lower extremities and in the esophagus.

Assessment

- Risk Factors

    - Venous thromboembolism – associated with Virchow's triad (hypercoagulability, impaired blood flow, damage to blood vessels)

        - Hip surgery, total-knee replacement, open prostate surgery

        - Heart failure

        - Immobility

        - Pregnancy

        - Oral contraceptives

    - Venous insufficiency

        - Sitting or standing in one position for a long period of time

- Obesity
- Pregnancy
- Thrombophlebitis
  - ○ Varicose veins
    - Sex (women)
    - Older than 30 years with an occupation requiring prolonged standing
    - Pregnancy
    - Obesity
    - Systemic diseases (heart disease)
    - Family history
- Subjective Data
  - ○ Limb pain – Aching pain and feeling of fullness or heaviness in the legs after standing
- Objective Data
  - ○ Physical Assessment Findings
    - Deep-vein thrombosis (DVT) and thrombophlebitis
      - □ Client may be asymptomatic.
      - □ Calf or groin pain, tenderness, and a sudden onset of edema of the extremity.
      - □ Warmth, edema, and induration and hardness over the involved blood vessel.
      - □ Changes in circumferences of right and left calf and thigh over time; localized edema over the affected area.
      - □ Shortness of breath and chest pain, which can indicate that the embolus has moved to the lungs (pulmonary embolism).
    - Venous insufficiency
      - □ Stasis dermatitis is a brown discoloration along the ankles that extends up the calf relative to the level of insufficiency.
      - □ Edema
      - □ Stasis ulcers (typically found around ankles)
    - Varicose veins
      - □ Distended, superficial veins that are visible just below the skin and are tortuous in nature.
      - □ Clients often report muscle cramping and aches, pain after sitting, and pruritus.
  - ○ Laboratory Tests
    - D-dimer test measures fibrin degradation products present in the blood produced from fibrinolysis. A positive test indicates that thrombus formation has possibly occurred.
  - ○ Diagnostic Procedures
    - DVT and thrombophlebitis
      - □ Venous duplex ultrasonography uses high-frequency sound waves to provide a real-time picture of the blood flow through a blood vessel.
      - □ Impedance plethysmography can be used to determine the variations of blood passing through a vein, thus identifying abnormal venous flow in the affected limb.

□ If the above tests are negative for a DVT, but one is still suspected, a venogram, which uses contrast material, or MRI may be needed for accurate diagnosis.

- Varicose veins – Trendelenburg test

  □ Nursing Actions

  ▸ Place the client in a supine position with legs elevated.

  ▸ When the client sits up, the veins will fill from the proximal end if varicosities are present (veins normally fill from the distal end).

Patient-Centered Care

- Nursing Care

  ○ DVT and thrombophlebitis

  - Encourage the client to rest.

    □ Facilitate bed rest and elevation of the extremity above the level of the heart as prescribed. (Avoid using a knee gatch or pillow under knees.)

    □ Administer intermittent or continuous warm moist compresses as prescribed.

    □ Do not massage the affected limb.

    □ Provide thigh-high compression or antiembolism stockings.

  - Prepare the client for an inferior vena cava interruption surgery (a filter traps emboli and prevents them from reaching the heart) as indicated.

  ○ Venous insufficiency

  - Elevate legs several times a day for at least 15 to 30 min.

  - Elevate feet approximately 6 inches at night.

  - Instruct client to avoid crossing legs and wearing constrictive clothing or stockings.

  - Instruct client to wear elastic compression stockings and apply them after the legs have been elevated and when swelling is at a minimum.

- Medications

  ○ DVT and thrombophlebitis – anticoagulants

  - Unfractionated heparin is given IV to prevent formation of other clots and to prevent enlargement of the existing clot. It has significant adverse effects and must be given in the facility. Prior to discharge, the client will be converted to oral anticoagulation therapy with warfarin (Coumadin).

    □ Nursing Actions

    ▸ Monitor aPTT to allow for adjustments of heparin dosage.   *30-40 seconds*

    1.5-2 x

    ▸ Monitor platelet counts for heparin-induced thrombocytopenia.   *= 45-90*

    ▸ Ensure that protamine sulfate, the antidote for heparin, is available if needed for excessive bleeding.

    ▸ Monitor for hazards and adverse effects associated with anticoagulant therapy.

    ↑ Bleeding

- Low-molecular weight heparin is given subcutaneously and is based on a client's weight. Enoxaparin (Lovenox) is used for the prevention and treatment of DVT. It is usually given in the facility, but the twice daily injections can be given in the home setting.

  □ Nursing Actions

    ▸ Instruct the client to observe for evidence of bleeding.

    ▸ Instruct the client on bleeding precautions that should be taken (use electric instead of bladed razor and brush teeth with a soft toothbrush).

- Warfarin inhibits synthesis of the four vitamin K-dependent clotting factors. The therapeutic effect takes 3 to 4 days to develop, so administration of the medication is begun while the client is still on heparin.

  □ Nursing Actions

    ▸ Monitor the client for bleeding.

    ▸ Monitor the client's PT and INR.

    ▸ Ensure that vitamin K (the antidote for warfarin) is available in case of excessive bleeding.

    ▸ Instruct the client about food sources of vitamin K (green leafy vegetables) and to avoid fluctuations in the amount and frequency of consumption.

    ▸ Instruct the client about observing for evidence of bleeding.

    ▸ Instruct the client on bleeding precautions that should be taken (use electric instead of bladed razor and brush teeth with soft toothbrush).

  ○ DVT and thrombophlebitis – thrombolytic therapy

    - Thrombolytic therapy dissolves clots that have already developed. Therapy must be started within 5 days after the development of the clot for the therapy to be effective. Tissue plasminogen activator, a thrombolytic agent, and platelet inhibitors such as abciximab (ReoPro), and eptifibatide (Integrilin) can be effective in dissolving a clot or preventing new clots during the first 24 hr. Administering the medication in a manner that provides direct contact with the thrombus can be more effective and lessen the chance of bleeding.

      □ Nursing Actions

        ▸ Monitor the client for bleeding (intracerebral bleeding).

        ▸ Instruct the client about bleeding precautions that should be taken. (Use electric instead of bladed razor and brush teeth with a soft toothbrush.)

- Teamwork and Collaboration

  ○ Venous insufficiency

    - Care of venous stasis ulcers requires long-term management.

    - Consultation with a dietitian and wound care specialist will facilitate the healing process.

[Handwritten margin notes: PT 11-12.5 therapeutic 1.5-2 =16.5-25; INR 2-3 therapeutic well]

- Therapeutic Procedures
  - ○ Varicose veins – sclerotherapy
    - ▪ A sclerosing irritating chemical solution is injected into the varicose vein to produce localized inflammation, which will, close the lumen of the vessel over time. For larger vessels, an incision and drainage of the trapped blood in a sclerosed vein may need to be performed 2 to 3 weeks after the injection. Pressure dressings are applied for approximately 1 week after each procedure to keep the vessel free of blood.
    - ▪ Client Education
      - □ Instruct the client to wear elastic stockings for prescribed time.
      - □ Mild analgesics such as acetaminophen (Tylenol) can be taken for discomfort.
- Surgical Interventions
  - ○ Varicose veins – vein stripping
    - ▪ Vein stripping is the removal of large varicose veins that cannot be treated with less-invasive procedures.
    - ▪ Nursing Actions
      - □ Preoperatively
        - ‣ Assist the provider with vein marking.
        - ‣ Evaluate the client's pulses as baseline for postoperative comparison.
      - □ Postoperatively
        - ‣ Maintain elastic bandages on the legs.
        - ‣ Monitor groin and leg for bleeding through the elastic bandages.
        - ‣ Monitor extremity for edema, warmth, color, and pulses.
        - ‣ Elevate legs above the level of the heart.
        - ‣ Encourage the client to engage in range-of-motion exercises of the legs.
        - ‣ Instruct the client to elevate the legs when sitting, and avoid dangling them over the side of the bed.
    - ▪ Client Education
      - □ Emphasize the importance of wearing elastic stockings after bandage removal.
  - ○ Varicose veins – endovenous laser treatment
    - ▪ This type of treatment uses a laser fiber that is inserted into the vessel proximal to the area to be treated and then threaded to the involved area where heat from the laser is used to close the dilated vein.
  - ○ Varicose veins – application of radio frequency energy
    - ▪ This type of treatment uses a small catheter with a radio frequency electrode, instead of a laser, that is inserted into the vessel proximal to the area to be treated that scars and closes a dilated vein.

Complications

- Ulcer Formation

  ○ Venous stasis ulcers often form over the medial malleolus. Venous ulcers are chronic, hard to heal, and often recur. They can lead to amputation and/or death.

  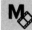 View Image: Venous Stasis Ulcer

  ○ Clients who also have neuropathy may not feel as much discomfort from the ulcer as its appearance may warrant.

  ○ Nursing Actions

    ▪ Administer and assist with treatments to improve circulation (wound vacuum, hyperbaric chamber).

    ▪ Assess and treat pain as prescribed.

    ▪ Apply oxygen-permeable polyethylene films to superficial ulcers.

    ▪ Apply occlusive, hydrocolloid dressings on deeper ulcers to promote granulation tissue and reepithelialization.

    ▪ Leave a dressing on for 3 to 5 days.

    ▪ If a wound needs chemical debridement, apply prescribed topical enzymatic agents to debride the ulcer, eliminate necrotic tissue, and promote healing.

    ▪ Administer systemic antibiotics as prescribed.

  ○ Client Education

    ▪ Recommend a diet high in zinc, protein, iron, and vitamins A and C.

    ▪ Instruct client on use of compression stockings.

- Pulmonary Embolism

  ○ A pulmonary embolism occurs when a thrombus is dislodged, becomes an embolus, and lodges in a pulmonary vessel. This can lead to obstruction of pulmonary blood flow, decreased systemic oxygenation, pulmonary tissue hypoxia, and possible death.

  ○ Nursing Actions

    ▪ Manifestations include sudden onset dyspnea, pleuritic chest pain, restlessness and apprehension, feelings of impending doom, cough and hemoptysis.

    ▪ Findings include tachypnea, crackles, pleural friction rub, tachycardia, S_3 or S_4 heart sounds, diaphoresis, a low-grade fever, petechiae over chest and axillae, and decreased arterial oxygen saturation.

    ▪ Notify the provider immediately, reassure the client, and assist to a position of comfort with the head of the bed elevated.

    ▪ Prepare for oxygen therapy and blood gas analysis while continuing to monitor and assess the client for other manifestations.

APPLICATION EXERCISES

1. A nurse is performing a physical assessment of a client who has chronic peripheral arterial disease (PAD). Which of the following is an expected finding?

    A. Edema around the client's ankles and feet

    B. Ulceration around the client's medial malleoli

    C. Scaling eczema of the client's lower legs with stasis dermatitis

    D. Pallor on elevation of the client's limbs and rubor when his limbs are dependent

2. A nurse is caring for a client who has severe peripheral arterial disease (PAD). The nurse should expect that the client will sleep most comfortably in which of the following positions?

    A. With the affected limb hanging from the bed

    B. With the affected limb elevated on pillows

    C. With the head of the bed raised

    D. In a side-lying, recumbent position

3. A nurse is teaching a client who has a new prescription for clopidogrel (Plavix). Which of the following should be included in the teaching? (Select all that apply.)

    _____ A. Effects may not be apparent for several weeks.

    _____ B. Monitor for the presence of black, tarry stools.

    _____ C. Instruct the client to use an electric razor.

    _____ D. Schedule a weekly PT test.

    _____ E. Advise the client about food sources containing vitamin K.

4. A nurse is caring for a client who has a deep-vein thrombosis (DVT) and has been taking unfractionated heparin for 1 week. Two days ago, the provider also prescribed warfarin (Coumadin). The client questions the nurse about receiving both heparin and warfarin at the same time. Which of the following is an appropriate response by the nurse?

    A. "I will remind your provider that you are already receiving heparin."

    B. "Laboratory findings indicated that two anticoagulants were needed."

    C. "It takes three or four days before the effects of warfarin are achieved and the heparin can be discontinued."

    D. "Only one of these medications is being given to treat your deep-vein thrombosis."

5. A nurse is caring for a client who has chronic venous insufficiency. The provider prescribed thigh-high compression stockings. The nurse should instruct the client to

    A. massage both legs firmly with lotion prior to applying the stockings.

    B. apply the stockings in the morning upon awakening and before getting out of bed.

    C. roll the stockings down to the knees if they will not stay up on the thighs.

    D. remove the stockings while out of bed for 1 hr, four times a day to allow the legs to rest.

6. A nurse is developing a poster presentation on peripheral arterial disease (PAD) for a community health fair. What content should the nurse include on the poster? Use ATI Active Learning Template: Systems Disorder to complete this item to include the following:

    A. Description of Disease Process

    B. Risk Factors: Describe at least six.

    C. Objective Data: Describe at least six findings.

    D. Client Education: Describe at least two actions by the client related to proper positioning and two actions related to promoting vasodilation.

APPLICATION EXERCISES KEY

1. A. INCORRECT: Edema around the ankles and feet is an expected finding in a client who has venous stasis.

   B. INCORRECT: Ulceration around the medial malleoli is an expected finding in a client who has venous stasis.

   C. INCORRECT: Scaling eczema of the lower legs with stasis dermatitis is an expected finding in a client who has venous stasis.

   D. **CORRECT:** In a client who has chronic PAD, pallor is seen in the extremities when the limbs are elevated, and rubor occurs when they are lowered.

    NCLEX® Connection: Physiological Adaptations, Pathophysiology

2. A. **CORRECT:** The client will prefer sleeping with the affected extremity in a dependent position because this relieves pain.

   B. INCORRECT: This sleeping position does not promote circulation in the lower extremity.

   C. INCORRECT: This sleeping position does not promote circulation in the lower extremity.

   D. INCORRECT: This sleeping position does not promote circulation in the lower extremity.

    NCLEX® Connection: Physiological Adaptations, Pathophysiology

3. A. **CORRECT:** Therapeutic benefits may not occur for several weeks when taking Plavix.

   B. **CORRECT:** Evidence of GI bleeding, such as abdominal pain, coffee-ground emesis, or black, tarry stools should be monitored and reported to the provider.

   C. INCORRECT: Bleeding precautions are required for a client taking anticoagulants, not antiplatelet medications.

   D. INCORRECT: PT and INR levels are monitored regularly in a client taking warfarin (Coumadin).

   E. INCORRECT: A client who is taking warfarin (Coumadin) should be advised about food sources containing vitamin K.

    NCLEX® Connection: Health Promotion and Maintenance, Health Promotion/Disease Prevention

4. A. INCORRECT: Warfarin is prescribed for 3 to 4 days before discontinuing IV heparin.

   B. INCORRECT: IV heparin is monitored to achieve adequate therapeutic levels in treating a DVT.

   C. **CORRECT:** Warfarin depresses synthesis of clotting factors but does not have an effect on clotting factors that are present. Therefore, it takes 3 to 4 days before the clotting factors that are present decay and the therapeutic effects of warfarin occur.

   D. INCORRECT: Heparin and warfarin are both effective in treating DVTs.

    NCLEX® Connection: Pharmacological and Parenteral Therapies, Medication Administration

5. A. INCORRECT: Massaging the affected area can dislodge a clot and cause embolism.

    B. **CORRECT:** Applying stockings in the morning upon awakening and before getting out of bed reduces venous stasis and assists in the venous return of blood to the heart. Legs are less edematous at this time.

    C. INCORRECT: Rolling stockings down can restrict circulation and cause edema.

    D. INCORRECT: Stockings should remain in place throughout the day and are removed before going to bed to provide continuous venous support. If the stockings are removed, such as for a bath or shower, then the legs should be elevated before the stockings are reapplied.

    Ⓝ NCLEX® Connection: Pharmacological and Parenteral Therapies, Medication Administration

6. *Using the ATI Active Learning Template: Systems Disorder*

    A. Description of Disease Process: PAD is inadequate blood flow of the lower extremities due to atherosclerosis. The intima and media of the arteries becomes thickened, and plaques may form on the walls of the arteries, making them rough and fragile. The arteries progressively stiffen and the lumen narrows, decreasing blood supply to tissues and increasing resistance to blood flow. It is classified as either an inflow or outflow type of PAD.

    B. Risk Factors

       - Hypertension
       - Hyperlipidemia
       - Diabetes mellitus
       - Cigarette smoking
       - Obesity
       - Sedentary lifestyle
       - Familial predisposition
       - Age

    C. Objective Data

       - Bruits over femoral and aortic arteries
       - Decreased capillary refill of toes (greater than 3 seconds)
       - Decreased or nonpalpable pulses
       - Loss of hair on the lower extremities
       - Dry, scaly mottled skin
       - Thick toenails
       - Cold, cyanotic extremity
       - Pallor of extremity with elevation
       - Dependent rubor
       - Muscle atrophy
       - Ulcers and possible gangrene of toes

    D. Client Education

       - Actions related to positioning
         - Avoid crossing the legs.
         - Avoid wearing restrictive garments.
         - Keep legs elevated to reduce swelling but not above the level of the heart.
       - Actions to promote vasodilation
         - Maintain a warm environment.
         - Wear insulated socks.
         - Avoid applying direct heat to the extremity.
         - Avoid exposure to cold.
         - Avoid stress, caffeine, and nicotine.

    Ⓝ NCLEX® Connection: Physiological Adaptations, Illness Management

chapter 36

Overview

- Hypertension occurs when systolic blood pressure is at or above 140 mm Hg or diastolic blood pressure is at or above 90 mm Hg. Normal adult blood pressure is less than 120 mm Hg systolic and 80 mm Hg diastolic.

- Essential hypertension, also called primary hypertension, accounts for most cases of hypertension. There is no known cause. Secondary hypertension can be caused by certain disease states, such as kidney disease, or as an adverse effect of some medications. Treatment for secondary hypertension occurs by removing the cause (adrenal tumor, medication).

- Four bodily mechanisms regulate blood pressure.

  ○ Arterial baroreceptors

    ▪ Baroreceptors are located in the carotid sinus, aorta, and left ventricle.

    ▪ They control blood pressure by altering the heart rate. They also cause vasoconstriction or vasodilation.

  ○ Regulation of body-fluid volume

    ▪ Properly functioning kidneys either retain fluid when a client is hypotensive or excrete fluid when a client is hypertensive.

  ○ Renin-angiotensin system

    ▪ Angiotensin II vasoconstricts and controls aldosterone release, which causes the kidneys to reabsorb sodium and inhibit fluid loss.

  ○ Vascular autoregulation

    ▪ This maintains consistent levels of tissue perfusion.

- Clients with a systolic blood pressure of 120 to 139 mm Hg or a diastolic blood pressure of 80 to 89 mm Hg are considered prehypertensive. Lifestyle changes are necessary for these clients to help prevent cardiovascular disease.

- Prolonged, untreated, or poorly controlled hypertension can cause peripheral vascular disease that primarily affects the heart, brain, eyes, and kidneys. The risk of developing complications increases as blood pressure increases.

- Hypertrophy of the left ventricle can develop as the heart pumps against resistance caused by the hypertension.

Health Promotion and Disease Prevention

- A client should maintain a body mass index of less than 30.
- Clients who have diabetes mellitus should keep blood glucose within a recommended reference range.
- A client should limit caffeine and alcohol intake.
- A client should use stress-management techniques during times of stress.
- A client should stop smoking. Nicotine patches or engaging in a smoking cessation class may be necessary.
- A client should engage in exercise that provides aerobic benefits at least 3 times a week.

Assessment

- Risk Factors
    - Essential hypertension
        - Positive family history
        - Excessive sodium intake
        - Physical inactivity
        - Obesity
        - High alcohol consumption
        - African American
        - Smoking
        - Hyperlipidemia
        - Stress
    - Secondary hypertension
        - Kidney disease
        - Cushing's disease (excessive glucocorticoid secretion)
        - Primary aldosteronism (causes hypertension and hypokalemia)
        - Pheochromocytoma (excessive catecholamine release)
        - Brain tumors, encephalitis
        - Medications such as estrogen, steroids, sympathomimetics
- Subjective Data
    - Clients who have hypertension can experience few or no symptoms. The nurse should monitor for:
        - Headaches, particularly in the morning.
        - Dizziness.
        - Fainting.
        - Retinal changes, visual disturbances.
        - Nocturia.

- Objective Data
  - Physical Assessment Findings
    - When a blood pressure reading is elevated, take it in both arms and with the client sitting and standing.
    - There are several levels of hypertension, as defined by the Joint National Committee on Prevention, Detection, Evaluation, and Treatment of High Blood Pressure.
      - Prehypertension – systolic 120 to 139 mm Hg; diastolic 80 to 89 mm Hg
      - Stage I hypertension – systolic 140 to 159 mm Hg; diastolic 90 to 99 mm Hg
      - Stage II hypertension – systolic greater than or equal to 160 mm Hg; diastolic greater than or equal to 100 mm Hg
  - Laboratory Tests
    - No laboratory tests exist to diagnose hypertension; however, several laboratory tests can identify the causes of secondary hypertension and target organ damage.
      - BUN, creatinine – elevation is indicative of kidney disease
      - Elevated serum corticoids to detect Cushing's disease
      - Blood glucose and cholesterol studies can identify contributing factors related to blood vessel changes.
  - Diagnostic Procedures
    - An ECG evaluates cardiac function.
      - Tall R-waves are often seen with left-ventricular hypertrophy.
    - A chest x-ray may show cardiomegaly.

Patient-Centered Care

- Nursing Care
  - Discuss factors with a client that increase the risk of hypertension and how he can manage them.
- Medications
  - Medications are added to treat hypertension that is not responsive to lifestyle changes alone. Diuretics are often first-line medications. However, clients can require a combination of medications to control hypertension.
  - Instruct clients who are taking antihypertensives to change positions slowly, be careful when getting out of bed, driving, and climbing stairs until the medication's effects are fully known.
  - Diuretics
    - Thiazide diuretics, such as hydrochlorothiazide (Microzide), inhibit water and sodium reabsorption, and increase potassium excretion.
    - The use of other diuretics may treat hypertension that's not responsive to the thiazide diuretics.
      - Loop diuretics, such as furosemide (Lasix), decrease sodium reabsorption and increase potassium excretion. Monitor the client closely for hypokalemia.
      - Potassium-sparing diuretics, such as spironolactone (Aldactone), affect the distal tubule and prevent reabsorption of sodium in exchange for potassium. Monitor the client closely for hyperkalemia.

- Nursing Considerations

  □ Monitor potassium levels and watch for muscle weakness, irregular pulse, and dehydration. Thiazide and loop diuretics can cause hypokalemia, and potassium-sparing diuretics can cause hyperkalemia.

- Client Education

  □ Encourage the client to keep all appointments with the provider to monitor efficacy of pharmacological treatment and possible electrolyte imbalance (hyponatremia, hyperkalemia).

  □ If the client is taking a potassium-depleting diuretic, encourage consumption of potassium-rich foods, such as bananas.

○ Calcium-channel blockers

- Verapamil hydrochloride (Calan), amlodipine (Norvasc), and diltiazem (Cardizem) alter the movement of calcium ions through the cell membrane, causing vasodilation and lowering blood pressure.

- Nursing Considerations

  □ Monitor blood pressure and pulse, and change the client's position slowly. Hypotension is a common side effect.

  □ Use calcium-channel blockers cautiously with clients who have heart failure.

- Client Education

  □ Constipation can occur with verapamil hydrochloride, so encourage intake of foods that are high in fiber.

  □ A decrease or increase in heart rate and atrioventricular (AV) block can occur. So, teach the client how to take her pulse and call the provider if it's irregular or lower than the established rate.

  □ Instruct the client to avoid grapefruit juice, which potentiates the medication's effects, increases hypotensive effects, and increases the risk of medication toxicity.

○ Angiotensin-converting enzyme (ACE) inhibitors

- ACE inhibitors prevent the conversion of angiotensin I to angiotensin II, which prevents vasoconstriction.

- Nursing Considerations

  □ Monitor blood pressure and pulse. Hypotension is a common adverse effect.

  □ Monitor for evidence of heart failure, such as edema. This medication may cause heart and kidney complications.

- Client Education

  □ Teach the client to report a cough, which is a side effect of ACE inhibitors. The client should notify the provider of this adverse effect, as the medication can be discontinued due to its persistent nature and occasional relationship to angioedema (swelling of the tissues in the throat that can progress to a life-threatening obstruction).

  □ Teach the client to reports manifestations of heart failure (edema).

- ○ Angiotensin-II receptor antagonists
  - Also called angiotensin-receptor blockers (ARBs), these medications, such as candesartan (Atacand), losartan (Cozaar), and telmisartan (Micardis), are a good option for clients taking ACE inhibitors who report cough and those who have hyperkalemia. Also, ARBs do not require a dosage adjustment for older adult clients.
  - Nursing Considerations
    - □ Monitor for manifestations of angioedema or heart failure. Angioedema is a serious, but uncommon adverse effect, and heart failure can result from taking this medication.
  - Client Education
    - □ Teach the client to change positions slowly.
    - □ Teach the client to report findings of angioedema (swollen lips or face) or heart failure (edema).
    - □ Teach the client to avoid foods that are high in potassium and to have serum potassium levels monitored because ARBS can cause hyperkalemia.
- ○ Aldosterone-receptor antagonists
  - Aldosterone-receptor antagonists, such as eplerenone (Inspra), block aldosterone action. The blocking effect of eplerenone on aldosterone receptors promotes the retention of potassium and excretion of sodium and water.
  - Nursing Considerations
    - □ Monitor kidney function, triglycerides, sodium, and potassium levels. The risk of adverse effects increases with deteriorating kidney function. Hypertriglyceridemia, hyponatremia, and hyperkalemia can occur as the dose increases.
      - ▸ Monitor potassium levels every 2 weeks for the first few months and every 2 months thereafter. The client should avoid taking potassium supplements or potassium-sparing diuretics.
  - Client Education
    - □ Teach the client about potential food, medication, and herbal interactions. Grapefruit juice and St. John's wort can increase adverse effects.
    - □ Instruct the client not to take salt substitutes with potassium or other foods that are rich in potassium.
- ○ Beta blockers
  - Beta blockers, such as metoprolol (Lopressor) and atenolol (Tenormin), are for clients who have unstable angina or MI. They decrease cardiac output and block the release of renin, subsequently decreasing vasoconstriction of the peripheral vasculature.
  - Nursing Considerations
    - □ Monitor blood pressure and pulse.
    - □ These medications can mask hypoglycemia in clients who have diabetes mellitus.
  - Client Education
    - □ Teach the client that these medications may cause fatigue, weakness, depression, and sexual dysfunction.
    - □ Advise the client not to suddenly stop taking the medication without consulting with the provider. Stopping suddenly can cause rebound hypertension.
    - □ Teach the client manifestations of hypoglycemia that do not include tachycardia, which beta blockers suppress.

- ○ Central-alpha agonists
  - Central-alpha agonists, such as clonidine (Catapres), reduce peripheral vascular resistance and decrease blood pressure by inhibiting the reuptake of norepinephrine.
  - Nursing Considerations
    - □ Monitor blood pressure and pulse.
    - □ This medication is not for first-line management of hypertension.
  - Client Education
    - □ Teach the client that adverse effects include sedation, orthostatic hypotension, and impotence.
- ○ Alpha-adrenergic Antagonists
  - Alpha-adrenergic antagonists, such as prazosin (Minipress), reduce blood pressure by causing vasodilation.
  - Nursing Considerations
    - □ Start treatment with a low dose of the medication, usually given at night.
    - □ Monitor blood pressure for 2 hr after initiation of treatment.
  - Client Education
    - □ Advise the client to rise slowly to prevent postural hypotension. Tell the client to use caution when driving until the effects of the medication are known.
- • Care After Discharge
  - ○ Instruct client to report manifestations of electrolyte imbalance (hyperkalemia, hypokalemia, hyponatremia).
  - ○ Express to the client and family the importance of adhering to the medication regimen, even if the client is asymptomatic.
  - ○ Provide verbal and written education to the client regarding medications and their side/adverse effects.
  - ○ Ensure that the client has the resources necessary to pay for and obtain prescribed antihypertensive medication.
  - ○ Encourage the client to schedule regular provider appointments to monitor hypertension and cardiovascular status.
  - ○ If the client has blood pressure that is difficult to manage, teach him or a significant other how to take blood pressure.
  - ○ Encourage the client to report findings and adverse effects, as they may be indicative of additional problems. Medications can often be changed to alleviate side or adverse effects.
    - Older adult clients are more likely to experience medication interactions.
    - Older adult clients are more likely to experience orthostatic hypotension.
  - ○ Treatment involves the client making lifestyle changes.
    - Nutrition
      - □ Monitor potassium with salt substitute use.
      - □ Consume less than 2.3 g/day of sodium.
      - □ Consume a diet low in fat, saturated fat, and cholesterol.

○ Control alcohol intake for men to 2 drinks per day and for women to 1 drink per day. Intake of 1 drink equals 12 oz beer, 4 oz wine, or 1 to 1.5 oz liquor.

○ Dietary approaches to stop hypertension (DASH) have been proven to be effective in the prevention and treatment of hypertension.

▸ The DASH diet should be high in fruits, vegetables, and low-fat dairy foods.

▸ Avoid foods high in sodium and fat (trans and saturated fat).

▸ Consume foods rich in potassium, calcium, and magnesium.

▪ Weight reduction and maintenance

○ Begin slowly and gradually advance the program with the guidance of the provider and physical therapist.

○ Exercise at least three times a week in a manner that provides aerobic benefits.

▪ Smoking cessation

○ There isn't a direct link between smoking and hypertension. But, the client should avoid it due to its association with the development of cardiovascular diseases.

▪ Stress reduction

○ Encourage the client to try yoga, massage, hypnosis, or other forms of relaxation.

Complications

- Hypertensive Crisis

  ○ Hypertensive crisis often occurs when clients do not follow the medication therapy regimen.

  ○ Nursing Actions

  ▪ Recognize clinical manifestations.

  ○ Severe headache

  ○ Extremely high blood pressure (generally, systolic blood pressure greater than 240 mm Hg, diastolic greater than 120 mm Hg)

  ○ Blurred vision, dizziness, and disorientation

  ○ Epistaxis

  ▪ Administer IV antihypertensive therapies, such as nitroprusside (Nitropress), nicardipine (Cardene IV), and labetalol hydrochloride as prescribed.

  ▪ Before, during, and after administration of IV antihypertensive, monitor blood pressure every 5 to 15 min.

  ▪ Assess neurological status such as pupils, level of consciousness, and muscle strength, to monitor for cerebrovascular change.

  ▪ Monitor the ECG to assess cardiac status.

APPLICATION EXERCISES

1. A nurse is screening a client for hypertension. Which of the following actions by the client increase his risk for hypertension? (Select all that apply.)

_____ A. Drinking 8 oz of nonfat milk daily

___X___ B. Eating popcorn at the movie theater

_____ C. Walking 1 mile daily at 12 min/mile pace

___X___ D. Consuming 36 oz of beer daily

_____ E. Getting a massage once a week

2. A nurse is caring for a client who is admitted to the emergency department with a blood pressure of 266/147 mm Hg. The client reports a headache and states that she is seeing double. The client states that she ran out of her diltiazem (Cardizem) 3 days ago, and she has not been able to purchase more. Which of the following nursing interventions should the nurse expect to perform first?

A. Administer acetaminophen for headache.

B. Provide teaching in regard to the importance of not abruptly stopping an antihypertensive.

C. Obtain IV access and prepare to administer an IV antihypertensive.

D. Call social services for a referral for financial assistance in obtaining prescribed medication.

3. A nurse is providing discharge teaching for a client who has a prescription for furosemide (Lasix) 40 mg PO daily. What time of day should the nurse encourage the client to take this medication?

A. Morning

B. Immediately after lunch

C. Immediately before dinner

D. Bedtime

4. A nurse is caring for a client who has a new diagnosis of hypertension and a new prescription for spironolactone (Aldactone) 25 mg/day. Which of the following statements by the client indicates a need for further teaching?

A. "I should eat a lot of fruits and vegetables, especially bananas and potatoes."

B. "I will report any changes in heart rate or rhythm."

C. "I should use a salt substitute that is low in potassium."

D. "I will continue to take this medication even if I am feeling better."

5. A nurse in an urgent care clinic is obtaining a history from a client who has type 2 diabetes mellitus and a recent diagnosis of hypertension. This is the second time in two weeks that the client experienced hypoglycemia. Which of the following data should the nurse report to the provider?

    A. Takes psyllium hydrophilic muccilloid (Metamucil) daily

    B. Drinks skim milk daily

    C. Takes metoprolol (Lopressor) daily

    D. Drinks grapefruit juice daily

6. A student nurse is preparing a post-conference presentation on hypertension. What should be included in the presentation? Use the ATI Active Learning Template: Systems Disorder to complete this item to include the following:

    A. Description of Disorder/Disease Process: Describe hypertension to include essential, secondary, and prehypertension.

    B. Risk Factors: Describe at least four risk factors for secondary hypertension.

    C. Objective and Subjective Data:
        • Describe at least three subjective data.
        • Describe the objective data stages of hypertension.

APPLICATION EXERCISES KEY

1. A. INCORRECT: Consuming low-fat beverages and foods lowers the risk for developing hypertension.

    B. **CORRECT:** Popcorn at a movie theater contains a large quantify of sodium and fat, which increases the risk for hypertension.

    C. INCORRECT: Engaging in regular exercise, such as walking, lowers the risk of developing hypertension.

    D. **CORRECT:** Consuming more than 24 oz of beer per day can contribute to weight gain, which increases the risk for hypertension.

    E. INCORRECT: Stress management activities, such as a massage, lowers the risk of hypertension.

    Ⓝ NCLEX® Connection: Health Promotion and Maintenance, High Risk Behaviors

2. A. INCORRECT: Administering acetaminophen is an appropriate action, but it is not the first action.

    B. INCORRECT: Providing teaching regarding medication administration is an appropriate action, but it is not the first action.

    C. **CORRECT:** The greatest risk to the client is injury due to a blood pressure of 266/147 mm Hg, which can be life-threatening and should be lowered as soon as possible. Obtaining IV access will permit administration of an IV hypertensive, which will act more rapidly than by the oral route.

    D. INCORRECT: Calling social services is an appropriate action, but it is not the first action.

    Ⓝ NCLEX® Connection: Pharmacological and Parenteral Therapies, Medication Administration

3. A. **CORRECT:** The client should take furosemide, a diuretic, in the morning so that the peak action and duration of the medication occurs during waking hours.

    B. INCORRECT: Taking furosemide, a diuretic, at this time increases the likelihood of interruption of the client's sleep due to the need to urinate.

    C. INCORRECT: Taking furosemide, a diuretic, at this time increases the likelihood of interruption of the client's sleep due to the need to urinate.

    D. INCORRECT: Taking furosemide, a diuretic, at this time increases the likelihood of interruption of the client's sleep due to the need to urinate.

    Ⓝ NCLEX® Connection: Physiological Adaptations, Hemodynamics

4. A. **CORRECT:** Potatoes and bananas are high in potassium, and spironolactone is a potassium-sparing diuretic. Consuming these foods can lead to hyperkalemia.

    B. INCORRECT: The client should report any changes in heart rate or rhythm.

    C. INCORRECT: Using salt substitutes that are low in potassium prevents hyperkalemia.

    D. INCORRECT: The client should be instructed to continue taking her medication even if she is symptom-free.

    Ⓝ NCLEX® Connection: Pharmacological and Parenteral Therapies, Medication Administration

5. A. INCORRECT: Adverse effects of Metamucil do not include hypoglycemia. This does not need to be reported to the provider.

   B. INCORRECT: Skim milk will increase blood glucose levels and lower cholesterol. This does not need to be reported to the provider.

   C. **CORRECT:** Lopressor can mask the effects of hypoglycemia in clients with diabetes mellitus. This should be reported to the provider.

   D. INCORRECT: Grapefruit juice will increase blood glucose levels. This does not need to be reported to the provider.

    NCLEX® Connection: Pharmacological and Parenteral Therapies, Adverse Effects/Contraindications/ Side Effects/Interactions

6. *Using the ATI Active Learning Template: Systems Disorder*

   A. Description of Disorder

   • Hypertension is when systolic blood pressure is at or above 140 mm Hg or diastolic blood pressure is at or above 90 mm Hg.

   • Essential, or primary hypertension, has no known cause.

   • Secondary hypertension is caused by certain diseases, such as kidney disorders, or as an adverse effect of a medication. Treatment occurs by removing the cause.

   • Prehypertension is when a client has a systolic blood pressure of 120 to 139 mm Hg or a diastolic blood pressure of 80 to 89 Hg.

   B. Risk Factors for Secondary Hypertension: kidney disease, Cushing's disease, primary aldosteronism (caused by hypertension and hypokalemia), pheochromocytoma (excessive catecholamine release), brain tumors, encephalitis, and medications such as estrogen, steroids, and sympathomimetics

   C. Objective and Subjective Data

   • Subjective Data: few or no symptoms; can include headaches, particularly in the morning; dizziness, fainting, retinal changes, visual disturbances, nocturia.

   • Objective Data

     ○ Obtain blood pressure readings in both arms with the client sitting and standing:

       ▪ Prehypertension – systolic 120 to 139 mm Hg, diastolic 80 to 89 mm Hg

       ▪ Stage I – systolic 140 to 159 mm Hg, diastolic 90 to 99 mm Hg

       ▪ Stage II – systolic greater than or equal to 160 mm Hg, diastolic greater than or equal to 100 mm Hg

    NCLEX® Connection: Physiological Adaptations, Illness Management

chapter 37

Overview

- Shock is a state of inadequate tissue perfusion that impairs cellular function and may lead to organ failure. Any condition that compromises the delivery of oxygen delivery to organs and tissues can lead to shock.

- Shock is a rapidly progressing, life-threatening process. Early detection with rapid response is necessary to improve client outcome.

- Ⓖ Older adult clients can have reduced compensatory mechanisms and rapidly progress through the stages of shock. Catecholamine secretions may not improve cardiac contractibility or cause vasoconstriction as in younger adults due to decreased baroreceptor response. Decreased ability to compensate can cause sustained low cardiac output and blood pressure.

- Shock is identified by its underlying cause
  - Cardiogenic – pump failure or heart failure
  - Hypovolemic – a decrease in intravascular volume of at least 10% to 15%
  - Obstructive – mechanical blockage in the heart or great vessels
  - Distributive – widespread vasodilation and increased capillary permeability

- All types of shock progress through the same stages and produce similar effects on body systems.
  - Initial – no visible changes in client parameters; only changes on the cellular level
  - Compensatory – measures to increase cardiac output to restore tissue perfusion and oxygenation.
  - Progressive – compensatory mechanisms begin to fail
  - Refractory – irreversible shock and total body failure

- The cause of shock, category of shock, and the stage of shock (initial, compensatory, progressive, or refractory) direct treatment.

Health Promotion and Disease Prevention

- Client Education

TYPE OF SHOCK	CLIENT EDUCATION
Cardiogenic	› Educate the client about ways to reduce the risk of an MI, such as exercise, diet, stress reduction and smoking cessation.
Hypovolemic	› Advise the client to drink plenty of fluids when exercising or when in hot weather. › Advise the client to obtain early medical attention with illness or trauma and with any evidence of dehydration or bleeding. › Educate the client about the manifestations of dehydration, including thirst, decreased urine output, and dizziness.

TYPE OF SHOCK	CLIENT EDUCATION
Obstructive/distributive/ hypovolemic	› Educate the client about wearing seatbelts, helmets, and the use of caution with dangerous equipment, machinery, or activities.
Septic shock	› Advise the client to obtain early medical attention with evidence of an infection, such as localized redness, swelling, drainage, fever, and urinary frequency and burning. › Advise the client to complete the entire course of antibiotics as directed.
Anaphylactic	› Advise the client to wear a medical identification wristband, avoid allergens, and to have an epinephrine pen available at all times. › Teach the client and family how to use the epinephrine pen and to be alert to early manifestations of an allergic reaction.

Assessment

- Risk Factors

  - Cardiogenic – cardiac pump failure due to MI, heart failure, cardiomyopathy, dysrhythmias, and valvular rupture or stenosis

    - Older adult clients are at increased risk for MI and cardiomyopathy.

  - Hypovolemic – excessive fluid loss from diuresis or vomiting/diarrhea, or blood loss secondary to surgery, trauma, gynecologic/obstetric causes, burns, and diabetic ketoacidosis.

    - Older adult clients are more prone to dehydration due to decreased fluid and protein intake and the use of medications, such as diuretics. Minimal amounts of fluid loss (vomiting, diarrhea) may cause the older adult client to become dehydrated.

  - Obstructive – blockage of great vessels, pulmonary artery stenosis, pulmonary embolism, cardiac tamponade, tension pneumothorax, and aortic dissection are among the causes

  - Distributive is divided into three types

    - Septic – endotoxins and other mediators causing massive vasodilation; most common cause is gram-negative bacteria

      - Urosepsis is more frequent in older adult clients due to increased use of catheters in extended care facilities and late detection of urinary tract infection (decreased sensation of burning, urgency).

    - Neurogenic – loss of sympathetic tone causing massive vasodilation; trauma, spinal shock, and epidural anesthesia are among the causes

    - Anaphylactic – antigen-antibody reaction causing massive vasodilation; allergens inhaled, swallowed, contacted, or introduced IV are causes

- Subjective Data

  - Manifestations can include chest pain, lethargy, somnolence, restlessness, anxiousness, dyspnea, diaphoresis, thirst, muscle weakness, nausea, and constipation

- Objective Data
  - Physical Assessment Findings
    - Hypoxia, tachypnea progressing to greater than 40/min, hypocarbia.
    - Skin may be pale, mottled or dusky in color, cool, diaphoretic, warm, flushed with fever (distributive shock), and exhibit a rash (anaphylactic and septic shock).
    - Angioedema (anaphylactic).
    - Wheezing.
    - Blood pressure may be within the expected reference range during the initial stage, but can increase during the progressive stage and then drop to less than 50 to 60 mm Hg.
    - Tachycardia progressing to greater than 140/min.
    - Pulse that is weak, thready, or bounding with distributive shock.
    - Decreased cardiac output.
    - Central venous pressure is decreased in hypovolemic shock.
    - Central venous pressure is increased with increased systemic vascular resistance in cardiogenic shock.
    - Decreased urine output.
    - Seizures.
  - Laboratory Tests
    - ABGs – decreased tissue oxygenation (decreased pH, decreased PaO_2, increased $PaCO_2$)
    - Serum lactic acid – increases due to anaerobic metabolism
    - Serum glucose and electrolytes – serum glucose can increase during shock
    - Cardiogenic shock
      - Cardiac enzymes – creatine phosphokinase, troponin
    - Hypovolemic shock
      - Hgb and Hct – decreased with hemorrhage, increased with dehydration
    - Septic shock
      - Cultures – blood, urine, wound
      - Coagulation tests – PT, INR, aPTT
  - Diagnostic Procedures
    - Hemodynamic monitoring
      - Arterial line insertion
        - Needed for continuous blood pressure monitoring and blood specimens for ABGs and other tests
      - Pulmonary artery catheter insertion
        - A pulmonary artery catheter is inserted to measure central venous pressure, pulmonary artery pressures, and cardiac output. Continuous hemodynamic monitoring is important to manage fluids and dosage of inotropic medications.

- Nursing Actions
  - Monitor ECG during catheter insertion.
  - Have resuscitation medications and equipment ready.
  - Monitor hemodynamic waveforms and readings.
  - Confirm catheter placement using a chest x-ray.
- Client Education
  - Explain all procedures to the client. The client may be anxious and scared.

- Cardiogenic and obstructive shock
  - ECG
    - Assess for ECG changes associated with MI and dysrhythmias.
  - Echocardiogram
    - Diagnostic procedure used for cardiomegaly, cardiomyopathy, the evaluation of cardiac contractility and function, ejection fraction, and valve function
  - Computerized tomography (CT)
    - Diagnostic procedure used for cardiomegaly, cardiac tamponade, pulmonary emboli, cardiomyopathy, aortic dissection or aneurysm, and pericardial effusion
  - Cardiac catheterization
    - Diagnostic procedure used to identify cardiac artery blockage
  - Chest x-ray
    - Diagnostic procedure used to diagnose cardiomegaly, pneumothorax, and to evaluate lungs
- Hypovolemic shock – miscellaneous diagnostic procedures
  - Investigate possible sources of bleeding
    - Blood in nasogastric drainage or stools
    - Esophagogastroduodenoscopy
    - CT scan of abdomen
  - Nursing Actions
    - Continuously monitor airway and vital signs.
    - Provide hemodynamic support by administration of fluids and medications because a client with suspected shock may be hemodynamically unstable.
    - Have resuscitation equipment available when transporting the client to and from procedures.
  - Client Education
    - Explain all procedures to the client.

Patient-Centered Care

- Nursing Care
  - Monitor
    - Oxygenation status (priority)
    - Vital signs
    - Cardiac rhythm with continuous cardiac monitoring
    - Urine output – hourly, report if less than 30 mL/hr
    - Level of consciousness
    - Skin color, temperature, moisture, capillary refill, turgor
  - Explain procedures and findings to the client and family while providing reassurance.
  - Place the client on high-flow oxygen, such as a 100% nonrebreather face mask.
    - If the client has COPD, insert a 2 L/min nasal cannula and increase the oxygen flow as needed.
  - Be prepared to intubate the client. Have emergency resuscitation equipment ready.
  - Maintain patent IV access.
  - For hypotension, place the client flat with his legs elevated to increase venous return.
  - If change in status occurs, notify the rapid response team and provider of the findings.
  - Initiate prescriptions to intervene during shock, including transfer to the intensive care unit, surgery, other specialty unit, or diagnostic area.
  - Prepare for and carry out hemodynamic monitoring.
    - Monitor central venous pressure, pulmonary artery pressures, cardiac output, and pulse pressure.
    - Titrate continuous IV drips to maintain hemodynamic parameters as prescribed.
- Medications

PHARMACOLOGICAL AGENTS	
INOTROPIC AGENTS – MILRINONE LACTATE (PRIMACOR)	
Actions	› Strengthens cardiac contraction and increases cardiac output
Nursing Considerations	› Administer by continuous IV infusion with constant hemodynamic monitoring.
	› Can titrate agent to maintain prescribed hemodynamic parameters.
	› Agent can cause vasodilation in some clients.
	› Agents are often administered in combination with a vasopressor.
VASOPRESSORS – DOBUTAMINE (DOBUTREX), DOPAMINE HYDROCHLORIDE (INTROPIN), NOREPHINEPHRINE (LEVOPHED)	
Actions	› Strengthens cardiac contraction and increases cardiac output
	› Increases kidney perfusion at low doses
	› Decreases kidney perfusion at high doses
Nursing Considerations	› Administer by continuous IV infusion with constant hemodynamic monitoring.
	› Can titrate vasopressor to maintain prescribed hemodynamic parameters.
	› Monitor urine output.
	› Administer through a central line to prevent extravasation. Rapid onset occurs in 5 min, and short duration occurs in 10 min.

PHARMACOLOGICAL AGENTS

PITUITARY HORMONE – VASOPRESSIN (PITRESSIN SYNTHETIC)

Actions	› Strengthens cardiac contraction › Causes vasoconstriction, increases systemic vascular resistance blood pressure, and increases cardiac output
Nursing Considerations	› Administer by continuous IV infusion with constant hemodynamic monitoring. › Can titrate vasopressor to maintain prescribed hemodynamic parameters. › Monitor urine output. › Administer through a central line to prevent extravasation. Rapid onset occurs in 5 min, and short duration occurs in 10 min.

SYMPATHOMIMETICS – EPINEPHRINE (ADRENALINE)

Actions	› Rapid-acting bronchodilator › Increases heart rate and cardiac output
Nursing Considerations	› Monitor blood pressure, pulse, and cardiac output. › Epinephrine can cause sloughing if infiltrates tissue.

OPIOID ANALGESICS – MORPHINE SULFATE, FENTANYL (SUBLIMAZE)

Actions	› Pain management
Nursing Considerations	› Monitor respirations of clients who are nonventilated. › Monitor blood pressure, heart rate, and SaO_2. › Monitor ABGs. › Use opioid analgesics cautiously in conjunction with hypnotic sedatives. › Assess and document the client's pain level and response to medication. › Use cautiously due to risk of increased vasodilation and hypotension. › Have naloxone (Narcan) and resuscitation equipment available for severe respiratory depression in a client who is nonventilated.

PROTON-PUMP INHIBITORS – PANTOPRAZOLE (PROTONIX)

Actions	› Protects against stress ulcer development
Nursing Considerations	› Do not mix with other medications.

ANTICOAGULANT – LOW-MOLECULAR WEIGHT HEPARIN, ENOXAPARIN SODIUM (LOVENOX)

Actions	› Deep vein thrombosis prophylaxis
Nursing Considerations	› Administer subcutaneously, usually in abdomen. › Do not rub injection site.

ISOTONIC CRYSTALLOIDS OR COLLOIDS (INCLUDING BLOOD PRODUCTS) – 0.9% SODIUM CHLORIDE OR LACTATED RINGER'S SOLUTION

Actions	› Hypovolemic shock – volume replacement
Nursing Considerations	› ALERT – During hypovolemic shock, replace volume first. › Use vasopressors only if blood pressure remains low after volume is replaced.

PHARMACOLOGICAL AGENTS	
ANTIHISTAMINES – DIPHENHYDRAMINE (BENADRYL)	
Actions	› Used to treat anaphylactic shock › Blocks histamine at receptor sites
Nursing Considerations	› Can cause drowsiness, hypotension, and tachycardia.
VASODILATOR – SODIUM NITROPRUSSIDE (NIPRIDE)	
Actions	› Used to treat cardiogenic shock › Reduces afterload and preload › Causes vasodilation › Decreases cardiac output and afterload
Nursing Considerations	› Assess blood pressure every 15 min. › Administer with caution because it is a potent vasodilator. › Protect the solution from light.
CORTICOSTEROIDS – HYDROCORTISONE (SOLU-CORTEF), METHYLPREDNISOLONE (SOLU-MEDROL)	
Actions	› Reduces WBC migration and decreases inflammation
Nursing Considerations	› Hydrocortisone can cause hypertension. › Discontinue medication gradually. › Administer hydrocortisone with an antiulcer medication to prevent peptic ulcer formation. › Monitor weight and blood pressure. › Monitor glucose and electrolytes.
ANTIBIOTICS SENSITIVE TO CULTURED ORGANISM(S) – VANCOMYCIN (VANCOCIN)	
Actions	› Used to treat septic shock › Inhibits cell growth or reproduction of undesired organism
Nursing Considerations	› Monitor for hypersensitivity reaction. › Administer IV vancomycin slowly. › Culture infected area prior to administration of the first dose of **vancomycin**. › Monitor the IV site for infiltration. › Do not administer **vancomycin** with other medications. › Monitor coagulopathy and renal function.

- Teamwork and Collaboration
  - Respiratory therapy
    - The respiratory therapist typically manages the ventilator, adjusts the settings, and provides chest physical therapy to improve ventilation and chest expansion. The respiratory therapist may also suction the endotracheal tube and administer inhalation medications such as bronchodilators.

- Therapeutic Procedures
  - ○ Intubation and mechanical ventilation: An artificial airway is inserted, and the client's respirations are controlled by mechanical ventilation.
    - Nursing Actions
      - □ Preintubation:
        - ▸ Monitor ECG, SaO_2, breath sounds, and color.
        - ▸ Sedate the client as needed.
        - ▸ Preoxygenate with 100% oxygen.
        - ▸ Assist with ventilation using a manual resuscitation bag and a face mask.
        - ▸ Have suction equipment, manual emergency resuscitation, and a face mask readily available.
        - ▸ Suction secretions as needed.
      - □ Postintubation:
        - ▸ Assess bilateral breath sounds, symmetrical chest movement, and a chest x-ray to confirm placement of the endotracheal tube.
        - ▸ Secure the endotracheal tube per facility guidelines.
        - ▸ Assess the balloon cuff for air leak periodically.
      - □ Positive end expiratory pressure (PEEP)
        - ▸ Positive pressure is applied at the end of expiration to keep the alveoli expanded.
        - ▸ PEEP is added to the ventilator setting to increase oxygenation and improve lung expansion.
    - Client Education
      - □ Explain all procedures to the client.
      - □ Provide reassurance to the client and family. Experiencing shock, as well as the treatments involved, can be frightening.
      - □ Explain to the client and family that the client will be unable to talk with the endotracheal tube in place.
  - ○ Needle decompression and chest tube insertion: This procedure is used to relieve pressure from a tension pneumothorax that may be causing obstructive shock.
    - Nursing Actions
      - □ Monitor ECG, SaO_2, breath sounds, and color.
      - □ Sedate as needed.
      - □ Set up a water seal chest-drainage system and attach it to suction.
      - □ Apply a dressing.
      - □ Assess the chest tube for air leaks.
      - □ Monitor and document the drainage.
      - □ Obtain a chest x-ray postprocedure.

- Client Education

  - Explain that needle decompression provides temporary relief while chest tube insertion allows for lung reinflation.

  - Provide reassurance to the client and family. Experiencing shock, as well as the treatments involved, can be frightening.

  ○ Pericardiocentesis: Pericardial fluid that is causing cardiac tamponade and obstructive shock is drained.

  - Nursing Actions

    - Monitor ECG, SaO$_2$, breath sounds, and color.

    - Sedate as needed.

    - Obtain a postprocedure chest x-ray.

  - Client Education

    - Explain that additional procedures are often necessary to resolve acute tamponade (pericardial window, pericardiectomy).

    - Provide reassurance to the client and family. Experiencing shock, as well as the treatments involved, can be frightening.

- Surgical Interventions: Surgery may be needed to correct the cause of shock, such as a hemorrhaging ulcer, wound, artery or vein.

  ○ Nursing Actions

    - Preprocedure

      - Manage the airway and provide supplemental oxygen and intubation if needed.

      - Provide hemodynamic support with fluids and medications to stabilize the client prior to surgical intervention, if possible.

    - Postprocedure

      - Continue to monitor blood pressure, ECG, pulmonary artery pressures, cardiac output, central venous pressure, and urine output.

      - Titrate and administer medications as prescribed.

      - Assess the surgical site for bleeding.

      - Monitor airway, breath sounds, and ABGs.

      - Monitor CBC.

  ○ Client Education

    - Explain all procedures to the client.

    - Provide reassurance and calm the client and family. Experiencing shock, as well as the treatments involved, can be frightening. The client may be awake.

Complications

- Multiple organ dysfunction syndrome (MODS)

  - MODS may develop from severe hypotension and reperfusion of ischemic cells causing further tissue injury. Inadequate tissue perfusion may cause organ failure in the lungs (adult respiratory distress syndrome), kidneys, heart (decreased coronary artery perfusion, decreased cardiac contractibility), and the gastrointestinal tract (necrosis).

  - Nursing Actions

    - Assess organ function and provide support measures that can increase tissue perfusion and improve organ function (ventilatory support, inotropic medications).

    - Implement measures to compensate for dysfunction (administration of clotting factors, dialysis).

- Disseminated Intravascular Coagulation (DIC)

  - DIC is a complication of septic shock. Thousands of small clots form within organ capillaries (liver, kidney, heart, brain), creating hypoxia and anaerobic metabolism. As a result of massive, multiple clot formation, platelets and other clotting factors such as fibrinogen are depleted and the client is at increased risk for hemorrhage. The client can develop diffuse petechiae and ecchymoses, and blood can leak from membranes and puncture sites.

  - Nursing Actions

    - Assess client preference related to transfusion of blood products. Some clients may not accept this treatment for various reasons (religion, fear of contamination).

    - Administer platelets and clotting factors and other blood products as prescribed.

    - Monitor hemodynamic levels.

    - Monitor results of laboratory tests (PT, PTT, serum fibrinogen, fibrin degradation).

    - Assess for further signs of bleeding.

    - Apply pressure to leaking IV/central line/arterial line sites.

  - Client Education

    - Explain procedures and care to the client and family.

APPLICATION EXERCISES

1. A nurse is caring for a client and reviewing a new prescription for an afterload-reducing medication. The nurse should recognize that this medication is administered for which of the following types of shock?

    A. Cardiogenic

    B. Obstructive

    C. Hypovolemic

    D. Distributive

2. A nurse is planning care for a client who has septic shock. Which of the following is the priority action for the nurse to take?

    A. Maintaining adequate fluid volume with IV infusions

    B. Administering antibiotic therapy

    C. Monitoring hemodynamic status

    D. Administering vasopressor medication

3. A nurse in the emergency department is caring for a client who has an allergic reaction to a bee sting. The client is experiencing wheezing and swelling of the tongue. Which of the following medications should the nurse expect to administer first?

    A. Methylprednisolone (Solu-Medrol) IV bolus

    B. Diphenhydramine (Benadryl) subcutaneously

    C. Epinephrine (Adrenaline) IV

    D. Albuterol (Proventil) inhaler

4. A nurse in the emergency department is completing an assessment of a client who is in shock. Which of the following findings should the nurse expect? (Select all that apply.)

    _____ A. Heart rate 60/min

    _____ B. Seizure activity

    _____ C. Respiratory rate 42/min

    _____ D. Increased urine output

    _____ E. Weak, thready pulse

5. A nurse in a cardiac unit is assisting with the admission of a client who is to undergo hemodynamic monitoring. Which of the following actions should the nurse anticipate performing?

    A. Administer large volumes of IV fluids.

    B. Assist with insertion of pulmonary artery catheter.

    C. Obtain Doppler pulses of the extremities.

    D. Gather supplies for insertion of a peripheral IV catheter.

6. A nurse educator is reviewing care of a client who is in shock with a group of newly hired nurse. What should be included in this discussion? Use the ATI Active Learning Template: Systems Disorder to complete this item to include the following sections:

    A. Description of Disorder: Describe each type of shock and at least one risk factor for each.

    B. Objective Data: Describe expected findings related to BP, pulse, respirations, and urine output.

APPLICATION EXERCISES KEY

1. A. **CORRECT:** Reducing afterload will allow the heart to pump more effectively, which is needed for the client who has cardiogenic shock.

    B. INCORRECT: In obstructive shock, the high afterload is due to obstruction of blood flow. Afterload-reducing agents will not remove the obstruction.

    C. INCORRECT: Fluid replacement and reduction of further fluid loss are the focus of management of hypovolemic shock.

    D. INCORRECT: Afterload-reducing medication is not administered to a client with distributive shock because the client already has decreased afterload.

    (N) NCLEX® Connection: Pharmacological and Parenteral Therapies, Expected Actions/Outcomes

2. A. INCORRECT: Maintaining the client's fluid volume by administration of IV fluids is an appropriate action, but it is not the priority action.

    B. **CORRECT:** Using the safety and risk reduction framework, administration of antibiotics is the priority action by the nurse. Eliminating endotoxins and mediators from bacteria will reduce the vasodilation that is occurring.

    C. INCORRECT: Monitoring the client's hemodynamic status is an appropriate action, but it is not the priority action.

    D. INCORRECT: Administering vasopressor medication is an appropriate action, but it is not the priority action.

    (N) NCLEX® Connection: Physiological Adaptations, Medical Emergencies

3. A. INCORRECT: Methylprednisolone may be administered, but it is not the first medication to be administered.

    B. INCORRECT: Diphenhydramine may be administered, but it is not the first medication to be administered

    C. **CORRECT:** Using the airway-breathing-circulation (ABC) priority-setting framework, epinephrine is administered first. It is a rapid-acting medication that promotes effective oxygenation and is used to treat anaphylactic shock.

    D. INCORRECT: Albuterol may be administered, but it is not the first medication to be administered.

    (N) NCLEX® Connection: Pharmacological and Parenteral Therapies, Adverse Effects/Contraindications/ Side Effects/Interactions

4. A. INCORRECT: Tachycardia is an expected finding in a client who is in shock.

    B. **CORRECT:** Seizure activity may be present in a client who is in shock.

    C. **CORRECT:** Tachypnea is an expected finding in a client who is in shock.

    D. INCORRECT: Decreased urine output is in expected finding in a client who is in shock.

    E. **CORRECT:** A weak, thready pulse is an expected finding in a client who is in shock.

    Ⓝ NCLEX® Connection: Physiological Adaptations, Medical Emergencies

5. A. INCORRECT: Patency of the catheter is maintained with a slow continuous infusion of 0.9% sodium chloride. The catheter is used for blood sampling and pressure monitoring, not fluid administration.

    B. **CORRECT:** A pulmonary artery catheter and pressure-monitoring system are inserted for hemodynamic monitoring of a client.

    C. INCORRECT: ECG monitoring is performed prior to hemodynamic monitoring.

    D. INCORRECT: An arterial line is needed to obtain blood samples for ABGs and other blood tests as part of hemodynamic monitoring.

    Ⓝ NCLEX® Connection: Physiological Adaptations, Hemodynamics

6. *Using the ATI Active Learning Template: Systems Disorder*

    A. Description of Disorder

    - Cardiogenic: Pump failure due to MI, heart failure, cardiomyopathy, dysrhythmia, and valvular rupture or stenosis
    - Hypovolemic: Excessive fluid loss from diuresis, vomiting/diarrhea, blood loss
    - Obstructive: Blockage of great vessels, pulmonary artery stenosis, pulmonary embolism, cardiac tamponade, tension pneumothorax and aortic dissection

    - Septic: Endotoxins (gram-negative bacteria) and mediators causing massive vasodilation
    - Neurogenic: Loss of sympathetic tone causing massive vasodilation due to trauma, spinal shock, epidural anesthesia
    - Anaphylactic: Antigen-antibody reaction causing massive vasodilation due to allergens (inhaled, swallowed, contacted, or introduced IV)

    B. Objective Data

    - BP – May be within the expected reference range during the initial stage, then can increase during the progressive stage and then drop to less than 50 to 60 mm Hg

    - Pulse: May be weak or thready; bounding with distributive shock
    - Respirations: Tachypnea progressing to greater then 40/min, hypocarbia, hypoxia
    - Urine output: Decreased

    Ⓝ NCLEX® Connection: Physiological Adaptations, Medical Emergencies

chapter 38

Overview

- A weakness in a section of a dilated artery that causes a widening or ballooning in the wall of the blood vessel is called an aneurysm.

- Aneurysms can occur in two forms. They can be saccular (only affecting one side of the artery), or they can be fusiform (involving the complete circumference of the artery).

- Seventy-five percent of aneurysms are abdominal aortic aneurysms.

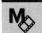   View Image: Common Aneurysm Sites

- Dissecting aneurysm (aortic dissection) can occur when blood accumulates within the artery wall (hematoma) following a tear in the lining of the artery (usually due to hypertension). This is a life-threatening condition.

Health Promotion and Disease Prevention

- Promote smoking cessation.

- Maintain appropriate weight for height and body frame.

- Encourage a healthy diet and physical activity.

- Control blood pressure with regular monitoring and medication if needed.

Assessment

- Risk Factors

  - Sex (male)

  - Atherosclerosis

  - Uncontrolled hypertension

  - Tobacco use

  - With age, arterial stiffening caused by loss of elastin in arterial walls, thickening of intima of arteries, and progressive fibrosis of media occurs; therefore, older adult clients are more prone to aneurysms and have a higher mortality rate from aneurysms than younger individuals.

- Subjective and Objective Data
  - Initially, clients are often asymptomatic.
  - Abdominal aortic aneurysm (AAA) – most common, related to atherosclerosis
    - Constant gnawing feeling in abdomen; flank or back pain
    - Pulsating abdominal mass (do not palpate; may cause rupture)
    - Bruit
    - Elevated blood pressure (unless in cardiac tamponade or rupture of aneurysm)
  - Aortic dissections (often associated with Marfan's syndrome)
    - Sudden onset of "tearing," "ripping," and "stabbing" abdominal or back pain
    - Hypovolemic shock
      - Diaphoresis, nausea, vomiting, faintness, apprehension
      - Decreased or absent peripheral pulses
      - Neurological deficits
      - Hypotension and tachycardia (initial)
  - Thoracic aortic aneurysm
    - Severe back pain (most common)
    - Hoarseness, cough, shortness of breath, and difficulty swallowing
    - Decrease in urinary output
  - Diagnostic procedures
    - X-ray
      - X-rays reveal the classic "eggshell" appearance of an aneurysm. Aneurysms are often discovered when examining a client for some other clinical possibility.
    - Computed tomography (CT) and ultrasonography
      - CT scans and ultrasonography are used to assess the size and location of aneurysms and are often repeated at periodic intervals to monitor the progression of an aneurysm.

Patient-Centered Care

- Nursing Care
  - Take vital signs every 15 min until stable, then every hour. Monitor for an increase in blood pressure.
  - Assess the onset, quality, duration, and severity of pain.
  - Assess temperature, circulation, and range of motion of extremities.
  - Continuously monitor the cardiac rhythm.
  - Monitor hemodynamic findings.
  - Monitor ABGs, SaO_2, electrolytes, and CBC laboratory findings.
  - Monitor hourly urine output – greater than 30 mL/hr indicates adequate kidney perfusion.
  - Administer oxygen as prescribed.
  - Obtain and maintain IV access.
  - Administer medications as prescribed.
    - Note – All aneurysms can be life-threatening and require medical attention.

- Medications
  - The priority intervention is to reduce systolic blood pressure between 100 and 120 mm Hg during an emergency. Long-term goal includes maintaining systolic blood pressure at or less than 130 to 140 mm Hg.
    - Administer antihypertensive agents as prescribed. Often more than one is prescribed (beta blockers and calcium blockers).
- Teamwork and Collaboration
  - Cardiology services may be consulted to manage and treat hypertension.
  - Radiology should be consulted for diagnostic studies to determine an aneurysm.
  - Vascular services may be consulted for surgical intervention.
- Surgical Interventions
  - Abdominal aortic aneurysm resection – excision of the aneurysm and the placement of a synthetic graft (elective or emergency)
    - Rupturing aneurysm requires prompt emergency surgery (50% mortality rate).
    - Elective surgery is used to manage AAA of 6 cm diameter or greater (2 to 5% mortality rate).
    - Risks include significant blood loss and the consequences of reduced cardiac output and tissue ischemia (MI, renal failure, respiratory distress, paralytic ileus).
    - Nursing Actions
      - Priority interventions include monitoring the arterial pressure, heart rhythm, and hemodynamic findings, as well as monitoring for evidence of graft occlusion or rupture postoperatively.
      - Monitor vital signs and circulation (pulses distal to graft) every 15 min.
      - Maintain the head of the bed below 45° to prevent flexion of the graft.
      - Report evidence of graft occlusion or rupture immediately (changes in pulses, coolness of extremity below graft, white or blue extremities or flanks, severe pain, abdominal distention, decreased urine output).
      - Monitor and maintain normal blood pressure. Prolonged hypotension can cause thrombi to form within the graft; severe hypertension can cause leakage or rupture at the arterial anastomosis suture line.
      - Maintain a warm environment to prevent temperature-induced vasoconstriction.
      - Administer IV fluids at prescribed rates to ensure adequate hydration and kidney perfusion.
      - Monitor for altered kidney perfusion and kidney failure caused by clamping aorta during surgery (urine output less than 50 mL/hr, weight gain, elevated BUN or serum creatinine).
      - Auscultate lung sounds. Encourage coughing and deep breathing every 2 hr. Encourage splinting with coughing.
      - Assess onset, quality, duration, and severity of pain.
        - ▸ Administer pain medication as prescribed.
      - Monitor bowel sounds and observe for abdominal distention. Maintain nasogastric suction as prescribed.
      - Prevent thromboembolism. Maintain sequential compression devices, early ambulation, administer antiplatelet or anticoagulant medications as prescribed.
      - Monitor for infection.
      - Administer antibiotics as prescribed to maintain adequate blood levels of the medication.

○ Percutaneous aneurysm repair – Insertion of endothelial stent grafts for aneurysm repair avoids abdominal incision and shortens the postoperative period (can be used to repair a thoracic aortic aneurysm).

- Nursing Actions
  - □ Nursing care after the procedure is similar to care following an arteriogram or cardiac catheterization (monitor pedal pulse). Refer to the chapter on *Invasive Cardiovascular Procedures*.

○ Thoracic aortic aneurysm repair

- Procedure similar to thoracic surgery, such as open heart. The course of action depends on the location of the aneurysm. Cardiopulmonary bypass is commonly used for this procedure.

- Nursing Actions
  - □ Nursing care after the procedure is similar to care following coronary artery bypass graft surgery (monitor respiratory status; respiratory distress is common after this type of procedure).

- Care After Discharge
  - □ Cardiac rehabilitation services may be consulted for prolonged weakness and assistance in increasing the client's level of activity.
  - □ Nutritional services may be consulted for food choices that are low in fat and cholesterol.

○ Client Education

- Monitor and maintain blood pressure. Emphasize importance of staying within parameters set by provider. Taking medications as prescribed prevents complications (rupture).

- Promote follow-up on scheduled CT scans to monitor aneurysm size (nonsurgical client). Collaborate with case management services to assist with transportation needs.

- Promote smoking cessation if the client smokes.

- Prevent infection (good hand hygiene, wound care management). Report evidence of infection (wound redness, edema, drainage; elevated temperature; surgical client).

- Encourage proper diet (low-fat, high-protein, vitamins A and C, zinc to promote wound healing).

- Review manifestations of aneurysm rupture (abdominal fullness or pain, chest or back pain, shortness of breath, cough, difficulty swallowing, hoarseness). Instruct client to report these immediately.

- Avoid strenuous activity and restrict heavy lifting to less than 15 lb (surgical client).

Complications

- Rupture
  - ○ Aneurysm rupture is a life-threatening emergency, often resulting in massive hemorrhage, shock, and death.
  - ○ Treatment requires simultaneous resuscitation and immediate surgical repair.
    - Aneurysms greater than 6 cm (2.4 inches) in diameter have a 50% chance of rupture within 1 year.
- Thrombus formation
  - ○ A thrombus may form inside the aneurysm. Emboli may be dislodged, blocking arteries distal to the aneurysm, which causes ischemia and shuts down other body systems.
  - ○ Assess circulation distal to aneurysm, including pulses and color and temperature of the lower extremities. Monitor the client's urine output.

APPLICATION EXERCISES

1. A nurse in the emergency department is assisting with the admission of a client who has a possible dissecting abdominal aortic aneurysm. Which of the following is the priority nursing intervention?

    A. Administer pain medication as prescribed.

    B. Ensure a warm environment.

    C. Administer IV fluids as prescribed.

    D. Initiate a 12-lead ECG.

2. A nurse is planning caring for a client who had a surgical placement of an synthetic graft to repair an aneurysm. Which of the following interventions should the nurse include in the plan of care?

    _____ A. Assess pedal pulses.

    _____ B. Monitor for an increase in pain below the graft site.

    _____ C. Maintain client in high Fowler's position.

    _____ D. Administer prescribed antiplatelet agents.

    _____ E. Report an hourly urine output of 60 mL.

3. A nurse is discussing a new diagnosis of an aneurysm with a client. The client asks the nurse to explain what causes an aneurysm to rupture. Which of the following is an appropriate response by the nurse?

    A. "The wall of an artery becomes thin and flexible."

    B. "It is due to turbulence in blood flow in the artery."

    C. "It is due to abdominal enlargement."

    D. "It is due to hypertension."

4. A nurse is admitting a client with a suspected occlusion of a graft of the abdominal aorta. Which of the following is an expected clinical finding?

    A. Increased urine output

    B. Bounding pedal pulse

    C. Increased abdominal girth

    D. Redness of the lower extremities

5. A nurse is reviewing clinical manifestations of a thoracic aortic aneurysm with a newly hired nurse. Which of the following should the nurse include in the discussion? (Select all that apply.)

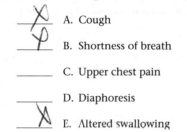

_____ A. Cough

_____ B. Shortness of breath

_____ C. Upper chest pain

_____ D. Diaphoresis

_____ E. Altered swallowing

6. A nurse educator is presenting a program to nurses on care of the client with an aneurysm. What should the educator include in this program? Use the ATI Active Learning Template: Systems Disorder to complete this item to include the following sections:

A. Risk Factors: Describe three.

B. Diagnostic Procedures: Describe two.

C. Nursing Interventions: Describe at least four.

APPLICATION EXERCISES KEY

1. A. INCORRECT: Administering pain mediation is important, but it is not the priority nursing intervention.

    B. INCORRECT: Ensuring a warm environment is important, but it is not the priority nursing intervention.

    C. **CORRECT:** Using the ABC priority-setting framework, the greatest risk to the client is inadequate circulatory volume. The priority nursing intervention is to administer IV fluids.

    D. INCORRECT: Initiating a 12-lead ECG is important, but it is not the priority nursing intervention.

    Ⓝ NCLEX® Connection: Physiological Adaptations, Medical Emergencies

2. A. **CORRECT:** Pulses distal to the graft site should be monitored to detect possible occlusion of the graft.

    B. **CORRECT:** Pain below the graft site can be an indication of graft occlusion or rupture.

    C. INCORRECT: The head of the bed should be maintained at less than 45° to prevent flexion of the graft.

    D. **CORRECT:** Antiplatelet agents and anticoagulants are prescribed to prevent thrombus formation.

    E. INCORRECT: An hourly urine output of 60 mL/hr is an expected finding.

    Ⓝ NCLEX® Connection: Reduction of Risk Potential, Therapeutic Procedures

3. A. INCORRECT: An aneurysm ruptures as a result of thickening in the intima of the artery and a lack of elasticity in the vessel wall, which is usually under pressure due to hypertension.

    B. INCORRECT: A bruit is objective data, which indicates the presence of an aneurysm, not the cause of rupture.

    C. INCORRECT: Abdominal distention may occur when an aneurysm ruptures, but it is not the cause of the rupture.

    D. **CORRECT:** Hypertension increases pressure within the arterial walls, resulting in rupture.

    Ⓝ NCLEX® Connection: Physiological Adaptations, Pathophysiology

4. A. INCORRECT: Decreased urine output is an expected finding with occlusion of a graft of the aorta.

    B. INCORRECT: Decreased or absent pedal pulse is an expected finding with occlusion of a graft of the aorta.

    C. **CORRECT:** Abdominal distention is an expected finding with occlusion of a graft of the aorta.

    D. INCORRECT: Pallor or cyanosis of the extremities is an expected finding with occlusion of a graft of the aorta.

    (N) NCLEX® Connection: Physiological Adaptations, Pathophysiology

5. A. **CORRECT:** Cough is a manifestation of a thoracic aortic aneurysm.

    B. **CORRECT:** Shortness of breath is a manifestation of a thoracic aortic aneurysm.

    C. INCORRECT: Report of severe back pain is a clinical finding of thoracic aortic aneurysm.

    D. INCORRECT: Diaphoresis is a clinical finding of dissecting aortic aneurysm.

    E. **CORRECT:** Difficulty swallowing is a manifestation of a thoracic aortic aneurysm.

    (N) NCLEX® Connection: Physiological Adaptations, Pathophysiology

6. *Using the ATI Active Learning Template: Systems Disorder*

    A. Risk Factors
    - Male sex
    - Atherosclerosis
    - Uncontrolled hypertension
    - Tobacco use
    - Age-related changes to the artery (loss of elastin, thickening of the intima, progressive fibrosis)

    B. Diagnostic Procedures
    - X-rays
    - CT scans
    - Ultrasonography

    C. Nursing Interventions
    - Take vital signs every 15 min until stable. Then, every hour, monitoring for increased blood pressure.
    - Assess pain (onset, quality, duration, severity).
    - Assess temperature, circulation, and range of motion of extremities.
    - Monitor cardiac rhythm continuously.
    - Monitor hemodynamic findings.
    - Monitor ABGs, Sa0$_2$, electrolytes, CBC laboratory findings.
    - Monitor hourly urine output.
    - Administer oxygen as prescribed.
    - Obtain and maintain IV access.
    - Administer medications as prescribed.

    (N) NCLEX® Connection: Physiological Adaptations, Illness Management

UNIT 5   Nursing Care of Clients with Hematologic Disorders

SECTIONS

› Diagnostic and Therapeutic Procedures
› Hematologic Disorders

NCLEX® CONNECTIONS

When reviewing the chapters in this unit, keep in mind the relevant sections of the NCLEX® outline, in particular:

Client Needs: Pharmacological and Parenteral Therapies	Client Needs: Reduction of Risk Potential	Client Needs: Physiological Adaptation
› Relevant topics/tasks include: » Blood and Blood Products › Identify the client according to facility policy prior to administration of red blood cells/blood products. › Check the client for appropriate venous access for red blood cell/blood product administration . › Administer blood products and evaluate the client's response.	› Relevant topics/tasks include: » Laboratory Values › Recognize deviations from normal for values of albumin (blood), ALT (SGPT), AST (SGOT), ammonia, bilirubin, bleeding time, calcium (total), cholesterol (HDL and LDL), digoxin, ESR, lithium, magnesium, phosphorous/phosphate, protein (total), urine (specific gravity, albumin, pH, WBC). › Educate the client about the purpose and procedure of prescribed laboratory tests.	› Relevant topics/tasks include: » Alterations in Body Systems › Assess the adaptation of the client to health alteration, illness and/or disease. » Fluid and Electrolyte Imbalances › Manage the care of the client with a fluid and electrolyte imbalance. » Hemodynamics › Intervene to improve the client's cardiovascular status.

chapter 39

Overview

- Hematologic assessment and diagnostic procedures evaluate blood function by testing indicators such as erythrocytes (RBC), leukocytes (WBC), platelets, and coagulation times.
- By testing the blood, diagnosis of a disease and efficacy of treatment can be determined.
- Bone marrow is responsible for the production of many blood cells including RBCs, WBCs, and platelets. A bone marrow biopsy provides diagnostic information about how the bone marrow is functioning.

Blood Collection/Testing

- Blood diagnostic procedures that nurses should be knowledgeable about:
  - Serum RBC count
  - Serum WBC count
  - Mean corpuscular volume (MCV)
  - Mean corpuscular Hgb (MCH)
  - Total iron-binding count (TIBC)
  - Iron
  - Platelets
  - Hgb
  - Hct
  - Coagulation studies
    - Prothrombin time (PT)
    - Partial thromboplastin time (aPTT)
    - International normalized ratio (INR)
    - D-dimer
    - Fibrinogen levels
    - Fibrin degradation products
- CBC is a series of tests that include RBC, WBC, MCV, MCH, Hgb, and Hct.
- Indications/interpretation of findings

TEST	EXPECTED REFERENCE RANGE	PURPOSE FOR TEST
RBC	Females: 4.2 to 5.4 million/uL Males: 4.7 to 6.1 million/uL	› Decreased level can be evidence of anemia.
WBC	5,000 to 10,000/uL	› Elevated level can be evidence of infection. › Decreased level can be evidence of immunosuppression.

TEST	EXPECTED REFERENCE RANGE	PURPOSE FOR TEST
MCV	80 to 95 mm³	› Elevated level can be evidence of macrocytic (large) cells, possible anemia. › Decreased level can be evidence of microcytic (small) cells, possible iron deficiency anemia.
MCH	27 to 31 pg/cell	› Same as above for MCV, but measures the amount of Hgb by weight per RBC.
TIBC	250 to 460 mcg/dL	› Elevated level can be evidence of iron deficiency. › Decreased level can be evidence of anemia, hemolysis, or hemorrhage.
Iron	Females: 60 to 160 mcg/dL Males: 80 to 180 mcg/dL	› Elevated level can be evidence of hemochromatosis, iron excess, liver disorder, or megaloblastic anemia. › Decreased level can be evidence of iron deficiency anemia, or hemorrhage.
Platelets	150,000 to 400,000 mm³	› Increased level can be evidence of malignancy or polycythemia vera. › Decreased level can be evidence of autoimmune disease, bone marrow suppression, or enlarged spleen.
Hgb	Females: 12 to 16 g/dL Males: 14 to 18 g/dL	› Decreased level can be evidence of anemia.
Hct	Females: 37 to 47% Males: 42 to 52%	› Decreased level can be evidence of anemia.
PT	11 to 12.5 seconds, 85 to 100%, or 1:1 client-control ratio	› Increased time can be evidence of deficiency or clotting. › Decreased time can be evidence of vitamin K excess.
aPTT	1.5 to 2 times normal range of 30 to 40 seconds (desired range for anticoagulation)	› Measures the intrinsic clotting factors. › Monitored for heparin therapy. › Increased time can be evidence of hemophilia, disseminated intravascular coagulation (DIC), or liver disease.
INR	2 to 3 on warfarin (Coumadin) therapy	› Measures the mean of PT. › Client's PT divided by average mean PT. › Monitored for warfarin therapy.
D-dimer	0.43 to 2.33 mcg/mL 0 to 250 ng/mL	› Measures hypercoagulability of the blood. › Elevated level indicates clot formation has occurred.
Fibrinogen levels	170 to 340 mg/dL	› Reflects available fibrinogen for clotting. › Decreased levels may indicate decreased ability to clot.
Fibrin degradation products	Less than 10 mcg/mL	› Increases when clot dissolving activity (fibrinolysis) is occurring. › Monitors efficacy of medications for DIC.

- Preprocedure
  - Nursing Actions
    - Use standard precautions in collecting and handling blood for specimen collection.
- Intraprocedure
  - Nursing Actions
    - Select the appropriate vial according to the test to be performed.
    - Collect a sufficient quantity of blood and fill to the indicated mark on the vial.
    - Properly label the specimen and deliver it to the laboratory promptly for appropriate storage and analysis. Check facility protocol regarding time frame within which the specimen must be delivered to the laboratory.
    - For coagulation studies, blood will be required to be drawn at specific times and sent to the laboratory immediately so that the nurse can adjust the dose of anticoagulant therapy based on the results.
- Postprocedure
  - Nursing Actions
    - Results of hematologic tests are usually available preliminarily within 24 to 48 hr, with final results in 72 hr.
    - If results are out of expected reference range, it is the nurse's responsibility to report the results to the provider for further intervention.

Bone Marrow Aspiration/Biopsy

- A biopsy is the extraction of a very small amount of tissue, such as bone marrow, to definitively diagnose cell type and to confirm or rule out malignancy. A bone marrow tissue sample is removed by needle aspiration for cytological (histological) examination.
  - Biopsies can be performed with local anesthesia or conscious sedation in an ambulatory setting, intraoperatively, or during scope procedures.

 View Image: Bone Marrow Biopsy

- Indications
  - A bone marrow biopsy is commonly performed to diagnose causes of blood disorders, such as anemia or thrombocytopenia, or to rule-out diseases, such as leukemia and other cancers, and infection.
- Interpretation of Findings
  - After a procedure is completed, the tissue sample is sent to pathology for interpretation.
- Preprocedure
  - Nursing Actions
    - Ensure that the client has signed the informed consent form.
    - Position the client in a prone or side lying position to expose the iliac crest for the procedure.
  - Client Education
    - Explain the procedure to the client. The biopsy site will be anesthetized with a local anesthetic, and the client may feel pressure and brief pain during the aspiration.

- Intraprocedure
  - Nursing Actions
    - Administer a sedative if prescribed.
      - Older adult clients are at greater risk for complications associated with sedation for biopsy procedures due to chronic illnesses.
      - An older adult's renal clearance also needs to be considered when using any analgesics for sedation.
    - Assist the provider with the test/procedure as needed.
    - As appropriate, apply pressure to the biopsy site to control bleeding.
    - As appropriate, place a sterile dressing over the biopsy site.
- Postprocedure
  - Nursing Actions
    - Monitor for evidence of infection (fever, increased WBCs, pain, and swelling at the site) and bleeding.
    - Apply ice to the biopsy site if prescribed.
    - Postprocedure discomfort is usually relieved by mild analgesics.
    - Avoid aspirin and other medications that affect clotting.
  - Client Education
    - Teach the client to report excessive bleeding and evidence of infection to the provider.
    - Teach the client to check the biopsy site daily. The site should be clean, dry, and intact.
    - If sutures are in place, remind the client to return in 7 to 10 days to have them removed.
- Complications
  - Infection
    - Infection can occur at the aspiration site.
    - Nursing Actions – Monitor the site and keep it clean and dry.
  - Bleeding
    - Bleeding can occur from the site.
    - Nursing Actions – Report bleeding to the provider immediately.

APPLICATION EXERCISES

1. A nurse in a clinic is caring for a client who has suspected anemia. The nurse should anticipate a prescription from the provider for which of the following tests?

    A. INR

    B. Platelet count

    C. WBC count

    D. Hgb

2. A nurse is caring for a client who has hemophilia. The nurse should anticipate a prescription from the provider for which of the following tests?

    A. RBC

    B. TIBC

    C. aPTT

    D. MCH

3. A nurse is providing teaching for a client who is to have a bone marrow biopsy of the iliac crest. Which of the following statements made by the client indicates a need for further teaching?

    A. "Cancer can be detected in the fluid being tested."

    B. "I will feel a heavy pressure sensation in my hip bone."

    C. "The type of antibiotic I need to take can be determined by this test."

    D. "I will be awake during the procedure."

4. A nurse is caring for a client who is having a bone marrow biopsy. What actions should the nurse take? Use the ATI Active Learning Template: Diagnostic Procedure to complete this item to include the following:

    A. Nursing Interventions: Describe two for each of the pre, intra, and postoperative periods.

    B. Potential Complications: Identify two.

    C. Client Education: Describe two teaching points.

APPLICATION EXERCISES KEY

1. A. INCORRECT: An INR test identifies the effectiveness of warfarin therapy.

    B. INCORRECT: A platelet count identifies an alteration in immune response.

    C. INCORRECT: A WBC count identifies the presence of an infection.

    D. **CORRECT:** An Hgb test is prescribed to confirm a diagnosis of anemia.

    Ⓝ NCLEX® Connection: Reduction of Risk Potential, Laboratory Values

2. A. INCORRECT: The RBC identifies the presence of anemia and is not indicated for a client who has a clotting disorder.

    B. INCORRECT: The TIBC identifies the presence of iron deficiency anemia and is not indicated for a client who has a clotting disorder.

    C. **CORRECT:** The aPTT checks the clotting factors in a client who has hemophilia.

    D. INCORRECT: The MCH indicates the presence of anemia and is not indicated for a client who has a clotting disorder.

    Ⓝ NCLEX® Connection: Reduction of Risk Potential, Laboratory Values

3. A. INCORRECT: The presence of cancer can be determined by this test.

    B. INCORRECT: The client will feel brief pain or pressure with this test.

    C. **CORRECT:** A culture and sensitivity test determines the type of antibiotics that a client who has an infection needs to take.

    D. INCORRECT: A client is awake during a bone marrow biopsy.

    Ⓝ NCLEX® Connection: Reduction of Risk Potential, Diagnostic Tests

4. *Using the ATI Active Learning Template: Diagnostic Procedure*

   A. Nursing Interventions
      - Pre
        - ○ Ensure that the client has signed the informed consent form.
        - ○ Position the client in a prone or side-lying position.
      - Intra
        - ○ Administer sedative medication.
        - ○ Assist with the procedure.
        - ○ Apply pressure to the biopsy site.
        - ○ Place a sterile dressing over the biopsy site.
      - Post
        - ○ Monitor for evidence of infection and bleeding.
        - ○ Apply ice to the biopsy site.
        - ○ Administer mild analgesics; avoid aspirin or medications that affect clotting.

   B. Potential Complications
      - Bleeding and infection

   C. Client Education
      - Explain the procedure to be performed: use of local anesthesia, sensation of pressure or brief pain.
      - Report excessive bleeding and evidence of infection to the provider.
      - Check the biopsy site daily. It should be clean, dry and intact.
      - If there are sutures, return in 7 to 10 days for removal.

   Ⓝ NCLEX® Connection: Reduction of Risk Potential, Diagnostic Tests

chapter 40

Overview

- Whole blood or components of whole blood can be transfused for clients who require replacement due to blood loss or blood disease.

- Blood components

  - Packed RBCs

  - Plasma

  - Albumin

  - Clotting factors

  - Prothrombin complex

  - Cryoprecipitate

  - Platelets

Transfusions

- Transfusion Types

  - Homologous transfusions – Blood from donors is used.

  - Autologous transfusions – The client's blood is collected in anticipation of future transfusions (elective surgery); this blood is designated for and can be used only by the client. Clients may donate blood 5 weeks in advance up to 72 hr prior to surgery.

    - Intraoperative blood salvage – blood loss during certain surgeries can be recycled through a cell-saver machine and transfused intraoperatively or postoperatively (orthopedic surgeries, CABG).

- Indications

  - Diagnoses

    - Excessive blood loss (Hgb 6 to 10 g/dL, depending on findings) – whole blood

    - Anemia (Hgb 6 to 10 g/dL, depending on findings) – packed RBCs

    - Kidney failure – packed RBCs

    - Coagulation factor deficiencies such as hemophilia – fresh frozen plasma

    - Thrombocytopenia/platelet dysfunction (platelets less than 20,000 or less than 80,000 and actively bleeding) – platelets

- Preprocedure

  - Incompatibility is a major concern when administering blood or blood products, and preventing incompatibility requires strict adherence to blood transfusion protocols.

    - Blood is typed based on the presence of antigens.

BLOOD TYPE	ANTIGEN	ANTIBODIES AGAINST	COMPATIBLE WITH
A	A	B	A, O
B	B	A	B, O
AB	AB	None	A, B, AB, O
O	None	A, B	O

    - Another consideration is the Rh factor – blood that contains D antigen makes the Rh factor positive. Rh-positive blood given to an Rh-negative person will cause hemolysis.

  - Nursing Actions

    - Assess laboratory values, such as Hgb and Hct. Packed RBCs are usually prescribed for clients who have an Hgb of less than 8 g/dL.

    - Verify the prescription for a specific blood product.

    - Obtain blood samples for compatibility determination, such as type and crossmatch.

    - Initiate large-bore IV access. A 20-gauge needle is standard for administering blood products.

      - For older adult clients, venous access for blood transfusions may be limited due to age-related vascular and skin changes.

    - Assess the client for a history of blood-transfusion reactions.

    - Obtain blood products from the blood bank. Inspect the blood for discoloration, excessive bubbles, or cloudiness.

    - Following facility protocol, confirm the client's identity, blood compatibility, and expiration time of the blood product with another nurse.

    - Prime the blood administration set with 0.9% sodium chloride. Blood products are infused only with 0.9% sodium chloride. Never add medications to blood products.

    - Ascertain whether a filter should be used.

    - Obtain the client's baseline vital signs.

    - Begin the transfusion, and use a blood warmer if indicated.

  - Client Education

    - Explain to the client the reason for the blood transfusion.

- Intraprocedure

  - Nursing Actions

    - Remain with the client for the first 15 to 30 min of the infusion (reactions occur most often during the first 15 min) and monitor:

      - Vital signs (then every hour afterward)

      - Rate of infusion

□ Respiratory status

□ Sudden increase in anxiety

□ Breath sounds

□ Neck-vein distention

- For older adult clients, assess vital signs more frequently because changes in pulse, blood pressure, and respiratory rate may indicate fluid overload, or may be the sole indicators of a transfusion reaction. Older adult clients who have cardiac or renal dysfunction are at an increased risk for heart failure and fluid-volume excess when receiving a blood transfusion.

- Notify the provider immediately if indications of a reaction occur.

- Complete the transfusion within a 2- to 4-hr time frame to avoid bacterial growth.

- Postprocedure

  - Nursing Actions

    - Obtain the client's vital signs upon completion of the transfusion.

    - Dispose of the blood-administration set appropriately (biohazard bags).

    - Monitor blood values as prescribed (CBC, Hgb, Hct).

      □ Hgb levels should rise by approximately 1 g/dL with each unit transfused.

    - Complete paperwork, and file in the appropriate places.

    - Document the client's response.

- Complications

TRANSFUSION REACTIONS	
ONSET	SIGNS AND SYMPTOMS
Acute hemolytic	
› Immediate	› This reaction may be mild or life-threatening. Clinical findings include chills, fever, low back pain, tachycardia, flushing, hypotension, chest tightening or pain, tachypnea, nausea, anxiety, and hemoglobinuria. › This reaction may cause cardiovascular collapse, kidney failure, disseminated intravascular coagulation, shock, and death.
Febrile	
› 30 min to 6 hr after transfusion	› Clinical findings include chills, fever, flushing, headache, and anxiety. › Use WBC filter. Administer antipyretics.
Mild allergic	
› During or up to 24 hr after transfusion	› Clinical findings include itching, urticaria, and flushing. › Administer antihistamines, such as diphenhydramine (Benadryl).
Anaphylactic	
› Immediate	› Clinical findings include wheezing, dyspnea, chest tightness, cyanosis, and hypotension. › Maintain airway; administer oxygen, IV fluids, antihistamines, corticosteroids, and vasopressors.

- Nursing Actions
  - Stop the transfusion immediately if a reaction is suspected.
  - Initiate an infusion of 0.9% sodium chloride. The infusion should be initiated with a separate line, so as not to infuse more blood from the transfusion tubing.
  - Save the blood bag with the remaining blood and the blood tubing for testing at the laboratory following facility protocol.
- Client Education
  - Explain to the client the reason that the blood is being discontinued.
- Circulatory overload
  - Clients who have impaired cardiac function can experience circulatory overload as a result of a transfusion.
    - Manifestations include dyspnea, chest tightness, tachycardia, tachypnea, headache, hypertension, jugular-vein distention, peripheral edema, orthopnea, sudden anxiety, and crackles in the base of the lungs.
  - Nursing Actions
    - Administer oxygen, monitor vital signs, slow the infusion rate, and administer diuretics as prescribed.
    - Notify the provider immediately.
- Sepsis and septic shock
  - Manifestations include fever, nausea, vomiting, abdominal pain, chills, and hypotension.
  - Nursing Actions
    - Maintain patent airway, and administer oxygen.
    - Administer antibiotic therapy as prescribed.
    - Obtain samples for blood cultures.
    - Administer vasopressors, such as dopamine, to combat vasodilation in the late phase.
    - Elevate the client's feet.
    - If disseminated intravascular coagulation (DIC) occurs:
      - Administer anticoagulants, such as heparin, in the early phase.
      - Administer clotting factors and blood products during the late phase (clotting factors are depleted in the early stage).

APPLICATION EXERCISES

1. A nurse should remain with a client during the first 15 min of a blood transfusion to

 A. verify the blood is being transfused.

 B. assess for an adverse reaction.

 C. explain the procedure to the client.

 D. obtain blood specimens.

2. A nurse is caring for a client who is receiving a blood transfusion. Which of the following actions should the nurse take when there is a transfusion reaction? (Select all that apply.)

 X____ A. Stop the transfusion.

 X____ B. Send the blood bag and IV tubing to the blood bank.

 X____ C. Maintain an IV infusion with 0.9% sodium chloride.

 _____ D. Elevate the client's feet.

 _____ E. Obtain blood cultures.

3. A nurse is monitoring a client who began receiving a unit of blood 10 min ago. Which of the following should pose an immediate concern for the nurse? (Select all that apply.)

 X____ A. Temperature change from 37° C (98.6° F) pretransfusion to 37.2° C (99.0° F) posttransfusion

 X____ B. Dyspnea

 _____ C. Heart rate increase from 74/min pretransfusion to 81/min posttransfusion

 X____ D. Client report of itching

 X____ E. Client appears flushed

4. A nurse is completing preoperative teaching with a client who will undergo an elective surgical procedure that will include a blood transfusion. Which of the following statements by the nurse should be included in the teaching?

 _too long

 A. "You should make an appointment to donate blood 8 weeks prior to the surgery."

 B. "If you need an autologous transfusion, the blood your brother donates can be used."

 C. "We will have you come in to donate your blood the day before surgery."

 D. "You will receive the blood you donated 4 weeks prior to the surgery."

5. A nurse is observing a newly hired nurse on the unit who is preparing to administer a blood transfusion. Which of the following actions by the newly hired nurse requires intervention by the nurse?

A. Inserts a large-bore IV catheter in the client

B. Verifies blood compatibility and expiration date of the blood with an assistive personnel (AP)

C. Administers 0.9% sodium chloride IV

D. Assesses for a history of blood-transfusion reactions

6. A nurse is caring for a client who is receiving a blood transfusion. What nursing actions should the nurse anticipate if a transfusion reaction is suspected? Use the ATI Active Learning Template: Nursing Skill to complete this item to include the following:

A. Indications:

- Describe the four types of reactions and the time of onset.

- Describe three medications that may be administered and for which reaction.

B. Potential Complications: Describe two nursing actions for each.

APPLICATION EXERCISES KEY

1.   A. INCORRECT: Verifying the blood being transfused occurs prior to blood administration.

   B. **CORRECT:** Assessment of the client during the first 15 min of the transfusion is important because this is when most blood reactions occur.

   C. INCORRECT: Explanation of the procedure should be done prior to blood administration.

   D. INCORRECT: Blood specimens are obtained only in the event of a blood reaction.

   (N) NCLEX® Connection: Pharmacological and Parenteral Therapies, Blood and Blood Products

2.   A. **CORRECT:** The first action is to stop the infusion.

   B. **CORRECT:** The blood bag and administration tubing are sent to the laboratory for analysis.

   C. **CORRECT:** 0.9% sodium chloride solution should be administered through new IV tubing.

   D. INCORRECT: The client's feet are elevated if sepsis or septic shock is suspected following a transfusion.

   E. INCORRECT: Blood specimens are not routinely obtained unless sepsis is suspected.

   (N) NCLEX® Connection: Pharmacological and Parenteral Therapies, Blood and Blood Products

3.   A. **CORRECT:** A slight increase in temperature is an expected finding.

   B. **CORRECT:** Dyspnea may indicate a transfusion reaction.

   C. INCORRECT: A slight increase in heart rate is an expected finding.

   D. **CORRECT:** A client's report of itching may indicate a transfusion reaction.

   E. **CORRECT:** A flushed appearance of the client may indicate a transfusion reaction.

   (N) NCLEX® Connection: Pharmacological and Parenteral Therapies, Blood and Blood Products

4.   A. INCORRECT: The client should donate blood for an autologous transfusion no sooner than 5 weeks in advance, up to 72 hr prior to surgery.

   B. INCORRECT: A homologous transfusion involves receiving a transfusion of blood from donors other than the recipient.

   C. INCORRECT: The client should donate blood for an autologous transfusion no sooner than 5 weeks in advance, up to 72 hr prior to surgery.

   D. **CORRECT:** An autologous transfusion involves collecting a client's blood no sooner than 5 weeks in advance, up to 72 hr prior to surgery so it can be transfused during an elective surgery.

   (N) NCLEX® Connection: Pharmacological and Parenteral Therapies, Blood and Blood Products

5.   A. INCORRECT: A large-bore IV catheter is used for administering blood products.

B. **CORRECT:** Verification of the client's identify, blood compatibility, and expiration date of the blood is done with another nurse. Assistive personnel cannot be asked to perform this task.

C. INCORRECT: Blood and blood products are infused with 0.9% sodium chloride. IV solutions containing dextrose cannot be used.

D. INCORRECT: The nurse should assess for a client history of blood-transfusion reactions to identify any potential risks for future reactions.

Ⓝ NCLEX® Connection: Pharmacological and Parenteral Therapies, Blood and Blood Products

6.   *Using the ATI Active Learning Template: Nursing Skill*

A. Indications

- Types of reactions and onset
    - Acute hemolytic – immediate
    - Febrile – 30 min to 6 hr after transfusion
    - Mild allergic – During or up to 24 hr after transfusion
    - Anaphylactic – immediate

- Medications
    - Antipyretics (acetaminophen [Tylenol]) – febrile
    - Antihistamines (diphenhydramine [Benadryl]) – mild allergic
    - Antihistamines, corticosteroids, vasopressors – anaphylactic

B. Potential Complications

- Circulatory overload
    - Administer oxygen.
    - Monitor vital signs.
    - Slow the infusion rate.
    - Administer diuretics as prescribed.
    - Notify the provider immediately.

- Sepsis and septic shock
    - Maintain patent airway.
    - Administer oxygen.
    - Administer antibiotics as prescribed.
    - Obtain blood samples for culture.
    - Administer vasopressors in late phase.
    - Elevate client's feet.
    - Assess for disseminated intravascular coagulation.

Ⓝ NCLEX® Connection: Physiological Adaptations, Unexpected Response to Therapies

chapter 41

Overview

- Anemia is an abnormally low amount of circulating RBCs, Hgb concentration, or both. It is an indicator of an underlying disease or disorder.

- Anemia results in diminished oxygen-carrying capacity and delivery to tissues and organs. The goal of treatment is to restore and maintain adequate tissue oxygenation.

- Anemias are due to:

  ○ Blood loss

  ○ Inadequate RBC production (hypoproliferative)

  ○ Increased RBC destruction (hemolytic)

  ○ Deficiency of necessary components such as folic acid, iron, erythropoietin, and/or vitamin B_{12}

- Iron-deficiency anemia due to inadequate intake is the most common cause of anemia in children, adolescents, and pregnant women.

- Iron-deficiency anemia due to blood loss (such as from a gastrointestinal ulcer) is the most common cause of anemia in women who are postmenopausal, as well as men. Women who are menstruating can develop anemia secondary to menorrhagia.

Health Promotion and Disease Prevention

- Women who are pregnant or menstruating should ensure that their diet contains adequate amounts of iron-rich foods. Otherwise, they should take an iron supplement.

- Individuals who are iron deficient, but have elevated cholesterol levels, should integrate iron-rich foods that are not red or organ meats into their diets (iron-fortified cereal and breads, fish and poultry, and dried peas and beans).

- Clients should regularly consume food sources high in folate (spinach, lentils, bananas) and folic acid fortified grains and juices.

Assessment

- Risk Factors

  ○ Acute or chronic blood loss

    ▪ Trauma

    ▪ Menorrhagia

    ▪ Gastrointestinal bleed (ulcers, tumor)

    ▪ Intra or postsurgical blood loss or hemorrhage

    ▪ Chemical or radiation exposure

- Increased hemolysis
  - Defective Hgb (sickle-cell disease) – RBCs become malformed during periods of hypoxia and obstruct capillaries in joints and organs
  - Impaired glycolysis – glucose-6-phosphate-dehydrogenase (G6PD) deficiency anemia
  - Immune disorder or destruction (transfusion reactions, autoimmune diseases)
  - Mechanical trauma to RBCs (mechanical heart valve, cardiopulmonary bypass)
- Inadequate dietary intake or malabsorption
  - Iron deficiency
  - Vitamin B_{12} deficiency – pernicious anemia due to deficiency of intrinsic factor produced by gastric mucosa, which is necessary for absorption of vitamin B_{12}
  - Folic acid deficiency
  - Pica, or a persistent eating of substances not normally considered food (nonnutritive substances), such as soil or chalk, for at least 1 month, may limit the amount of healthy food choices a client makes
- Bone-marrow suppression
  - Exposure to radiation or chemicals (such as insecticides or solvents)
  - Aplastic anemia results in a decreased number of RBCs as well as decreased platelets and WBCs.
- Older adult clients are at risk for nutrition-deficient anemias (iron, vitamin B_{12}, folate).
- Anemia may be misdiagnosed as depression or debilitation in older adult clients.
- Gastrointestinal bleeding is a common cause of anemia in older adult clients.
- Subjective Data
  - May be asymptomatic in mild cases
  - Pallor
  - Fatigue
  - Irritability
  - Numbness and tingling of extremities
  - Dyspnea on exertion
  - Sensitivity to cold
  - Pain and hypoxia with sickle-cell crisis
- Objective Data
  - Physical Assessment Findings
    - Shortness of breath/fatigue, especially upon exertion
    - Tachycardia and palpitations
    - Dizziness or syncope upon standing or with exertion
    - Pallor with pale nail beds and mucous membranes
    - Nail bed deformities
    - Smooth, sore, bright-red tongue (vitamin B_{12} deficiency)

- ○ Laboratory Tests
  - ▪ CBC count
    - □ RBCs are the major carriers of hemoglobin in the blood.
    - □ Hgb transports oxygen and carbon dioxide to and from the cells and can be used as an index of the oxygen-carrying capacity of the blood.
    - □ Hct is the percentage of RBCs in relation to the total blood volume.
  - ▪ RBC indices are used to determine the type and cause of most anemias.
    - □ Mean corpuscular volume (MCV) – Size of red blood cells
      - ▸ Normocytic – Normal size
      - ▸ Microcytic – Small cells
      - ▸ Macrocytic – Large cells
  - ▪ Mean corpuscular Hgb (MCH) determines the amount of Hgb per RBC
    - □ Normochromic – normal amount of Hgb per cell
    - □ Hypochromic – decreased Hgb per cell
  - ▪ Mean corpuscular Hgb concentration (MCHC) indicates Hgb amount relative to the size of the cell

RBC INDICES			
	NORMAL MCV, MCH, MCHC	DECREASED MCV, MCH, MCHC	INCREASED MCV
Classification	› Normocytic, normochromic anemia	› Microcytic, hypochromic anemia	› Macrocytic anemia
Possible causes	› Acute blood loss › Sickle-cell disease	› Iron-deficiency anemia › Anemia of chronic illness › Chronic blood loss	› Vitamin B_{12} deficiency › Folic acid deficiency

- ▪ Iron studies
  - □ Total iron-binding capacity (TIBC) reflects an indirect measurement of serum transferrin, a protein that binds with iron and transports it for storage.
  - □ Serum ferritin is an indicator of total iron stores in the body.
  - □ Serum iron measures the amount of iron in the blood. Low serum iron and elevated TIBC indicates iron-deficiency anemia.
- ▪ Hgb electrophoresis separates normal Hgb from abnormal. It is used to detect thalassemia and sickle-cell disease.
- ▪ A sickle-cell test evaluates the sickling of RBCs in the presence of decreased oxygen tension.

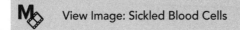
View Image: Sickled Blood Cells

- ▪ A Schilling test measures vitamin B_{12} absorption with and without intrinsic factor. It is used to differentiate between malabsorption and pernicious anemia.
- ○ Diagnostic Procedures
  - ▪ Bone-marrow aspiration/biopsy is used to diagnose aplastic anemia (failure of bone marrow to produce RBCs as well as platelets and WBCs).

Patient-Centered Care

- Nursing Care

    ○ Encourage increased dietary intake of the deficient nutrient (iron, vitamin B_{12}, folic acid).

    ○ Administer medications, as prescribed, at the proper time for optimal absorption, and using an appropriate technique.

    ○ Teach the client and family about energy conservation in the client and the risk of the client experiencing dizziness upon standing.

    ○ Teach the client about the time frame for resolution.

- Medications

    ○ Iron supplements – ferrous sulfate (Feosol), ferrous fumarate (Feostat), ferrous gluconate (Fergon)

        ▪ Oral iron supplements are used to replenish serum iron and iron stores. Iron is an essential component of Hgb, and subsequently, oxygen transport.

        ▪ Parenteral iron supplements (iron dextran) are only given for severe anemia.

        ▪ Nursing Considerations

            □ Administer parenteral iron using the Z-track method.

        ▪ Client Education

            □ Instruct to have hemoglobin checked in 4 to 6 weeks to determine efficacy.

            □ Vitamin C may increase oral iron absorption.

            □ Instruct the client to take iron supplements between meals to increase absorption, if tolerated.

    ○ Erythropoietin – epoetin alfa (Epogen, Procrit)

        ▪ A hematopoietic growth factor used to increase production of RBCs

        ▪ Nursing Considerations

            □ Monitor for an increase in blood pressure.

            □ Monitor Hgb and Hct twice a week.

            □ Monitor for a cardiovascular event if Hgb increases too rapidly (greater than 1 g/dL in 2 weeks).

        ▪ Client Education

            □ Reinforce the importance of having Hgb and Hct evaluated on a twice-a-week basis.

    ○ Vitamin B_{12} supplementation (cyanocobalamin)

        ▪ Vitamin B_{12} is necessary to convert folic acid from its inactive form to its active form. All cells rely on folic acid for DNA production.

        ▪ Vitamin B_{12} supplementation can be given orally if the deficit is due to inadequate dietary intake. However, if deficiency is due to lack of intrinsic factor being produced by the parietal cells of the stomach or malabsorption syndrome, it must be administered parenterally or intranasally to be absorbed.

- Nursing Considerations
  - Administer vitamin B$_{12}$ according to appropriate route related to cause of vitamin B$_{12}$ anemia (parenteral versus oral).
  - Administer parenteral forms of vitamin B$_{12}$ intramuscularly or deep subcutaneous to decrease irritation. Do not mix other medications in the syringe.
- Client Education
  - Clients who lack intrinsic factor or have an irreversible-malabsorption syndrome should be informed that this therapy must be continued for the rest of their life.
  - A client should receive vitamin B$_{12}$ injections on a monthly basis.

  ○ Folic acid supplements
    - Folic acid is a water-soluble, B-complex vitamin. It is necessary for the production of new RBCs.
    - Nursing Considerations
      - Folic acid can be given orally or parenterally.
    - Client Education
      - Large doses of folic acid may mask vitamin B$_{12}$ deficiency.
      - Large doses of folic acid will turn the client's urine dark yellow.

- Therapeutic Procedures
  ○ Blood transfusions lead to an immediate improvement in blood-cell counts and manifestations of anemia.
    - Typically only used when the client has significant manifestations of anemia, because of the risk of blood-borne infections.

Complications

- Heart failure
  ○ Heart failure can develop due to the increased demand on the heart to provide oxygen to tissues. A low Hct decreases the amount of oxygen carried to tissues in the body, which makes the heart work harder and beat faster (tachycardia, palpitations).
  ○ Nursing Actions
    - Administer oxygen and monitor oxygen saturation.
    - Monitor cardiac rhythm.
    - Obtain daily weight.
    - Administer blood transfusion as prescribed.
    - Administer cardiac medications as prescribed (diuretics, antidysrhythmics).
    - Administer antianemia medications as prescribed.

APPLICATION EXERCISES

1. A nurse is planning care for a client who has a Hgb of 7.5 and a Hct of 21.5. Which of the following should the nurse include in the plan of care? (Select all that apply.)

___X___ A. Provide assistance with ambulation.

___X___ B. Monitor oxygen saturation.

_____ C. Weigh the client weekly.

___X___ D. Obtain stool specimen for occult blood.

___X___ E. Schedule daily rest periods.

2. A nurse is teaching a client who has a new prescription for ferrous sulfate (Feosol). Which of the following should be included in the teaching?   IRON

A. Stools will be dark red in color.

B. Take with a glass of milk if gastrointestinal distress occurs.

C. Foods high in vitamin C will promote absorption.

D. Take for 14 days.

3. A nurse is providing discharge teaching to a client who had a gastrectomy for stomach cancer. Which of the following information should be included in the teaching? (Select all that apply.)

___X___ A. "You will need a monthly injection of vitamin B_{12} for the rest of your life."

___X___ B. "Using the nasal spray form of vitamin B_{12} on a daily basis may be an option."

_____ C. "An oral supplement of vitamin B_{12} taken on a daily basis may be an option."

_____ D. "You should increase your intake of animal proteins, legumes, and dairy products to increase vitamin B_{12} in your diet."

_____ E. "Add soy milk fortified with vitamin B_{12} to your diet to decrease the risk of pernicious anemia."

4. A nurse is completing an integumentary assessment of a client who has anemia. Which of the following is an expected finding?

A. Absent turgor

B. Spoon-shaped nails

C. Shiny, hairless legs

D. Yellow mucous membranes

5. A nurse in a clinic receives a phone call from a client seeking information about his new prescription for erythropoietin (Epogen). Which of the following information should be reviewed with the client?

    A. The client needs an erythrocyte sedimentation rate (ESR) test weekly.

    B. The client should have his hemoglobin checked twice a week.

    C. Oxygen saturation levels should be monitored.

    D. Folic acid production will increase.

6. A nurse educator is presenting a community education program on anemia to a group of clients. What should be included in this presentation? Use the ATI Active Learning Template: Systems Disorder to complete this item to include the following:

    A. Description of Disorder/Disease Process: Describe and identify at least three causes.

    B. Objective and Subjective Data: Identify at least three of each form of data.

    C. Laboratory Tests: Describe the importance of the TIBC test.

APPLICATION EXERCISES KEY

1. A. **CORRECT:** A client who has anemia may experience dizziness and should be assisted when ambulating to prevent a fall.

    B. **CORRECT:** Oxygen saturation should be monitored in a client who has anemia due to the decreased oxygen-carrying capacity of the blood.

    C. INCORRECT: The client should be weighed daily.

    D. **CORRECT:** Stool testing is performed to identify a possible cause of anemia due to gastrointestinal bleeding.

    E. **CORRECT:** A client who has anemia may experience fatigue, and rest periods should be planned to conserve energy.

    Ⓝ NCLEX® Connection: Safety and Infection Control, Accident/Error/Injury Prevention

2. A. INCORRECT: Stools will be dark green to black in color when taking iron.

    B. INCORRECT: Milk binds with iron and decreases its absorption.

    C. **CORRECT:** Vitamin C enhances the absorption of iron by the intestinal tract.

    D. INCORRECT: Iron therapy usually takes 4 to 6 weeks for Hgb and Hct to return to the normal reference range.

    Ⓝ NCLEX® Connection: Pharmacological and Parenteral Therapies, Medication Administration

3. A. **CORRECT:** A client who had a gastrectomy will require monthly injections of vitamin B_{12} for the rest of his life.

    B. **CORRECT:** Cyanocobalamin nasal spray used daily is an option for a client who had a gastrectomy.

    C. INCORRECT: Oral supplements of vitamin B_{12} will not be absorbed due to the lack of intrinsic factor produced by the stomach.

    D. INCORRECT: Dietary sources of vitamin B_{12} will not be absorbed due to the lack of intrinsic factor produced by the stomach.

    E. INCORRECT: Dietary sources of vitamin B_{12} will not be absorbed due to the lack of intrinsic factor produced by the stomach.

    Ⓝ NCLEX® Connection: Basic Care and Comfort, Nutrition and Oral Hydration

4.   A. INCORRECT: Absent skin turgor is a finding in a client who has dehydration.

    B. **CORRECT:** Deformities of the nails, such as being spoon-shaped, are a finding in a client who has anemia.

    C. INCORRECT: These findings are present in a client who has peripheral vascular disease.

    D. INCORRECT: The client who has anemia will have pale nail beds and mucous membranes.

    Ⓝ NCLEX® Connection: Reduction of Risk Potential, Potential for Complications from Surgical Procedures and Health Alterations

5.   A. INCORRECT: The effectiveness of erythropoietin is evaluated by changes in the hematocrit.

    B. **CORRECT:** Hemoglobin and hematocrit are monitored twice a week.

    C. INCORRECT: Blood pressure is monitored for an increase.

    D. INCORRECT: Erythropoietin promotes increased production of RBCs.

    Ⓝ NCLEX® Connection: Pharmacological and Parenteral Therapies, Medication Administration

6.   *Using the ATI Active Learning Template: Systems Disorder*

    A. Description of Disorder
- Anemia is an abnormally low amount of circulating red blood cells, hemoglobin concentration, or both. It may be due to blood loss, inadequate production or increased destruction of red blood cells, and dietary deficiencies of folic acid, iron, erythropoietin, and/or vitamin B_{12}.

    B. Objective and Subjective Data
- Objective Data
  - Shortness of breath and fatigue with exertion
  - Tachycardia, palpitations, dizziness, or syncope upon standing or with exertion
  - Pallor, pale nail beds, pale mucous membranes, nail bed deformities
  - Smooth, sore, bright-red tongue
- Subjective Data
  - May be asymptomatic, pallor, fatigue, irritability, numbness and tingling of extremities, dyspnea on exertion, sensitivity to cold, pain, and hypoxia with sickle-cell crisis

    C. Laboratory Tests
- This test is an indirect measurement of serum transferrin, a protein that binds with iron and transports it for storage. Serum transferrin is an indicator of the total iron stores in the body.

    Ⓝ NCLEX® Connection: Physiological Adaptations, Alterations in Body Systems

chapter 42

Overview

- Coagulation disorders occur secondary to an alteration in platelets, clotting factors, or both. Coagulopathy is the term for any condition that affects an individual's ability to coagulate. Coagulopathies are suspected when the usual measures used to stop bleeding fail.

- Coagulopathy may occur secondary to an autoimmune disorder or extensive blood loss in which platelets and clotting factors are lost. In some cases, the development of microemboli in the circulatory system paradoxically "uses up" the clotting factors that cause hemorrhages to occur at the same time intravascular clotting occurs.

- Coagulation disorders include the following:

  - Idiopathic thrombocytopenic purpura (ITP) – A coagulopathy that is an autoimmune disorder in which the life span of platelets is decreased by antiplatelet antibodies although platelet production is normal. This can result in severe hemorrhage following a cesarean birth or lacerations.

  - Disseminated intravascular coagulation (DIC) – A life-threatening coagulopathy in which clotting and anticlotting mechanisms occur at the same time.

    - The client who has DIC is at risk for both internal and external bleeding, as well as damage to organs resulting from ischemia caused by microclots.

Risk Factors

- Risk factors for ITP
  - Female (ages 20 to 40 years)
  - Autoimmune disorder
  - Recent virus (children only)
- Risk factors for DIC that occur secondary to other complications
  - Septicemia
  - Cardiopulmonary arrest
  - Hemorrhage

Assessment

- Objective Data
  - Physical Assessment Findings
    - Unusual spontaneous bleeding from the client's gums and nose (epistaxis)
    - Oozing, trickling, or flow of blood from incisions or lacerations
    - Petechiae and ecchymoses

- Excessive bleeding from venipuncture, injection sites, or slight traumas
- Tachycardia, hypotension, and diaphoresis
- Organ failure secondary to microemboli
  - Laboratory Tests
    - Hemoglobin (decreased with DIC and ITP)
    - Platelet levels (thrombocytopenia) (decreased with DIC and ITP)
    - Fibrinogen levels (decreased with DIC)
    - Prothrombin time (increased with DIC)
    - Partial thromboplastin (increased with DIC)
    - Fibrin split product levels/fibrin degradation products (increased with DIC)
    - D-dimer (increased with DIC)
    - Blood typing and crossmatch

Patient-Centered Care

- Nursing Care
  - DIC
    - Nursing interventions for DIC initially focus on assessing for and correcting the underlying cause (sepsis, hemorrhage). The focus then turns to preventing organ damage secondary to microemboli and replacing the blood's clotting components.
    - Monitor for signs of microemboli (cyanotic nail beds, pain).
  - DIC and ITP
    - Regularly take vital signs, and assess hemodynamic status.
    - Monitor for signs of organ failure or intracranial bleed (oliguria, decreased level of consciousness).
    - Monitor laboratory values for clotting factors.
    - Administer fluid volume replacement.
    - Transfuse blood, platelets, and other clotting products.
    - Monitor for complications from the administration of blood and blood products.
    - Avoid use of NSAIDs.
    - Administer supplemental oxygen.
    - Provide protection from injury.
    - Instruct client to avoid Valsalva maneuver (could cause cerebral hemorrhage).
    - Implement bleeding precautions (avoid use of needles).
- Medications
  - ITP – Corticosteroids and immunosuppressants
  - DIC – Anticoagulants (heparin)
    - May be used to decrease microclots from forming and using up clotting factors
- Surgical Interventions
  - ITP – Splenectomy may be performed by the provider if client does not respond to medical management.

APPLICATION EXERCISES

1. A nurse is caring for a client who has disseminated intravascular coagulation (DIC). Which of the following indicates that the client's clotting factors are becoming depleted? (Select all that apply.)

_____ A. Platelets 100,000/mm³

_____ B. Fibrinogen levels 97 mg/dL

_____ C. Fibrin degradation products 4.3 mcg/mL

_____ D. D-dimer 179 ng/mL

_____ E. Sedimentation rate 38 mm/hr

2. A nurse is assessing a client and suspects the client is experiencing disseminated intravascular coagulation (DIC). Which of the following physical findings should the nurse anticipate?

A. Bradycardia

B. Hypertension

C. Epistaxis

D. Xerostomia

3. A nurse is caring for a client who has idiopathic thrombocytopenic purpura (ITP). The nurse should notify the provider and report possible small-vessel clotting when which of the following is assessed?

A. Petechiae on the upper chest

B. Hypotension

C. Cyanotic nail beds

D. Severe headache

4. A nurse is caring for a client who has disseminated intravascular coagulation (DIC). Which of the following medications should the nurse anticipate administering to the client?

A. Heparin

B. Vitamin K

C. Antibiotic

D. Antilipemic

5. A nurse is developing a plan of care for a client who has disseminated intravascular coagulation (DIC). Which interventions should the nurse include in the plan of care? Use the ATI Active Learning Template: Systems Disorder to complete this item to include Patient-Centered Care: Describe five interventions.

APPLICATION EXERCISES KEY

1. A. **CORRECT:** In DIC, platelet levels are decreased, causing clotting factors to become depleted. Clotting times are increased, which raises the risk for fatal hemorrhage.

    B. **CORRECT:** In DIC, fibrinogen levels are decreased, causing clotting factors to become depleted. Clotting times are increased, which raises the risk for fatal hemorrhage.

    C. INCORRECT: Fibrin degradation products are increased when DIC occurs.

    D. INCORRECT: A D-dimer level is increased when DIC occurs.

    E. INCORRECT: The sedimentation rate is increased, but it is not an indicator of DIC.

    Ⓝ NCLEX® Connection: Reduction of Risk Potential, Laboratory Values

2. A. INCORRECT: Tachycardia is a finding that is indicative of DIC.

    B. INCORRECT: Hypotension is a finding that is indicative of DIC.

    C. **CORRECT:** Epistaxis is unexpected bleeding of the gums and nose and is a finding indicative of DIC.

    D. INCORRECT: Xerostomia is dryness of the mouth and is not indicative of DIC.

    Ⓝ NCLEX® Connection: Physiological Adaptations, Pathophysiology

3. A. INCORRECT: Petechiae on the upper chest can indicate impaired clotting.

    B. INCORRECT: Hypotension can indicate impaired clotting.

    C. **CORRECT:** Cyanotic nail beds indicate microvascular clotting is occurring and should be immediately reported to avoid ischemic loss of the fingers or toes.

    D. INCORRECT: Severe headache can indicate cerebral bleeding.

    Ⓝ NCLEX® Connection: Physiological Adaptations, Unexpected Response to Therapies

4. A. **CORRECT:** Heparin may be administered to decrease the formation of microclots, which deplete clotting factors.

    B. INCORRECT: Vitamin K promotes blood coagulation and is not a medication that is prescribed for a client who has DIC.

    C. INCORRECT: An antibiotic is given to treat bacterial infections and is not a medication that the nurse should anticipate being administered to a client who has DIC.

    D. INCORRECT: An antilipemic is given to treat hyperlipidemia and is not a medication that the nurse should anticipate being administered to a client who has DIC.

    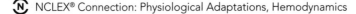 NCLEX® Connection: Physiological Adaptations, Hemodynamics

5. *Using ATI Active Learning Template: Systems Disorder*
    - Patient-Centered Care
        ○ Monitor for signs of microemboli (cyanotic nail beds, pain).
            ▪ Regularly take vital signs and assess hemodynamic status.
        ○ Monitor for signs of organ failure or intracranial bleed (oliguria, decreased level of consciousness).
        ○ Monitor laboratory values for clotting factors.
        ○ Administer fluid volume replacement.
        ○ Transfuse blood, platelets, and other clotting products.
        ○ Monitor for complications from the administration of blood and blood products.
        ○ Avoid use of NSAIDs.
        ○ Administer supplemental oxygen.
        ○ Provide protection from injury.
        ○ Instruct client to avoid Valsalva maneuver (could cause cerebral hemorrhage).
        ○ Implement bleeding precautions (avoid use of needles).

    NCLEX® Connection: Physiological Adaptations, Hemodynamics

UNIT 6 · Nursing Care of Clients with Fluid/Electrolyte/Acid-Base Imbalances

CHAPTERS

› Fluid Imbalances
› Electrolyte Imbalances
› Acid-Base Imbalances

NCLEX® CONNECTIONS

When reviewing the chapters in this unit, keep in mind the relevant sections of the NCLEX® outline, in particular:

Client Needs: Physiological Adaptation

› Relevant topics/tasks include:

» Fluid and Electrolyte Imbalances

› Evaluate the client's response to interventions to correct fluid or electrolyte imbalance.

» Hemodynamics

› Apply knowledge of pathophysiology to interventions in response to the client's abnormal hemodynamics.

» Medical Emergencies

› Evaluate and document the client's response to emergency interventions.

chapter 43

Overview

- Body fluids are distributed between intracellular (ICF), which is two thirds of body water, and extracellular (ECF), which is one third of body water, fluid compartments.

- Fluid can move between compartments (through selectively permeable membranes) by a variety of methods (diffusion, active transport, filtration, osmosis) to maintain homeostasis.

- Balance is maintained through input and output.

- Intake is regulated by thirst.

- Output is regulated by the kidneys, skin, lungs, and GI tract.

- Fluid imbalances that nurses should be familiar with are

  ○ Fluid volume deficits

  ○ Fluid volume excess

FLUID VOLUME DEFICITS

Overview

- Fluid volume deficits (FVDs) include hypovolemia-isotonic (loss of water and electrolytes from the ECF) and dehydration-osmolar (loss of water with no loss of electrolytes).

- Hemoconcentration occurs with dehydration, resulting in increases in Hct, serum electrolytes, and urine specific gravity.

- Note: Compensatory mechanisms include sympathetic nervous system responses of increased thirst, antidiuretic hormone (ADH) release, and aldosterone release.

- Hypovolemia can lead to hypovolemic shock.

Health Promotion and Disease Prevention

- Increase fluid intake with vigorous exercise.

- Increase fluid intake in high altitudes and dry climates to promote hydration.

- Avoid drinking fluids that contain alcohol or caffeine. This increases fluid excretion.

Ⓖ   • Older adults have an increased risk for dehydration due to a decrease in total body mass, which includes total body water content. The thirst mechanism is less sensitive in older adults.

Assessment

- Risk Factors
  - Causes of Hypovolemia
    - Abnormal gastrointestinal (GI) losses – Vomiting, nasogastric suctioning, diarrhea
    - Abnormal skin losses – Diaphoresis
    - Abnormal renal losses – Diuretic therapy, diabetes insipidus, renal disease, adrenal insufficiency, osmotic diuresis
    - Third spacing – Peritonitis, intestinal obstruction, ascites, burns
    - Hemorrhage
    - Altered intake, such as nothing by mouth (NPO)
  - Causes of Dehydration
    - Hyperventilation
    - Diabetic ketoacidosis
    - Enteral feeding without sufficient water intake
- Subjective Data and Objective Data
  - Vital signs – Hyperthermia, tachycardia, thready pulse, hypotension, orthostatic hypotension, decreased central venous pressure, tachypneic (increased respirations), hypoxia
    - Tachycardia occurs in an attempt to maintain a normal blood pressure.
  - Neuromusculoskeletal – Dizziness, syncope, confusion, weakness, fatigue
  - Gastrointestinal – Thirst, dry furrowed tongue, nausea/vomiting, anorexia, acute weight loss
  - Renal – Oliguria (decreased production and concentration of urine)
  - Other signs – Diminished capillary refill, cool clammy skin, diaphoresis, sunken eyeballs, flattened neck veins, poor skin turgor, and tenting.
  - Laboratory Tests
    - Hematocrit (Hct)
      - Hypovolemia – Increased Hct
    - Serum osmolarity
      - Dehydration – Increased (hemoconcentration) osmolarity (greater than 300 mOsm/L), — increased protein, blood urea nitrogen (BUN), electrolytes, glucose
    - Urine specific gravity and osmolarity
      - Dehydration – Increased (concentration)
    - Serum sodium
      - Dehydration – Increased (hemoconcentration)

Patient-Centered Care

- Nursing Care

  - Check urinalysis, oxygen saturation (SaO$_2$), and CBC and electrolytes.

  - Administer supplemental oxygen as prescribed.

  - Monitor vital signs and heart rhythm.

  - Auscultate lung sounds.

  - Initiate and maintain IV access.

  - Place the client in shock position (on back with legs elevated).

  - Fluid replacement – Administer IV fluids as prescribed (isotonic solutions, such as lactated Ringer's, normal saline, blood transfusions).

  - Monitor intake and output. Alert the provider for urine output less than 30 cc/hr.

  - Monitor level of consciousness, and maintain client safety.

  - Assess level of gait stability. Encourage client to use call light and ask for assistance.

  - Initiate fall precautions.

  - Encourage the client to change positions, slowly rolling from side to side, or standing up.

- Teamwork and Collaboration

  - Respiratory services may be consulted for oxygen management.

- Care After Discharge

  - Client Education

    - Encourage the client to drink plenty of liquids to promote hydration.

    - Educate the client regarding causes of dehydration, such as nausea/vomiting.

Complications

- Hypovolemic Shock

  - Vital organ hypoxia/anoxia – Decreased hemoglobin oxygen saturation and pulse pressure (systolic-diastolic blood pressure)

  - Nursing Actions

    - Administer oxygen.

    - Provide fluid replacement with the following:

      □ Colloids (whole blood, packed RBCs, plasma, synthetic plasma expanders)

      □ Crystalloids (Ringer's lactate, normal saline)

    - Administer vasoconstrictors, such as dopamine (Intropin) and norepinephrine (Levophed); coronary vasodilators, such as sodium nitroprusside (Nipride); and/or positive inotropic medications, such as dobutamine (Dobutrex).

    - Perform hemodynamic monitoring.

FLUID VOLUME EXCESSES

Overview

- Fluid volume excesses (FVEs) include hypervolemia-isotonic (water and sodium are retained in abnormally high proportions) and overhydration-osmolar (more water is gained than electrolytes).

- Note: Severe hypervolemia can lead to pulmonary edema and heart failure.

- Note: Compensatory mechanisms include increased release of natriuretic peptides, resulting in increased loss of sodium and water by the kidneys and the decrease in the release of aldosterone.

Health Promotion and Disease Prevention

- Consume a diet low in sodium. Consult with provider regarding diet restrictions.

- Promote fluid restriction intake. Consult with provider regarding prescribed restrictions.

Assessment

- Risk Factors

  - Causes of Hypervolemia

    - Chronic stimulus to the kidney to conserve sodium and water (heart failure, cirrhosis, increased glucocorticosteroids)

    - Abnormal renal function with reduced excretion of sodium and water (renal failure)

    - Interstitial to plasma fluid shifts (hypertonic fluids, burns)

    - Age-related changes in cardiovascular and renal function

    - Excessive sodium intake

  - Causes of Overhydration

    - Water replacement without electrolyte replacement (strenuous exercise with profuse diaphoresis)

- Subjective Data and Objective Data

  - Vital signs – Tachycardia, bounding pulse, hypertension, tachypnea, increased central venous pressure

  - Neuromusculoskeletal – Confusion, muscle weakness, headache

  - Gastrointestinal – Weight gain, ascites

  - Respiratory – Dyspnea, orthopnea, crackles, diminished breath sounds

  - Other signs – Edema, distended neck veins, pale and cool skin.

View Media
- › Crackles (Audio)
- › Pitting Edema (Image)

○ Laboratory Findings

■ Hematocrit

□ Hypervolemia – Decreased hematocrit (Hct)

■ Serum osmolarity

□ Overhydration – Decreased (hemodilution) osmolarity (less than 270 mOsm/L)

■ Serum sodium

□ Hypervolemia – Sodium within expected reference range

■ Electrolytes, BUN, and creatinine

□ Overhydration/hypervolemia – Decreased electrolytes, BUN, and creatinine

■ Arterial Blood Gases

■ Respiratory alkalosis – Decreased $PaCO_2$ (less than 35 mm Hg), increased PH (greater than 7.45)

○ Diagnostic Procedures

■ Chest x-ray – Reveals possible pulmonary congestion

Patient-Centered Care

- Nursing Care

  ○ Check ABGs, SaO_2, CBC, and chest x-ray results.

  ○ Position the client in a semi-Fowler's position.

  ○ Obtain daily weight.

  ○ Monitor intake and output.

  ○ Administer supplemental oxygen as prescribed.

  ○ Reduce IV flow rates.

  ○ Administer diuretics (osmotic, loop) as prescribed.

  ○ Limit fluid and sodium intake as prescribed.

  ○ Monitor and document presence of edema (pretibial, sacral, periorbital).

  ○ Reposition the client at least every 2 hr.

  ○ Support arms and legs to decrease dependent edema as appropriate.

  ○ Monitor vital signs and heart rhythm.

  ○ Auscultate lung sounds (listen for crackles).

- Teamwork and Collaboration

  ○ Respiratory services may be consulted for oxygen management.

  ○ Pulmonology may be consulted if fluid moves into lungs.

- Care After Discharge
  - Client Education
    - Encourage client to weigh himself daily. Notify provider if there is a 1- to 2-lb gain in 24 hr, or a 3-lb gain in a week.
    - Instruct the client to consume a low-sodium diet, read food labels to check sodium content, and keep a record of daily sodium intake.
    - Promote fluid restriction intake. Consult with provider regarding prescribed restrictions.

Complications

- Pulmonary Edema
  - Pulmonary edema can be caused by severe fluid overload.
    - Symptoms include anxiety, tachycardia, acute respiratory distress, increased vein distention, dyspnea at rest, change in level of consciousness, and ascending crackles (fluid level within lungs) and cough, productive of frothy pink-tinged sputum.
  - Nursing Actions
    - Position the client in high-Fowler's position to maximize ventilation.
    - Administer oxygen, positive airway pressure, and/or possible intubation and mechanical ventilation.
    - Administer morphine and diuretic as prescribed.

APPLICATION EXERCISES

1. A nurse is admitting a client who reports nausea, vomiting, and weakness. Upon assessment, the client has dry oral mucous membranes, temperature 38.5° C (101.3° F), pulse 92/min, respirations 24/min, skin cool with tenting present, and blood pressure 102/64 mm Hg. His urine is concentrated with a high specific gravity. Which of the following are clinical manifestations of fluid volume deficit? (Select all that apply.)

_____X_____ A. Decreased skin turgor

_____X_____ B. Concentrated urine

_____ C. Bradycardia

_____X_____ D. Low-grade fever

_____X_____ E. Tachypnea

2. A nurse is admitting an older adult client who is experiencing dyspnea, weakness, and weight gain of 2 lb, with 1+ bilateral edema of the lower extremities. Upon assessment, the client has a temperature 37.2° C (99° F), pulse 96/min, respirations 26/min, oxygen saturation 94% on 3 L oxygen via nasal cannula, and blood pressure 152/96 mm Hg. Which of the following clinical manifestations are indicative of fluid volume excess? (Select all that apply.)

_____X_____ A. Dyspnea

_____X_____ B. Edema

_____ C. Bradycardia

_____X_____ D. Hypertension

_____X_____ E. Weakness

3. A nurse is caring for a client who is dehydrated. Which of the following clinical manifestations should the nurse assess for that is indicative of fluid volume deficit?

A. Moist skin

B. Distended neck veins

C. Increased urinary output

(D.) Tachycardia

4. A nurse is caring for an older adult client in a long-term care facility. The client has become weak and confused. He ate 40% of his breakfast and lunch. Upon assessment, the client's temperature is 38.3° C (100.9° F), pulse rate 92/min, respirations 20/min, and blood pressure 108/60 mm Hg. He has lost ¾ lb and reports dizziness when assisted to the bathroom. He also has a nonproductive cough with diminished breath sounds in the right lower lobe. Which of the following actions should the nurse take?

   A. Initiate fluid restrictions to limit intake.

   B. Observe for signs of hypertension.

   C. Encourage the client to ambulate to promote oxygenation.

   D. Monitor respirations for shortness of breath.

5. A nurse is planning caring for a client who is experiencing fluid volume excess. Which nursing actions should the nurse include in the plan of care? Use the ATI Active Learning Template: Systems Disorder to complete this item to include the following section: Patient-Centered Care: Describe three interventions the nurse should take.

APPLICATION EXERCISES KEY

1. A. **CORRECT:** Decreased skin turgor is a clinical manifestation present with fluid volume deficit. Skin turgor is decreased to due to the lack of fluid within the body and results in dryness of the skin.

    B. **CORRECT:** Concentrated urine is a clinical manifestation present with fluid volume deficit. The urine is concentrated due to urinary output being decreased.

    C. INCORRECT: Bradycardia is not a clinical manifestation present with fluid volume deficit.

    D. **CORRECT:** Low-grade fever is a clinical manifestation present with fluid volume deficit. Low-grade fever is one of the body's ways to maintain homeostasis to compensate for lack of fluid within the body.

    E. **CORRECT:** Tachypnea is a clinical manifestation present with fluid volume deficit. Increased respirations are the body's way to obtain oxygen due to the lack of fluid volume within the body.

     NCLEX® Connection: Physiological Adaptations, Fluid and Electrolyte Imbalances

2. A. **CORRECT:** Dyspnea is a clinical manifestation present with fluid volume excess. Dyspnea is due to an excess of fluids within the body and lungs, and the client is struggling to breath to obtain oxygen.

    B. **CORRECT:** Edema is a clinical manifestation present with fluid volume excess. Edema is due to the excess of fluid within the body. Weight gain can be a result of edema.

    C. INCORRECT: Bradycardia is not a clinical manifestation related to fluid volume excess.

    D. **CORRECT:** Hypertension is a clinical manifestation related to fluid volume excess. Blood pressure rises as the heart must work harder due to the excess fluid.

    E. **CORRECT:** Weakness is a clinical manifestation present with fluid volume excess. Weakness is due to the excess fluid that is retained, which depletes energy and increases the workload for the body.

    NCLEX® Connection: Physiological Adaptations, Fluid and Electrolyte Imbalances

3. A. INCORRECT: Moist skin is a clinical manifestation indicative of fluid volume excess.

    B. INCORRECT: Distended neck veins is a clinical manifestation indicative of fluid volume excess.

    C. INCORRECT: Increased urinary output is a clinical manifestation indicative of fluid volume excess.

    D. **CORRECT:** Tachycardia is an attempt to maintain blood pressure, a clinical manifestation indicative of fluid volume deficit.

    NCLEX® Connection: Physiological Adaptations, Fluid and Electrolyte Imbalances

4.   A. INCORRECT: The nurse should not initiate fluid restrictions to limit intake. This would be an appropriate action for a client who has fluid volume excess. The client is dehydrated, and fluids should be encouraged.

B. INCORRECT: The nurse should not be monitoring for signs of hypertension. This would be an appropriate action for a client who has fluid volume excess. The client is hypotensive due to fluid volume depletion. The nurse should monitor the client for hypotension.

C. INCORRECT: The nurse should not encourage the client to ambulate to promote oxygenation. This would be an appropriate action for a client who has fluid volume excess. The client is experiencing dizziness due to dehydration and is at risk for falling. The nurse should keep the client in bed and assist him to the bathroom as needed.

D. **CORRECT:** It is an appropriate action for the nurse to monitor the client's respiratory status and for shortness of breath. The client has a nonproductive cough with diminished breath sounds in the right lower lobe. This client is dehydrated and has fluid volume deficit.

(N) NCLEX® Connection: Physiological Adaptations, Fluid and Electrolyte Imbalances

5.   *Using the ATI Active Learning Template: Systems Disorder*
   • Patient-Centered Care: Nursing Care
     ○ Check ABGs, SaO_2, CBC, and chest x-ray results.
     ○ Position the client in a semi-Fowler's position.
     ○ Obtain daily weight.
     ○ Monitor intake and output.
     ○ Administer supplemental oxygen as prescribed.
     ○ Reduce IV flow rates.
     ○ Administer diuretics (osmotic, loop) as prescribed.
     ○ Limit fluid and sodium intake as prescribed.
     ○ Monitor and document presence of edema (pretibial, sacral, periorbital).
     ○ Reposition the client at least every 2 hr.
     ○ Support arms and legs to decrease dependent edema as appropriate.
     ○ Monitor vital signs and heart rhythm.
     ○ Auscultate lung sounds (listen for crackles).

(N) NCLEX® Connection: Physiological Adaptations, Fluid and Electrolyte Imbalances

chapter 44

Overview

- Electrolytes are minerals (sometimes called salts) that are present in all body fluids. They regulate fluid balance and hormone production, strengthen skeletal structures, and act as catalysts in nerve response, muscle contraction, and the metabolism of nutrients.

- When dissolved in water or other solvent, electrolytes separate into ions and conduct either a positive (cations – magnesium, potassium, sodium, calcium) or negative (anions – phosphate, sulfate, chloride, bicarbonate) electrical current.

- Electrolytes are distributed between intracellular (ICF) and extracellular (ECF) fluid compartments. Although laboratory tests can accurately reflect the electrolyte concentrations in plasma, it is not possible to directly measure electrolyte concentrations within cells.

ELECTROLYTE EXPECTED REFERENCE RANGES			
Sodium	136 to 145 mEq/L	Calcium	9.0 to 10.5 mg/dL
Potassium	3.5 to 5.0 mEq/L	Magnesium	1.3 to 2.1 mEq/L
Chloride	98 to 106 mEq/L	Phosphorus	3.0 to 4.5 mg/dL

SODIUM IMBALANCES

Overview

- Sodium (Na^+) is the major electrolyte found in extracellular fluid.

- Sodium is essential for maintaining acid-base balance, active and passive transport mechanisms, and maintaining irritability and conduction of nerve and muscle tissue.

- The expected reference range for serum sodium levels is 136 to 145 mEq/L.

  - Decreased sodium levels are referred to as hyponatremia.

  - Elevated sodium levels are referred to as hypernatremia.

Hyponatremia

- Hyponatremia is a net gain of water or loss of sodium-rich fluids that results in sodium levels less than 136 mEq/L.
  - Hyponatremia delays and slows the depolarization of membranes.
  - Water moves from the ECF into the ICF, causing cells to swell (cerebral edema).
  - Compensatory mechanisms include the renal excretion of sodium-free water.
- Assessment
  - Risk Factors
    - Causes of hyponatremia
      - Deficient ECF volume
        - Abnormal gastrointestinal (GI) losses – vomiting, nasogastric suctioning, diarrhea, tap water enemas, gastrointestinal obstructions
        - Kidney losses – diuretics, kidney disease, adrenal insufficiency
        - Skin losses – excessive sweating, burns, wound drainage, ascites (as it relates to cirrhosis)
      - Increased or normal ECF volume
        - Excessive oral water intake
        - Syndrome of inappropriate antidiuretic hormone (SIADH) – excess secretion of antidiuretic hormone (ADH)
      - Edematous states – heart failure, cirrhosis, nephrotic syndrome
      - Excessive hypotonic IV fluids
      - Inadequate sodium intake (nothing by mouth status [NPO])
    - Older adult clients are at a greater risk due to the increased incidence of chronic illnesses, use of diuretic medications, and risk for insufficient sodium intake.
  - Subjective Data and Objective Data
    - Clinical indicators depend on whether it is associated with a normal (euvolemic), decreased (hypovolemic), or increased ECF (hypervolemic) volume.
    - Vital signs – hypothermia, tachycardia, rapid thready pulse, hypotension, orthostatic hypotension (vital signs can vary based on state of ECF volume)
    - Neuromusculoskeletal – headache, confusion, lethargy, muscle weakness to the point of possible respiratory compromise, fatigue, decreased deep-tendon reflexes, seizures
    - Gastrointestinal – increased motility, hyperactive bowel sounds, abdominal cramping, nausea
    - Laboratory Tests
      - Serum sodium
        - Decreased: less than 136 mEq/L
      - Serum osmolarity
        - Decreased: less than 270 mOsm/L

- Patient-Centered Care
  - Nursing Care
    - Report abnormal laboratory findings to the provider.
    - Fluid overload: Restrict water intake as prescribed by the provider.
    - For clients who have heart failure and hyponatremia, provide loop diuretics and ACE inhibitors as prescribed.
    - Acute hyponatremia
      - Administer hypertonic oral and IV fluids as prescribed.
      - Administer 3% sodium chloride slowly, and monitor sodium levels frequently.
      - Encourage foods and fluids high in sodium (cheeses, milk, condiments).
    - Restoration of normal ECF volume: Administer isotonic IV therapy (0.9% sodium chloride, lactated Ringer's).
    - Monitor intake and output, and daily weight.
    - Monitor vital signs and level of consciousness; report abnormal findings to the provider.
    - Encourage the client to change positions slowly.
  - Teamwork and Collaboration
    - Nephrology may be consulted for electrolyte and fluid replacement.
    - Respiratory services may be consulted for oxygen management.
    - Nutritional services may be consulted for food choices high in sodium and restricting fluid intake.
  - Care After Discharge
    - Client Education
      - Encourage the client to weigh daily and to notify the provider of a 1- to 2-lb gain in 24 hr, or 3-lb (1.4 kg) gain in a week.
      - Instruct the client to consume a high-sodium diet, including reading food labels to check sodium content, and keeping a daily record of sodium intake.
- Complications
  - Acute Hyponatremia
    - Complications (coma, seizures, respiratory arrest) can result from acute hyponatremia if not treated immediately.
    - Nursing Actions
      - Maintain an open airway, and monitor client's vital signs.
      - Implement seizure precautions, and take appropriate action if seizures occur.
      - Monitor the client's level of consciousness.

Hypernatremia

- Increased sodium causes hypertonicity of the serum. This causes a shift of water out of the cells, resulting in dehydrated cells.

  ○ Hypernatremia is a serum sodium level greater than 145 mEq/L.

  ○ Hypernatremia is a serious electrolyte imbalance. It can cause significant neurological, endocrine, and/or cardiac disturbances.

Assessment

- Risk Factors

  ○ Causes of hypernatremia (loss of water)

    ▪ Water deprivation (NPO)

    ▪ Excessive sodium intake – dietary sodium intake, hypertonic IV fluids, bicarbonate intake

    ▪ Excessive sodium retention – kidney failure, Cushing's syndrome, aldosteronism, some medications (glucocorticosteroids)

    ▪ Fluid losses – fever, diaphoresis, burns, respiratory infection, diabetes insipidus, hyperglycemia, watery diarrhea

    ▪ Age-related changes, specifically decreased total body water content and inadequate fluid intake related to an altered thirst mechanism

    ▪ Compensatory mechanisms include increased thirst and production of ADH.

- Subjective Data and Objective Data

  ○ Vital signs – hyperthermia, tachycardia, orthostatic hypotension

  ○ Neuromusculoskeletal – restlessness; irritability; muscle twitching to the point of muscle weakness, including respiratory compromise; decreased deep-tendon reflexes (DTR) to the point of absent DTRs; seizures; coma

  ○ Gastrointestinal – thirst, dry mucous membranes, increased motility, hyperactive bowel sounds, abdominal cramping, nausea

  ○ Other signs – edema, warm flushed skin, oliguria (decreased production of urine)

  ○ Laboratory Tests

    ▪ Serum sodium – increased: greater than 145 mEq/L

    ▪ Serum osmolarity – increased: greater than 300 mOsm/L

- Patient-Centered Care

  ○ Nursing Care

    ▪ Report abnormal laboratory findings to the provider.

    ▪ Fluid loss

      □ Based on serum osmolarity and hemodynamic stability

        ▸ Administer hypotonic IV fluids (0.45% sodium chloride).

        ▸ Administer isotonic IV fluids (0.9% sodium chloride).

- Excess sodium
    - Encourage water intake, and discourage sodium intake.
    - Administer diuretics (loop diuretics) for clients who have poor kidney excretion.
- Monitor level of consciousness, and ensure safety.
- Monitor the client's vital signs and heart rhythm.
- Auscultate lung sounds.
- Provide oral hygiene and other comfort measures to decrease thirst.
- Monitor intake and output, and alert the provider of inadequate renal output.
  - Teamwork and Collaboration
    - Nephrology may be consulted for electrolyte and fluid management.
    - Respiratory services may be consulted for oxygen management.
    - Nutritional services may be consulted for food choices low in sodium and to restrict fluid intake.
  - Care After Discharge
    - Client Education
      - Encourage the client to weigh daily. Notify the provider of a 1- to 2-lb gain in 24 hr, or 3-lb (1.4 kg) gain in a week.
      - Encourage the client to consume a low-sodium diet, read food labels to check sodium content, and keep a record of daily sodium intake.
      - Encourage fluids as prescribed by the provider.
- Complications
  - Acute Hypernatremia
    - Complications (seizures, convulsion, death) can result from acute hypernatremia if not treated immediately.
    - Nursing Actions
      - Maintain open airway, and monitor the client's vital signs.
      - Implement seizure precautions, and take appropriate action if seizures occur.
      - Monitor the client's level of consciousness.

POTASSIUM IMBALANCES

Overview

- Potassium (K^+) is the major cation in the intracellular fluid (ICF).
- Potassium plays a vital role in cell metabolism; transmission of nerve impulses; functioning of cardiac, lung, and muscle tissues; and acid-base balance.
- Potassium has a reciprocal action with sodium.
- The expected reference range for serum potassium levels is 3.5 to 5.0 mEq/L.
  - Decreased potassium levels are referred to as hypokalemia.
  - Elevated potassium levels are referred to as hyperkalemia.

Hypokalemia

- Hypokalemia is the result of an increased loss of potassium from the body or movement of potassium into the cells, resulting in a serum potassium less than 3.5 mEq/L.
- Assessment
  - Risk Factors
    - Causes of hypokalemia
      - □ Decreased total body potassium
        - ▸ Abnormal GI losses – vomiting, nasogastric suctioning, diarrhea, inappropriate laxative use
        - ▸ Kidney losses – excessive use of diuretics (furosemide [Lasix], corticosteroids)
        - ▸ Skin losses – diaphoresis, wound losses
      - □ Insufficient potassium
        - ▸ Inadequate dietary intake (rare)
        - ▸ Prolonged administration of nonelectrolyte-containing IV solutions (5% dextrose in water)
      - □ Intracellular shift – metabolic alkalosis, after correction of acidosis, during periods of tissue repair (burns, trauma, starvation), total parenteral nutrition
    - Older adult clients are at greater risk due to increased use of diuretics and laxatives.
  - Subjective Data and Objective Data
    - Vital signs – weak, irregular pulse, hypotension, respiratory distress
    - Neuromusculoskeletal – weakness to the point of respiratory collapse and paralysis, muscle cramping, decreased muscle tone and hypoactive reflexes, paresthesias, mental confusion
    - ECG – premature ventricular contractions (PVCs), bradycardia, blocks, ventricular tachycardia, inverted T waves, ST depression
    - Gastrointestinal – decreased motility, abdominal distention, constipation, ileus, nausea, vomiting, anorexia
    - Other signs – polyuria (dilute urine)
    - Laboratory Tests
      - □ Serum potassium: decreased (less than 3.5 mEq/L)
      - □ Arterial blood gases: metabolic alkalosis (pH greater than 7.45)
    - Diagnostic Procedures
      - □ Electrocardiogram (ECG)
        - ▸ ECG will show findings of dysrhythmias (premature ventricular contractions [PVCs], ventricular tachycardia, inverted T waves, ST depression).
- Patient-Centered Care
  - Nursing Care
    - Report abnormal findings to the provider.
    - Replacement of potassium
      - □ Encourage foods high in potassium (avocados, broccoli, dairy products, dried fruit, cantaloupe, bananas).
      - □ Provide oral potassium supplementation.

- IV potassium supplementation
  - □ Never administer by IV bolus (high risk of cardiac arrest).
  - □ The maximum recommended rate is 5 to 10 mEq/hr.
- Assess for phlebitis (tissue irritant).
- Monitor and maintain adequate urine output.
- Observe for shallow ineffective respirations and diminished breath sounds.
- Monitor the client's cardiac rhythm, and intervene promptly as needed.
- Monitor clients receiving digoxin (Lanoxin). Hypokalemia increases the risk for digoxin toxicity.
- Monitor level of consciousness, and maintain client safety.
- Monitor bowel sounds and abdominal distention, and intervene as needed.
- Monitor kidney function (BUN, GFR, creatinine).
- Monitor magnesium, calcium, and phosphorus.
- Provide assistance with ADLs (weakness is usually pronounced if the client has a K^+ less than 2.5).

○ Teamwork and Collaboration
  - Nephrology may be consulted for electrolyte and fluid management.
  - Respiratory services may be consulted for oxygen management.
  - Nutritional services may be consulted for food choices and potassium-rich foods.
  - Cardiology may be consulted for dysrhythmias.

○ Care After Discharge
  - Client Education
    - □ Educate the client regarding potassium-rich foods to consume.
    - □ Teach the client ways to prevent a decrease in potassium by excessive use of diuretics and laxatives.

- Complications
  - ○ Respiratory Failure
    - Nursing Actions
      - □ Maintain an open airway, and monitor the client's vital signs.
      - □ Monitor the client's level of consciousness.
      - □ Monitor for hypoxemia and hypercapnia.
      - □ Assist with intubation and mechanical ventilation if indicated.
  - ○ Cardiac Arrest
    - Nursing Actions
      - □ Perform continuous cardiac monitoring.
      - □ Treat dysrhythmias.

Hyperkalemia

- Hyperkalemia is the result of an increased intake of potassium, movement of potassium out of the cells, or inadequate renal excretion resulting in a serum potassium level greater than 5.0 mEq/L.

- Assessment

  - Risk Factors

    - Causes of hyperkalemia

      - Increased total body potassium – PO and IV potassium administration, salt substitute

      - Extracellular shift – decreased insulin, acidosis (diabetic ketoacidosis), tissue catabolism (sepsis, trauma, surgery, fever, myocardial infarction)

      - Hypertonic states – uncontrolled diabetes mellitus

      - Decreased excretion of potassium – renal failure, severe dehydration, potassium-sparing diuretics, angiotensin-converting enzyme inhibitors, NSAIDs, adrenal insufficiency

    - Older adult clients are at a greater risk due to the increased use of salt substitutes, ACE inhibitors, and potassium-sparing diuretics.

  - Subjective Data and Objective Data

    - Vital signs – slow, irregular pulse, hypotension

    - Neuromusculoskeletal – restlessness, irritability, weakness to the point of ascending flaccid paralysis, paresthesias

    - ECG – premature ventricular contractions, ventricular fibrillation, peaked T waves, widened QRS

    - Gastrointestinal – nausea, vomiting, increased motility, diarrhea, hyperactive bowel sounds

    - Other signs – oliguria

    - Laboratory Tests

      - Serum potassium: increased (greater than 5.0 mEq/L)

      - Arterial blood gases: metabolic acidosis (pH less than 7.35)

    - Diagnostic Procedures

      - Electrocardiogram

        ‣ Will show dysrhythmias (ventricular fibrillation, peaked T waves, widened QRS)

- Patient-Centered Care

  - Nursing Care

    - Report abnormal findings to the provider.

    - Cardiac protection: Prepare to administer calcium gluconate or calcium chloride.

    - Decrease potassium intake

      - Stop the infusion of IV potassium.

      - Withhold oral potassium.

      - Provide a potassium-restricted diet (avoid foods high in potassium [avocados, broccoli, dairy products, dried fruit, cantaloupe, bananas]).

- Promote movement of potassium from ECF to ICF
  - Administer IV fluids with dextrose and regular insulin.
  - Administer sodium bicarbonate to reverse acidosis.
- Monitor the client's cardiac rhythm, and intervene promptly as needed.
- Medications (to increase potassium excretion)
  - Administer loop diuretics (furosemide [Lasix]) if kidney function is adequate.
    - Loop diuretics increase the depletion of potassium from the renal system.
    - Nursing Considerations
      - Maintain IV access.
    - Client Education
      - Educate the client on a potassium-restricted diet.
      - Instruct the client to hold oral potassium supplements until further advised by the provider.
  - Administer cation exchange resins (sodium polystyrene sulfonate [Kayexalate]).
    - Works as a laxative and excretes excess potassium from the body. Can be used with clients who have renal disorders.
    - Nursing Considerations
      - If potassium levels are extremely high, dialysis may be required.
    - Client Education
      - Educate the client on a potassium-restricted diet.
      - Instruct the client to hold oral potassium supplements until advised by the provider.
- Teamwork and Collaboration
  - Nephrology may be consulted if dialysis is needed and for electrolyte and fluid management.
  - Nutritional services may be consulted for food choices containing potassium-restricted foods.
  - Cardiology may be consulted for dysrhythmias.
- Care After Discharge
  - Client Education
    - Educate the client about potassium-restricted foods to consume.
    - Teach the client ways to prevent an increase in potassium by reading food labels and avoiding salt substitutes containing potassium.
- Complications
  - Cardiac Arrest
    - Nursing Actions
      - Treat dysrhythmias.
      - Perform continuous cardiac monitoring.

OTHER ELECTROLYTE IMBALANCES

Overview

- Other electrolyte imbalances
  - Calcium
    - Hypocalcemia
    - Hypercalcemia
  - Chloride
    - Hypochloremia
    - Hyperchloremia
  - Magnesium
    - Hypomagnesemia
    - Hypermagnesemia
  - Phosphorus
    - Hypophosphatemia
    - Hyperphosphatemia
- In particular, nurses should be aware of the implications of hypocalcemia and hypomagnesemia.

Hypocalcemia

- Hypocalcemia is a serum calcium less than 9.0 mg/dL or ionized calcium less than 4.5 mg/dL.
- Assessment
  - Risk Factors
    - Lactose intolerance
    - Malabsorption syndromes (Crohn's disease)
    - Hypoalbuminemia
    - End-stage kidney disease (ESKD)
    - Post thyroidectomy
    - Hypoparathyroidism
    - Inadequate intake of calcium
    - Vitamin D deficiency (becoming more common today) or lack of 25-hydroxy vitamin D related to ESKD
    - Pancreatitis
    - Hyperphosphatemia
    - Medications that block parathyroid function, cause hyperphosphatemia, chelate calcium, or prevent absorption of calcium
    - Sepsis

○ Subjective Data and Objective Data

- Paresthesia of the fingers and lips (early symptom)

- Muscle twitches/tetany

- Frequent, painful muscle spasms at rest

- Hyperactive deep-tendon reflexes

- Positive Chvostek's sign (tapping on the facial nerve triggering facial twitching)

- Positive Trousseau's sign (hand/finger spasms with sustained blood pressure cuff inflation)

- Cardiovascular – decreased myocardial contractility (decreased heart rate and hypotension)

- Gastrointestinal – hyperactive bowel sounds, diarrhea, abdominal cramping

- Laboratory Tests

  □ Calcium level less than 9.0 mg/dL

- Diagnostic Procedures

  □ Electrocardiogram

    ‣ ECG changes – prolonged QT interval and prolonged ST interval

- Patient-Centered Care

  ○ Nursing Care

  - Administer oral or IV calcium supplements.

  - Implement seizure precautions.

  - Have emergency equipment on standby.

  - Encourage foods high in calcium, including dairy products and dark green vegetables.

  ○ Teamwork and Collaboration

  - Endocrinology may be consulted for electrolyte and fluid management.

  - Respiratory services may be consulted for oxygen management.

  - Nutritional services may be consulted for food choices high in calcium.

  - Cardiology may be consulted for dysrhythmias.

  ○ Care After Discharge

  - Client Education

    □ Educate the client about consuming foods high in calcium (yogurt, milk).

    □ Teach the client ways to increase calcium in diet by reading food labels.

Hypomagnesemia

- Hypomagnesemia is a serum magnesium level less than 1.3 mg/dL.
- Assessment
  - ○ Risk Factors
    - Causes of hypomagnesemia
      - □ Malnutrition (insufficient magnesium intake)
      - □ Alcohol ingestion (magnesium excretion)
    - Subjective and Objective Data
      - □ Neuromuscular – increased nerve impulse transmission (hyperactive deep-tendon reflexes, paresthesias, muscle tetany), positive Chvostek's and Trousseau's signs
      - □ Gastrointestinal – hypoactive bowel sounds, constipation, abdominal distention, paralytic ileus
- Patient-Centered Care
  - ○ Nursing Care
    - Discontinue magnesium-losing medications (e.g., loop diuretics).
    - Administer oral or IV magnesium sulfate following safety protocols. IV route is used because IM can cause pain and tissue damage. Oral magnesium can cause diarrhea and increase magnesium depletion. Monitor the client closely.
    - Encourage foods high in magnesium, including dairy products and dark green vegetables.
  - ○ Teamwork and Collaboration
    - Endocrinology may be consulted for electrolyte and fluid management.
    - Respiratory services may be consulted for oxygen management.
    - Nutritional services may be consulted for food choices high in magnesium.
    - Cardiology may be consulted for dysrhythmias.
  - ○ Care After Discharge
    - Client Education
      - □ Educate the client regarding foods that are high in magnesium.
      - □ Teach the client ways to increase magnesium in diet by reading food labels.

APPLICATION EXERCISES

1. A nurse is caring for a client who has laboratory findings of serum Na⁺ 133 mEq/L and K⁺ 3.4 mEq/L. Which of the following treatments can result in these laboratory findings?

    A. Three tap water enemas

    B. 0.9% sodium chloride solution IV at 50 mL/hr

    C. 5% dextrose in water solution with 20 mEq of K⁺ IV at 80 mL/hr

    D. Administration of glucocorticoids

2. A nurse is caring for a client who has a laboratory finding of serum potassium 5.4 mEq/L. The nurse should assess for which of the following clinical manifestations?

    A. ECG changes

    B. Constipation

    C. Polyuria

    D. Hypotension

3. A nurse is caring for a client who has a nasogastric tube attached to low intermittent suctioning. The nurse should monitor for which of the following electrolyte imbalances?

    A. Hypercalcemia

    B. Hyponatremia

    C. Hyperphosphatemia

    D. Hypomagnesemia

4. A nurse is assessing a client for Chovstek's sign. Which of the following techniques should the nurse use to perform this test?

    A. Apply a blood pressure cuff to the client's arm.

    B. Place the stethoscope bell over the client's carotid artery.

    C. Tap lightly on the client's cheek.

    D. Ask the client to lower his chin to his chest.

5. A nurse is assessing a client who has hyperkalemia. Which of the following conditions is associated with this electrolyte imbalance?

A. Diabetic ketoacidosis

B. Heart failure

C. Cushing's syndrome

D. Thyroidectomy

6. A nurse is caring for a client who has hypokalemia. Use the ATI Active Learning Template: Systems Disorder to complete this item to include the following sections:

A. Description of Disorder

B. Patient-Centered Care:
- Nursing Care: Describe at least six actions.
- Teamwork and Collaboration: Describe one action.
- Care after Discharge: Describe one action.

C. Complications: Describe one.

APPLICATION EXERCISES KEY

1. A. **CORRECT:** Receiving three tap water enemas can result in a decrease in serum sodium and potassium in the client. Tap water is hypotonic, and gastrointestinal losses are isotonic. This creates an imbalance and solute dilution.

    B. INCORRECT: Receiving 0.9% sodium chloride solution IV at 50 mL/hr would not produce these results.

    C. INCORRECT: Receiving 5% dextrose in water solution with 20 mEq of K⁺ at 80 mL/hr would not produce these results.

    D. INCORRECT: Receiving glucocorticoids would not produce these results.

    Ⓝ NCLEX® Connection: Physiological Adaptations, Fluid and Electrolyte Imbalances

2. A. **CORRECT:** The nurse should assess the client for ECG changes. Potassium levels can affect the heart and result in arrhythmias.

    B. INCORRECT: Constipation is a clinical manifestation of hypokalemia.

    C. INCORRECT: Polyuria is a clinical manifestation of hypokalemia.

    D. INCORRECT: Hypotension is a clinical manifestation of hypokalemia.

    Ⓝ NCLEX® Connection: Physiological Adaptations, Fluid and Electrolyte Imbalances

3. A. INCORRECT: An increase in calcium is not indicated with nasogastric losses due to suctioning.

    B. **CORRECT:** The nurse should monitor the client for hyponatremia. Nasogastric losses are isotonic and contain sodium.

    C. INCORRECT: An increase in phosphatemia is not indicated with nasogastric losses due to suctioning.

    D. INCORRECT: A decrease in magnesium is not indicated with nasogastric losses due to suctioning.

    Ⓝ NCLEX® Connection: Physiological Adaptations, Fluid and Electrolyte Imbalances

4. A. INCORRECT: This is performed to assess for Trousseau's sign.

   B. INCORRECT: This is performed to auscultate a carotid bruit.

   C. **CORRECT:** The nurse taps the client's cheek over the facial nerve just below and anterior to the ear to elicit Chvostek's sign. A positive response is indicated when the client exhibits facial twitching on this side of his face.

   D. INCORRECT: This is performed to assess for range of motion of the neck.

   Ⓝ NCLEX® Connection: Reduction of Risk Potential, Diagnostic Tests

5. A. **CORRECT:** Hyperkalemia, an increase in serum potassium, is a laboratory finding associated with diabetic ketoacidosis.

   B. INCORRECT: Hyponatremia, a decrease in serum sodium, is a laboratory finding associated with heart failure.

   C. INCORRECT: Hypernatremia, an increase in serum sodium, is a laboratory finding associated with Cushing's syndrome.

   D. INCORRECT: Hypocalcemia, a decrease in serum calcium, is a laboratory finding is found in clients following a thyroidectomy.

   Ⓝ NCLEX® Connection: Physiological Adaptations, Fluid and Electrolyte Imbalances

6. *Using the ATI Active Learning Template: Systems Disorder*

A. Description of Disorder

- Hypokalemia is the result of an increased loss of potassium from the body or movement of potassium into the cells, resulting in a serum potassium less than 3.5 mEq/L.

B. Patient-Centered Care

- Nursing Care

  ○ Report abnormal findings to the provider.

  ○ Replacement of potassium

  ○ Encourage foods high in potassium (avocados, broccoli, dairy products, dried fruit, cantaloupe, bananas).

  ○ Provide oral potassium supplementation.

  ○ IV potassium supplementation

  ○ Never administer by IV bolus (high risk of cardiac arrest).

  ○ The maximum recommended rate is 5 to 10 mEq/hr.

  ○ Assess for phlebitis (tissue irritant).

  ○ Monitor and maintain adequate urine output.

  ○ Observe for shallow ineffective respirations and diminished breath sounds.

  ○ Monitor the client's cardiac rhythm, and intervene promptly as needed.

  ○ Monitor clients receiving digoxin (Lanoxin). Hypokalemia increases the risk for digoxin toxicity.

  ○ Monitor level of consciousness, and maintain client safety.

  ○ Monitor bowel sounds and abdominal distention, and intervene as needed.

  ○ Monitor kidney function (BUN, GFR, creatinine).

  ○ Monitor magnesium, calcium, and phosphorus.

  ○ Provide assistance with ADLs (weakness is usually pronounced if the client has a K^+ less than 2.5).

- Teamwork and Collaboration

  ○ Nephrology may be consulted for electrolyte and fluid management.

  ○ Respiratory services may be consulted for oxygen management.

  ○ Nutritional services may be consulted for food choices and potassium-rich foods.

  ○ Cardiology may be consulted for dysrhythmias.

- Care After Discharge

  ○ Client Education

    ▪ Educate the client regarding potassium-rich foods to consume.

    ▪ Teach the client ways to prevent a decrease in potassium by excessive use of diuretics and laxatives.

C. Complications

- Respiratory failure

- Cardiac arrest

Ⓝ NCLEX® Connection: Physiological Adaptations, Fluid and Electrolyte Imbalances

chapter 45

Overview

- For cells to function optimally, metabolic processes must maintain a steady balance between the acids and bases found in the body.

  ○ Acid-base balance represents homeostasis of hydrogen (H^+) ion concentration in body fluids. Hydrogen shifts between the extracellular and intracellular compartments to compensate for acid-base imbalances.

  ○ Minor changes in hydrogen concentration have major effects on normal cellular function.

- Arterial pH is an indirect measurement of hydrogen ion concentration and is a result of respiratory and renal compensational function. Arterial blood gases (ABGs) are most commonly used to evaluate acid-base balance.

  ○ The pH is the expression of the balance between carbon dioxide (CO_2), which is regulated by the lungs, and bicarbonate (HCO_3^-), a base regulated by the kidneys.

    - The greater the concentration of hydrogen, the more acidic the body fluids and the lower the pH.

    - The lower the concentration of hydrogen, the more alkaline the body fluids and the higher the pH.

Maintenance of Acid-Base Balance

- Acid-base balance is maintained by chemical, respiratory, and renal processes.

  ○ Chemical and protein buffers

    - Are the first line of defense

    - Either bind or release hydrogen ions as needed

    - Respond quickly to changes in pH

  ○ Respiratory buffers

    - Are the second line of defense

    - Control the level of hydrogen ions in the blood through the control of CO_2 levels

    - When a chemoreceptor senses a change in the level of CO_2, a signal is sent to the brain to alter the rate and depth of respirations.

      □ Hyperventilation = decrease in hydrogen ions

      □ Hypoventilation = increase in hydrogen ions

- ○ Renal buffers

  - ▪ The kidneys are the third line of defense.

  - ▪ This buffering system is much slower to respond, but it is the most effective buffering system with the longest duration.

  - ▪ The kidneys control the movement of bicarbonate in the urine. Bicarbonate can be reabsorbed into the bloodstream or excreted in the urine in response to blood levels of hydrogen.

  - ▪ The kidneys may also produce more bicarbonate when needed.

    - □ High hydrogen ions = bicarbonate reabsorption and production

    - □ Low hydrogen ions = bicarbonate excretion

- Compensation refers to the process by which the body attempts to correct changes and imbalances in pH levels.

  - ○ Full compensation occurs when the pH level of the blood returns to normal (7.35 to 7.45).

  - ○ If the pH level is not able to normalize, then it is referred to as partial compensation.

- Metabolic alkalosis, metabolic acidosis, respiratory alkalosis, and respiratory acidosis are examples of acid-base imbalances.

- Acid-base imbalances are a result of insufficient compensation. Respiratory and renal function plays a large role in the body's ability to effectively compensate for acid-base alterations. Organ dysfunction negatively affects acid-base compensation.

Respiratory Compensation　　Metabolic Compensation

$$H_2O + CO_2 \longleftrightarrow H_2CO_3 \longleftrightarrow H^+ + HCO_3^-$$

Water　Carbon dioxide　　Carbonic acid　　Hydrogen ion　Bicarbonate

Expelled by lungs　　　　　　Expelled by kidneys

Health Promotion and Disease Prevention

- Encourage a healthy diet and physical activity.

- Limit the consumption of alcohol.

- Encourage drinking six to eight glasses of water daily.

- Maintain an appropriate weight for height and body frame.

- Promote smoking cessation.

Assessment

- Risk Factors/Causes of Acid-Base Imbalances

RESPIRATORY ACIDOSIS – HYPOVENTILATION		
Results from	› Respiratory depression from poisons, anesthetics, trauma, or neurological diseases (myasthenia gravis, Guillain-Barré) › Inadequate chest expansion due to muscle weakness, pneumothorax/hemothorax, flail chest, obesity, tumors, or deformities	› Airway obstruction that occurs in laryngospasm, asthma, and some cancers › Alveolar-capillary blockage secondary to a pulmonary embolus, thrombus, cancer, or pulmonary edema › Inadequate mechanical ventilation
Results in	› Increased CO_2	› Increased H^+ concentration

RESPIRATORY ALKALOSIS – HYPERVENTILATION		
Results from	› Hyperventilation due to fear, anxiety, intracerebral trauma, salicylate toxicity, or excessive mechanical ventilation.	› Hypoxemia from asphyxiation, high altitudes, shock, or early-stage asthma or pneumonia.
Results in	› Decreased CO_2	› Decreased H^+ concentration

METABOLIC ACIDOSIS		
Results from	› Excess production of hydrogen ions » Diabetic ketoacidosis (DKA) » Lactic acidosis » Starvation » Heavy exercise » Seizure activity » Fever » Hypoxia » Intoxication with ethanol or salicylates	› Inadequate elimination of hydrogen ions » Kidney failure › Inadequate production of bicarbonate » Kidney failure » Pancreatitis » Liver failure » Dehydration › Excess elimination of bicarbonate » Diarrhea, ileostomy
Results in	› Decreased HCO_3^-	› Increased H^+ concentration

METABOLIC ALKALOSIS		
Results from	› Base excess » Oral ingestion of bases (antacids) » Venous administration of bases (blood transfusions, total parenteral nutrition [TPN], or sodium bicarbonate)	› Acid deficit » Loss of gastric secretions (through prolonged vomiting, NG suction) » Potassium depletion (due to thiazide diuretics, laxative abuse, Cushing's syndrome)
Results in	› Increased HCO_3^-	› Decreased H^+ concentration

- Subjective and Objective Data

RESPIRATORY ACIDOSIS – HYPOVENTILATION

› Vital signs: tachycardia (severe acidosis may lead to bradycardia), tachypnea
› Dysrhythmias
› Neurological: anxiety, irritability, confusion, coma
› Respiratory: ineffective, shallow, rapid breathing
› Skin: pale or cyanotic

RESPIRATORY ALKALOSIS – HYPERVENTILATION

› Vital signs: tachypnea
› Neurological: anxiety, tetany, convulsions, tingling, numbness
› Cardiovascular: palpitations, chest pain, dysrhythmias
› Respiratory: Rapid, deep respirations

METABOLIC ACIDOSIS

› Vital signs: bradycardia, weak peripheral pulses, hypotension, tachypnea
› Dysrhythmias
› Neurological: muscle weakness, hyporeflexia, flaccid paralysis, fatigue, confusion
› Respiratory: rapid, deep respirations (Kussmaul respirations)
› Skin: warm, dry, flushed

METABOLIC ALKALOSIS

› Vital signs: tachycardia, normotensive or hypotensive
› Dysrhythmias
› Neurological: numbness, tingling, tetany, muscle weakness, hyperreflexia, confusion, convulsion
› Respiratory: depressed skeletal muscles resulting in ineffective breathing

- ○ Laboratory Tests and Diagnostic Procedures
    - To determine the type of imbalance, follow these steps:
        - Step 1: Look at pH.
            - ▸ If less than 7.35, diagnose as acidosis.
            - ▸ If greater than 7.45, diagnose as alkalosis.
        - Step 2: Look at $PaCO_2$ and HCO_3^- simultaneously.
            - ▸ Determine which is in the expected reference range.
            - ▸ Conclude that the other is the indicator of imbalance.
            - ▸ Diagnose less than 35 or greater than 45 $PaCO_2$ as respiratory in origin.
            - ▸ Diagnose less than 22 or greater than 26 HCO_3^- as metabolic in origin.
        - Step 3: Combine diagnoses of Steps 1 and 2 to name the type of imbalance.

- Step 4: Evaluate the PaO_2 and the SaO_2.
  - ▸ If the results are below the expected reference range, the client is hypoxic.
- Step 5: Determine compensation as follows:
  - ▸ Uncompensated: The pH will be outside the expected reference range, and either the HCO_3^- or the $PaCO_2$ will be outside the expected reference range.
  - ▸ Partially compensated: The pH, HCO_3^-, and $PaCO_2$ will be outside the expected reference range.
  - ▸ Fully compensated: The pH will be within the expected reference range, but the $PaCO_2$ and HCO_3^- will both be outside the expected reference range. Looking back at the pH will provide a clue as to which system initiated the problem, respiratory or metabolic. If the pH is less than 7.40, think "acidosis," and determine which system has the acidosis value. If the pH is greater than 7.40, think "alkalosis," and determine which system has the alkalosis value.

- The following are the five classic types of ABG results demonstrating balance and imbalance.

STEP 1	STEP 2		STEP 3
If pH is:	Determine which is in normal range		Combine names
	$PaCO_2$	HCO_3^-	Diagnosis
7.35 to 7.45	35 to 45	22 to 26	Homeostasis
less than 7.35	greater than 45	22 to 26	Respiratory acidosis
less than 7.35	35 to 45	less than 22	Metabolic acidosis
greater than 7.45	less than 35	22 to 26	Respiratory alkalosis
greater than 7.45	35 to 45	greater than 26	Metabolic alkalosis

Patient-Centered Care

- Nursing Care
  - For all acid-base imbalances, it is imperative to treat the underlying cause.
  - Respiratory acidosis: Oxygen therapy, maintain patent airway, and enhance gas exchange (positioning and breathing techniques, ventilatory support, bronchodilators, mucolytics).
  - Respiratory alkalosis: Oxygen therapy, anxiety reduction interventions, and rebreathing techniques.
  - Metabolic acidosis: Varies with causes (if DKA, administer insulin; if related to GI losses, administer antidiarrheals and provide rehydration; if serum bicarbonate is low, administer sodium bicarbonate [1 mEq/kg]).
  - Metabolic alkalosis: Varies with causes (if GI losses, administer antiemetics, fluids, and electrolyte replacements; if related to potassium depletion, discontinue causative agent).
- Teamwork and Collaboration
  - Respiratory services can be consulted for oxygen therapy, breathing treatments, and ABGs.
  - Pulmonology services can be consulted for respiratory management.

- Care after Discharge
  - Client Education
    - Education may vary in relation to the client's condition.
    - Encourage adherence to the prescribed diet and dialysis regimen for clients who have kidney dysfunction.
    - Encourage the client to weigh self daily and notify the provider if there is a 1- to 2-lb (0.5 to 0.9 kg) gain in 24 hr or a 3-lb (1.4 kg) gain in 1 week.
    - Promote smoking cessation if the client is a smoker.
    - Teach the client to take medication as prescribed. Encourage adherence to the medication regimen for clients who have COPD.
  - Set up referral services (home oxygen).

Complications

- Convulsions, Coma, and Respiratory Arrest
  - Nursing Actions
    - Implement seizure precautions, and perform management interventions if necessary.
    - Provide life-support interventions if necessary.

APPLICATION EXERCISES

1. A nurse is caring for a client admitted with confusion and lethargy. The client was found at home unresponsive with an empty bottle of aspirin lying next to her bed. Vital signs reveal a blood pressure of 104/72 mm Hg, heart rate of 116 beats/min with a regular rhythm, and a respiratory rate of 42/min and deep. Which of the following arterial blood gases findings should the nurse expect?

    A. pH 7.68, PaO_2 96 mm Hg, $PaCO_2$ 38 mm Hg, HCO_3^- 24 mEq/L

    B. pH 7.48, PaO_2 100 mm Hg, $PaCO_2$ 28 mm Hg, HCO_3^- 23 mEq/L

    C. pH 6.98, PaO_2 100 mm Hg, $PaCO_2$ 30 mm Hg, HCO_3^- 18 mEq/L

    D. pH 7.58, PaO_2 96 mm Hg, $PaCO_2$ 38 mm Hg, HCO_3^- 29 mEq/L

2. A nurse is caring for a client who was in a motor-vehicle accident. He is reporting chest pain and difficulty breathing. A chest x-ray reveals the client has a pneumothorax, and arterial blood gases are obtained. Which of the following findings should the nurse expect?

    A. pH 7.06, PaO_2 86 mm Hg, $PaCO_2$ 52 mm Hg, HCO_3^- 24 mEq/L

    B. pH 7.42, PaO_2 100 mm Hg, $PaCO_2$ 38 mm Hg, HCO_3^- 23 mEq/L

    C. pH 6.98, PaO_2 100 mm Hg, $PaCO_2$ 30 mm Hg, HCO_3^- 18 mEq/L

    D. pH 7.58, PaO_2 96 mm Hg, $PaCO_2$ 38 mm Hg, HCO_3^- 29 mEq/L

3. A nurse is admitting a client who has been vomiting for 24 hr. Arterial blood gases are obtained. Based on the laboratory findings, which of the following conditions should the nurse expect?

    A. Respiratory acidosis

    B. Respiratory alkalosis

    C. Metabolic acidosis

    D. Metabolic alkalosis

4. A nurse is orienting a newly licensed nurse on conditions related to metabolic acidosis. Which of the following statements by the new nurse indicates the teaching has been effective?

    A. "Metabolic acidosis can occur due to diabetic ketoacidosis."

    B. "Metabolic acidosis can occur in a client who has myasthenia gravis."

    C. "Metabolic acidosis can occur in a client who has asthma."

    D. "Metabolic acidosis can occur due to cancer."

5. A nurse is assessing a client who has pancreatitis. His arterial blood gases reveal metabolic acidosis. Which of the following is an expected finding? (Select all that apply.)

_____ A. Tachycardia

___X___ B. Hypertension

___X___ C. Bounding pulses

___X___ D. Hyperreflexia

___X___ E. Dysrhythmia

___X___ F. Tachypnea

6. A nurse is caring for a client who has liver cancer. The client's arterial blood gases reveal metabolic acidosis. Use the ATI Active Learning Template: Systems Disorder to complete this item to include the following:

A. Risk Factors: Include three conditions related to metabolic acidosis.

B. Patient-Centered Care: Include two nursing care actions.

C. Complications: Identify one.

APPLICATION EXERCISES KEY

1. A. INCORRECT: These arterial blood gases indicate metabolic alkalosis.

    B. INCORRECT: These arterial blood gases indicate metabolic alkalosis.

    C. **CORRECT:** An aspirin overdose would result in arterial blood gas findings of metabolic acidosis.

    D. INCORRECT: These arterial blood gases indicate respiratory alkalosis.

    (N) NCLEX® Connection: Reduction of Risk Potential, Laboratory Values

2. A. **CORRECT:** A pneumothorax can cause alveolar hyperventilation and increased carbon dioxide levels, resulting in a state of respiratory acidosis.

    B. INCORRECT: Arterial blood gases reflecting respiratory acidosis is not indicated for this client.

    C. INCORRECT: Arterial blood gases reflecting metabolic acidosis is not indicated for this client.

    D. INCORRECT: Arterial blood gases reflecting metabolic alkalosis is not indicated for this client.

    (N) NCLEX® Connection: Reduction of Risk Potential, Laboratory Values

3. A. INCORRECT: Respiratory acidosis would not be indicated for this client.

    B. INCORRECT: Respiratory alkalosis would not be indicated for this client.

    C. INCORRECT: Metabolic acidosis would not be indicated for this client.

    D. **CORRECT:** Excessive vomiting causes a loss of gastric acids and an accumulation of bicarbonate in the blood, resulting in metabolic alkalosis.

    (N) NCLEX® Connection: Physiological Adaptations, Fluid and Electrolyte Imbalances

4. A. **CORRECT:** Metabolic acidosis results from an excess production of hydrogen ions, which occurs in diabetic ketoacidosis.

    B. INCORRECT: Respiratory acidosis can occur in a client who has myasthenia gravis.

    C. INCORRECT: Respiratory acidosis can occur in a client who has asthma.

    D. INCORRECT: Respiratory acidosis can occur due to cancer.

    (N) NCLEX® Connection: Physiological Adaptations, Fluid and Electrolyte Imbalances

5. A. INCORRECT: Tachycardia is not an expected finding in a client who has pancreatitis and metabolic acidosis.

    B. **CORRECT:** Hypotension is an expected finding of metabolic acidosis.

    C. **CORRECT:** Weak peripheral pulses is an expected finding of metabolic acidosis.

    D. **CORRECT:** Hyporeflexia is an expected finding of metabolic acidosis.

    E. **CORRECT:** Dysrhythmia is an expected finding in a client who has pancreatitis and metabolic acidosis.

    F. **CORRECT:** Tachypnea is an expected finding in a client who has pancreatitis and metabolic acidosis.

    Ⓝ NCLEX® Connection: Physiological Adaptations, Fluid and Electrolyte Imbalances

6. *Using ATI Active Learning Template: Systems Disorder*

    A. Risk Factors

    • Metabolic acidosis results from

      ○ Excess production of hydrogen ions

        ▪ DKA   ▪ Heavy exercise   ▪ Hypoxia
        ▪ Lactic acidosis   ▪ Seizure activity   ▪ Intoxication with
        ▪ Starvation   ▪ Fever   ethanol or salicylates

      ○ Inadequate elimination of hydrogen ions – Renal failure

      ○ Inadequate production of bicarbonate

        ▪ Renal failure   ▪ Liver failure
        ▪ Pancreatitis   ▪ Dehydration

      ○ Excess elimination of bicarbonate – Diarrhea, ileostomy

    • Metabolic acidosis results in

      ○ Decreased HCO_3^-

      ○ Increased H^+ concentration

    B. Patient-Centered Care: Nursing Actions

    • For all acid-base imbalances, it is imperative to treat the underlying cause.

    • Respiratory acidosis – Oxygen therapy, maintain patent airway, and enhance gas exchange (positioning and breathing techniques, ventilatory support, bronchodilators, mucolytics).

    • Respiratory alkalosis – Oxygen therapy, anxiety reduction interventions, and rebreathing techniques.

    • Metabolic acidosis – Varies with causes (if DKA, administer insulin; if related to GI losses, administer antidiarrheals and provide rehydration; if serum bicarbonate is low, administer sodium bicarbonate [1 mEq/kg]).

    • Metabolic alkalosis – Varies with causes (if GI losses, administer antiemetics, fluids, and electrolyte replacements; if related to potassium depletion, discontinue causative agent).

    C. Complications

    • Convulsions, coma, and respiratory arrest

    • Nursing Actions

      ○ Implement seizure precautions, and perform management interventions if necessary.

      ○ Provide life-support interventions if necessary.

    Ⓝ NCLEX® Connection: Physiological Adaptations, Fluid and Electrolyte Imbalances

UNIT 7   Nursing Care of Clients with Gastrointestinal Disorders

SECTIONS

› Diagnostic and Therapeutic Procedures
› Upper Gastrointestinal Disorders
› Lower Gastrointestinal Disorders
› Gallbladder and Pancreas Disorders
› Liver Disorders

NCLEX® CONNECTIONS

When reviewing the chapters in this unit, keep in mind the relevant sections of the NCLEX® outline, in particular:

Client Needs: Basic Care and Comfort	Client Needs: Pharmacological and Parenteral Therapies	Client Needs: Reduction of Risk Potential

› Relevant topics/tasks include:
» Elimination
  › Assess and manage the client with an alteration in elimination.
  › Evaluate whether the client's elimination is restored/maintained.
» Nutrition and Oral Hydration
  › Provide/maintain special diets based on the client's diagnosis/nutritional needs and cultural considerations.
	› Relevant topics/tasks include:
	» Blood and Blood Products
	  › Document necessary information on the administration of red blood cells/blood products.
	» Pharmacological Pain Management
	  › Assess the client's need for administration of a PRN pain medication.
	» Total Parenteral Nutrition (TPN)
	  › Administer parenteral nutrition and evaluate the client's response.
		› Relevant topics/tasks include:
		» Diagnostic Tests
		  › Perform diagnostic testing.
		» Potential for Complications of Diagnostic Tests/Treatments/Procedures
		  › Insert, maintain, and remove nasogastric tubes and/or urethral catheters.
		» Therapeutic Procedures
		  › Manage the client during and following a procedure with moderate sedation.

chapter 46

Overview

- Gastrointestinal diagnostic procedures often involve scopes and x-rays to visualize parts of the gastrointestinal system and to evaluate gastrointestinal contents.

- Gastrointestinal diagnostic procedures that nurses should be knowledgeable about
  - Liver function tests and other blood tests
  - Urine bilinogen
  - Fecal occult blood test (FOBT) and stool samples
  - Endoscopy
  - Gastrointestinal (GI) series

Liver Function Tests and Other Blood Tests

- Liver function tests are aspartate aminotransferase (AST), alanine aminotransferase (ALT), alkaline phosphatase (ALP), bilirubin, and albumin.

- Other blood tests that provide information on the functioning of the gastrointestinal system include amylase, lipase, alpha-fetoprotein, and ammonia.

- Indications – suspected liver, pancreatic, or biliary tract disorder

- Interpretation of Findings

BLOOD TEST	EXPECTED REFERENCE RANGE	INTERPRETATION OF FINDINGS
Aspartate aminotransferase (AST)	5 to 40 units/L	› Elevation occurs with hepatitis or cirrhosis.
Alanine aminotransferase (ALT)	8 to 20 units/L 3 to 35 IU/L	› Elevation occurs with hepatitis or cirrhosis.
Alkaline phosphatase (ALP)	30 to 120 units/L 30 to 85 IU/L	› Elevation indicates liver damage.
Amylase	56 to 90 IU/L	› Elevation occurs with pancreatitis.
Lipase	0 to 110 units/L	› Elevation occurs with pancreatitis.
Total bilirubin	0.1 to 1.0 mg/dL	› Elevations indicate altered liver function, bile duct obstruction, or other hepatobiliary disorder.
Direct (conjugated) bilirubin	0.1 to 0.3 mg/dL	› Elevations indicate altered liver function, bile duct obstruction, or other hepatobiliary disorder.

BLOOD TEST	EXPECTED REFERENCE RANGE	INTERPRETATION OF FINDINGS
Indirect (unconjugated) bilirubin	0.2 to 0.8 mg/dL	› Elevations indicate altered liver function, bile duct obstruction, or other hepatobiliary disorder.
Albumin	3.5 to 5.0 g/dL	› Decrease may indicate hepatic disease.
Alpha-fetoprotein	Less than 40 mcg/L	› Elevated in liver cancer.
Ammonia	15 to 110 mcg/dL	› Elevated in liver disease.

- Preprocedure – Explain to the client how blood is obtained and what information this will provide.
- Postprocedure – Inform the client when and how results are provided.

Urine Bilirubin

- Also known as urobilinogen, this is a urine test to determine the presence of bilirubin in the urine.
- Indications – Suspected liver or biliary tract disorder
- Interpretation of Findings – A positive or elevated finding indicates possible liver disorder (cirrhosis, hepatitis) or biliary obstruction.
- Preprocedure
  - Nursing Actions – The test may be performed by using a dipstick (urine bilirubin) or a 24-hr urine collection (urobilinogen).
  - Client Education – Teach the client how to collect urine and provide proper collection container.
- Postprocedure
  - Nursing Actions – Inform the client when and how results are provided.

Fecal Occult Blood Test and Stool Samples

- A stool sample is collected and tested for blood, ova and parasites (*Giardia lamblia*), and bacteria (*Clostridium difficile*). Stool also may be collected to assess for DNA changes in the vimentin gene.
- Indications
  - Client Presentation
    - Gastrointestinal bleeding
    - Unexplained diarrhea
- Interpretation of Findings
  - A positive finding for blood is indicative of gastrointestinal bleeding (ulcer, colitis, cancer).
  - A positive finding for ova and parasites is indicative of a gastrointestinal parasitic infection.
  - A positive finding for *Clostridium difficile* is indicative of this opportunistic infection, which usually becomes established secondary to use of broad-spectrum antibiotics.
  - A change in the vimentin gene can be an indicator of colorectal cancer.

- Preprocedure
  - Nursing Actions
    - Occult blood – Provide the client with cards impregnated with guaiac that can be mailed to provider or with a specimen collection cup. If the cards are used, three samples are usually required.
    - Stool for ova and parasites and bacteria – Provide the client with a specimen collection cup.
  - Client Education
    - Occult blood – Instruct the client about proper collection technique. The client may also need to be instructed about dietary and medication restrictions to follow prior to obtaining samples (red meat, anticoagulants).
    - Stool for ova and parasites and bacteria – Instruct the client about proper collection technique (time frame for submission to laboratory, need for refrigeration).
- Postprocedure
  - Nursing Actions – Inform the client when and how the results are provided.

Endoscopy

- Endoscopic procedures allow direct visualization of body cavities, tissues, and organs through the use of a flexible, lighted tube (endoscope). They are performed for diagnostic and therapeutic purposes.

 View Image: Endoscope

  - Endoscopic procedures are performed in a variety of facilities. The provider can perform biopsies, remove abnormal tissue, and perform minor surgery, such as cauterizing a bleeding ulcer. A contrast medium may be injected to allow visualization of structures beyond the capabilities of the scope.
  - Gastrointestinal scope procedures
    - Colonoscopy
    - Esophagogastroduodenoscopy (EGD)
    - Endoscopic retrograde cholangiopancreatography (ERCP)
    - Sigmoidoscopy
- Indications
  - Potential Diagnoses
    - Gastrointestinal bleeding, ulcerations or inflammation, polyps, malignant tumors
  - Client Presentation
    - Anemia (secondary to bleeding)
    - Abdominal discomfort
    - Abdominal distention or mass
- Interpretation of findings may indicate a need for medication or surgical removal of a lesion.

- General endoscopic procedures
  - ○ Preprocedure
    - ▪ Nursing Actions
      - ▫ Evaluate the client's understanding of the procedure.
      - ▫ Verify that a consent form has been signed.
      - ▫ Assess vital signs and verify the client's allergies.
      - ▫ Evaluate baseline laboratory tests and report unexpected findings to the provider (CBC, electrolyte panel, BUN, creatinine, PT, aPTT, and liver function studies). Evaluate chest x-ray, ECG, and ABGs, as indicated.
      - ▫ Evaluate the client's medical history for increased risk of complications.
        - ▸ Age can influence the client's ability to understand the procedures, tolerance of the required positioning, and compliance with pretest preparation.
          - ▹ Current health status – Consider conditions and medications that can affect the client's tolerance of and recovery from the procedure.
          - ▹ Cognitive status – Determine the client's understanding of the procedure and baseline mental status.
          - ▹ Support system – Determine whether a support person will assist the client after the procedure.
        - ▸ Recent food or fluid intake – May affect the provider's ability to visualize key structures and increase the client's risk for complications (aspiration). Notify the provider if dietary restrictions were not followed.
        - ▸ Medications – Some medications place the client at risk for complications (NSAIDs, warfarin, aspirin). Notify the provider if medication restrictions were not followed.
        - ▸ Previous radiographic examinations – Any recent radiographic examinations using barium may affect the provider's ability to view key structures. Notify the provider if contrast has been recently used.
        - ▸ Ensure that the client followed proper bowel preparation (laxatives, enemas). Inadequate bowel preparation can result in cancellation and delays the examination. This can also lead to the client experiencing extended periods of being NPO or on a liquid diet.
        - ▸ Electrolyte and fluid status – Imbalances secondary to repeated enemas may affect the client's ability to tolerate bowel preparation.
        - ▸ Ensure that the client is NPO for the prescribed period prior to the examination.
    - ▪ Client Education
      - ▫ Provide instructions regarding medication and food restrictions.
      - ▫ Provide prescriptions for medications used for the bowel prep.
      - ▫ Instruct the client about the number and type of enemas, if prescribed.
  - ○ Postprocedure
    - ▪ Nursing Actions
      - ▫ Monitor vital signs.
      - ▫ Assess for complications.
    - ▪ Client Education
      - ▫ If a biopsy was performed, food restrictions may be prescribed.

- Specific Endoscopic Procedures

COLONOSCOPY	
Definition	› Use of a flexible fiber-optic colonoscope, entering through the anus, to visualize the rectum and the sigmoid, descending, transverse, and ascending colon.
Anesthesia	› Moderate sedation – midazolam (Versed) usually with an opiate analgesic
Positioning	› Left side with knees to chest

Preparation	› Bowel prep
	  » May include laxatives, such as bisacodyl (Dulcolax) and polyethylene glycol (GOLYTELY)
	  » Clear liquid diet (avoid red, purple, orange fluids); NPO after midnight
	› The client must avoid medications indicated by provider.

Postprocedure	› Notify the provider of severe pain (possible perforation) or sign of hemorrhage. › Monitor for rectal bleeding. › Monitor vital signs and respiratory status. › Resume normal diet as prescribed. › Encourage increased fluid intake. › Instruct the client that there may be increased flatulence due to air instillation during the procedure.
EGD	
Definition	› Insertion of endoscope through the mouth into the esophagus, stomach, and duodenum.
Anesthesia	› Moderate sedation – topical anesthetic
Positioning	› Left side-lying
Preparation	› NPO 6 to 8 hr; remove dentures prior to procedure.
Postprocedure	› Monitor vital signs and respiratory status. › Notify the provider of bleeding, abdominal or chest pain, and any evidence of infection. › Withhold fluids until return of gag reflex.
ERCP	
Definition	› Insertion of a endoscope through the mouth into the biliary tree via the duodenum. Allows visualization of the biliary ducts, gall bladder, liver, and pancreas.
Anesthesia	› Conscious sedation – topical anesthetic
Positioning	› Initially semi-prone with repositioning throughout procedure
Preparation	› NPO 6 to 8 hr; remove dentures prior to procedure › Explain the procedure and the need to change positions during the procedure.
Postprocedure	› Monitor vital signs and respiratory status. › Notify the provider of bleeding, abdominal or chest pain, and any evidence of infection. › Withhold fluids until return of gag reflex.

SIGMOIDOSCOPY	
Definition	› Scope is shorter than colonoscope, allowing visualization of the anus, rectum, and sigmoid colon.
Anesthesia	› None required
Positioning	› On left side
Preparation	› Bowel prep, which may include laxatives, such as bisacodyl (Dulcolax) and polyethylene glycol (GOLYTELY) › Clear liquid diet › NPO after midnight › The client must avoid medications indicated by the provider.
Postprocedure	› Monitor vital signs and respiratory status. › Monitor for rectal bleeding. › Resume normal diet as prescribed. › Encourage increased fluid intake. › Instruct the client that there may be increased flatulence due to air instillation during the procedure.

- Complications
  - Oversedation – Use of moderate sedation places the client at risk for oversedation.
    - Manifestations of oversedation – Difficult to arouse, poor respiratory effort, evidence of hypoxemia, tachycardia, and elevated or low blood pressure
    - Nursing Actions
      - Be prepared to administer antidotes for the sedatives administered prior to and during the procedure, maintain an open airway, administer oxygen, and monitor vital signs.
      - Notify the provider immediately and call for assistance.
    - Client Education
      - Driving and major decision making are restricted until the effects of the sedation have worn off, and this varies with the type of agents used.
  - Hemorrhage
    - Manifestations of hemorrhage include bleeding, cool and clammy skin, hypotension, tachycardia, dizziness, and tachypnea.
    - Nursing Actions
      - Assess for hemorrhage from the site, monitor vital signs, and monitor diagnostic test results (particularly Hgb and Hct).
      - Notify the provider immediately.
    - Client Education – Report fever, pain, and bleeding to the provider.

- Aspiration – Using moderate sedation or topical anesthesia may affect the gag reflex.

  - Manifestations of aspiration include dyspnea, tachypnea, adventitious breath sounds, tachycardia, and fever.

  - Nursing Actions

    - Keep the client NPO until the gag reflex returns. Ensure that the client is awake and alert prior to consuming food or fluid. Encourage the client to deep breathe and cough to promote removal of secretions.

    - Notify the provider if there is a delay in gag reflex return.

  - Client Education – Report any respiratory congestion or compromise to the provider.

- Perforation of the gastrointestinal tract

  - Manifestations include chest or abdominal pain, fever, nausea, vomiting, and abdominal distention.

  - Nursing Actions – Monitor diagnostic tests for evidence of infection, including elevated WBC, and notify the provider of unexpected findings.

  - Client Education – Report fever, pain, and bleeding to the provider.

Gastrointestinal Series

- Gastrointestinal studies are done with or without contrast and help define anatomic or functional abnormalities.

  - These include radiographic imaging of the esophagus, stomach, and entire intestinal tract.

  - Upper gastrointestinal imaging is done by having the client drink a radiopaque liquid (barium). For small bowel follow-through, barium is traced through the small intestine to the ileocecal junction.

  - A barium enema is done by instilling a radiopaque liquid into the rectum and colon.

- Indications

  - Potential Diagnoses – gastric ulcers, peristaltic disorders, tumors, varices, and intestinal enlargements or constrictions

  - Client Presentation – abdominal pain, altered elimination habits (constipation, diarrhea), or gastrointestinal bleeding

- Interpretation of findings include altered bowel shape and size, increased motility, or obstruction.

- Preprocedure

  - Nursing Actions

    - Inform the client about medications, food and fluid restrictions (clear liquid and/or low residue diet, NPO after midnight), and avoiding smoking or chewing gum (increases peristalsis).

    - Assess the client's understanding of bowel preparation (laxatives, enemas), so the image will not be distorted by feces.

    - Barium enema studies must be scheduled prior to upper gastrointestinal studies.

    - Assess for contraindications to bowel preparation (possible bowel perforation or obstruction, inflammatory disease).

- ○ Client Education
  - Tell the client to restrict food and fluids for bowel preparation.
  - Inform the client that if the small intestine is to be visualized additional radiographs will be done over the next 24 hr.
- Postprocedure
  - ○ Nursing Actions
    - Monitor elimination of contrast material and administer a laxative if prescribed.
    - Increase fluid intake to promote elimination of contrast material.
  - ○ Client Education
    - Instruct the client to monitor elimination of contrast material and to report retention of contrast material (constipation) or diarrhea accompanied by weakness.
    - Discuss the possible need for an over-the-counter medication to prevent constipation resulting from the barium.
    - Instruct the client that stools will be white for 24 to 72 hr until barium clears. The client should report abdominal fullness, pain, or delay in return to brown stool.

APPLICATION EXERCISES

1. A nurse is reviewing the bowel prep using polyethylene glycol (GOLYTELY) with a client scheduled for a colonoscopy. Which of the following should be included in the teaching?

    A. Check with the provider about taking current medications when consuming bowel prep.

    B. Consume a normal diet until starting the bowel prep.

    C. The bowel prep will not begin acting until the day after it is consumed.

    D. The bowel prep may be discontinued once feces start to be expelled.

2. A nurse is having difficulty arousing a client following an esophagogastroduodenoscopy (EGD). Which of the following is the priority action by the nurse?

    A. Assess the client's airway.

    B. Allow the client to sleep.

    C. Increase the rate of IV fluid administration.

    D. Evaluate preprocedure laboratory findings.

3. A nurse in a clinic is instructing a client about a fecal occult blood test, which requires mailing three specimens. Which of the following statements by the client indicates understanding of the teaching?

    A. "I will continue taking my Coumadin while I complete these tests."

    B. "I'm glad I don't have to follow any special diet at this time."

    C. "This test determines if I have parasites in my bowel."

    D. "This is an easy way to rule out having colon cancer."

4. A nurse is completing preprocedure teaching for a client who will undergo a sigmoidoscopy. Which of the following should be included in the teaching? (Select all that apply.)

    _____ A. Increased flatulence can occur following the procedure.

    _____ B. NPO status should be maintained preprocedure.

    _____ C. Conscious sedation is used.

    _____ D. Repositioning will occur throughout the procedure.

    _____ E. Fluid intake is limited the day after the procedure.

5. A nurse is reviewing the health record of a client who is being admitted with a suspected tumor of the jejunum. The nurse should anticipate a prescription for which of the following tests?

    A. Serum alpha-fetoprotein

    B. Endoscopic retrograde cholangiopancreatography (ERCP)

    C. Gastrointestinal x-ray with contrast

    D. Urine bilirubin

6. A nurse in a clinic is reviewing teaching with a client who will undergo a gastrointestinal series of x-rays. What should be included in the teaching? Use the ATI Active Learning Template: Diagnostic Procedure to complete this item to include the following sections:

    A. Procedure Name: Describe the procedure and technique involved.

    B. Indications: Identify at least three potential diagnoses and two clinical manifestations.

    C. Client Education: Describe three teaching points.

APPLICATION EXERCISES KEY

1. A. **CORRECT:** Some medications may be withheld when taking GOLYTELY due to their lack of absorption. This should be discussed with the provider.

   B. INCORRECT: The client is instructed to consume a clear liquid diet prior to starting the bowel prep.

   C. INCORRECT: The actions of GOLYTELY begin within 2 to 3 hr after consumption.

   D. INCORRECT: The client is instructed to consume the full amount prescribed.

   Ⓝ NCLEX® Connection: Reduction of Risk Potential, Therapeutic Procedures

2. A. **CORRECT:** Using the airway, breathing, and circulation (ABC) priority-setting framework, the priority intervention is airway maintenance.

   B. INCORRECT: Allowing the client to rest is an appropriate action but not the priority at this time.

   C. INCORRECT: Increasing the rate of IV fluid administration is an appropriate action but not the priority at this time.

   D. INCORRECT: Evaluating preprocedure laboratory findings is an appropriate action but not the priority at this time.

   Ⓝ NCLEX® Connection: Reduction of Risk Potential, Therapeutic Procedures

3. A. INCORRECT: Clients are instructed to stop taking anticoagulants prior to obtaining stool specimens for fecal occult blood testing because they can interfere with the results.

   B. INCORRECT: Clients are instructed to avoid consuming red meat prior to obtaining stool specimens for fecal occult blood testing because this can interfere with the results.

   C. INCORRECT: Fecal occult blood testing does not identify parasites present in stool.

   D. **CORRECT:** Fecal occult blood testing is a screening procedure for colon cancer.

   Ⓝ NCLEX® Connection: Reduction of Risk Potential, Therapeutic Procedures

4. A. **CORRECT:** Increased flatulence can occur due to the instillation of air during the procedure.

   B. **CORRECT:** The client is instructed to remain NPO after midnight the night before the procedure.

   C. INCORRECT: No sedation is provided during a sigmoidoscopy.

   D. INCORRECT: The client is placed on the left side for this procedure.

   E. INCORRECT: The client is instructed to increase fluid intake following the procedure.

   Ⓝ NCLEX® Connection: Reduction of Risk Potential, Therapeutic Procedures

5. A. INCORRECT: Serum alpha-fetoprotein is a laboratory test used in cases of suspected liver cancer.

    B. INCORRECT: An ERCP is used to visualize the duodenum, biliary ducts, gall bladder, liver, and pancreas.

    C. **CORRECT:** A gastrointestinal x-ray with contrast involves the client drinking barium, which is then traced through the small intestine to the junction with the colon. This would identify a tumor in the jejunum.

    D. INCORRECT: Urine bilirubin is a laboratory test used in cases of a possible liver disorder or biliary tract obstruction.

    (N) NCLEX® Connection: Reduction of Risk Potential, Diagnostic Tests

6. *Using the ATI Active Learning Template: Diagnostic Procedure*

    A. Procedure Name
      - Radiographic images used to define anatomic or functional abnormalities of the esophagus, stomach and intestinal tract. These can include an upper GI image, which includes the client drinking radiopaque barium liquid, which is traced through the small intestine, or a barium enema, in which liquid barium is instilled into the rectum and colon.

    B. Indications
      - Diagnoses: Gastric ulcers, peristaltic disorders, tumors, varices, intestinal enlargements or constrictions
      - Manifestations: Abdominal pain, altered elimination habits (constipation, diarrhea), gastrointestinal bleeding

    C. Client Education
      - Follow fluid and food restrictions for bowel preparation.
      - Additional radiographs may be done over a 24 hr period.
      - Monitor elimination of contrast media and report retention of contrast media (constipation) or diarrhea accompanied by weakness. Over-the-counter medication may be used to prevent constipation.
      - Stool may be white for 24 to 72 hr until barium clears the system. Report abdominal fullness, pain, or a delay in a return to brown stool.

    (N) NCLEX® Connection: Reduction of Risk Potential, Therapeutic Procedures

chapter 47

Overview

- Gastrointestinal therapeutic procedures are performed for maintenance of nutritional intake, treatment of gastrointestinal obstructions and other disorders, and treatment of obesity.
- Gastrointestinal therapeutic procedures that nurses should be knowledgeable about
  - Enteral feedings
  - Total parenteral nutrition (TPN)
  - Paracentesis
  - Nasogastric decompression
  - Bariatric surgeries
  - Ostomies

Enteral Feedings

- Enteral feedings are instituted when a client can no longer take adequate nutrition orally.
- Indications
  - Diagnoses
    - Clients who are intubated
    - Pathologies that cause difficulty swallowing and/or increase risk of aspiration (stroke, advanced Parkinson's disease, and multiple sclerosis)
    - Clients who cannot maintain adequate oral nutritional intake and need supplementation
  - Client Presentation
    - Malnutrition
    - Aspiration pneumonia
- Complications
  - Overfeeding results from infusion of greater quantity of feeding than can be readily digested by the client, resulting in abdominal distention, nausea, and vomiting.
    - Nursing Actions
      - Check residual every 4 to 6 hr.
      - Follow protocol for withholding excess residual volumes as directed (typically 100 to 200 mL).
      - Withhold feeding as prescribed and resume at reduced rate as prescribed.

○ Diarrhea occurs secondary to concentration of feeding or its constituents.

   ▪ Nursing Actions

      ▫ Slow rate of feeding and notify the provider.

      ▫ Confer with the dietitian.

      ▫ Provide skin care and protection.

○ Aspiration pneumonia

   ▪ Pneumonia can occur secondary to aspiration of feeding.

      ▫ Tube displacement is the primary cause of aspiration of feeding.

   ▪ Nursing Actions

      ▫ Stop the feeding.

      ▫ Turn the client to his side and suction the airway. Administer oxygen if indicated.

      ▫ Monitor vital signs for an elevated temperature.

      ▫ Auscultate breath sounds for increased congestion.

      ▫ Notify the provider and obtain a chest x-ray if prescribed.

Total Parenteral Nutrition

- Total parenteral nutrition (TPN) is a hypertonic intravenous (IV) bolus solution. The purpose of TPN administration is to prevent or correct nutritional deficiencies and minimize the adverse effects of malnourishment.

   ○ TPN administration is usually through a central line, such as a tunneled triple lumen catheter or a single- or double-lumen peripherally inserted central (PICC) line.

   ○ TPN contains complete nutrition, including calories (in a high concentration [20% to 50%] of dextrose), lipids/essential fatty acids, protein, electrolytes, vitamins, and trace elements. Standard IV bolus therapy is typically less than or equal to 700 calories/day.

   ○ Partial parenteral nutrition or peripheral parenteral nutrition (PPN) is less hypertonic, intended for short-term use, and administered in a large peripheral vein. Usual dextrose concentration is 10% or less. Risks include phlebitis.

- Indications

   ○ Potential indications for TPN include any condition that

      ▪ Affects the ability to absorb nutrition.

      ▪ Has a prolonged recovery.

      ▪ Creates a hypermetabolic state.

      ▪ Creates a chronic malnutrition.

   ○ Diagnoses

      ▪ Chronic pancreatitis

      ▪ Diffuse peritonitis

      ▪ Short bowel syndrome

      ▪ Gastric paresis from diabetes mellitus

      ▪ Severe burns

- ○ Client Presentation
  - ▪ Basic guidelines regarding when to initiate TPN
    - ▢ A weight loss of 7% body weight and NPO for 5 days or more
    - ▢ A hypermetabolic state
- • Nursing Actions
  - ○ Preparation of the Client

  - ▪ Determine the client's readiness for TPN.
    - ▢ Obtain daily laboratory values, including electrolytes. Solutions are customized for each client according to daily laboratory results.
  - ○ Ongoing Care
    - ▪ The flow rate is gradually increased and gradually decreased to allow body adjustment (usually no more than a 10% hourly increase in rate).
      - ▢ Never abruptly stop TPN. Speeding up/slowing down the rate is contraindicated. An abrupt rate change can alter blood glucose levels significantly.
    - ▪ Monitor vital signs every 4 to 8 hr.
    - ▪ Follow sterile procedures to minimize the risk of sepsis.
      - ▢ TPN solution is prepared by the pharmacy using aseptic technique with a laminar flow hood.
      - ▢ Change tubing and solution bag (even if not empty) every 24 hr.
      - ▢ A filter is added to the tubing to collect particles from the solution.
      - ▢ Do not use the line for other IV bolus solutions (prevents contamination and interruption of the flow rate).
      - ▢ Do not add anything to the solution due to risks of contamination and incompatibility.
      - ▢ Use sterile procedures, including a mask, when changing the central line dressing (per facility procedure).
  - ○ Interventions
    - ▪ Check capillary glucose every 4 to 6 hr for at least the first 24 hr.
      - ▢ Clients receiving TPN frequently need supplemental regular insulin until the pancreas can increase its endogenous production of insulin.
      - ▢ Keep dextrose 10% in water at the bedside in case the solution is unexpectedly ruined or the next bag is not available. This will minimize the risk of hypoglycemia with abrupt changes in dextrose concentrations.
      - ▢ Older adult clients have an increased incidence of glucose intolerance.
- • Complications
  - ○ Metabolic complications include hyperglycemia, hypoglycemia, and vitamin deficiencies.
    - ▪ Nursing Actions
      - ▢ Daily laboratory tests are prescribed and results obtained before a new solution is prepared.
      - ▢ Fluid needs are typically replaced with a separate IV bolus to prevent fluid volume excess.
      - ▢ Monitor for hyperglycemia.

- ○ Air embolism – A pressure change during tubing changes can lead to an air embolism.
    - ▪ Nursing Actions
        - □ Monitor for manifestations of an air embolism (sudden onset of dyspnea, chest pain, anxiety, hypoxia).
        - □ Clamp the catheter immediately and place the client on his left side in Trendelenburg position to trap air. Administer oxygen and notify provider so trapped air can be aspirated.
- ○ Infection – Concentrated glucose is a medium for bacteria.
    - ▪ Nursing Actions
        - □ Observe the central line insertion site for local infection (erythema, tenderness, exudate).
        - □ Change the sterile dressing on a central line per protocol (typically every 48 to 72 hr).

        - □ Change IV tubing per protocol (typically every 24 hr).
        - □ Observe the client for manifestations of systemic infection (fever, increased WBC, chills, malaise).
        - □ Do NOT use TPN line for other IV bolus fluids and medications (repeated access increases the risk for infection).
- ○ Fluid Imbalance
    - ▪ TPN is a hyperosmotic solution (three to six times the osmolarity of blood), which poses a risk for fluid shifts, placing client at increased risk of fluid volume excess.
        - □ Older adult clients are more vulnerable to fluid and electrolyte imbalances. Clients who have a history of heart failure may need a more concentrated solution to avoid fluid overload.
    - ▪ Nursing Actions
        - □ Assess lungs for crackles and monitor for respiratory distress.
        - □ Monitor daily weight and I&O.
        - □ Use a controlled infusion pump to administer TPN at the prescribed rate.
        - □ Do not speed up the infusion to "catch up."
        - □ Gradually increase the flow rate until the prescribed infusion rate is achieved.

Paracentesis

- A paracentesis is performed by inserting a needle or trocar through the abdominal wall into the peritoneal cavity. The therapeutic goal is relief of abdominal ascites pressure.
    - ○ A paracentesis can be performed in a provider's office, outpatient center, or acute care setting at the bedside.
    - ○ Once drained, ascitic fluid may be sent for laboratory culture.
- Indications
    - ○ Abdominal ascites
        - ▪ Ascites is an abnormal accumulation of protein-rich fluid in the abdominal cavity most often caused by cirrhosis of the liver. The result is increased abdominal girth and distention.
        - ▪ Respiratory distress is the determining factor in the use of a paracentesis to treat ascites, and in the evaluation of treatment effectiveness.
    - ○ Client Presentation – compromised lung expansion

- Preprocedure
  - Nursing Actions
    - Determine the client's readiness for the procedure.
      - Variables such as the age of the client and chronic and acute diseases can influence the client's ability to tolerate and recover from this procedure.
    - Assess pertinent lab results (serum albumin, protein, glucose, amylase, BUN, and creatinine).
    - Verify that the client has signed the informed consent form.
    - Gather equipment for the procedure.
    - Have the client void, or insert an indwelling urinary catheter.
    - Position the client as tolerated. Clients with ascites are typically more comfortable sitting up.
    - Review baseline vital signs, record weight, and measure abdominal girth.
    - Administer sedation as prescribed.
    - Administer prescribed IV bolus fluids or albumin, prior to or after a paracentesis, to restore fluid balance.
  - Client Education
    - Explain the procedure and its purpose to the client.
    - Instruct the client that local anesthetics will be used at the insertion site.
    - Explain that there may be pressure or pain with needle insertion.
    - Assess the client's knowledge of the procedure.
- Intraprocedure
  - Nursing Actions
    - Monitor vital signs.
    - Adhere to standard precautions.
    - Label laboratory specimens and send to the laboratory.
    - Between 4 and 6 L of fluid is slowly drained from the abdomen by gravity. The nurse is responsible for monitoring the amount of drainage and notifying the provider of any evidence of complications.
- Postprocedure
  - Nursing Actions
    - Maintain pressure at the insertion site for several minutes. Apply a dressing to the site.
    - If the insertion site continues to leak after holding pressure for several minutes, dry sterile gauze dressings should be applied and changed as often as necessary.
    - Check vital signs, record weight, and measure abdominal girth. Document and compare to preprocedure measurements.
    - Continue to monitor vital signs and insertion site per facility protocol.
    - Monitor temperature every 4 hr for a minimum of 48 hr.
    - Assess I&O every 4 hr.

- Administer medication, as prescribed.

  □ Diuretics such as spironolactone (Aldactone) and furosemide (Lasix) may be prescribed to control fluid volume.

  □ Potassium supplements may be necessary when a loop diuretic such as furosemide has been administrated.

- Administer IV bolus fluids or albumin as prescribed.

- Assist the client into a position of comfort with the head of the bed elevated to promote lung expansion.

- Document color, odor, consistency, and amount of fluid removed; location of insertion site; evidence of leakage at the insertion site; manifestations of hypovolemia; and changes in mental status.

- Continue monitoring of serum albumin, protein, glucose, amylase, BUN, and creatinine levels.

- Complications

  ○ Hypovolemia

    - Albumin levels can drop dangerously low because the peritoneal fluid removed contains a large amount of protein. The removal of this protein-rich fluid can cause shifting of intravascular volume, resulting in hypovolemia.

    - Nursing Actions

      □ Preventive measures include slow drainage of fluid and administration of plasma expanders, such as albumin, to counter albumin losses.

      □ Monitor for evidence of hypovolemia, such as tachycardia, hypotension, pallor, diaphoresis, and dizziness.

      □ Any unexpected findings should be reported to the provider.

  ○ Bladder perforation

    - Bladder perforation is a rare but possible complication.

    - Manifestations of bladder perforation include hematuria, low or no urine output, suprapubic pain and/or distention, symptoms of cystitis, and fever.

    - Nursing Actions – If a bladder perforation is suspected, notify the provider immediately.

    - Client Education – Inform the client to report manifestations of bladder perforation as described above.

  ○ Peritonitis

    - Peritonitis can occur as a result of injury to the intestines during needle insertion. Manifestations of peritonitis include sharp, constant abdominal pain, fever, nausea, vomiting, and diminished or absent bowel sounds.

    - Nursing Actions – Notify the provider immediately.

    - Client Education – Inform the client to report findings listed above.

Bariatric Surgeries

- Bariatric surgeries are a treatment for morbid obesity when other weight control methods have failed.

  - Bariatric surgeries reduce the functional size of the stomach (vertical banded gastroplasty). This is the least common type of bariatric surgery due to the risk of complications.

  - There are several surgical procedures that can be done laparoscopically.

    - Vertical banded gastroplasty involves stapling a portion of the stomach to decrease its functional size.

    - Adjustable banded gastroplasty involves constricting the functional size of the stomach.

    - Intestinal bypass includes bypassing the stomach and part of the small intestine to decrease the absorption of nutrients and calories.

      - This surgery involves removal of a portion of the stomach and creating a pouch or sleeve with the remaining portion (sleeve gastrectomy).

      - Sleeve gastrectomy may be used as a first step in weight loss. If needed, the client may then have a second surgery to complete the intestinal bypass.

  - Some procedures combine more than one of these approaches.

  - Many clients will undergo plastic surgery to remove excess skin following weight loss.

> **M** View Images
> › Vertical Banded Gastroplasty   › Adjustable Band Gastroplasty
> › Intestinal Bypass

- Indications

  - Diagnosis – History of morbid obesity

  - Client Presentation – BMI greater than 40, or BMI greater than 35 with comorbidities

- Preprocedure

  - Nursing Actions

    - Encourage client to express emotions about eating behaviors, weight, and weight loss to identify psychosocial factors related to obesity.

    - Ensure that the client understands changes to diet and lifestyle that are needed.

    - Prepare the client for postoperative course and potential complications.

    - Arrange for availability of a bariatric bed and mechanical lifting devices to prevent client/staff injury.

- Postprocedure

  - Nursing Actions

    - Monitor for leak of anastomosis (increasing back, shoulder, abdominal pain; restlessness; tachycardia; oliguria) and notify the provider immediately. This is a life-threatening emergency.

    - Notify the provider for suspected nasogastric (NG) tube displacement. The NG tube is typically sutured in place following stomach surgery; do not attempt to manipulate the tube.

    - Provide postoperative care and prevent postoperative complications.

- Monitor for the development of postoperative complications that are at increased risk due to obesity (atelectasis, thromboemboli, incisional hernia, peritonitis).
- Assess the airway and oxygen saturation per facility protocol. Maintain the client in a semi-Fowler's position for lung expansion.
- Monitor bowel sounds.
- Apply an abdominal binder as prescribed to prevent dehiscence if there is an abdominal incision.
- Ambulate the client as soon as possible.
- Resume fluids as prescribed. The first fluids may be restricted to 30 mL and increased in frequency and volume.
- Provide six small meals a day when the client can resume oral nutrients. Observe for indications of dumping syndrome (cramps, diarrhea, tachycardia, dizziness, fatigue).

- Collaborate with case management and mental health resources to assist with long-term behavior modification.
  - ○ Client Education
    - Instruct the client on limitations regarding liquids or pureed foods for the first 6 weeks, as well as the volume that can be consumed (often not to exceed 1 cup).
    - Client is instructed to walk daily for at least 30 min.
    - Remind the client that overeating can dilate the surgically created pouch causing weight to be regained.
    - Instruct the client to take vitamin and mineral supplements.
- Complications
  - ○ Dehydration
    - Warn the client that excessive thirst or concentrated urine may be an indication of dehydration and the surgeon should be notified.
    - Work with the client to establish goals and schedule for adequate daily fluid intake.
  - ○ Malabsorption/malnutrition
    - Because bariatric surgeries reduce the size of the stomach or bypass portions of the intestinal tract, fewer nutrients will be ingested and absorbed.
    - Nursing Actions
      - □ Monitor the client's tolerance of increasing amounts of food and fluids.
      - □ Refer the client for dietary management.
    - Client Education
      - □ Tell the client to eat two servings of protein a day.
      - □ Tell the client to eat only nutrition-dense foods. Avoid empty calories, such as colas and fruit juice drinks.

Nasogastric Decompression

- Clients who have an intestinal obstruction require NG decompression. An NG tube is inserted, then suction is applied to relieve abdominal distention. Treatment continues until the obstruction resolves or is removed. The obstruction can be mechanical (tumors, adhesions, fecal impaction) or functional (paralytic ileus).
- Indications
  - Diagnoses – Any disorder that causes a mechanical or functional intestinal obstruction
  - Client Presentation
    - Vomiting (begins with stomach contents and continues until fecal material is also being regurgitated)
    - Bowel sounds may be absent (paralytic ileus) or hyperactive and high-pitched (obstruction).
    - Intermittent, colicky abdominal pain and distention; hiccups
- Preprocedure
  - Nursing Actions – Gather necessary equipment and supplies.
  - Client Education – Instruct the client on the purpose of the NG tube and the client's role in its placement.
- Postprocedure
  - Nursing Actions
    - Assess and maintain proper function of the NG tube and suction equipment.
    - Maintain accurate I&O.
    - Assess bowel sounds and abdominal girth; return of flatus.
    - Monitor tube for displacement (decrease in drainage, increased nausea, vomiting, distention).
  - Client Education – Instruct the client to maintain NPO status.
- Complications
  - Fluid/electrolyte imbalance
  - Skin breakdown
    - Nursing Actions
      - Monitor for fluid and electrolyte imbalance (metabolic acidosis – low obstruction; alkalosis – high obstruction).
      - Monitor I&O, observing for discrepancies.
      - Assess nasal skin for irritation.

Ostomies

- An ostomy is a surgical opening from the inside of the body to the outside and can be located in various areas of the body. Ostomies can be permanent or temporary.
  - A stoma is the artificial opening created during the ostomy surgery.
  - The main types of ostomies performed in the abdominal area
    - Ileostomy – a surgical opening into the ileum to drain stool
    - Colostomy – a surgical opening into the large intestine to drain stool

View Images
  › Colostomy   › Healthy Stoma

- Indications
  - Diagnoses
    - Ileostomy is performed when the entire colon must be removed due to disease (Crohn's disease).
    - Colostomy is performed when a portion of the bowel must be removed (cancer, ischemic injury) or requires rest for healing (diverticulitis, trauma).

ILEOSTOMY	TRANSVERSE COLOSTOMY	SIGMOID COLOSTOMY
Normal postoperative output		
› Less than 1,000 mL/day › May be bile-colored and liquid	› Small semi-liquid with some mucus 2 to 3 days after surgery › Blood may be present in the first few days after surgery	› Small to moderate amount of mucus with semi-formed stool 4 to 5 days after surgery
Postoperative changes in output		
› After several days to weeks, the output will decrease to approximately 500 to 1,000 mL/day › Becomes more paste-like as the small intestine assumes the absorptive function of the large intestine	› After several days to weeks, output will become more stool-like, semi-formed, or formed	› After several days to weeks, output will resemble semi-formed stool
Pattern of output		
› Continuous output	› Resumes a pattern similar to the preoperative pattern	› Resumes a pattern similar to the preoperative pattern

- Preprocedure
  - Nursing Actions – Determine the client's readiness for the procedure. Assess visual acuity, manual dexterity, cognitive status, cultural influences, and support systems.
  - Client Education – Instruct the client and a support person regarding care and management of an ostomy.
- Postprocedure
  - Nursing Actions
    - Assess the type and fit of the ostomy appliance. Monitor for leakage (risk to skin integrity). Fit the ostomy appliance based on:
      - Type and location of the ostomy
      - Visual acuity and manual dexterity of the client
    - Assess peristomal skin integrity and appearance of the stoma. The stoma should appear pink and moist.
    - Apply skin barriers and creams (adhesive paste) to peristomal skin and allow to dry before applying a new appliance.
    - Evaluate stoma output. Output should be more liquid and more acidic the closer the ostomy is to the proximal small intestine.
    - Empty the ostomy bag when it is ¼ to ½ full of drainage.
    - Assess for fluid and electrolyte imbalances, particularly with a new ileostomy.

- ○ Client Education
  - ▪ Educate the client regarding dietary changes and ostomy appliances that can help manage flatus and odor.
    - ▫ Foods that can cause odor include fish, eggs, asparagus, garlic, beans, and dark green leafy vegetables.
    - ▫ Foods that can cause gas include dark green leafy vegetables, beer, carbonated beverages, dairy products, and corn. Yogurt can be ingested to decrease gas.
    - ▫ After an ostomy involving the small intestine is placed, the client should be instructed to avoid high-fiber foods for the first 2 months after surgery, chew food well, increase fluid intake, and evaluate for evidence of blockage when slowly adding high-fiber foods to the diet.
    - ▫ Proper appliance fit and maintenance prevent odor when pouch is not open. Filters, deodorizers, or placement of a breath mint in the pouch can minimize odor while the pouch is open.

  - ▪ Provide opportunities for the client to discuss feelings about the ostomy and concerns about its impact on the client's life. Encourage the client to look at and touch the stoma.
  - ▪ Refer the client to a local ostomy support group.
- • Complications
  - ○ Stomal ischemia/necrosis
    - ▪ The stomal appearance should normally be pink or red and moist.
      - ▫ Signs of stomal ischemia are pale pink or bluish/purple in color and dry in appearance.
      - ▫ If the stoma appears black or purple in color, this indicates a serious impairment of blood flow and requires immediate intervention.
    - ▪ Nursing Actions – Obtain vital signs, oxygen saturation, and current laboratory results. Notify the provider or surgeon of unexpected findings.
    - ▪ Client Education – Teach the client to watch for indications of stomal ischemia/necrosis.
  - ○ Intestinal obstruction can occur for a variety of reasons.
    - ▪ Nursing Actions
      - ▫ Monitor and record output from the stoma.
      - ▫ Assess for manifestations of obstruction, including abdominal pain, hypoactive or absent bowel sounds, distention, nausea, and vomiting. Notify the surgeon of unexpected findings.
    - ▪ Client Education – Note indications of an intestinal obstruction following discharge.

APPLICATION EXERCISES

1. A nurse is caring for a client who had a paracentesis. Which of the following findings indicate the bowel was perforated during the procedure?

    A. Client report of upper chest pain

    B. Decreased urine output

    C. Pallor

    D. Temperature elevation

2. A nurse is providing care to a client who is 1 day postoperative paracentesis. The nurse observes clear, pale-yellow fluid leaking from the operative site. Which of the following is an appropriate nursing intervention?

    A. Place a clean towel near the drainage site.

    B. Apply a dry, sterile dressing.

    C. Attach an ostomy bag.

    D. Place the client in a supine position.

3. A nurse is planning care for a client who has a new prescription for total parenteral nutrition (TPN). Which of the following interventions should be included in the plan of care? (Select all that apply.)

    _____ A. Obtain a capillary blood glucose four times daily.

    _____ B. Administer prescribed medications through a secondary port on the TPN IV tubing.

    _____ C. Monitor vital signs three times during the 12-hr shift.

    _____ D. Change the TPN IV tubing every 24 hr.

    _____ E. Ensure a daily aPTT is obtained.

4. A nurse is completing discharge teaching with a client who is 3 days postoperative for a transverse colostomy. Which of the following should be included in the teaching?

    A. Mucus will be present in stool for 5 to 7 days after surgery.

    B. Expect 500 to 1,000 mL of semi-liquid stool after 2 weeks.

    C. Stoma should be moist and pink.

    D. Change the ostomy bag when it is ¾ full.

5. A nurse is caring for a client who is receiving TPN solution. It has been 24 hr since the current bag of solution was hung, and 400 mL remains to infuse. Which of the following is the appropriate action for the nurse to take?

   A. Remove the current bag and hang a new bag.

   B. Infuse the remaining solution at the current rate and then hang a new bag.

   C. Increase the infusion rate so the remaining solution is administered within the hour and hang a new bag.

   D. Remove the current bag and hang a bag of lactated Ringer's solution.

6. A nurse educator is reviewing care of a client having bariatric surgery with a group of newly hired nurses. What should be included in this discussion? Use the ATI Active Learning Template: Therapeutic Procedure to complete this to include the following sections.

   A. Description of Procedure: Describe three types of bariatric surgery.

   B. Nursing Interventions: Describe at least five, to include equipment needed to promote client/staff safety.

   C. Client Education: Describe postoperative pattern of food and fluid consumption.

APPLICATION EXERCISES KEY

1. A. INCORRECT: A report of sharp, constant abdominal pain is associated with bowel perforation.

    B. INCORRECT: Decreased urine output is associated with bladder perforation during a paracentesis.

    C. INCORRECT: Pallor is not a finding indicating bowel perforation.

    D. **CORRECT:** Fever is an indication of bowel perforation during a paracentesis.

     NCLEX® Connection: Reduction of Risk Potential, Potential for Complications of Diagnostic Tests/Treatments/Procedures

2. A. INCORRECT: Sterile dressings should be applied to the operative site to prevent infection and allow for assessment of drainage.

    B. **CORRECT:** Application of a sterile dressing will contain the drainage and allow continuous assessment of color and quantity.

    C. INCORRECT: Application of an ostomy bag is not appropriate and does not allow for assessment of ongoing drainage.

    D. INCORRECT: The client should be placed with the head of the bed elevated to promote lung expansion.

     NCLEX® Connection: Reduction of Risk Potential, Therapeutic Procedures

3. A. **CORRECT:** The client is at risk for hyperglycemia during the administration of TPN and may require supplemental insulin.

    B. INCORRECT: No other medications or fluids should be administered through the same IV tubing being used to administer TPN due to the increased risk of infection and disruption of the rate of TPN infusion.

    C. **CORRECT:** Vital signs are recommended every 4 to 8 hr to assess for fluid volume excess and infection.

    D. **CORRECT:** It is recommended to change the IV tubing that is used to administer TPN every 24 hr.

    E. INCORRECT: The aPTT measures the coagulability of the blood, which is unnecessary during the administration of TPN.

     NCLEX® Connection: Pharmacological and Parenteral Therapies, Total Parenteral Nutrition (TPN)

4. A. INCORRECT: Mucus and blood may be present for 2 to 3 days after surgery.

    B. INCORRECT: Output should become stool-like, semi-formed, or formed within days to weeks.

    C. **CORRECT:** A pink, moist stoma is an expected finding with a transverse colostomy.

    D. INCORRECT: The ostomy bag should be changed when it is ¼ to ½ full.

     NCLEX® Connection: Pharmacological and Parenteral Therapies, Total Parenteral Nutrition (TPN)

5. A. **CORRECT:** The current bag of TPN should not hang more than 24 hr due to the risk of infection.

   B. INCORRECT: The current bag of TPN should not hang more than 24 hr due to the risk of infection.

   C. INCORRECT: The rate of infusion of TPN infusion should never be increased abruptly due to the risk of hyperglycemia.

   D. INCORRECT: Administration of TPN should never be discontinued abruptly due to the sudden change in blood glucose that can occur.

   Ⓝ NCLEX® Connection: Physiological Adaptations, Alterations in Body Systems

6. *Using the ATI Active Learning Template: Therapeutic Procedure*

   A. Description of Procedure
      • Vertical banded gastroplasty involves stapling a portion of the stomach to decrease its functional size.
      • Adjustable banded gastroplasty involves constricting the functional size of the stomach.
      • Intestinal bypass involves bypassing the stomach and part of the small intestine to decrease the absorption of nutrients and calories.

   B. Nursing Interventions
      • Encourage client to express emotions related to weight, weight loss, and eating behaviors to identify related psychosocial concerns.
      • Ensure the client understands required dietary and lifestyle changes.
      • Arrange for availability of a bariatric bed and mechanical lifting device to prevent client/staff injury.
      • Monitor for leak of anastomosis and notify provider immediately if this occurs.
      • Assess airway and oxygen saturation. Maintain client in semi-Fowler's position for lung expansion.
      • Monitor bowel sounds.
      • Apply abdominal binder if prescribed.
      • Ambulate client as soon as possible.
      • Monitor intake and output.
      • Monitor NG tube placement and function, as well as function of suction equipment.

   C. Client Education
      • Fluids will be allowed beginning with 30 mL and gradually increase in volume and frequency.
      • Food will be allowed beginning with six small meals.
      • Volume may be limited to 1 cup of liquid or pureed foods.

   Ⓝ NCLEX® Connection: Reduction of Risk Potential, Therapeutic Procedures

chapter 48

Overview

- The esophagus is a tube that consists of smooth muscle and leads from the throat to the stomach. Esophageal disorders can affect any part of the esophagus.

- There are two sphincters (upper esophageal [UES], lower esophageal [LES]) that prevent the reflux of food and fluids into the mouth or esophagus.

> **M**   View Image: Esophageal Sphincters

- Contractions of the esophagus propel food and fluids toward the stomach, while relaxation of the lower esophageal sphincter allows them to pass into the stomach.

- Esophageal disorders that nurses should be knowledgeable about include:

  - Gastroesophageal reflux disease (GERD)

  - Esophageal varices

GERD

Overview

- Gastroesophageal reflux disease (GERD) is a common condition characterized by gastric content and enzyme backflow into the esophagus. These corrosive fluids irritate the esophageal tissue, causing delay in their clearance. This further exposes esophageal tissue to the acidic fluids, causing more irritation.

- The primary treatment of GERD is diet and lifestyle changes, advancing to medication use (antacids, H_2-receptor antagonists, proton pump inhibitors) and surgery.

- Untreated GERD leads to inflammation, breakdown, and long-term complications, including adenocarcinoma of the esophagus.

Health Promotion and Disease Prevention

- Maintain a weight below BMI of 30.

- Stop smoking.

- Limit or avoid alcohol and tobacco use.

Assessment

- Risk Factors
  - Obesity
  - Older age (delayed gastric emptying and weakened LES tone)
  - Sleep apnea
  - Nasogastric tube
  - Contributing factors
    - Excessive ingestion of foods that relax the LES include fatty and fried foods, chocolate, caffeinated beverages (coffee), peppermint, spicy foods, tomatoes, citrus fruits, and alcohol
    - Prolonged or frequent abdominal distention (from overeating or delayed emptying)
    - Increased abdominal pressure from obesity, pregnancy, bending at the waist, ascites, or tight clothing at the waist
    - Medications that relax the LES (theophylline, nitrates, calcium channel blockers, anticholinergics, and diazepam [Valium])
    - Increased gastric acid caused by medications (NSAIDs) or stress (environmental)
    - Debilitation resulting in weakened LES tone
    - Hiatal hernia (LES displacement into the thorax with delayed esophageal clearance)
    - Lying flat
- Subjective Data
  - Classic report of: dyspepsia after eating an offending food or fluid, and regurgitation.
  - Pain is "wavelike" and may radiate (neck, jaw, or back). The client reports feeling of having a heart attack.
  - Pain worsens with position (bending, straining, laying down).
  - Pain occurs after eating and may last 20 min to 2 hr.
  - Throat irritation (chronic cough, laryngitis), hypersalivation, bitter taste in mouth (caused by regurgitation). Chronic GERD can lead to dysphagia.
  - Atypical chest pain (from esophageal spasm).
  - Increased flatus and eructation (burping).
  - Pain is relieved (almost immediately) by drinking water, sitting upright, or taking antacids.
  - Manifestations occurring four to five times per week on a consistent basis are considered diagnostic.
- Objective Data
  - Physical Assessment Findings
    - Tooth erosion
    - Hoarseness
  - Diagnostic Procedures
    - Esophagogastroduodenoscopy (EGD) is done under moderate sedation to observe for tissue damage (present in 60% of clients who have GERD) and possibly to dilate structures.
      - EGD allows visualization of the esophagus, revealing esophagitis or Barrett's epithelium (premalignant cells).
      - Nursing Actions: Verify gag response has returned prior to providing oral fluids or food following the procedure.

- 24-hr ambulatory esophageal pH monitoring – A small catheter is placed through the nose and into the distal esophagus, where pH readings are taken in relation to food, position, and activity.

    □ Most accurate method of diagnosing GERD.

    □ Especially helpful in diagnosis for clients who have atypical manifestations.

    □ Nursing Actions: Instruct client to keep a journal of foods and beverages consumed as well as activity during the 24-hr test period.

- Esophageal manometry records lower esophageal sphincter pressure.

    □ Nursing Actions: Instruct the client to keep a diary of manifestations related to food, position, and activity throughout the day.

- Barium swallow to identify a hiatal hernia, which would contribute to or cause GERD.

Patient-Centered Care

- Medications
    - Antacids
        - Antacids (aluminum hydroxide [Mylanta]) neutralize excess acid.
        - Nursing Considerations – Ensure there are no contraindications with other prescribed medications (levothyroxine).
        - Client Education – Instruct the client to take antacids when acid secretion is the highest (1 to 3 hr after eating and at bedtime), and to separate from other medications by at least 1 hr.
    - Histamine$_2$ Receptor Antagonists
        - Histamine$_2$ receptor antagonists (ranitidine [Zantac], famotidine [Pepcid], nizatidine [Axid]) reduce the secretion of acid. The onset is longer than antacids, but the effect has a longer duration.
            □ Cimetidine (Tagamet) is no longer first-line as it has a higher risk profile in older adult clients and interacts with more than 60 other medications.
        - Nursing Considerations – Use cautiously in clients who have kidney disease.
        - Client Education
            □ Take with meals and at bedtime.
            □ Do not mix nizatidine (Axid) with vegetable-based juices.
    - Proton Pump Inhibitors (PPIs)
        - PPIs (pantoprazole [Protonix], omeprazole [Prilosec], esomeprazole [Nexium], and lansoprazole [Prevacid]) reduce gastric acid by inhibiting the cellular pump necessary for gastric acid secretion.
        - Nursing Considerations – Sustained release capsules may be opened and sprinkled on food or mixed with applesauce (clients who have swallowing difficulty) or mixed with juice (for clients who have an NG tube).
        - Client Education – Clients who are prescribed rabeprazole (Aciphex) should wear sunscreen daily.
    - Prokinetics
        - Prokinetic medications (metoclopramide hydrochloride [Reglan]) increase the motility of the esophagus and stomach.
        - Nursing Considerations – Monitor the client for extrapyramidal side effects.
        - Client Education – Instruct the client to report abnormal, involuntary movement.

- Therapeutic Procedures – Stretta procedure uses radiofrequency energy, applied by an endoscope, to decrease vagus nerve activity. This causes the LES muscle tissue to contract and tighten.
- Surgical Interventions
  - Fundoplication may be indicated for clients who fail to respond to other treatments. The fundus of the stomach is wrapped around and behind the esophagus through a laparoscope to create a physical barrier.
  - Client Education
    - Diet
      - Avoid offending foods.
      - Avoid large meals.
      - Remain upright after eating.
      - Avoid eating before bedtime.
    - Lifestyle
      - Avoid clothing that is tight-fitting around the abdomen.
      - Lose weight, if applicable.
      - Elevate the head of the bed 15.2 to 20.3 cm (6 to 8 in) with blocks. The use of pillows is not recommended because this rounds the back, bringing the stomach contents up and closer to the chest.
      - Sleep on the right side.

Complications

- Aspiration of gastric secretion
  - Causes
    - Reflux of gastric fluids into the esophagus can be aspirated into the trachea.
    - Risks associated with aspiration include:
      - Asthma exacerbations from inhaled aerosolized acid.
      - Frequent upper respiratory, sinus, or ear infections.
      - Aspiration pneumonia.
- Barrett's epithelium (premalignant) and esophageal adenocarcinoma.
  - Cause – Reflux of gastric fluids leads to esophagitis. In chronic esophagitis, the body continuously heals inflamed tissue, eventually replacing normal esophageal epithelium with premalignant tissue (Barrett's epithelium) or malignant adenocarcinoma.
  - Nursing Actions – Determine the cause of GERD with the client and review lifestyle changes that can decrease gastric reflux.

ESOPHAGEAL VARICES

Overview

- Esophageal varices are swollen, fragile blood vessels in the esophagus.

 View Image: Varices

- When esophageal varices hemorrhage, it is often a medical emergency associated with a high mortality rate. Reoccurrence of esophageal bleeding is common.

Health Promotion and Disease Prevention

- Avoid alcohol consumption.

Assessment

- Risk Factors
  - Portal hypertension (elevated blood pressure in veins that carry blood from the intestines to the liver) is caused by impaired circulation of blood through the liver. Collateral circulation subsequently develops, creating varices in the upper stomach and esophagus. Varices are fragile and can bleed easily.
    - Portal hypertension is the primary risk factor for the development of esophageal varices.
  - Alcoholic cirrhosis.
  - Viral hepatitis.

  - Older adult clients frequently have depressed immune function, decreased liver function, and cardiac disorders that make them especially vulnerable to bleeding.
- Subjective Data
  - The client may experience no manifestations until the varices begin to bleed.
    - Hematemesis and melena
  - Activities that precipitate bleeding are the Valsalva maneuver, lifting heavy objects, coughing, sneezing, and alcohol consumption.
- Objective Data
  - Physical Assessment Findings (Bleeding Esophageal Varices)
    - Hypotension
    - Tachycardia
  - Laboratory Tests
    - Liver function tests indicate a liver disorder.
    - Hemoglobin and hematocrit tests can indicate anemia secondary to occult bleeding or overt bleeding.
  - Diagnostic Procedures
    - Endoscopy – Therapeutic interventions can be performed during the endoscopy.
      - Nursing Actions: Administer preprocedure sedation. After the procedure, monitor vital signs and take measures to prevent aspiration.

Patient-Centered Care

- Nursing Care

  - If bleeding is suspected, establish IV access with a large bore needle, monitor vital signs and hematocrit, type and crossmatch for possible blood transfusions, and monitor for overt and occult bleeding.

- Medications

  - Nonselective Beta-Blockers

    - Nonselective beta-blockers (propranolol [Inderal]) are prescribed to decrease heart rate and consequently reduce hepatic venous pressure.

    - Used prophylactically (not for emergency hemorrhage).

  - Vasoconstrictors

    - IV terlipressin (synthetic vasopressin) and natural somatostatin have been proven most effective to increase portal inflow.

    - Vasopressin (Desmopressin) and octreotide (Sandostatin) are avoided due to multiple adverse effects.

    - Nursing Considerations – Vasopressin cannot be given to clients who have coronary artery disease due to resultant coronary constriction. Potent vasoconstriction may also cause problems with peripheral and cerebral circulation.

- Teamwork and Collaboration – alcohol recovery program (varices secondary to alcohol use disorder)

- Therapeutic Procedures

  - Endoscopic injection sclerotherapy or variceal band ligation

    - Ligating bands can be placed, and/or injection sclerotherapy can be performed during an endoscopic procedure. Used only for active bleeding and not prophylactically.

    - Nursing Actions: Administer preprocedure sedation. After the procedure, monitor vital signs and take measures to prevent aspiration.

    - Sclerotherapy carries a greater risk of postoperative hemorrhage.

    - Antacids and/or H_2 receptor blockers are administered postoperatively.

  - Transjugular Intrahepatic Portal-Systemic Shunt (TIPS)

    - While the client is under sedation or general anesthesia, a catheter is passed into the liver via the jugular vein in the neck. A stent is then placed between the portal and hepatic veins bypassing the liver. Portal hypertension is subsequently relieved.

    - Nursing Actions – Monitor vital signs. Keep the head of the bed elevated.

  - Esophagogastric balloon tamponade

    - An esophagogastric tube with esophageal and gastric balloons is used to compress blood vessels in the esophagus and stomach. Traction is applied after balloons are inflated to desired pressure. When the bleeding is stopped, the traction is released and the pressure in the balloons is reduced gradually. Reserved for clients who have unsuccessful TIPS procedures. Clients are typically intubated and placed on mechanical ventilation prior to the procedure to prevent aspiration.

    - Nursing Actions

      - Check balloons for leaks prior to insertion.

      - Monitor placement of the tube and observe for possible obstruction of airway.

      - Monitor for aspiration into the lungs and secretions or blood from the esophagus.

     □ Provide oral suction as needed.

     □ Maintain balloon pressure at prescribed pressure for prescribed time to decrease risk of esophageal or gastric necrosis from ischemia.

     □ Irrigate the tube as prescribed and document color of return (clear vs. bloody).

     □ Monitor the client who has decreased mentation or confusion and who may pull on the tube.

- Surgical Interventions – considered as a last resort
  - Bypass procedures establish a venous shunt that bypasses the liver, decreasing portal hypertension.
    - Common shunts include splenorenal (splenic, left renal veins), mesocaval (mesenteric vein, vena cava), and portacaval (portal vein, inferior vena cava).
    - Clients commonly have a nasogastric tube inserted during surgery to monitor for hemorrhage.
    - Nursing Actions (pre, post)
      - □ Monitor for an increase in liver dysfunction or encephalopathy.
      - □ Monitor nasogastric tube secretions for bleeding.
      - □ Monitor PT, aPTT, platelets, and INR.

Complications

- Hypovolemic Shock – due to hemorrhage from varices
  - Nursing Actions
    - Observe for manifestations of hemorrhage and shock (tachycardia, hypotension).
    - Monitor vital signs, Hgb, Hct, and coagulation studies.
    - Replace losses and support therapeutic procedures to stop and control bleeding.

APPLICATION EXERCISES

1. A nurse is caring for a client who has a new diagnosis of gastroesophageal reflux disease (GERD). The nurse should anticipate prescriptions by the provider for which of the following medications? (Select all that apply.)

_____X_____ A. Antacids

_____X_____ B. Histamine₂ receptor antagonists

_____ C. Opioid analgesics

_____ D. Fiber laxatives

_____X_____ E. Proton pump inhibitors

2. A nurse is admitting a client who has bleeding esophageal varices. The nurse should anticipate a prescription for which of the following medications?

A. Propranolol (Inderal)

B. Metoclopramide (Reglan)

C. Ranitidine (Zantac)

D. Terlipressin (synthetic vasopressin)

3. A nurse is completing an assessment of a client who has GERD. Which of the following is an expected finding?

A. Absence of saliva

B. Loss of tooth enamel

C. Client reports sweet taste in mouth

D. Client reports absence of eructation

4. A nurse is teaching a client who has GERD. Which of the following should the client be instructed to limit in his diet? (Select all that apply.)

_____X_____ A. Coffee

_____X_____ B. Tomatoes

_____ C. Bananas

_____X_____ D. Chocolate

_____ E. Pasta

5. A nurse is completing discharge teaching to a client who is postoperative following fundoplication. Which of the following statements by the client indicates understanding of the teaching?

    A. "When sitting in my lounge chair after a meal, I will lower the back of it."

    B. "I will try to eat three large meals a day."

    C. "I will elevate the head of my bed on blocks."

    D. "When sleeping, I will lay on my left side."

6. A nurse is preparing a poster on GERD to be displayed at a community health fair. What should be included in the poster? Use the ATI Active Learning Template: Systems Disorder to complete this item to include the following sections:

    A. Description of Disorder/Disease Process

    B. Risk Factors: Describe at least eight.

    C. Subjective Data: Describe at least eight.

APPLICATION EXERCISES KEY

1. A. **CORRECT:** Antacids neutralize gastric acid which irritates the esophagus during reflux.

    B. **CORRECT:** Histamine$_2$ receptor antagonists decrease acid secretion, which contributes to reflux.

    C. INCORRECT: Opioid analgesics are not effective in treating GERD.

    D. INCORRECT: Fiber laxatives are not effective in treating GERD.

    E. **CORRECT:** Proton pump inhibitors decrease gastric acid production, which contributes to reflex.

    Ⓝ NCLEX® Connection: Physiological Adaptations, Alterations in Body Systems

2. A. INCORRECT: Propranolol is not used for clients who are actively bleeding. It may be given prophylactically to decrease portal hypertension.

    B. INCORRECT: Metoclopramide decreases motility of the esophagus and stomach.

    C. INCORRECT: Histamine$_2$-receptor antagonists are administered following surgical procedures for bleeding esophageal varices.

    D. **CORRECT:** Terlipressin constricts blood vessels and is used to treat bleeding esophageal varices.

    Ⓝ NCLEX® Connection: Physiological Adaptations, Alterations in Body Systems

3. A. INCORRECT: Hypersalivation is an expected finding in a client who has GERD.

    B. **CORRECT:** Tooth erosion is an expected finding in a client who has GERD.

    B. INCORRECT: A client who has GERD would report a bitter taste in the mouth.

    D. INCORRECT: Increased burping is an expected finding in a client who has GERD.

    Ⓝ NCLEX® Connection: Physiological Adaptations, Pathophysiology

4. A. **CORRECT:** Coffee relaxes the lower esophageal sphincter and should be avoided by a client who has GERD.

    B. **CORRECT:** Tomatoes relax the lower esophageal sphincter and should be avoided by a client who has GERD.

    C. INCORRECT: Bananas do not affect the client who has GERD and do not need to be limited.

    D. **CORRECT:** Chocolate relaxes the lower esophageal sphincter and should be avoided by a client who has GERD.

    E. INCORRECT: Pasta does not affect the client who has GERD and does not need to be limited.

    Ⓝ NCLEX® Connection: Basic Care and Comfort, Nutrition and Oral Hydration

5.   A. INCORRECT: The client is instructed to remain upright after eating following a fundoplication.

B. INCORRECT: The client is instructed to avoid large meals after a fundoplication.

C. **CORRECT:** After a fundoplication, the client is instructed to elevate the head of the bed to limit reflux.

D. INCORRECT: After a fundoplication, the client is instructed to sleep on the right side.

(N) NCLEX® Connection: Reduction of Risk Potential, Therapeutic Procedures

6.   *Using the ATI Active Learning Template: Systems Disorder*

A. Description of Disorder/Disease Process
   • Gastroesophageal reflux disease (GERD) is a common condition characterized by gastric content and enzyme backflow into the esophagus. These fluids are corrosive to esophageal tissue, causing a delay in their clearance. This further exposes esophageal tissue to the acidic fluids, increasing tissue irritation.

B. Risk Factors
   • Obesity
   • Older age
   • Sleep apnea
   • Excessive ingestion of foods that relax the lower esophageal sphincter (fatty and fried foods, chocolate, caffeinated beverages, peppermint, spicy foods, tomatoes, citrus fruits, and alcohol)
   • Pregnancy
   • Bending at the waist, wearing tight clothing at the waist
   • Medications (theophylline, nitrates, calcium channel blockers, anticholinergics, NSAIDs)
   • Stress
   • Hiatal hernia
   • Lying flat

C. Subjective Data
   • Dyspepsia after eating and regurgitation (classic)
   • Throat irritation (chronic cough, laryngitis)
   • Hypersalivation
   • Bitter taste in mouth
   • Chest pain due to esophageal spasm
   • Increased flatus and eructation (burping)
   • Pain relieved by drinking water, sitting upright or taking antacids

(N) NCLEX® Connection: Health Promotion and Maintenance, Health Promotion/Disease Prevention

chapter 49

Overview

- A peptic ulcer is an erosion of the mucosal lining of the stomach or duodenum. The mucous membranes can become eroded to the point that the epithelium is exposed to gastric acid and pepsin, which can precipitate bleeding and perforation. Perforation that extends through all the layers of the stomach or duodenum can cause peritonitis. An individual who has a peptic ulcer has peptic ulcer disease (PUD).
- There are gastric ulcers, duodenal ulcers, and stress ulcers (which occur after major stress or trauma).

Health Promotion and Disease Prevention

- Drink alcohol in moderation.
- Stop smoking and use of tobacco products.
- Use stress management techniques.
- Avoid NSAIDS as indicated.
- Limit caffeine-containing beverages.

Assessment

- Risk Factors
  - Causes of peptic ulcers:
    - *Helicobacter pylori (H. pylori)* infection
    - Nonsteroidal anti-inflammatory drug (NSAID) and corticosteroid use
    - Severe stress
    - Hypersecretory states
    - Type O blood
    - Excess alcohol ingestion
    - Chronic pulmonary or kidney disease
    - Zollinger-Ellison syndrome (combination of peptic ulcers, hypersecretion of gastric acid, and gastrin secreting tumors)
- Subjective Data
  - Dyspepsia – heartburn, bloating, nausea, and vomiting (may be perceived as uncomfortable fullness or hunger)
  - Pain

GASTRIC ULCER	DUODENAL ULCER
30 to 60 min after a meal	1.5 to 3 hr after a meal.
Rarely occurs at night	Often occurs at night.
Pain exacerbated by ingestion of food	Pain may be relieved by ingestion of food or antacid.

- Objective Data

  ○ Physical Assessment Findings

    ▪ Epigastric pain upon palpation. Pain that radiates to the back may indicate perforation is imminent. May be left upper epigastrium (gastric) or right epigastrium (duodenal).

    ▪ Bloody emesis (hematemesis) or stools (melena).

    ▪ Weight loss.

  ○ Laboratory Tests

    ▪ *H. pylori* testing

      □ Gastric samples are collected via an endoscopy to test for *H. pylori*.

      □ C 13 urea breath testing is when the client exhales into a collection container (baseline), drinks carbon-enriched urea solution, and is asked to exhale into a collection container. The client should take nothing by mouth (NPO) prior to the test. If *H. pylori* is present, the solution will break down and carbon dioxide will be released. The two collections are compared to confirm the presence of *H. pylori*.

      □ IgG serologic testing documents the presence of *H. pylori* based on antibody assays.

      □ Stool sample tests for the presence of the *H. pylori* antigen.

    ▪ Hemoglobin and hematocrit (unexpected findings secondary to bleeding)

    ▪ Stool sample for occult blood

  ○ Diagnostic Procedures

    ▪ Esophagogastroduodenoscopy (EGD) – refer to the chapter on *Gastrointestinal Diagnostic Procedures*

      □ An EGD provides a definitive diagnosis of peptic ulcers and may be repeated to evaluate the effectiveness of treatment. Gastric samples are obtained to test for *H. pylori*.

      □ Nursing Actions – Medications (bismuth, misoprostol, sucralfate, histamine$_2$ antagonists) can interfere with testing for *H. pylori* (false negatives). Therefore, a complete medication history should be reviewed prior to testing.

      □ Client Education – Avoid taking the medications listed above prior to the test.

Patient-Centered Care

- Nursing Care

  ○ Instruct client to avoid foods that cause distress.

  ○ Monitor for orthostatic changes in vital signs and tachycardia as these findings are suggestive of gastrointestinal bleeding.

  ○ Administer saline lavage via nasogastric tube, if prescribed.

  ○ Administer medication as prescribed.

  ○ Decrease environmental stress.

  ○ Encourage rest periods.

  ○ Encourage smoking cessation and avoiding alcohol consumption.

- Medications
  - Antibiotics: metronidazole (Flagyl), amoxicillin (Amoxil), clarithromycin (Biaxin), tetracycline (Achromycin V)
    - Eliminate *H. pylori* infection.
    - Nursing Considerations – A combination of two to three different antibiotics may be administered.
    - Client Education – Instruct the client to complete a full course of medication.
  - Histamine$_2$-receptor antagonists: ranitidine hydrochloride (Zantac), famotidine (Pepcid)
    - Suppress the secretion of gastric acid by selectively blocking H$_2$ receptors in parietal cells lining the stomach.
    - Used in conjunction with antibiotics to treat ulcers caused by *H. pylori*.
    - Used to prevent stress ulcers in clients who are NPO after major surgery, have large areas of burns, are septic, or have increased intracranial pressure.
    - Nursing Considerations
      - Ranitidine and famotidine can be administered IV in acute situations.
      - Ranitidine can be taken with or without food.
      - Treatment of peptic ulcer disease is usually started as an oral dose twice a day until the ulcer is healed, followed by a maintenance dose usually taken once a day at bedtime.
    - Client Education – Instruct clients to notify the provider of obvious or occult GI bleeding (coffee-ground emesis).
  - Proton pump inhibitors: pantoprazole (Protonix), esomeprazole (Nexium)
    - Reduce gastric acid secretion by irreversibly inhibiting the enzyme that produces gastric acid.
    - Reduce basal and stimulated acid production.
    - Nursing Considerations – Insignificant side/adverse effects with short-term treatment.
    - Client Education
      - Instruct the client not to crush, chew, or break sustained-release capsules.
      - Instruct the client to take omeprazole once a day prior to eating in the morning.
      - Encourage the client to avoid alcohol and irritating medications (NSAIDs).
  - Antacids: aluminum carbonate, magnesium hydroxide (Milk of Magnesia)
    - Antacids are given 1 to 3 hr after meals to neutralize gastric acid, which occurs with food ingestion and at bedtime.
    - Nursing Considerations – Give 1 hr apart from other medications to avoid reducing the absorption of other medications.
    - Client Education
      - Encourage compliance by reinforcing the intended effect of the antacid (relief of pain, healing of ulcer).
      - Teach clients to take all medications at least 1 hr before or after taking an antacid.
  - Mucosal protectant: sucralfate (Carafate)
    - Nursing Considerations
      - Give 1 hr before meals and at bedtime.
      - Monitor for adverse effect of constipation.

- Teamwork and Collaboration
    - Nutrition consult – diet that restricts acid-producing foods (milk products, caffeine, decaffeinated coffee, spicy foods, medications [NSAIDs])
- Therapeutic Procedures
    - Esophagogastroduodenoscopy (EGD) – Areas of bleeding may be treated with epinephrine or laser coagulation.
- Surgical Interventions
    - Gastric surgeries include:
        - Gastrectomy – All or part of the stomach is removed with laparoscopic or open approach.
            - Antrectomy – The antrum portion of the stomach is removed.
            - Gastrojejunostomy (Billroth II procedure) – The lower portion of the stomach is excised, the remaining stomach is anastomosed to the jejunum, and the remaining duodenum is surgically closed.
        - Vagotomy – A highly selective vagotomy severs only the nerve fibers that disrupt acid production. Often done laparoscopically to reduce postoperative complications.
        - Pyloroplasty – The opening between the stomach and small intestine is enlarged to increase the rate of gastric emptying.
    - Nursing Actions
        - Monitor incision for evidence of infection.
        - Place the client in a semi-Fowler's position to facilitate lung expansion.
        - Monitor nasogastric tube drainage. Scant blood may be seen in first 12 to 24 hr.
        - Notify the provider before repositioning or irrigating the nasogastric tube (disruption of sutures).
        - Monitor bowel sounds.
        - Advance diet as tolerated to avoid undesired effects (abdominal distention, diarrhea).
        - Administer medication as prescribed (analgesics, stool softeners).

    - Client Education
        - Educate the client to take vitamin and mineral supplements due to decreased absorption after a gastrectomy, including vitamin B_{12}, vitamin D, calcium, iron, and folate.
        - Consume small, frequent meals while avoiding large quantities of carbohydrates as directed.

Complications

- Perforation/Hemorrhage
  - When peptic ulcers perforate or bleed, it is an emergency situation.
    - Perforation presents as severe epigastric pain spreading across the abdomen. The abdomen is rigid, board-like, hyperactive to diminished bowel sounds, and there is rebound tenderness. Perforation is a surgical emergency.
    - Gastrointestinal bleeding in the form of hematemesis or melena may cause manifestations of shock (hypotension, tachycardia, dizziness, confusion), and decreased hemoglobin.
  - Nursing Actions
    - Perform frequent assessments of pain and vital signs to detect subtle changes that may indicate perforation or bleeding.
    - Report findings, prepare the client for endoscopic or surgical intervention, replace fluid and blood losses to maintain blood pressure, insert nasogastric tube, and provide saline lavages.
- Pernicious anemia occurs due to a deficiency of the intrinsic factor normally secreted by the gastric mucosa.
  - Manifestations include pallor, glossitis, fatigue, and paresthesias.
  - Client Education – Monthly lifelong vitamin B_{12} injections will be necessary.
- Dumping syndrome is a group of manifestations that occur following eating. A shift of fluid to the abdomen is triggered by rapid gastric emptying or high-carbohydrate ingestion.
  - In response to the sudden influx of a hypertonic fluid, the small intestine pulls fluid from the extracellular space to convert the hypertonic fluid to an isotonic fluid. This fluid shift causes a decrease in circulating volume, resulting in vasomotor symptoms (syncope, pallor, palpitations, dizziness, headache).
  - Gastric surgery, especially gastrojejunostomy (Billroth II), poses the greatest risk for dumping syndrome. Following gastric surgery, the reduced stomach has less ability to control the amount and rate of chyme that enters the small intestine after a meal.
  - Nursing Actions
    - Monitor for vasomotor manifestations:

	EARLY MANIFESTATIONS	LATE MANIFESTATIONS
Onset	Within 30 min after eating	1.5 to 3 hr after eating
Cause	› Rapid emptying	› Excessive insulin release
Symptoms	› Nausea, vomiting, and dizziness › Tachycardia › Palpitations	› Hunger, dizziness, and sweating › Tachycardia and palpitations › Shakiness and feelings of anxiety › Confusion

- Assist/instruct the client to lie down when vasomotor manifestations occur.
- Administer medications.
  - Administration of powdered pectin or octreotide (Sandostatin) subcutaneously may be prescribed if manifestations are severe and not effectively controlled with dietary measures. Pectin slows the absorption of carbohydrates. Octreotide blocks gastric and pancreatic hormones, which can lead to findings of dumping syndrome.
  - Antispasmodic medications (dicyclomine [Bentyl]).
  - Acarbose (Prandase) slows the absorption of carbohydrates.
  - Malnutrition and fluid electrolyte imbalances may occur due to altered absorption. Monitor intake and output, laboratory values, and weight.
- Client Education
  - Lying down after a meal slows the movement of food within the intestines.
  - Limit the amount of fluid ingested at one time.
  - Eliminate liquids with meals, for 1 hr prior to, and following a meal.
  - Consume a high-protein, high-fat, low-fiber, and low- to moderate-carbohydrate diet.
  - Avoid milk, sweets, or sugars (fruit juice, sweetened fruit, milk shakes, honey, syrup, jelly).
  - Consume small, frequent meals rather than large meals.

APPLICATION EXERCISES

1. A nurse in the emergency department is completing an assessment of a client who has suspected stomach perforation due to a peptic ulcer. Which of the following are expected findings? (Select all that apply.)

___X___ A. Rigid abdomen

___X___ B. Tachycardia

_____ C. Elevated blood pressure

_____ D. Circumoral cyanosis

___X___ E. Rebound tenderness

2. A nurse is providing teaching for a client who has a new diagnosis of dumping syndrome following gastric surgery. Which of the following should be included in the teaching?

A. Eat three moderate-sized meals a day.

B. Drink at least one glass of water with each meal.

C. Eat a bedtime snack that contains a milk product.

D. Increase protein in the diet.

3. A nurse is teaching a client who has a duodenal ulcer and a new prescription for esomeprazole (Nexium). Which of the following should be included in the teaching? (Select all that apply.)

___X___ A. Take the medication 1 hr before a meal.

___X___ B. Limit NSAIDs when taking this medication.

_____ C. Expect skin flushing when taking this medication.

_____ D. Increase fiber intake when taking this medication.

_____ E. Chew the medication thoroughly before swallowing.

4. A nurse is completing discharge teaching for a client who has an infection due to *Helicobacter pylori* (*H. pylori*). Which of the following statements by the client indicates understanding of the teaching?

A. "I will continue my prescription for corticosteroids."

B. "I will schedule a CT scan to monitor improvement."

C. "I will take a combination of medications for treatment."

D. "I will have my throat swabbed to recheck for this bacteria."

5. A nurse is completing an assessment of a client who has a gastric ulcer. Which of the following are expected findings? (Select all that apply.)

_____ A. Client reports pain relieved by eating.

_____ B. Client states that pain often occurs at night.

__✗__ C. Client reports a sensation of bloating.

__✗__ D. Client states that pain occurs ½ to 1 hr after a meal.

__✗__ E. Client experiences pain upon palpation of the epigastric region.

6. A nurse is preparing a poster about peptic ulcer disease to be displayed at a community health fair. What should be included in the poster? Use the ATI Active Learning Template: Systems Disorder to complete this item to include the following sections:

A. Description of Disorder/Disease Process: Include the types of ulcers.

B. Client Education:
   - Describe at least three prevention activities.
   - Describe four risk factors for peptic ulcers.

APPLICATION EXERCISES KEY

1. A. **CORRECT:** Manifestations of perforation include a rigid, board-like abdomen.

    B. **CORRECT:** Tachycardia occurs due to gastrointestinal bleeding that accompanies a perforation.

    C. INCORRECT: Hypotension is an expected finding in a client who has a perforation and bleeding.

    D. INCORRECT: Circumoral cyanosis is not a manifestation of perforation.

    E. **CORRECT:** Rebound tenderness is an expected finding in a client who has a perforation.

    (N) NCLEX® Connection: Physiological Adaptations, Unexpected Response to Therapies

2. A. INCORRECT: The client should consume small, frequent meals rather than moderate-sized meals.

    B. INCORRECT: The client should eliminate liquids with meals and for 1 hr prior to and following meals.

    C. INCORRECT: The client should avoid milk products.

    D. **CORRECT:** The client should eat a high-protein, high-fat, low-fiber, and moderate- to low-carbohydrate diet.

    (N) NCLEX® Connection: Basic Care and Comfort, Nutrition and Oral Hydration

3. A. **CORRECT:** The client is instructed to take the medication 1 hr before meals.

    B. **CORRECT:** The client is instructed to limit taking NSAIDs when on this medication.

    C. INCORRECT: Skin flushing is not an adverse effect of this medication.

    D. INCORRECT: Fiber intake does not need to be increased when taking this medication.

    E. INCORRECT: The client is instructed to swallow the capsule whole. It should not be crushed or chewed.

    (N) NCLEX® Connection: Pharmacological and Parenteral Therapies, Medication Administration

4.   A. INCORRECT: Corticosteroid use is a contributing factor to an infection caused by *H. pylori*.

   B. INCORRECT: An esophagogastroduodenoscopy (EGD) is done to evaluate for the presence of *H. pylori* and to evaluate effectiveness of treatment.

   C. **CORRECT:** A combination of antibiotics and a histamine₂ receptor antagonist is used to treat an infection caused by *H. pylori*.

   D. INCORRECT: *H. pylori* is evaluated by obtaining gastric samples, not a throat swab.

   Ⓝ NCLEX® Connection: Physiological Adaptations, Alterations in Body Systems

5.   A. INCORRECT: A client who has a duodenal ulcer will report that pain is relieved by eating.

   B. INCORRECT: Pain that rarely occurs at night is an expected finding.

   C. **CORRECT:** A client report of a bloating sensation is an expected finding.

   D. **CORRECT:** A client who has a gastric ulcer will often report pain 30 to 60 min after a meal.

   E. **CORRECT:** Pain in the epigastric region upon palpation is an expected finding.

   Ⓝ NCLEX® Connection: Physiological Adaptations, Pathophysiology

6.   *Using the ATI Active Learning Template: Systems Disorder*

   A. Description of Disorder/Disease Process
   - An erosion of the mucosal lining of the stomach or duodenum. Mucous membranes can become eroded to the point that the epithelium is exposed to gastric acid and pepsin, which can precipitate bleeding and perforation. Types of ulcers include gastric, duodenal, and stress ulcers.

   B. Client Education
   - Prevention Activities
     - Drink alcohol in moderation.
     - Stop smoking and use of tobacco products.
     - Use stress management strategies.
     - Avoid NSAIDs.
     - Limit caffeine-containing beverages.
   - Risk Factors
     - *Helicobacter pylori (H. pylori)*
     - NSAID and corticosteroid use
     - Severe stress
     - Hypersecretory conditions
     - Blood type O
     - Excess alcohol ingestion
     - Chronic pulmonary or kidney disease
     - Zollinger-Ellison syndrome

   Ⓝ NCLEX® Connection: Health Promotion and Maintenance, Health Promotion/Disease Prevention

CHAPTER 50   Acute and Chronic Gastritis

Overview

- Cox 1 enzymes produce mucosal prostaglandins that form a protective layer over the lining of the stomach.
- Gastritis is an inflammation in the lining of the stomach.

 View Image: *H. pylori* Gastritis

- Acute gastritis has sudden onset, is of short duration, and may result in gastric bleeding if severe.
- Chronic gastritis has a slow onset and, if profuse, may damage parietal cells resulting in pernicious anemia.
- Extensive gastric mucosal wall damage may cause erosive gastritis (ulcers) and increase the risk of stomach cancer.

Health Promotion and Disease Prevention

- Follow a prescribed diet.
- Watch for indications of GI bleeding.
- Follow the prescribed medication regimen.
- Eat small, frequent meals, avoiding foods and beverages that cause irritation.
- Report constipation, nausea, vomiting, or bloody stools.
- Stop smoking.

Assessment

- Risk Factors
  - Bacterial infection: *Helicobacter pylori (H. pylori), Salmonella, Streptococci, Staphylococci,* or *Escherichia coli*
  - Family member with *H. pylori* infection
  - Family history of gastritis
  - Prolonged use of NSAIDs, corticosteroids (stops prostaglandin synthesis)
  - Excessive alcohol use
  - Bile reflux disease
  - Autoimmune diseases (systemic lupus, rheumatoid arthritis)
  - Advanced age
  - Radiation therapy

- ○ Smoking
- ○ Caffeine
- ○ Excessive stress
- ○ Exposure to contaminated food or water
- Subjective Data
  - ○ Dyspepsia, general abdominal discomfort, indigestion
  - ○ Upper abdominal pain or burning may increase or decrease after eating
  - ○ Nausea
  - ○ Reduced appetite
  - ○ Abdominal bloating or distention
  - ○ Hematemesis (bloody emesis)
  - ○ Erosive gastritis
    - ▪ Black, tarry stools; coffee-ground emesis
    - ▪ Acute abdominal pain
- Objective Data
  - ○ Physical Assessment Findings
    - ▪ Vomiting
    - ▪ Weight loss
    - ▪ Stools or vomitus test positive for occult blood
  - ○ Laboratory Tests
    - ▪ Noninvasive tests
      - ▫ CBC to check for anemia (in women, Hgb less than 12 g/dL and RBC less than 4.2 cells/mcL; in men, Hgb less than 14 g/dL and RBC less than 4.7 cells/mcL)
      - ▫ Serum and stool antibody/antigen test for presence of *H. pylori*
      - ▫ C 13 urea breath test – used to measure *H. pylori*
  - ○ Diagnostic Procedures
    - ▪ Upper endoscopy
      - ▫ A small flexible scope is inserted through the mouth into the esophagus, stomach, and duodenum to visualize the upper digestive tract. This procedure allows for a biopsy, cauterization, removal of polyps, dilation, or diagnosis. (See the chapter on *Gastrointestinal Diagnostic Procedures*.)
    - ▪ Client Education
      - ▫ Instruct the client to maintain NPO status 6 to 8 hr prior to procedure.
      - ▫ Advise the client to have a ride home available after the procedure.
      - ▫ Inform the client that a local anesthetic will be sprayed onto the back of the throat, but throat may be sore following the procedure.
      - ▫ Instruct the client to monitor for indications of perforation (chest or abdominal pain, fever, nausea, vomiting, and abdominal distention) and have emergency contact numbers available.

Collaborative Care

- Nursing Care
  - Monitor fluid intake and urine output.
  - Administer IV fluids as prescribed.
  - Monitor electrolytes (diarrhea and vomiting may deplete electrolytes and cause dehydration).
  - Assist the client in identifying foods that are triggers.
  - Provide small, frequent meals and encourage the client to eat slowly.
  - Advise the client to avoid alcohol, caffeine, and foods that may cause gastric irritation.
  - Assist the client in identifying ways to reduce stress.
  - Monitor for indications of gastric bleeding (coffee-ground emesis; black, tarry stools).
  - Monitor for findings of anemia (tachycardia, hypotension, fatigue, shortness of breath, pallor, feeling light-headed or dizzy, chest pain).
- Medications

HISTAMINE$_2$ ANTAGONISTS	
Action	› Decreases gastric acid output by blocking gastric histamine$_2$ receptors
Medications	› Nizatidine (Axid) › Famotidine (Pepcid) › Ranitidine (Zantac)
Nursing Interventions	› Allow 1 hr before or after to administer antacid. › Monitor for neutropenia and hypotension. › Administer IV slowly, too quickly may cause bradycardia and hypotension.
Client Education	› Advise not to smoke or drink alcohol. › Advise to take oral dose with meals. › Advise to wait 1 hr prior to or following H$_2$ receptor antagonist to take an antacid. › Advise to monitor for indications of GI bleeding (black stools, coffee-ground emesis).
ANTACIDS	
Action	› Increases gastric pH and neutralizes pepsin › Improves mucosal protection
Medications	› Aluminum hydroxide (Amphojel) › Magnesium hydroxide with aluminum hydroxide (Maalox, Mylanta)
Nursing Interventions	› Do not give to clients with kidney failure or renal dysfunction. › Monitor aluminum antacids for aluminum toxicity and constipation; magnesium antacids for diarrhea or hypermagnesemia.
Client Education	› Advise to take on an empty stomach. › Advise to wait 1 hr to take other medications.

PROTON PUMP INHIBITORS	
Action	› Reduces gastric acid by stopping acid-producing proton pump
Medications	› Omeprazole (Prilosec) › Lansoprazole (Prevacid) › Rabeprazole sodium (Aciphex) › Pantoprazole (Protonix) › Esomeprazole (Nexium)
Nursing Interventions	› Can cause nausea, vomiting, and abdominal pain. › Use filter for IV administration.
Client Education	› Advise to allow 30 min before eating and not to crush or chew pills. › It can take up to 4 days to see the effects. › Advise to take on an empty stomach.
PROSTAGLANDINS	
Action	› Reduces gastric acid secretion
Medications	› Misoprostol (Cytotec)
Nursing Interventions	› May be given with NSAIDs to prevent gastric mucosal damage. › May cause abdominal pain and diarrhea.
Client Education	› Advise to use contraceptives. › Advise not to take if there is a chance of becoming pregnant. › Advise to take with food to reduce gastric effects.
ANTI-ULCER/MUCOSAL BARRIERS	
Action	› Inhibits acid and forms a protective coating over mucosa
Medications	› Sucralfate (Carafate)
Nursing Interventions	› Allow 30 min before or after to give antacid.
Client Education	› Advise to take on an empty stomach. › Advise not to smoke or drink alcohol. › Advise to continue to take medication even if manifestations subside. › Advise to notify the provider of tinnitus.
ANTIBIOTICS	
Action	› Eliminates *H. pylori* infection
Medications	› Clarithromycin (Biaxin) › Amoxicillin (Amoxil) › Tetracycline (Achromycin V) › Metronidazole (Flagyl)
Nursing Interventions	› Monitor for increased abdominal pain and diarrhea. › Monitor electrolytes and hydration if fluid is depleted.
Client Education	› Advise to complete prescribed dosage. › Advise to notify the provider of persistent diarrhea.

- Teamwork and Collaboration
  - A nutritionist may be necessary to assist in the alterations to diet.
  - Supportive care may be needed to reduce stress, increase exercise, and stop smoking.
- Therapeutic Procedures – upper endoscopy
- Surgical Interventions (see the chapter on *Peptic Ulcer Disease*.)
  - Surgery is prescribed for clients who have ulcerations or significant bleeding or when nonsurgical interventions are ineffective.
  - Vagotomy or highly selective vagotomy – A highly selective vagotomy severs only the nerve fibers that control gastric acid secretion, and often is done laparoscopically to reduce postoperative complications.
  - Pyloroplasty is usually done at the same time as the vagotomy.
  - Partial gastrectomy – Removal of the involved portion of the stomach.

Complications

- Gastric bleeding may be caused by:
  - Severe acute gastritis with deep tissue inflammation extending into the stomach muscle.
  - In chronic erosive gastritis, bleeding may be slow or profuse as in a perforation of the stomach wall.
  - Nursing Actions
    - Monitor vital signs and airway.
    - Provide fluid replacement and blood products.
    - Monitor CBC and clotting factors.
    - Insert a nasogastric (NG) tube for gastric lavage (irrigate with normal saline or water to stop active gastric bleed) as indicated.
      - Obtain an x-ray to confirm placement of NG tube prior to fluid instillation to prevent aspiration.
    - Monitor NG tube output.
    - Administer IV medications (proton-pump inhibitors, H_2-receptor antagonists) as prescribed.
  - Client Education
    - Instruct the client to monitor for signs of slow gastric bleeding (coffee-ground emesis; black, tarry stools). Seek immediate medical attention with severe abdominal pain or vomiting blood. Take medications as directed.
- Gastric outlet obstruction caused by severe acute gastritis with deep tissue inflammation extending into the stomach muscle
  - Nursing Actions
    - Monitor fluids and electrolytes because continuous vomiting results in loss of chloride (metabolic alkalosis) and severe fluid and electrolyte depletion.
    - Provide fluid and electrolyte replacement, and monitor I&O.
    - Prepare to insert a NG tube to empty stomach contents if prescribed.
    - Prepare for a diagnostic endoscopy.
  - Client Education – Instruct the client to seek medical attention for continuous vomiting, bloating, and nausea.

- Dehydration
  - Causes – loss of fluid due to vomiting or diarrhea
  - Nursing Actions
    - Monitor fluid intake and urine output.
    - Provide IV fluids if needed.
    - Monitor electrolytes.
  - Client Education – Instruct the client to contact a provider for vomiting and diarrhea.
- Pernicious anemia
  - Causes
    - Chronic gastritis may damage the parietal cells. This may lead to reduced production of intrinsic factor, which is necessary for the absorption of vitamin B_{12}.
    - Insufficient vitamin B_{12} may lead to pernicious anemia.
  - Nursing Actions – Instruct the client of the need for monthly vitamin B_{12} injections.
- Dumping syndrome
  - Causes – Dumping syndrome is a vasomotor response to food ingestion, resulting in syncope, pallor, palpitations, dizziness, and headache. Gastric surgery increases the risk of dumping syndrome. (See the chapter on *Peptic Ulcer Disease*.)
  - Nursing Actions
    - Instruct client to lay down following meals to slow movement of food through intestine and prevent injury.
    - Instruct client on self-administration of octreotide (Sandostatin) subcutaneous injection two to three times daily before meals, as prescribed.

APPLICATION EXERCISES

1. A nurse is teaching a client who has a new diagnosis of pernicious anemia due to chronic gastritis. Which of the following should be included in the teaching?

    A. Cells producing gastric acid have been damaged.

    B. A monthly injection of medication is required.

    C. Vitamin K supplements will be administered.

    D. Increased production of intrinsic factor is occurring.

2. A nurse is providing discharge teaching to a client who has a new prescription for aluminum hydroxide (Amphojel). The nurse should advise the client to

    A. take the medication with food.

    B. monitor for diarrhea.

    C. wait 1 to 2 hr before taking other oral medications.

    D. maintain a low-fiber diet.

3. A nurse is planning care for a client who has acute gastritis. Which of the following nursing interventions should the nurse include in the plan of care? (Select all that apply.)

    ____X____ A. Evaluate intake and output.

    ____X____ B. Monitor laboratory reports of electrolytes.

    _____ C. Provide three large meals a day.

    _____ D. Administer ibuprofen for pain.

    ____X____ E. Observe stool characteristics.

4. A nurse is caring for a client who has chronic gastritis and is scheduled for a selective vagotomy. The purpose of this procedure is to

    A. increase duodenal gastric emptying.

    B. reduce gastric acid secretions.

    C. increase gastric mucus secretion.

    D. reduce histamine secretion.

5. A nurse is completing teaching to a client who has a new prescription for famotidine (Pepcid). Which of the following statements by the client indicates understanding of the teaching?

    A. "This medicine coats the lining of my stomach."

    B. "This should stop the pain right away."

    C. "I will take my pill at meal time."

    D. "I will monitor for bleeding from my nose."

6. A nurse is reviewing acute and chronic gastritis with a group of clients. What should be included in this discussion? Use the ATI Active Learning Template: Systems Disorder to complete this item to include the following:

    A. Alteration in Health:

        • Describe gastritis.

        • Compare/contrast acute vs. chronic gastritis.

    B. Pathophysiology: Describe as related to client problem.

    C. Risk Factors: Describe six.

APPLICATION EXERCISES KEY

1. A. INCORRECT: Damage to parietal cells has occurred, which leads to pernicious anemia.

    B. **CORRECT:** A monthly injection of vitamin B_{12} is necessary to treat pernicious anemia.

    C. INCORRECT: Vitamin K supplements are given to clients who have a bleeding disorder.

    D. INCORRECT: Parietal cell damage results in insufficient production of intrinsic factor.

    Ⓝ NCLEX® Connection: Physiological Adaptations, Alterations in Body Systems

2. A. INCORRECT: The client is advised to take aluminum hydroxide on an empty stomach.

    B. INCORRECT: Aluminum hydroxide may cause constipation.

    C. **CORRECT:** The client is advised not to take oral medications within 1 to 2 hr of an antacid.

    D. INCORRECT: The client is advised to increase dietary fiber, due to the constipating effect of the medication.

    Ⓝ NCLEX® Connection: Pharmacological and Parenteral Therapies, Medication Administration

3. A. **CORRECT:** Intake and output should be evaluated to prevent electrolyte loss and dehydration.

    B. **CORRECT:** Laboratory findings of electrolytes should be monitored to prevent fluid loss and dehydration.

    C. INCORRECT: Small, frequent meals should be included in the plan of care.

    D. INCORRECT: Ibuprofen, an NSAID, should be avoided in the client who has acute gastritis.

    E. **CORRECT:** The presence of blood in the stools may indicate gastrointestinal bleeding and should be monitored.

    Ⓝ NCLEX® Connection: Physiological Adaptations, Illness Management

4. A. INCORRECT: A pyloroplasty is performed to widen the opening from the stomach to the duodenum, which increases gastric emptying.

    B. **CORRECT:** A selective vagotomy reduces gastric acid secretions.

    C. INCORRECT: A selective vagotomy does not increase gastric mucus secretion.

    D. INCORRECT: A selective vagotomy does not reduce histamine secretion.

    Ⓝ NCLEX® Connection: Physiological Adaptations, Alterations in Body Systems

5. A. INCORRECT: Famotidine decreases gastric acid output. It does not have a protective coating action.

    B. INCORRECT: It may take several days before pain relief occurs when starting this therapy.

    C. **CORRECT:** Famotidine can be taken with fluid or food of the client's choice.

    D. INCORRECT: The client is instructed to monitor for GI bleeding when taking famotidine.

    (N) NCLEX® Connection: Pharmacological and Parenteral Therapies, Medication Administration

6. *Using the ATI Active Learning Template: Systems Disorder*

    A. Alteration in Health

    - Gastritis is an inflammation of the lining of the stomach as a result of irritation to the mucosa.
      - Acute – Sudden onset, short duration, may result in gastric bleeding.
      - Chronic – Slow onset; when profuse, it may damage parietal cells, resulting in pernicious anemia.

    B. Pathophysiology

    - Gastric acid overwhelms the production of Cox 1 enzymes, which provide mucosal prostaglandins that line the stomach. This results in an erosion of the mucosa and increases the risk for ulcers and stomach cancer.

    C. Risk Factors

    - Bacterial infection (*H. pylori, Salmonella, Streptococci, Staphylococci, E. coli*)
    - Family history of *H. pylori* or family member with *H. pylori*
    - Prolonged use of NSAIDs or corticosteroids
    - Excessive alcohol use
    - Bile reflux disease
    - Autoimmune diseases
    - Advanced age
    - Radiation therapy
    - Smoking
    - Caffeine
    - Excessive stress
    - Exposure to contaminated food or water

    (N) NCLEX® Connection: Physiological Adaptations, Alterations in Body Systems

CHAPTER 51 Noninflammatory Bowel Disorders

Overview

- Noninflammatory bowel disorders can cause pain, changes in bowel pattern, bleeding, and malabsorption. This group of disorders includes hemorrhoids, cancer, hernia, irritable bowel syndrome (IBS), and intestinal obstruction.

  - Hemorrhoids are distended or edematous intestinal veins resulting from increased intra-abdominal pressure (straining, obesity). Pregnancy increases the risk of hemorrhoids.

  - Cancer of the small or large intestine can be caused by age-related changes, genetic influence, or chronic bowel disease.

- Nurses should be knowledgeable about noninflammatory bowel disorders and treatments. Topics to be reviewed include:

  - Hernia

  - Irritable bowel syndrome

  - Intestinal obstruction

HERNIA

Overview

- Bowel herniation is the displacement of the bowel through the abdominal muscle into other areas of the abdominal cavity.

- Incisional hernias can occur as a post-surgical complication.

- A hernia that cannot be moved back into place with gentle palpation is considered irreducible and should be treated surgically.

Assessment

- Risk Factors

  - Male sex (indirect hernia)

  - Advanced age (direct hernia)

  - Increased intra-abdominal pressure due to pregnancy, obesity (femoral, adult-acquired umbilical hernia)

  - Genetics (congenital umbilical hernia)

- Physical Findings

  - Protrusion or "lump" at involved site (groin area, umbilicus, healed incision)

- Nursing Actions
  - Instruct client to wear truss pad with hernia belt during waking hours and to inspect skin daily (nonsurgical client).
  - Instruct client to avoid increased intra-abdominal pressure for 2 to 3 weeks postoperatively (avoid coughing, straining, heavy lifting).

IRRITABLE BOWEL SYNDROME

Overview

- Irritable bowel syndrome (IBS) is a disorder of the gastrointestinal system. IBS causes changes in bowel function (chronic diarrhea, constipation, or abdominal pain).
- IBS severity depends upon the cause; food intolerances worsen the clinical manifestations.

Health Promotion and Disease Prevention

- Avoid foods that contain dairy, eggs, and wheat products.
- Avoid alcoholic and caffeinated beverages and other fluids containing fructose and sorbitol.
- Drink 2 to 3 L of fluid per day from food and fluid sources.
- Increase the amount of daily fiber intake (approximately 30 to 40 g/day).

Assessment

- Risk Factors
  - Female sex
  - Stress
  - Eating large meals containing a large amount of fat
  - Caffeine
  - Alcohol

Subjective and Objective Data

- Cramping pain in abdomen
- Abdominal pain due to changes in bowel pattern and consistency
- Nausea with meals or passing stool
- Anorexia
- Abdominal bloating
- Belching
- Diarrhea
- Constipation

Laboratory Tests

- CBC, serum albumin, erythrocyte sedimentation rate (ESR), and occult stools are all typically within the expected reference range.

Diagnostic Tests

- IBS is difficult to diagnose with specific tests and is usually based on the presence of specific characteristic, including abdominal pain accompanied by changes in bowel patterns, abdominal distention, feeling that defecation is not complete, and the presence of mucus with stools.

- Hydrogen breath test – The client is asked to exhale into a hydrogen analyzer before and after ingesting test sugar (lactose or lactulose, dependent on the suspected problem). Positive test results indicate excess hydrogen in the bloodstream from bacterial overgrowth or malabsorption.

  - Client education – Instruct client to remain NPO at least 12 hr prior to test, except for sips of water.

Patient-Centered Care

- Nursing Care

  - Review strategies to reduce stress.

  - Instruct the client to limit the intake of irritating agents (gas-forming foods, caffeine, alcohol).

  - Encourage a diet high in fiber.

  - Instruct client to keep a food diary to record intake and bowel patterns (to refine diet and prevent exacerbations).

Medications

- Alosetron (Lotronex)

  - An IBS-specific medication that selectively blocks 5-HT4 receptors that innervate the viscera. The expected result is increased firmness in stools, and decreased urgency and frequency of defecation.

  - Indicated for irritable bowel syndrome with diarrhea (IBS-D) in women that has lasted more than 6 months and is resistant to conventional management.

  - Nursing Considerations

    - Contraindicated for clients who have chronic constipation, history of bowel obstruction, Crohn's disease, ulcerative colitis, impaired intestinal circulation, or thrombophlebitis.

    - The dosage will start as once a day and may be increased to twice a day.

  - Client Education

    - Instruct the client that manifestations should resolve within 1 to 4 weeks, but will return 1 week after medication is discontinued.

    - Teach client to report constipation, fever, malaise, darkened urine, or bleeding from rectum or in stool immediately.

- Lubiprostone (Amitiza)
  - An IBS specific medication that increases fluid secretion in the intestine to promote intestinal motility. This is indicated for irritable bowel syndrome with constipation (IBS-C).
  - Nursing Considerations
    - Contraindicated for clients who have known or possible bowel obstruction.
    - Not effective for treatment of men with IBS.
  - Client Education – Instruct the client to take with food to decrease nausea.

INTESTINAL OBSTRUCTION

Overview

- Intestinal obstruction can result from mechanical (90%) or nonmechanical (10%) causes. Mechanical obstruction usually requires surgery.
- Manifestations vary according to type.
  - Mechanical obstructions have colicky, intermittent pain that is milder.
  - Nonmechanical obstructions tend to have vague, diffuse, constant pain and significant abdominal distention.
- Bowel sounds are hyperactive above the obstruction and hypoactive below.
- Obstructions of the small intestine are the most common.
- Treatment focuses on fluid and electrolyte balance, decompressing the bowel, and relief/removal of the obstruction.

Assessment

- Risk Factors
  - Mechanical obstructions result from:
    - Encirclement or compression of intestine by adhesions, tumors, fibrosis (endometriosis), or strictures (Crohn's disease, radiation).
      - Postsurgical adhesions are the most common cause of small bowel obstructions.
      - Carcinomas are the most common cause of large intestine obstructions.
      - Diverticulitis and tumors are common causes of obstruction in older adult clients.
    - Volvulus (twisting) or intussusception (telescoping) of bowel segments.
    - Hernia (bowel becomes trapped in weakened area of abdominal wall).
    - Fecal impactions.
      - Older adult clients are at a greater risk for fecal impactions. Bowel regimens can be effective in preventing impactions.

View Images

› Bowel Intussusception   › Volvulus   › Hernia

○ Nonmechanical obstructions (paralytic ileus) result from decreased peristalsis secondary to:

  ▪ Neurogenic disorders (manipulation of the bowel during major surgery and spinal fracture)

  ▪ Vascular disorders (vascular insufficiency and mesenteric emboli)

  ▪ Electrolyte imbalances (hypokalemia)

  ▪ Inflammatory responses (peritonitis or sepsis)

• Subjective and Objective Data

  ○ Clinical manifestations vary depending on the location of the obstruction.

SMALL BOWEL AND LARGE INTESTINE OBSTRUCTIONS	SMALL BOWEL OBSTRUCTIONS	LARGE INTESTINE OBSTRUCTIONS
› Obstipation – the inability to pass a stool and/or flatus for more than 8 hr despite feeling the urge to defecate › Abdominal distention › High-pitched bowel sounds above site of obstruction (borborygmi) with hypoactive bowel sounds below, or overall hypoactive; absent bowel sounds later in process	› Severe fluid and electrolyte imbalance › Metabolic alkalosis › Visible peristaltic waves (possible) › Abdominal pain, discomfort › Profuse, sudden projectile vomiting with fecal odor; vomiting relieves pain	› Minor fluid and electrolyte imbalance › Metabolic acidosis (possible) › Significant abdominal distention › Intermittent abdominal cramping › Infrequent vomiting › Diarrhea or "ribbon-like" stools around an impaction

  ○ Laboratory Tests

    ▪ Increased hemoglobin, BUN, creatinine, and hematocit may indicate dehydration.

    ▪ Increased serum amylase and WBC count may be due to strangulating obstructions.

    ▪ Arterial blood gases (ABGs) indicate metabolic imbalance, depending on obstruction type.

    ▪ Chemistry profiles reveal decreased sodium, chloride, and potassium.

  ○ Diagnostic Procedures

    ▪ X-ray: Flat plate and upright abdominal x-rays evaluate the presence of free air and gas patterns.

    ▪ Endoscopy determines the cause of obstruction.

    ▪ CT scan determines the cause and exact location of the obstruction.

 View Image: Radiograph of Abdominal Obstruction

Patient-Centered Care

• Nursing Care

  ○ Nonmechanical cause of obstruction

    ▪ Nothing by mouth with bowel rest.

    ▪ Assess bowel sounds.

    ▪ Provide oral hygiene.

- Administer IV fluid and electrolyte replacement (particularly potassium).
- Pain management, as prescribed (once diagnosis identified).
- Encourage ambulation.
  - ○ Mechanical cause of obstruction
    - Prepare for surgery and provide preoperative nursing care.
    - Withhold intake until peristalsis resumes.
- Therapeutic Procedures
  - ○ Nasogastric tube inserted to decompress the bowel
    - Nursing Actions
      - □ Maintain intermittent suction as prescribed.
      - □ Assess NG tube patency and irrigate every 4 hr, or as prescribed.
      - □ Monitor and assess gastric output.
      - □ Monitor nasal area for skin breakdown.
      - □ Provide oral hygiene every 2 hr.
      - □ Monitor vital signs, skin integrity, weight, and I&O.
      - □ Clamp the NG tube during ambulation.
- Medications
  - ○ Prokinetics to promote gastric motility (octreotide [Sandostatin]) in paralytic ileus or partial obstruction.
  - ○ Broad spectrum antibiotics, especially with suspected bowel strangulation.
- Surgical Interventions
  - ○ Procedure varies based on cause of obstruction. May include lysis of adhesions, colon resection, colostomy creation (temporary or permanent), embolectomy, thrombectomy, resection of gangrenous intestinal tissue, or complete colectomy.
  - ○ Exploratory laparotomy – Determine the cause of obstruction and rectify if possible.
    - Nursing Actions
      - □ Ensure the client understands the type of procedure (open or laparoscopic).
      - □ Monitor for hemodynamic instability.
      - □ Administer IV fluid replacement and maintenance as prescribed.
      - □ Monitor bowel sounds.
      - □ Maintain NG tube patency and measure output.
      - □ Clamp NG tube as prescribed to assess the client's tolerance prior to removal.
      - □ Advance diet as tolerated when prescribed, beginning with clear liquids – clamp tube after eating for 1 to 2 hr.
      - □ Instruct client to report intolerance of intake following NG tube removal (nausea, vomiting, increasing distention).

Complications

- Dehydration (potential hypotension; small bowel obstruction)
  - Cause – persistent vomiting
  - Nursing Actions
    - Assess the client's hydration through evaluation of hematocrit, BUN, orthostatic vital signs, skin turgor/mucous membranes, urine output, and specific gravity. Notify the provider of a fluid imbalance.
    - Administer IV fluids as prescribed.
- Electrolyte Imbalance (small bowel obstruction)
  - Cause – persistent vomiting
  - Nursing Actions
    - Monitor electrolytes, especially potassium levels.
    - Notify the provider of an electrolyte imbalance.
    - Administer IV fluids as prescribed to replace electrolytes.
- Metabolic Alkalosis
  - Cause – Small intestinal obstruction causes vomiting, leading to a loss of gastric hydrochloride.
  - Nursing Actions
    - Monitor for hypoventilation (confusion, hypercarbia), which is a compensatory action by the lungs.
    - Obtain arterial blood gas.
    - Notify the provider of unexpected laboratory findings.
    - Replace fluid and electrolytes as prescribed.
    - Provide oral hygiene to alleviate client's increased thirst response.
      - Thirst response is decreased in the older adult. Provide oral hygiene routinely to ensure maintenance of moist mucous membranes.
- Metabolic Acidosis
  - Cause – a lower level obstruction due to nonreabsorption of alkaline fluids
  - Nursing Actions
    - Monitor for deep, rapid respirations (compensatory action by the lungs), confusion, hypotension, and flushed skin.
    - Obtain arterial blood gas.
    - Notify the provider of unexpected laboratory findings.

APPLICATION EXERCISES

1. A nurse is completing an admission assessment of a client who has a small bowel obstruction. Which of the following findings should the nurse report to the provider? (Select all that apply.)

_____ A. Profuse emesis prior to insertion of the nasogastric tube

___X___ B. Urine specific gravity 1.040

___X___ C. Hematocrit 60%

___X___ D. Serum potassium 3.0 mEq/L

_____ E. WBC 10,000/uL

2. A nurse is planning care for a client who has a small bowel instruction and a nasogastric (NG) tube in place. Which of the following nursing interventions should be included in the plan of care? (Select all that apply.)

_____ A. Subtract the NG drainage from the client's output.

_____ B. Irrigate the NG tube every 8 hr.

___X___ C. Assess bowel sounds.

___X___ D. Provide oral hygiene every 2 hr.

___X___ E. Clamp the NG tube during ambulation.

3. A nurse is caring for a client who has a small bowel obstruction from adhesions. Which of the following findings are consistent with this diagnosis? (Select all that apply.)

___X___ A. Emesis greater than 500 mL with a fecal odor

___X___ B. Report of spasmodic abdominal pain

___X___ C. Pain relieved with vomiting

_____ D. Abdomen flat with rebound tenderness to palpation

_____ E. Laboratory findings indicating metabolic acidosis

4. A nurse is caring for an older adult client in an extended care facility. Which of the following indicates the client has a stool impaction causing a large intestine obstruction?

A. The client reports he had a bowel movement yesterday.

B. The client is having small, frequent liquid stools.

C. The client is flatulent.

D. The client indicates he vomited once this morning.

5. A nurse is completing discharge teaching to a client who has irritable bowel syndrome (IBS). Which of the following should be included in the teaching?

    A. Increase dietary intake of dairy products.

    B. Consume 15 to 20 g of fiber daily.

    C. Plan three moderate to large meals per day.

    D. Drink at least 2 L of fluids each day.

6. A nursing student is preparing a poster for display in the nursing lab on caring for a client who has a bowel obstruction. What information should be included in this poster? Use the ATI Active Learning Template: Systems Disorder to complete this item to include the following sections:

    A. Risk Factors: Identify at least two for each form of obstruction.

    B. Objective and Subjective Data: Compare and contrast the types of obstructions.

    C. Diagnostic Procedures: Identify at least two.

APPLICATION EXERCISES KEY

1. A. INCORRECT: Profuse emesis is an expected finding in a client who has a small bowel obstruction.

    B. **CORRECT:** This finding indicates significant dehydration in the client, is outside the expected reference range, and should be reported to the provider.

    C. **CORRECT:** This finding indicates significant dehydration in the client, is outside the expected reference range, and should be reported to the provider.

    D. **CORRECT:** This finding indicates significant dehydration in the client, is outside the expected reference range, and should be reported to the provider.

    E. INCORRECT: This finding is within the expected reference range and does not need to be reported to the provider.

    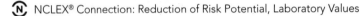 NCLEX® Connection: Reduction of Risk Potential, Laboratory Values

2. A. INCORRECT: NG drainage is included as output and must be considered when planning fluid replacement.

    B. INCORRECT: The NG tube is irrigated every 4 hr to maintain patency.

    C. **CORRECT:** Bowel sounds should be assessed to evaluate treatment and resolution of the obstruction.

    D. **CORRECT:** An NG tube promotes mouth breathing. Frequent oral hygiene should be included in the plan of care.

    E. **CORRECT:** The client can tolerate clamping of the NG tube for short periods, such as during ambulation. Scheduled clamping should be included in the plan of care prior to removal of the NG tube.

    NCLEX® Connection: Reduction of Risk Potential, Therapeutic Procedures

3. A. **CORRECT:** Large emesis with a fecal odor is a finding in a client who has a small bowel obstruction.

    B. **CORRECT:** Report of abdominal pain is a finding in a client who has a small bowel obstruction.

    C. **CORRECT:** Relief of pain after vomiting is a finding in a client who has a small bowel obstruction.

    D. INCORRECT: Abdominal distention is a finding in a client who has a small bowel obstruction.

    E. INCORRECT: Metabolic alkalosis due to the loss of gastric acid is a finding in a client who has a small bowel obstruction.

    NCLEX® Connection: Physiological Adaptations, Pathophysiology

4. A. INCORRECT: A report of a bowel movement yesterday is unlikely in a client who has a suspected impaction.

    B. **CORRECT:** Small, frequent liquid stools can be passed around an impaction.

    C. INCORRECT: The presence of flatus does not indicate an obstruction of the large intestine.

    D. INCORRECT: A report of a single episode of vomiting does not indicate an obstruction of the large intestine.

     NCLEX® Connection: Physiological Adaptations, Pathophysiology

5. A. INCORRECT: Dairy products should be limited or avoided by a client who has IBS due to their higher fat content.

    B. INCORRECT: A client who has IBS should increase their daily fiber intake to 30 to 40 g.

    C. INCORRECT: A client who has IBS should eat small frequent meals.

    D. **CORRECT:** A client who has IBS should drink 2 to 3 L of fluids a day to promote a consistent bowel pattern.

     NCLEX® Connection: Basic Care and Comfort, Nutrition and Oral Hydration

6. *Using the ATI Active Learning Template: Systems Disorder*

    A. Risk Factors

    - Mechanical
      - Encirclement or compression of intestines by adhesions, tumors, fibrosis, or strictures
      - Volvulus, intussusception
      - Hernia, fecal impaction

    - Nonmechanical – decreased peristalsis due to neurogenic or vascular disorders, electrolyte imbalances, and inflammatory responses
    - Small bowel – postsurgical adhesions
    - Large bowel – carcinoma

    B. Objective and Subjective Data

    - Mechanical – mild, colicky, intermittent pain
    - Nonmechanical – vague, diffuse, constant pain; significant abdominal distention
    - Small bowel obstruction
      - Visible peristaltic waves possible
      - Profuse, sudden projectile vomiting with fecal odor, which relieves pain
      - Severe fluid and electrolyte imbalance, metabolic alkalosis

    - Large bowel obstruction – significant abdominal distention, infrequent vomiting, diarrhea or "ribbon-like" stools around an impaction, minor fluid and electrolyte imbalance, metabolic acidosis (possible)
    - Bowel sounds – hyperactive above and hypoactive below the obstruction, inability to pass a stool, and/or flatus for more than 8 hr despite urge to defecate

    C. Diagnostic Procedures

    - X-rays (flat plate, upright abdominal)
    - Endoscopy
    - CT scan

     NCLEX® Connection: Physiological Adaptations, Alterations in Body Systems

chapter 52

CHAPTER 52   Inflammatory Bowel Disease

Overview

- Inflammatory bowel disease (IBD) can affect structures or segments along the gastrointestinal tract. The term includes both acute and chronic disorders.
- Acute IBD includes:
  - Appendicitis, or inflammation of the appendix related to obstruction. Adolescents and young adults are at increased risk. (Refer to the *Gastrointestinal Structural and Inflammatory Disorders* chapter in the *Nursing Care of Children Review Module*.)
  - Peritonitis, or inflammation of the peritoneum. Peritonitis results from infection of the peritoneum due to puncture (surgery or trauma), septicemia, or rupture of part of the gastrointestinal tract.
  - Gastroenteritis, or inflammation of the stomach and small intestine, is triggered by infection. Vomiting and frequent, watery stools place the client at increased risk for fluid and electrolyte imbalance and impaired nutrition.
- Chronic IBD includes ulcerative colitis, Crohn's disease, and diverticulitis. Chronic IBD is characterized by diarrhea (up to 20 stools during acute exacerbation), crampy abdominal pain, and exacerbations ("flare-ups")/remissions.
- Diverticulitis is inflammation and infection of the bowel mucosa caused by bacteria or fecal matter trapped in one or more diverticula (pouches in the intestine). Diverticulitis is not to be confused with diverticulosis, which is the presence of many small pouches in the colon with or without inflammation. Many clients who have diverticulosis never develop diverticulitis.

DISORDER	DESCRIPTION OF DISEASE PROCESS	RELEVANT INFORMATION
Ulcerative colitis	› Edema and inflammation of the rectum and sigmoid colon. › May expand the length of the colon. › Mucosa and submucosa are affected and may abscess.	› Bowel obstruction may occur; intestinal mucosal cell changes may cause colon cancer or insufficient production of intrinsic factor, resulting in insufficient absorption of vitamin B_{12} (pernicious anemia).
Crohn's disease	› Inflammation and ulceration of the gastrointestinal tract, often at the distal ileum. › All bowel layers may become involved; lesions are sporadic. › Fistulas are common.	› Can involve the entire GI tract from the mouth to the anus. › Malabsorption and malnutrition may develop when the jejunum and ileum become involved. Supplemental vitamins and minerals including vitamin B_{12} injections may be necessary.
Diverticulitis	› Inflammation of the diverticula (hernia in intestinal wall) that frequently occurs in the colon.	› About 10% of clients who have diverticula develop diverticulitis. Frequent episodes may lead to bleeding and infection. › Diverticula may bleed and the loss of blood may be minimal or severe. › Diverticula may perforate and cause peritonitis.

Assessment

- Risk Factors
  - Genetics – Ulcerative colitis and Crohn's disease
  - Culture – Caucasians (ulcerative colitis) and Jewish heritage (ulcerative colitis and Crohn's disease)
  - Gender and age – The incidence of ulcerative colitis peaks at adolescence to young adulthood (more often in females) and older adulthood (more often in males).
    - Crohn's disease may be diagnosed at any age.
    - Diverticulitis occurs more often in older adults and affects men more frequently than women.
  - Diet – A diet low in fiber may predispose a client to ulcerative colitis and the development of diverticula.
  - Smoking – Smokers (Crohn's disease) and nonsmokers (ulcerative colitis)
  - Other factors – Stress, autoimmunity, and infection may be causative agents for both ulcerative colitis and Crohn's disease.

- Physical Assessment Findings

PHYSICAL ASSESSMENT FINDINGS BY DISORDER		
ULCERATIVE COLITIS		
Subjective Data	› Abdominal pain/cramping: often left-lower quadrant pain › Anorexia and weight loss	
Objective Data	› Fever › Diarrhea: up to 15 to 20 liquid stools/day › Mucus, blood, or pus can be present	› Abdominal distention, tenderness, and/or firmness upon palpation › High-pitched bowel sounds › Rectal bleeding
CROHN'S DISEASE		
Subjective Data	› Abdominal pain/cramping: often right-lower quadrant pain › Anorexia and weight loss	
Objective Data	› Fever › Diarrhea: five loose stools/day with mucus or pus	› Abdominal distention, tenderness and/or firmness upon palpation › High-pitched bowel sounds › Steatorrhea
DIVERTICULITIS		
Subjective Data	› Abdominal pain in left-lower quadrant › Nausea and vomiting	
Objective Data	› Fever › Chills › Tachycardia	

LABORATORY FINDINGS			
	Ulcerative colitis	Crohn's disease	Diverticulitis
Hematocrit and hemoglobin	Decreased	Decreased	Decreased
Erythrocyte sedimentation rate (ESR)	Increased	Increased	—
WBC	Increased	Increased	Increased
C-reactive protein	Increased	Increased	—
Platelet count	Increased	Increased	—
Serum albumin	Decreased	Decreased	—
Folic acid and B_{12}	—	Decreased	—
pANCA (perinuclear anti-neutrophil cytoplasmic antibody)	Increased	—	—
Antiglycan antibody	—	Increased	—
Stool for occult blood	May be positive	May be positive	May be positive
Urinalysis	—	WBC	May be positive for RBCs
K^+, Mg, and Ca	Decreased	Decreased	—

- ○ Diagnostic Procedures
  - Abdominal x-ray and CT scan
  - Barium enema: Barium is inserted into the rectum as a contrast medium for x-rays. This allows for the rectum and large intestine to be visualized, and is used to diagnose ulcerative colitis. A barium enema may show the presence of diverticulosis and is contraindicated in the presence of diverticulitis due to the risk of perforation.
  - Colonoscopy and sigmoidoscopy: A lighted, flexible scope is inserted into the rectum to visualize the rectum and large intestine.
- ○ Nursing Actions – Monitor postprocedure for manifestations of bowel perforations (rectal bleeding, firm abdomen, tachycardia, hypotension).
- ○ Findings
  - Small intestine ulcerations and narrowing may be consistent with Crohn's disease.
  - Ulcerations and inflammation of the sigmoid colon and rectum may be significant for ulcerative colitis.
- ○ Client Education
  - Instruct the client to remain NPO after midnight and provide bowel preparation instructions.
  - Inform the client of possible abdominal discomfort and cramping during the barium enema.

Patient-Centered Care

- Nursing Care
  - Ulcerative colitis and Crohn's disease
    - Instruct the client to seek emergency care for signs of bowel obstruction or perforation (fever, severe abdominal pain, vomiting).
    - Instruct clients who have extreme or long exacerbations that NPO status and administration of TPN promotes bowel rest while providing adequate nutrition.
    - Educate the client to eat foods that are high in protein and calories, and low in fiber.
    - Assist the client in identifying foods that trigger clinical manifestations.
    - Instruct the client to avoid caffeine and alcohol, and take a multivitamin that contains iron.
    - Advise the client that small frequent meals may reduce the occurrence of manifestations.
    - Inform the client that dietary supplements that are high in protein and low in fiber (elemental and semielemental products, canned nutrition beverages) may be used.
    - Monitor for electrolyte imbalance, especially potassium. Diarrhea can cause a loss of fluids and electrolytes.
    - Monitor I&O and assess for dehydration.
    - Educate the client regarding the use of vitamin supplements and B_{12} injections, if needed.
  - Diverticulitis
    - The client is hospitalized when clinical findings are more severe (severe pain, high fever). The client is NPO, has nasogastric suctioning, is receiving IV fluids, IV antibiotics, total parenteral nutrition, and opioid analgesics for pain.
    - Instruct the client who has mild diverticulitis on self-care at home. The client should take medications as prescribed (antibiotics, analgesics, antispasmodics) and get adequate rest.
    - Educate the client to consume a clear liquid diet until manifestations subside. The client may progress to a low-fiber diet as tolerated.
    - Instruct the client to add fiber to the diet once solid foods are tolerated without other manifestations. The client should slowly advance to a high-fiber diet as tolerated.
    - Teach client to avoid seeds or indigestable material, which can block diverticulum (nuts, popcorn, seeds).
    - Instruct client to avoid irritating the bowel (avoid alcohol, limit fat to 30% of daily calorie intake).
    - Provide client with instructions to promote normal bowel function and consistency (may take bulk-forming laxatives only, drink adequate fluids, avoid use of enemas).

- Medications

CLASSIFICATION/THERAPEUTIC INTENT	NURSING CONSIDERATIONS/CLIENT EDUCATION
Ulcerative colitis and Crohn's disease	

› 5-aminosalicylic acid (5-ASA)
  » Anti-inflammatory
    › Reduces inflammation of the intestinal mucosa
› Medications: sulfonamides
  » Sulfasalazine (Azulfidine)
  » Olsalazine (Dipentum) for clients intolerant to sulfasalazine
	› These medications may be contraindicated if the client has a sulfa allergy.
	› Monitor CBC, renal, and hepatic function.
	› Sulfasalazine is given orally.
	› Advise the client of the following:
	  » Take with food.
	  » Avoid sun exposure.
	  » Increase fluid intake.
	  » Urine and skin may appear yellow or brown.
	  » Color may damage soft contact lenses. Notify the provider if sore throat, rash, bruising, and/or fever occur.

› 5-ASA
  » Anti-inflammatory
› Medication: nonsulfonamides
  » Mesalamine (Asacol, Pentasa, Rowasa)
	› The adverse effects are not as serious as sulfasalazine.
	› These medications may be contraindicated if the client has a sulfa allergy.
	› Monitor CBC, renal, and hepatic function.
	› Asacol and Pentasa may be given orally.
	› Rowasa is given by retention enema or rectal suppository.
	› The client should retain rectal suspension for at least 4 hr.
	› The suppository should be firm at the time of insertion and should be retained for at least 1 hr.
	› Inform the client to report headache or gastrointestinal problems (abdominal discomfort, diarrhea).

› Corticosteroids
  » Reduces inflammation and pain
› Medications
  » Prednisone (Delta-son)
  » Budesonide (Entocort)
  » Hydrocortisone enema (Cortenema)
  » Rectal foam (Cortifoam)
  » IV corticosteroids for fulminant disease (occurring suddenly)
	› Use corticosteroids in low doses to minimize adverse effects.
	› Monitor blood pressure.
	› Reduce systemic dose slowly.
	› Monitor electrolytes and glucose.
	› May slow healing.
	› Advise the client to:
	  » Take oral dose with food.
	  » Avoid discontinuing dose suddenly.
	  » Report unexpected increase in weight or other signs of fluid retention.
	  » Avoid crowds and other exposures to infectious diseases.
	  » Report evidence of infection (clients who have Crohn's disease; may mask infection).

CLASSIFICATION/THERAPEUTIC INTENT	NURSING CONSIDERATIONS/CLIENT EDUCATION
Ulcerative colitis and Crohn's disease	

› Immunosuppressants
  » Mechanism of action in treatment of IBD is unknown.
› Medications
  » Cyclosporine (Sandimmune) and methotrexate (Rheumatrex) for severe refractory disease (resistant to treatment)
	› Teach clients to avoid crowds and other chances of exposures to infectious diseases and to report evidence of infection.
	› Advise the client to monitor for indications of bleeding, bruising, or infection.
	› Monitor kidney and hepatic function.

› Immunomodulators
  » Suppress the immune response
  » An antibody used to reduce tumor necrosis factor
› Medications
  » Infliximab (Remicade)
  » Certolizumab (Cimzia)
	› Follow directions for IV use with care and in accordance with facility policy.
	› Many adverse effects are possible, including chills, fever, hypertension, dysrhythmias, and low levels of blood cells.
	› Monitor liver enzymes and hemoglobin and hematocrit.
	› Teach clients to avoid crowds and other chances of exposures to infectious diseases, and to report indications of infection. The client is at risk for development or reactivation of tuberculosis.
	› Advise the client to monitor for evidence of bleeding, bruising, or infection.

› Antidiarrheals
  » Suppress the number of stools
› Medications
  » Diphenoxylate hydrochloride and atropine (Lomotil)
  » Loperamide (Imodium)
	› Used to decrease risk of fluid volume deficit and electrolyte imbalance. They also reduce discomfort.
	› Observe for indications of respiratory depression, especially in the older adult client.
	› Observe for manifestations of toxic megacolon (hypotension, abdominal distention, decrease or absence of bowel sounds).
	› Due to the central nervous system effects, the client should be taught to avoid hazardous activities until the response to the medication is established.

Diverticulitis	

› Antimicrobials
  » Treat infection (decrease inflammation)
› Medications
  » Ciprofloxacin (Cipro)
  » Metronidazole (Flagyl)
	› May cause suprainfection. Instruct client to observe for findings of thrush or vaginal yeast infection.
	› Not appropriate for children less than 18 years of age (risk of Achilles tendon rupture).
	› Decreased dose should be used for clients who have impaired renal function.
	› Instruct client that urine may darken (expected, harmless side effect).
	› Teach client to monitor for manifestations of CNS effect (numbness of extremities, ataxia, and seizures) and to notify provider immediately.

- Teamwork and Collaboration
  - Refer the client for nutritional counseling.
  - The client may benefit from complementary therapy (biofeedback, massage, yoga).
  - The client may need a mental health referral for assistance with coping.
- Surgical Interventions
  - Clients who do not have success with medical treatment or who have complications (bowel perforation, colon cancer) are candidates for surgery.
  - Surgical Procedure for Ulcerative Colitis
    - Colectomy with or without ileostomy
  - Surgical Procedures for Crohn's Disease
    - Stricturoplasty may be performed laparoscopically in some cases.
    - Surgical repair of fistulas or in response to other complications related to the disease (perforation)
  - Surgical Procedures for Diverticulitis (dependent on problem type)
    - Colon resection
    - Double-barrel colostomy, but may be temporary
    - Treatment of complications (peritonitis, abscess, obstruction, fistula, bleeding)
  - Preoperative Care
    - Preoperative care is similar to care for clients who have other abdominal surgeries.
    - Reinforce teaching on the type of surgery to be performed.
    - If the creation of a stoma is planned, collaborate with an enterostomal therapy nurse regarding care related to the stoma.
    - Administer antibiotic bowel prep (neomycin sulfate), if prescribed.
    - Administer cleansing enema or laxative, if prescribed.
  - Postoperative Care
    - Postoperative care is similar to care for clients who have other types of abdominal surgery.
    - The client should be NPO and have a nasogastric tube to suction, unless the surgery was performed laparoscopically.
    - An ileostomy may drain as much as 1,000 mL/day. Prevent fluid volume deficit (Administer IV fluids if the client is NPO. Oral hydration may be administered later in the course of recovery).
- Care After Discharge – Refer the client who has an ostomy to an enterostomal therapist and to an ostomate support group.

Complications

- Complications of ulcerative colitis, Crohn's disease, and diverticulitis include bleeding and fluid and electrolyte imbalance. Peritonitis may occur due to perforation of the bowel. Abscess formation may occur as a complication of diverticular disease and Crohn's disease.

- Peritonitis is a life threatening inflammation of the peritoneum and lining of the abdominal cavity. It is most often caused by bacteria in the peritoneal cavity.

  - Assessment Findings
    - Rigid, boardlike abdomen (hallmark sign)
    - Nausea, vomiting
    - Rebound tenderness
    - Tachycardia
    - Fever

  - Nursing Actions
    - Place the client in Fowler or semi-Fowler's position. (This promotes comfort and allows for the client to breathe easier.)
    - Administer oxygen as prescribed. Turn, cough, deep breathe. Mechanical ventilation may be required in severe cases.
    - Maintain and monitor nasogastric suction.
    - Keep the client NPO.
    - Monitor fluid and electrolyte status (be alert for evidence of hypovolemia).
    - Administer IV antibiotics as prescribed.
    - If surgery is performed:
      - I&O may be monitored every hour immediately after surgery.
      - Use sterile technique to irrigate the peritoneal area via a catheter or drain (if ordered by the provider).

  - Client Education
    - Provide client education related to short-term hemodialysis, if prescribed.
    - Instruct client to maintain adequate rest and resume home activity slowly, as tolerated. No heavy lifting for at least 6 weeks.
    - Teach client to monitor for evidence of return infection; notify provider immediately.
    - Collaborate with case management to determine home care and wound management needs.

- Bleeding due to deterioration of the bowel.
  - Nursing Actions
    - Observe for indications of rectal bleeding.
    - Monitor vital signs.
    - Check laboratory values, especially hematocrit, hemoglobin, and coagulation factors.

  - Client Education
    - Instruct the client to report rectal bleeding.
    - Explain to the client the importance of bed rest.

- Fluid and electrolyte imbalance occurs due to loss of fluid through diarrhea and vomiting, and may occur with nasogastric suctioning.
  - Nursing Actions
    - Monitor laboratory values and provide replacement therapy.
    - Monitor weight.
    - Assess for indications of fluid volume deficit (loss of or absent skin turgor).
  - Client Education
    - Instruct the client to record and report the number of loose stools.
    - Encourage the client to obtain adequate fluid intake.
    - Advise the client to follow the prescribed diet.
- Abscess and fistula formation occurs due to the destruction of the bowel wall, leading to an infection.
  - Nursing Actions
    - Monitor fluid and electrolytes.
    - Observe for manifestations of dehydration.
    - Provide a diet high in protein and calories (at least 3,000 calories/day), and low in fiber.
    - Administer a vitamin supplement.
    - Consult with an enterostomal therapist to develop a plan to prevent skin breakdown and promote wound healing.
    - Monitor for evidence of infection, which may indicate abdominal abscesses or sepsis.
    - Ensure the function of drainage devices if used.
- Toxic megacolon occurs due to inactivity of the colon. Massive dilation of the colon occurs and the client is at risk for perforation.
  - Nursing Actions
    - Maintain nasogastric suction.
    - Administer IV fluids and electrolytes.
    - Administer prescribed medications (antibiotics, corticosteroids).
    - Prepare the client for surgery (usually an ileostomy) if the client does not begin to show signs of improvement within 72 hr or less.

APPLICATION EXERCISES

1. A nurse is reviewing the laboratory findings of a client who has an acute exacerbation of Crohn's disease. Which of the following laboratory findings is indicative of Crohn's disease? (Select all that apply.)

_____ A. Increased hematocrit

___X___ B. Increased erythrocyte sedimentation rate (ESR)

___X___ C. Increased WBC

_____ D. Increased folic acid

_____ E. Increased serum albumin

2. A nurse is assessing a client who has been taking prednisone following an exacerbation of inflammatory bowel disease (IBD). Which of the following assessment findings is the highest priority?

A. Client reports difficulty sleeping.

B. Blood glucose at 0800 is 140 mg/dL.

C. Client reports having a sore throat.

D. Client reports gaining 4 lb in last 6 months.

3. A nurse is reinforcing teaching for a client who has a prescription for sulfasalazine (Azulfidine). Which of the following should the nurse include in the teaching?

A. "Take the medication 1 or 2 hr after eating."

B. "This medication may cause yellowing of the sclera."

C. "Notify the provider if you experience a sore throat."

D. "This medication may cause your stools to turn black."

4. A nurse in a clinic is teaching a client who has ulcerative colitis. Which of the following statements by the client indicates understanding of the teaching?

A. "I will plan to limit fiber in my diet."

B. "I will eat my meals and plan fluid intake between meals."

C. "I will switch to black tea instead of drinking coffee."

D. "I will try to eat three moderate to large meals a day."

5. A nurse is completing discharge teaching to a client who has Crohn's disease. Which of the following should be included in the teaching?

    A. Decrease intake of calorie-dense foods.

    B. Drink canned protein supplements.

    C. Take calcium supplements daily.

    D. Take a bulk-forming laxative daily.

6. A nurse is teaching a client who has diverticulitis. What should be included in the teaching? Use the ATI Active Learning Template: Systems Disorder to complete this item to include the following:

    A. Pathophysiology

    B. Risk Factors: Identify two.

    C. Laboratory Data: Identify two findings.

    D. Diagnostic Procedures: Identify three.

    E. Client Education: Describe dietary teaching.

APPLICATION EXERCISES KEY

1. A. INCORRECT: Hematocrit is decreased as a result of chronic blood loss.

    B. **CORRECT:** Increased ESR is a clinical finding in a client who has Crohn's disease.

    C. **CORRECT:** Increased WBC is a clinical finding in a client who has Crohn's disease.

    D. INCORRECT: A decrease in folic acid level is indicative of malabsorption.

    E. INCORRECT: A decrease in serum albumin is indicative of malabsorption.

    Ⓝ NCLEX® Connection: Physiological Adaptations, Pathophysiology

2. A. INCORRECT: Difficulty sleeping is an important finding but not the priority finding.

    B. INCORRECT: A blood glucose slightly above the expected reference range is an important finding but not the priority finding.

    C. **CORRECT:** The greatest risk to the client who is taking prednisone is an infection due to immunosuppression. This is the priority finding.

    D. INCORRECT: Weight gain is an important finding but not the priority finding.

    Ⓝ NCLEX® Connection: Pharmacological and Parenteral Therapies, Adverse Effects/Contraindications/ Side Effects/Interactions

3. A. INCORRECT: Sulfasalazine should be taken with food.

    B. INCORRECT: Sulfasalazine does not cause yellowing of the sclera.

    C. **CORRECT:** A client who is taking sulfasalazine may have a depressed immune system and be more vulnerable to infection. The provider should be notified of this finding.

    D. INCORRECT: Sulfasalazine does not change the color of stools.

    Ⓝ NCLEX® Connection: Pharmacological and Parenteral Therapies, Medication Administration

4.   A. **CORRECT:** A low-fiber diet is recommended for the client who has ulcerative colitis to reduce inflammation.

B. INCORRECT: A client who has dumping syndrome should avoid fluids with meals.

C. INCORRECT: Caffeinated beverages, such as black tea, should be avoided by the client who has ulcerative colitis.

D. INCORRECT: Small frequent meals are recommended for the client who has ulcerative colitis.

Ⓝ NCLEX® Connection: Basic Care and Comfort, Nutrition and Oral Hydration

5.   A. INCORRECT: A high-protein diet is recommended for the client who has Crohn's disease.

B. **CORRECT:** A high-protein diet is recommended for the client who has Crohn's disease, and canned protein supplements are encouraged.

C. INCORRECT: Vitamin supplements, not calcium, are recommended for the client who has Crohn's disease.

D. INCORRECT: Bulk-forming laxatives are recommended for the client who has diverticulitis.

Ⓝ NCLEX® Connection: Physiological Adaptations, Illness Management

6.   *Using the ATI Active Learning Template: Systems Disorder*

A. Pathophysiology
   - Inflammation and infection of the bowel mucosa caused by bacteria or fecal matter trapped in one or more diverticula (pouches in the intestine).

B. Risk Factors
   - Older adults
   - More often in men

C. Laboratory Data
   - Decreased hemoglobin and hematocrit.
   - Stool may be positive for occult blood.
   - Urine may be positive for RBCs.

D. Diagnostic Procedures
   - Abdominal x-ray
   - CT scan
   - Colonoscopy
   - Sigmoidoscopy

E. Client Education
   - Consume clear liquid until manifestations subside. Progress to a low fiber diet as tolerated. Add fiber once solid foods are tolerated. Slowly advance to a high-fiber diet.
   - Avoid seeds or indigestible material (nuts, popcorn, seeds).
   - Avoid alcohol. Limit fat to 30% of daily caloric intake.

Ⓝ NCLEX® Connection: Physiological Adaptations, Illness Management

CHAPTER 53   Cholecystitis and Cholelithiasis

Overview

- Cholecystitis is an inflammation of the gallbladder wall.

- Cholecystitis is most often caused by gallstones (cholelithiasis) obstructing the cystic and/or common bile ducts (bile flows from the gallbladder to the duodenum) causing bile to back up and the gall bladder to become inflamed.

- Cholelithiasis is the presence of stones in the gall bladder related to either the precipitation of bile or cholesterol into stones.

- Bile is used for the digestion of fats. It is produced in the liver and stored in the gall bladder.

- Cholecystitis can be acute or chronic, and can obstruct the pancreatic duct, causing pancreatitis. It can also cause the gall bladder to rupture, resulting in secondary peritonitis.

Health Promotion and Disease Prevention

- Consume a low-fat diet rich in HDL sources (seafood, nuts, olive oil).

- Participate in a regular exercise program.

- Do not smoke.

Assessment

- Risk Factors

  - More common in females

    - Hormone therapy and use of some oral contraceptives

  - High-fat diet

  - Obesity (impaired fat metabolism, high cholesterol)

  - Genetic predisposition

  - Older than 60 years of age (decreased contractility, more likely to develop gallstones)

  - Individuals who have type 1 diabetes mellitus (high triglycerides)

  - Low-calorie, liquid protein diets

  - Rapid weight loss (increases cholesterol)

- Subjective Data

  - Sharp pain in the right upper quadrant, often radiating to the right shoulder

  - Pain with deep inspiration during right subcostal palpation (Murphy's sign)

  - Intense pain (increased heart rate, pallor, diaphoresis) with nausea and vomiting after ingestion of high-fat food caused by biliary colic

- ○ Rebound tenderness (Blumberg's sign; performed by the provider only)
- ○ Dyspepsia, eructation (belching), and flatulence
- ○ Fever
- Objective Data
  - ○ Physical Assessment Findings
    - Jaundice, clay-colored stools, steatorrhea (fatty stools), dark urine, and pruritus (accumulation of bile salts in the skin) in clients who have chronic cholecystitis (due to biliary obstruction).
    - Older adult clients who have diabetes mellitus may have atypical presentation of cholecystitis (absence of pain or fever).
  - ○ Laboratory Tests
    - WBC increased with left shift indicates inflammation
    - Direct, indirect, and total serum bilirubin (increased if bile duct obstructed)
    - Amylase and lipase (increased with pancreatic involvement)
    - Aspartate aminotransferase (AST), lactate dehydrogenase (LDH), and alkaline phosphatase (ALP) (increased with liver dysfunction) may indicate the common bile duct is obstructed.
    - Serum cholesterol (greater than 200 mg/dL)
  - ○ Diagnostic Procedures
    - Ultrasound visualizes gall stones and a dilated common bile duct.
    - An abdominal x-ray or CT scan can visualize calcified gallstones and an enlarged gall bladder.
    - A hepatobiliary scan (HIDA) assesses the patency of the biliary duct system after an IV injection of contrast.
    - An endoscopic retrograde cholangiopancreatography (ERCP) allows for direct visualization using an endoscope that is inserted through the esophagus and into the common bile duct via the duodenum. A sphincterotomy with gall stones removal may be done during this procedure. (Refer to the chapter on *Gastrointestinal Diagnostic Procedures*.)
    - A percutaneous transhepatic cholangiography (PTC) involves the direct injection of contrast into the biliary tract through the use of a flexible needle. The gallbladder and ducts can be visualized.

Patient-Centered Care

- Nursing Care – Administer analgesics as needed and prescribed.
- Medications
  - ○ Analgesics – Morphine sulfate or hydromorphone (Dilaudid) are preferred over meperidine (Demerol), which can cause seizures, especially in older adults.
  - ○ Bile Acid – chenodiol (Chenix), ursodiol (ursodeoxycholic acid)
    - Bile acid gradually dissolves cholesterol-based gall stones, with few adverse effects.
    - Nursing Considerations – Use caution in clients who have liver conditions or disorders with varices.

- Therapeutic Procedures
  - ○ Extracorporeal shock wave lithotripsy (ESWL) – Shock waves are used to break up stones. This may be used more on nonsurgical candidates of normal weight who have small, cholesterol-based stones.
  - ○ Nursing Actions
    - ▪ Instruct and assist client to lay on fluid-filled bag for delivery of shock waves.
    - ▪ Administer analgesia, as prescribed.
  - ○ Client Education – Inform the client that several procedures may be required to break up all stones.
- Surgical Interventions
  - ○ Cholecystectomy – removal of the gallbladder with a laparoscopic or open approach
  - ○ The client usually is discharged within 24 hr if a laparoscopic approach is used. An open approach requires the client to be hospitalized for 2 to 3 days.
    - ▪ Nursing Actions
      - □ Laparoscopic approach – Provide immediate postoperative care.
      - □ Natural orifice transluminal endoscopic surgery (NOTES) – Surgery is performed through entry of the mouth, vagina, or rectum. This approach decreases the risk of complications for the client.
      - □ Open approach
        - ▸ A T-tube may be placed in the common bile duct. This is only required when there is exploration of the common bile duct intraoperatively.
        - ▸ The use of T-tubes has significantly decreased due to the laparoscopic approach.
      - □ Care of the T-tube
        - ▸ Monitor and record drainage (initially bloody, then green-brown bile).
        - ▸ Expect more than 400 mL of drainage in 24 hr initially, with gradual decrease in amount.
        - ▸ Instruct client to report an absence of drainage with manifestations of nausea and pain (may indicate obstruction in the T-tube).
        - ▸ Instruct client to report sudden increases in drainage or amounts exceeding 1,000 mL/day.
        - ▸ Inspect the surrounding skin for evidence of infection or bile leakage.
        - ▸ Maintain flow by gravity and do not raise drainage bag above level of gallbladder.
        - ▸ Empty the drainage bag every 8 hr.
        - ▸ Clamp the tube 1 to 2 hr before and after meals to assess tolerance to food post cholecystectomy, and prior to removal.
        - ▸ Assess stools for color (stools clay-colored until biliary flow is reestablished).
        - ▸ Monitor for bile peritonitis (pain, fever, jaundice).
        - ▸ Monitor and document response to food.
    - ▪ Client Education
      - □ Laparoscopic or NOTES approach
        - ▸ Ambulate frequently to minimize free air pain, common following laparoscopic surgery (under the right clavicle, shoulder, scapula).
        - ▸ Monitor incision for evidence of infection or wound dehiscence (laparoscopic approach).

▸ Educate the client regarding pain control.

▸ Report indications of bile leak (pain, vomiting, abdominal distention) to the provider.

▸ Activities are often resumed in 1 week.

▫ Open approach

▸ Resume activity gradually. Avoid heavy lifting for 4 to 6 weeks.

▸ Report sudden increase in drainage, foul odor, pain, fever, or jaundice.

▸ The T-tube is usually left in 1 to 2 weeks postoperatively.

▸ Take showers instead of baths until T-tube is removed.

▸ Clamp T-tube 1 to 2 hr before and after meals to prepare for removal.

▸ The color of stools should return to brown in about a week, and diarrhea is common.

▪ Dietary Counseling

▫ Encourage a low-fat diet (reduce dairy products and avoid fried foods, chocolate, nuts, gravies). Small, frequent meals may be more easily tolerated.

▫ Avoid gas-forming foods (beans, cabbage, cauliflower, broccoli).

▫ Promote weight reduction.

▫ Instruct client to take fat-soluble vitamins or bile salts as prescribed to enhance absorption and aid with digestion.

Complications

- Obstruction of the bile duct

  ○ This can cause ischemia, gangrene, and a rupture of the gallbladder wall. A rupture of the gallbladder wall can cause a local abscess or peritonitis (rigid, board-like abdomen, guarding), which requires a surgical intervention and administration of broad spectrum antibiotics.

- Bile peritonitis

  ○ This can occur if adequate amounts of bile are not drained from the surgical site. This is a rare complication, but it may be fatal.

  ○ Nursing Actions

    ▪ Monitor for pain, fever, and jaundice.

    ▪ Report to the provider immediately.

- Postcholecystectomy syndrome (PCS)

  ○ Manifestations of gallbladder disease can continue after surgery. The client will report findings similar to those experienced prior to surgery related to pain and nausea. Manifestations can recur immediately or years later.

  ○ Nursing Actions

    ▪ Assess pain characteristics and other reported findings.

    ▪ Instruct client that further diagnostic evaluation may be necessary.

APPLICATION EXERCISES

1. A nurse is providing discharge teaching to a client who is postoperative following open cholecystectomy with T-tube placement. Which of the following instructions should the nurse include in the teaching? (Select all that apply.)

_____ A. Take baths rather than showers.

_____ B. Clamp T-tube for 1 to 2 hr before and after meals.

_____ C. Keep the drainage system above the level of the gallbladder.

_____ D. Expect to have constipation.

_____ E. Empty drainage bag every 8 hr.

2. A nurse is reviewing nutrition teaching for a client who has cholecystitis. Which of the following food choices can trigger cholecystitis?

A. Brownie with nuts

B. Bowl of mixed fruit

C. Grilled turkey

D. Baked potato

3. A nurse is completing preoperative teaching for a client who will undergo a laparoscopic cholecystectomy. Which of the following should be included in the teaching?

A. "The scope will be passed through your rectum."

B. "You may have shoulder pain after surgery."

C. "The T-tube will remain in place for 1 to 2 weeks."

D. "You should limit how often you walk for 1 to 2 weeks."

4. A nurse is reviewing a new prescription for ursodiol (Ursodeoxycholic Acid) with a client who has cholelithiasis. Which of the following should be included in the teaching?

A. This medication reduces biliary spasms.

B. This medication reduces inflammation in the biliary tract.

C. This medication dilates the bile duct to promote passage of bile.

D. This medication dissolves gall stones.

5. A nurse in a clinic is reviewing the laboratory reports of a client who has suspected cholelithiasis. Which of the following is an expected finding?

    A. Serum albumin 4.1 g/dL

    B. WBC 9,511/uL

    C. Direct bilirubin 2.1 mg/dL

    D. Serum cholesterol 171 mg/dL

6. A nurse is presenting a program on gall bladder disease to a group of clients at a health fair. What should be included in the program? Use the ATI Active Learning Template: Systems Disorder to complete this item to include the following sections:

    A. Risk Factors: Describe at least four.

    B. Subjective Data: Describe at least four findings.

    C. Objective Data: Describe at least four findings.

    D. Client Education: Describe three preventative activities.

APPLICATION EXERCISES KEY

1. A. INCORRECT: Soaking in bath water is contraindicated due to the increased risk for introduction of organisms and infection.

   B. **CORRECT:** The T-tube should be clamped 1 to 2 hr before and after meals to assess tolerance to food postcholecystectomy, and prior to removal.

   C. INCORRECT: The drainage system should not be placed above the level of the gallbladder due to the risk of infection from the reflux of drainage from the tube into the wound bed.

   D. INCORRECT: Diarrhea is common and stools will return to brown color in a week.

   E. **CORRECT:** The drainage bag attached to the T-tube should be emptied every 8 hr.

   N NCLEX® Connection: Reduction of Risk Potential, Therapeutic Procedures

2. A. **CORRECT:** Foods that are high in fat, such as a brownie with nuts, can cause cholecystitis.

   B. INCORRECT: Fruits are low in fat and not associated with cholecystitis.

   C. INCORRECT: Turkey is low in fat and not associated with cholecystitis.

   D. INCORRECT: Baked potatoes are low in fat and not associated with cholecystitis.

   N NCLEX® Connection: Basic Care and Comfort, Nutrition and Oral Hydration

3. A. INCORRECT: Surgery is performed through the rectum during the natural orifice transluminal endoscopic surgery (NOTES) approach.

   B. **CORRECT:** Shoulder pain occurs due to free air that is introduced into the abdomen during laparoscopic surgery.

   B. INCORRECT: A T-tube is placed during the open surgery approach when the common bile duct is explored.

   D. INCORRECT: The client is instructed to ambulate frequently following a laparoscopic surgical approach to minimize the free air that has been introduced.

   N NCLEX® Connection: Reduction of Risk Potential, Therapeutic Procedures

4. A. INCORRECT: Ursodiol is used to dissolve gall stones.

   B. INCORRECT: Ursodiol does not reduce inflammation in the biliary tract.

   C. INCORRECT: Ursodiol dissolves gall stones to allow passage of bile in the bile duct.

   D. **CORRECT:** Ursodiol is a bile acid that gradually dissolves cholesterol-based gall stones.

   N NCLEX® Connection: Pharmacological and Parenteral Therapies, Medication Administration

5.   A. INCORRECT: Serum albumin is within the expected reference range and is not an indicator of cholelithiasis.

   B. INCORRECT: An expected finding would be an increased WBC due to inflammation. This finding is within the expected reference range.

   C. **CORRECT:** This finding is outside the expected reference range and is increased in the client who has cholelithiasis.

   D. INCORRECT: An expected finding for a client who has cholelithiasis is a serum cholesterol greater than 200 mg/dL.

   Ⓝ NCLEX® Connection: Reduction of Risk Potential, Laboratory Values

6.   *Using the ATI Active Learning Template: Systems Disorder*

   A. Risk Factors

   - Female sex, use of hormone therapy, and some oral contraceptives
   - High-fat or low-calorie, liquid protein diets
   - Obesity
   - Genetic predisposition
   - Age over 60 years
   - Type 1 diabetes mellitus
   - Rapid weight loss

   B. Subjective Data

   - Sharp pain in the right upper quadrant that often radiates to the right shoulder
   - Pain upon deep inspiration during right subcostal palpation
   - Intense pain with nausea and vomiting after ingestion of high-fat food
   - Dyspepsia
   - Eructation (belching)
   - Flatulence
   - Fever

   C. Objective Data

   - Jaundice
   - Clay-colored stools
   - Steatorrhea (fatty stools)
   - Dark urine
   - Pruritus

   D. Client Education

   - Get regular exercise.
   - Stop smoking.
   - Consume a low-fat diet rich in HDL sources (seafood, nuts, olive oil).

   Ⓝ NCLEX® Connection: Physiological Adaptations, Pathophysiology

chapter 54

Overview

- The islets of Langerhans in the pancreas secrete insulin and glucagon. The pancreatic tissues secrete digestive enzymes that break down carbohydrates, proteins, and fats.

- Pancreatitis is an autodigestion of the pancreas by pancreatic digestive enzymes that activate prematurely before reaching the intestines. The mechanism of action is unknown. Pancreatitis can result in inflammation, necrosis, and hemorrhage.

- Classic presentation of an acute attack includes severe, constant, knifelike pain (left upper quadrant, mid-epigastric, and/or radiating to the back) that is unrelieved by nausea and vomiting.

- Acute pancreatitis is an inflammatory process due to activated pancreatic enzymes autodigesting the pancreas. Severity varies, but overall mortality is 10% to 20%.

- Chronic pancreatitis is a progressive, destructive disease with the development of calcification and necrosis, possibly resulting in hemorrhagic pancreatitis. Mortality can be as high as 50%.

Health Promotion and Disease Prevention

- Avoid excessive alcohol consumption.
- Eat a diet low-fat diet.

Assessment

- Risk Factors
  - Biliary tract disease (gallstones can cause a blockage where the common bile duct and pancreatic duct meet)
  - Alcohol use
    - The primary cause of chronic pancreatitis is alcohol use disorder. This may occur more often in older adults as age-related changes reduce the ability to physiologically handle alcohol.
  - Endoscopic retrograde cholangiopancreatography (ERCP) (postprocedure complication)
  - Gastrointestinal surgery
  - Metabolic disturbances (hyperlipidemia, hyperparathyroidism, hypercalcemia)
  - Kidney failure or transplant
  - Genetic predisposition
  - Trauma
  - Penetrating ulcer (gastric or duodenal)
  - Medication/drug toxicity

- Subjective Data
  - Sudden onset of severe, boring pain
    - Epigastric, radiating to back, left flank, or left shoulder
    - Worse when lying down or while eating
    - Worse after consumption of alcohol or high-fat foods
    - Not relieved with vomiting
  - Pain relieved somewhat by fetal position
  - Nausea and vomiting
  - Weight loss
- Objective Data
  - Physical Assessment Findings
    - Seepage of blood-stained exudates into tissue as a result of pancreatic enzyme actions
      - Ecchymoses on the flanks (Turner's sign)
      - Bluish-grey periumbilical discoloration (Cullen's sign)

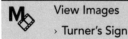

M⬥	View Images	
	› Turner's Sign	› Cullen's Sign

    - Generalized jaundice
    - Absent or decreased bowel sounds (possible paralytic ileus)
    - Warm, moist skin; fruity breath (evidence of hyperglycemia)
    - Ascites
    - Tetany
      - Trousseau's sign (hand spasm when blood pressure cuff is inflated)
      - Chvostek's sign (facial twitching when facial nerve is tapped)
  - Laboratory Tests
    - Serum amylase (increases within 12 hr, remains increased for 4 days) and serum lipase (increases slowly but remains increased for up to 2 weeks)
      - Urine amylase remains increased for up to 2 weeks.
      - Increases in enzymes indicate pancreatic cell injury.
      - Memory aid: In pancreatitis, the "ases" (aces) are high.
      - For amylase and lipase to be considered positive, the enzyme increases must be significant (two to three times greater than the expected value for amylase, and three to five times greater than the expected value for lipase). The degree of enzyme elevation does not directly correlate with the severity of the disease.
    - WBC count: increased due to infection and inflammation
    - Platelets: decreased
    - Serum calcium and magnesium: decreased due to fat necrosis with pancreatitis
    - Serum liver enzymes and bilirubin: increased with associated biliary dysfunction
    - Serum glucose: increased due to a decrease in insulin production by the pancreas
  - Diagnostic Procedures – Computed tomography (CT) scan with contrast is reliably diagnostic of acute pancreatitis.

Patient-Centered Care

- Nursing Care
  - Rest the pancreas.
    - NPO – no food until pain-free
    - Total parenteral nutrition (TPN) or jejunal feedings (less risk of hyperglycemia)
    - When diet is resumed: bland, low-fat diet with no stimulants (caffeine); small, frequent meals
    - Administer antiemetic as needed, as prescribed
    - Nasogastric tube – gastric decompression
    - No alcohol consumption
    - No smoking
    - Limit stress
    - Pain management
  - Position the client for comfort (fetal, side-lying, the head of the bed elevated, sitting up or leaning forward).
  - Administer analgesics and other medications as prescribed.
  - Monitor blood glucose and provide insulin as needed (potential for hyperglycemia).
  - Monitor hydration status (orthostatic blood pressure, intake and output, laboratory values).
  - Administer IV fluids and electrolyte replacement as prescribed.
- Medications
  - Opioid analgesics: morphine sulfate for acute pain
    - Nursing Considerations
      - Large doses of IV opioids often are needed for pain management.
      - Meperidine (Demerol) is discouraged in older adult clients due to the risk of seizures.
  - Antibiotics: imipenem (Primaxin)
    - Antibiotics may be used, but are generally indicated for clients who have acute necrotizing pancreatitis.
    - Nursing Considerations
      - Monitor for evidence of infection.
      - Monitor for seizures.
  - Anticholinergics (dicyclomine [Bentyl]) decrease intestinal motility and the flow of pancreatic enzymes.
    - Nursing Considerations – Use with caution in clients who have cardiac problems or ulcerative colitis.
  - Spasmolytics (papaverine [Pavabid]) relax smooth muscle.
    - Nursing Considerations
      - Monitor for jaundice.
      - May cause orthostatic hypotension.

- ○ Histamine receptor antagonists (ranitidine [Zantac]) and proton pump inhibitors (omeprazole [Prilosec]) decrease gastric acid secretion.

- ○ Pancreatic enzymes (pancrelipase [Viokase]) aid with digestion of fats and proteins when taken with meals and snacks.

  - ▪ Nursing Considerations

    - □ Client may sprinkle contents of capsules on nonprotein foods.

    - □ Client should drink a full glass of water following pancrelipase.

    - □ Clients should wipe lips and rinse mouth after taking (to prevent skin breakdown or irritation).

- • Teamwork and Collaboration – Dietary referral for postpancreatitis diet and nutritional supplements when oral intake resumed

- • Therapeutic Procedures – ERCP to create an opening in the sphincter of Oddi if pancreatitis is caused by gallstones

- • Surgical Interventions

  - ○ Cholecystectomy if pancreatitis is a result of cholecystitis and gallstones

  - ○ Pancreaticojejunostomy (Roux-en-Y) reroutes drainage of pancreatic secretions into jejunum

- • Care After Discharge

  - ○ Home health services may be indicated for clients regarding nutritional needs, possible wound care, and assistance with ADLs.

  - ○ Alcoholics Anonymous (AA) may be indicated for the client or family member who has an alcohol use disorder.

Complications

- • Hypovolemia – up to 6 L of fluid can be third-spaced; caused by retroperitoneal loss of protein-rich fluid from proteolytic digestion. The client can develop hypovolemic shock.

  - ○ Nursing Actions – Monitor vital signs, electrolytes, and provide IV fluid and electrolyte replacement.

- • Chronic pancreatitis due to alcohol use

  - ○ Client Education – Encourage the client to avoid alcohol intake and caffeinated beverages, and to participate in support groups for individuals who have alcohol use disorder.

- • Pancreatic infection: pseudocyst (outside pancreas); abscess (inside pancreas)

  - ○ Cause – leakage of fluid out of damaged pancreatic duct

  - ○ Nursing Actions

    - ▪ Monitor for rupture and hemorrhage.

    - ▪ Maintain sump tube if placed for drainage of cyst.

    - ▪ Monitor skin around tube for breakdown secondary to corrosive enzymes.

- Type 1 diabetes mellitus
  - Cause – lack or absence of insulin (due to destruction of pancreatic beta cells)
  - Nursing Actions
    - Monitor blood glucose.
    - Administer insulin as prescribed.
  - Client Education – Inform the client about long-term diabetes management.

- Left lung effusion and atelectasis – more common complication in older adults and may precipitate pneumonia
  - Causes
    - Splinting of chest due to pain upon coughing and deep breathing
    - Pancreatic ascites
  - Nursing Actions – Monitor for hypoxia and provide ventilatory support.
- Coagulation defects (disseminated intravascular coagulopathy)
  - Causes – release of thromboplastic endotoxins secondary to necrotizing hemorrhagic pancreatitis (NHP)
  - Nursing Actions – Monitor bleeding times.
- Multi-system organ failure – Inflammation of pancreas is believed to trigger systemic inflammation.
  - Cause – necrotizing hemorrhagic pancreatitis
  - Nursing Actions
    - Administer treatments as prescribed.
    - Monitor for evidence of organ failure (respiratory distress, jaundice, oliguria).
    - Report unexpected findings to provider.

APPLICATION EXERCISES

1. A nurse is completing the admission assessment of a client who has acute pancreatitis. Which of the following findings is the priority to be reported to the provider?

    A. History of cholelithiasis

    B. Serum amylase levels three times greater than the expected value

    C. Client report of severe pain radiating to the back that is rated at an "8"

    D. Hand spasms present when blood pressure is checked

2. A nurse is preparing to administer pancrelipase (Viokase) to a client who has pancreatitis. Which of the following is an appropriate nursing action?

    A. Administer medication 30 min after a snack.

    B. Offer a glass of water following medication administration.

    C. Administer the medication 30 min before meals.

    D. Sprinkle the contents on peanut butter.

3. A nurse is completing an admission assessment of a client who has pancreatitis. Which of the following is an expected finding?

    A. Pain in right upper quadrant radiating to right shoulder

    B. Report of pain being worse when sitting upright

    C. Pain relieved with defecation

    D. Epigastric pain radiating to left shoulder

4. A nurse is reviewing the health record of a client who has pancreatitis. The physical exam report by the provider indicates the presence of Cullen's sign. Which of the following is an appropriate action by the nurse to identify this finding?

    A. Tap lightly at the costovertebral margin on the client's back.

    B. Palpate the client's right lower quadrant.

    C. Inspect the skin around the umbilicus.

    D. Auscultate the area below the client's scapula.

5. A nurse is completing nutrition teaching for a client who has pancreatitis. Which of the following statements by the client requires further teaching?

    A. "I plan to eat small, frequent meals."

    B. "I will eat easy-to-digest foods with limited spice."

    C. "I will use skim milk when cooking."

    D. "I plan to drink regular cola."

6. A nurse is reviewing the plan of care for a client who has pancreatitis. What should be included in the plan? Use the ATI Active Learning Template: Systems Disorder to complete this item to include the following sections:

    A. Client Problem Related to Alteration in Health: Describe the classic presentation of pancreatitis.

    B. Laboratory Data: Describe four tests and expected findings.

    C. Nursing Interventions: Describe at least six.

APPLICATION EXERCISES KEY

1. A. INCORRECT: A history of cholelithiasis is important but not the priority finding the nurse should report to the provider.

   B. INCORRECT: Increased serum amylase is important but not the priority finding the nurse should report to the provider.

   C. INCORRECT: A report of pain is important but not the priority finding the nurse should report to the provider.

   D. **CORRECT:** The greatest risk to the client is hypocalcemia due to the risk of cardiac dysrhythmia. Hand spasms when taking a blood pressure is an indication of hypocalcemia and is the priority finding to report to the provider.

   Ⓝ NCLEX® Connection: Physiological Adaptations, Medical Emergencies

2. A. INCORRECT: Pancrelipase should be administered with meals and snacks.

   B. **CORRECT:** The client should drink a full glass of water following administration of pancrelipase.

   C. INCORRECT: Pancrelipase should be administered with meals and snacks.

   D. INCORRECT: The contents of the pancrelipase capsule may be sprinkled on nonprotein foods, and peanut butter is a protein food.

   Ⓝ NCLEX® Connection: Pharmacological and Parenteral Therapies, Medication Administration

3. A. INCORRECT: A client who has cholecystitis will report pain in the right upper quadrant radiating to the right shoulder.

   B. INCORRECT: A client who has pancreatitis will report pain being worse when lying down or when eating.

   C. INCORRECT: A client who has pancreatitis will report that pain is relieved with vomiting.

   D. **CORRECT:** A client who has pancreatitis will report severe, boring epigastric pain that radiates to the back, left flank, or left shoulder.

   Ⓝ NCLEX® Connection: Physiological Adaptations, Pathophysiology

4.   A. INCORRECT: This action assesses for pain which may indicate pyelonephritis.

      B. INCORRECT: This action assesses for the presence of rebound tenderness.

      C. **CORRECT:** Cullen's sign is indicated by a bluish-grey discoloration in the periumbilical area.

      D. INCORRECT: Lung sounds are assessed by auscultating the area below the client's scapula.

      (N) NCLEX® Connection: Reduction of Risk Potential, Diagnostic Tests

5.   A. INCORRECT: Small, frequent meals are recommended for the client who has pancreatitis.

      B. INCORRECT: Bland, easy-to-digest foods are recommended for the client who has pancreatitis.

      C. INCORRECT: Low-fat foods are recommended for the client who has pancreatitis.

      D. **CORRECT:** Caffeine-free beverages are recommended for the client who has pancreatitis. Regular cola contains caffeine.

      (N) NCLEX® Connection: Basic Care and Comfort, Nutrition and Oral Hydration

6.   *Using the ATI Active Learning Template: Systems Disorder*

      A. Client Problem Related to Alteration in Health
- Severe, constant, knife-like pain (left upper quadrant, mid-epigastric, and/or radiating to the back) that is unrelieved by nausea and vomiting.

      B. Laboratory Data
- Serum amylase two to three times greater than expected value (increases within 12 hr, remains increased for 4 days)
- Serum lipase two to three times greater than expected value (increases slowly and remains increased for up to 2 weeks)
- Urine amylase remains increased for up to 2 weeks
- Increased WBC count due to inflammation/infection
- Decreased serum calcium and magnesium
- Serum liver enzymes and bilirubin increased with associated biliary dysfunction
- Serum glucose increased

      C. Nursing Interventions
- Maintain NPO status until pain-free.
- Administer TPN or jejunal feedings.
- Maintain NG tube.
- Resume diet beginning with bland, low-fat foods, and no caffeine.
- Plan small, frequent meals.
- Administer antiemetics as needed.
- Limit stress.
- Provide pain management.
- Do not consume alcohol or smoke.

      (N) NCLEX® Connection: Physiological Adaptations, Alterations in Body Systems

chapter 55

Overview

- Hepatitis is an inflammation of liver cells.

- Hepatitis can be caused by a viral or toxic agent, or as a secondary infection in conjunction with another virus. It is classified as acute or chronic.

- Cirrhosis is permanent scarring of the liver that is usually caused by chronic inflammation.

HEPATITIS

Overview

- Viral hepatitis is the most common type of hepatitis.

- Toxic and drug-induced hepatitis occurs secondary to an exposure to a chemical or medication agent such as alcohol, industrial toxins, ephedra, or acetaminophen.

- Hepatitis can occur in conjunction with other viruses such as varicella-zoster, cytomegalovirus, or herpes simplex.

- There are five major categories of viral hepatitis.

  ○ Hepatitis A virus (HAV)

  ○ Hepatitis B virus (HBV)

  ○ Hepatitis C virus (HCV)

  ○ Hepatitis D virus (HDV)

  ○ Hepatitis E virus (HEV)

- After exposure to a virus or toxin, the liver becomes enlarged from the inflammatory process. As the disease progresses, there is an increase in inflammation and necrosis, interfering with blood flow to the liver.

- Individuals can be infected with hepatitis and remain symptom-free, and therefore are unaware that they could be contagious.

Health Promotion and Disease Prevention

- Encourage hepatitis prevention activities:
  - ○ Community health educational interventions on transmission and exposure.
  - ○ Follow vaccination recommendations according to the CDC.
  - ○ Follow isolation precautions according to the CDC.
  - ○ Reinforce and use safe injection practices.
    - ▪ Aseptic technique for the preparation and administration of parenteral medications.
    - ▪ Sterile, single-use, disposable needle and syringe for each injection.
    - ▪ Use single-dose vials as often as possible.
    - ▪ Use needleless systems or safety caps.
  - ○ Use personal protective equipment, such as gown, gloves, and goggles, appropriate to the type of exposure.
    - ▪ Hepatitis A: Incontinent clients.
    - ▪ Hepatitis B or C: Exposure to blood.
- Proper hand hygiene (before preparing and eating food, after using the toilet or changing a diaper).
- When traveling to underdeveloped countries, drink purified water, and avoid sharing eating utensils and bed linens.

Assessment

- Risk Factors

TYPE	ROUTE OF TRANSMISSION	RISK FACTORS
Hepatitis A (HAV)	› Fecal-oral route	› Ingestion of contaminated food or water › Close personal contact with an infected individual
Hepatitis B (HBV)	› Blood	› Unprotected sex with infected individual › Infants born to infected mothers › Contact with infected blood › Injection drug users
Hepatitis C (HCV)	› Blood	› Drug abuse › Sexual contact
Hepatitis D (HDV)	› Coinfection with HBV	› Injection drug users › Unprotected sex with infected individual
Hepatitis E (HEV)	› Fecal-oral route	› Ingestion of contaminated food or water

- ○ High-risk behaviors
  - ▪ Unscreened blood transfusions (prior to 1992)
  - ▪ Hemodialysis
  - ▪ Percutaneous exposure (dirty needles, sharp instruments, body piercing, tattooing, use of another person's drug paraphernalia or personal hygiene tools)
  - ▪ Unprotected sexual intercourse with a hepatitis-infected person, sex with multiple partners, and/or anal sex
  - ▪ Ingestion of food prepared by a hepatitis-infected person who does not practice proper sanitation precautions
  - ▪ Travel/residence in underdeveloped country (using tap water to clean food products, drinking contaminated water)
  - ▪ Eating and/or living in crowded environments (correctional facilities, dormitories, universities, long-term care facilities, military base housing)
- • Subjective Data
  - ○ Failure to take personal precautions with blood and body fluid
  - ○ Influenzalike symptoms
    - ▪ Fatigue
    - ▪ Decreased appetite with nausea
    - ▪ Abdominal pain
    - ▪ Joint pain
- • Objective Data
  - ○ Physical Assessment Findings
    - ▪ Fever
    - ▪ Vomiting
    - ▪ Dark-colored urine
    - ▪ Clay-colored stool
    - ▪ Jaundice
  - ○ Laboratory Tests
    - ▪ Hepatitis A
      - □ Elevated alanine aminotransferase (ALT): Expected reference range 3 to 35 IU/L or 8 to 20 units/L.
      - □ Elevated aspartate aminotransferase (AST): Expected reference range 5 to 40 units/L.
      - □ Normal or elevated alkaline phosphatase (ALP): Expected reference range 30 to 120 units/L.
      - □ Elevated total bilirubin level: Expected reference range 0.1 to 1.0 mg/dL.
      - □ Presence of hepatitis A virus antibodies (anti-HAV) indicates the presence of hepatitis A.
      - □ Presence of immunoglobulin M antibodies (IgM) indicates inflammation of the liver.
      - □ Presence of immunoglobulin G antibodies (IgG) indicates permanent immunity to hepatitis A.

- Hepatitis B
  - □ Elevated alanine aminotransferase (ALT): Expected reference range 3 to 35 IU/L or 8 to 20 units/L.
  - □ Elevated aspartate aminotransferase (AST): Expected reference range 5 to 40 units/L.
  - □ Normal or elevated alkaline phosphatase (ALP): Expected reference range 30 to 120 units/L.
  - □ Elevated total bilirubin level: Expected reference range 0.1 to 1.0 mg/dL.
  - □ Presence of hepatitis B surface antigen (HBsAg) indicates that the individual is infectious.
  - □ Presence of hepatitis B surface antibody (anti-HBs) indicates recovery and immunity from HBV infection.
  - □ Presence of hepatitis B core antibody (anti-HBc) indicates previous or ongoing infection.
  - □ Presence of IgM antibody to hepatitis B core antigen (IgM anti-HBc) indicates acute infection.
  - □ Presence of hepatitis B e antigen (HBeAg) indicates that the virus is replicating.
  - □ Presence of hepatitis B e antibody (anti-HBe) is a predictor of long-term clearance of the virus.
- Hepatitis C
  - □ Elevated alanine aminotransferase (ALT): Expected reference range 3 to 35 IU/L or 8 to 20 units/L.
  - □ Elevated aspartate aminotransferase (AST): Expected reference range 5 to 40 units/L.
  - □ Normal or elevated alkaline phosphatase (ALP): Expected reference range 30 to 120 units/L.
  - □ Elevated total bilirubin level: Expected reference range 0.1 to 1.0 mg/dL.
  - □ Presence of hepatitis C virus antibodies (anti-HCV) detects hepatitis C infection.
  - □ Presence of enzyme immunoassay (EIA) detects hepatitis C infection.
  - □ Presense of enhanced chemiluminescence immunoassay (CIA) detects hepatitis C infection.
  - □ Presence of recombinant immunoblot assay (RIBA) detects hepatitis C infection.
  - □ Presence of HCV RNA polymerase chain reaction (PCR) is a qualitative test to detect the presence and amount of hepatitis C virus.
- Hepatitis D
  - □ Identification of intrahepatic delta antigen.
  - □ Presence of hepatitis D virus antibodies (anti-HDV) indicates the presence of hepatitis D virus.
- Hepatitis E
  - □ Presence of hepatitis E virus antibodies (anti-HEV) indicates the presence of hepatitis E virus.

○ Diagnostic Procedures

- Liver biopsy: This is the most definitive diagnostic approach, and it is used to identify the intensity of the infection, and the degree of liver damage.

  □ Nursing Actions

  ▸ Before the procedure

  ▷ Explain the procedure.

  ▷ Witness informed consent.

  ▷ Ensure the client fasts for at least 2 hr.

  ▷ Administer preprocedural medications as prescribed.

  ▸ During the procedure

  ▷ Assist the client into the supine position with the upper right quadrant of the abdomen exposed.

  ▷ Assist client with relaxation techniques.

  ▷ Instruct client to exhale breath and hold for at least 10 seconds while the needle is inserted.

  ▷ Instruct client to resume breathing once the needle is withdrawn.

  ▷ Apply pressure to the puncture site.

  ▸ After the procedure

  ▷ Assist client to a right side-lying position and maintain for several hours.

  ▷ Monitor the client's vital signs.

  ▷ Assess for abdominal pain.

  ▷ Assess for bleeding from puncture site.

Patient-Centered Care

- Nursing Care

  ○ Most clients will be cared for in the home unless they are acutely ill.

  ○ Enforce contact precautions if indicated.

  ○ Limit the client's activity in order to promote hepatic healing.

  ○ Provide a high-carbohydrate, high-calorie, low- to moderate-fat, and low- to moderate-protein diet, and small, frequent meals to promote nutrition and healing.

  ○ To promote hepatic rest and the regeneration of tissue, administer only necessary medications.

  ○ Educate the client and family regarding measures to prevent the transmission of the disease with others at home (avoid sexual intercourse until hepatitis antibody testing is negative, avoid alcohol, avoid over-the-counter medications or herbal medications, use proper hand hygiene).

  ○ Provide culturally sensitive care.

- Medications
  - Hepatitis A
    - Hepatitis A vaccination is recommended for postexposure protection.
    - Immunoglobulin is recommended for postexposure protection for people older than 40 yr, children younger than 12 months old, people who have chronic liver disease, immunosuppressed clients, or people allergic to the vaccination.
  - Hepatitis B
    - Acute infection
      - No medications, supportive care.
    - Chronic infection
      - Antiviral medications: adefovir dipivoxil (Hepsera), interferon alfa-2b (Intron A), peginterferon alfa-2a (Pegasys), lamivudine (Epivir-HBV), entecavir (Baraclude), and telbivudine (Tyzeka).
  - Hepatitis C
    - Combination therapy with peginterferon and ribavirin (Virazole) is the preferred treatment.
  - Hepatitis D
    - Same as for hepatitis B.
  - Hepatitis E
    - No medications, supportive care.
- Teamwork and Collaboration
  - Possible consults with infection control, social worker, primary care provider, and/or community resources.

Complications

- Chronic hepatitis
  - Ongoing inflammation of the liver cells.
  - Results from hepatitis B, C, or D.
  - Increases the client's risk for liver cancer.
- Fulminating hepatitis
  - Extremely progressive form of viral hepatitis.
  - Clients develop symptoms of viral hepatitis, then within hours or days develop severe liver failure.
  - Prevention of viral hepatitis.
  - No medications, supportive care.
- Cirrhosis of the liver (See next section in this chapter.)
  - Permanent scarring of the liver that is usually caused by chronic inflammation.
- Liver cancer
- Liver failure
  - Irreversible damage to liver cells, with decreased ability to function adequately to meet the body's needs.

CIRRHOSIS

Overview

- Cirrhosis is extensive scarring of the liver caused by necrotic injury or a chronic reaction to inflammation over a prolonged period of time. Normal liver tissue is replaced with fibrotic tissue that lacks function.

- Portal and periportal areas of the liver are primarily involved, affecting the liver's ability to handle the flow of bile. The development of new bile channels causes an overgrowth of tissue and liver scarring/enlargement. Jaundice is often the result.

Health Promotion and Disease Prevention

- The three types of cirrhosis

  ○ Postnecrotic: caused by viral hepatitis or certain medications or toxins.

  ○ Laennec's: caused by chronic alcoholism.

  ○ Biliary: caused by chronic biliary obstruction or autoimmune disease.

- Stay current on immunizations.

- Encourage the client to avoid drinking alcohol, and to engage in an alcohol recovery program.

Assessment

- Risk Factors

  ○ Alcohol abuse

  ○ Chronic viral hepatitis (hepatitis B, C, or D)

  ○ Autoimmune hepatitis (destruction of the liver cells by the immune system)

  ○ Steatohepatitis (fatty liver disease causing chronic inflammation)

  ○ Damage to the liver caused by drugs, toxins, and other infections

  ○ Chronic biliary cirrhosis (bile duct obstruction, bile stasis, hepatic fibrosis)

  ○ Cardiac cirrhosis resulting from severe right heart failure inducing necrosis and fibrosis due to lack of blood flow

- Subjective Data

  ○ Fatigue

  ○ Weight loss, abdominal pain, distention

  ○ Pruritus (severe itching of skin)

  ○ Confusion or difficulty thinking (due to the buildup of waste products in the blood and brain that the liver is unable to get rid of)

  ○ Personality and mentation changes, emotional lability, euphoria, sometimes depression

- Objective Data
  - Physical Assessment Findings
    - Cognitive changes
    - Altered sleep/wake pattern
    - Depression, emotional lability, euphoria
    - Gastrointestinal bleeding (enlarged veins [varices] develop and burst, causing vomiting and passing of blood in bowel movements)
    - Ascites (bloating or swelling due to fluid buildup in abdomen and legs)
    - Jaundice (yellowing of skin) and icterus (yellowing of the eyes)
    - Petechiae (round, pinpoint, red-purple lesions), ecchymoses (large yellow and purple-blue bruises), nosebleeds, hematemesis, melena (decreased synthesis of prothrombin, deteriorating hepatic function)
    - Palmar erythema (redness, warmth of the palms of the hands)
    - Spider angiomas (red lesions, vascular in nature with branches radiating on the nose, cheeks, upper thorax, shoulders)
    - Dependent peripheral edema of extremities and sacrum
    - Asterixis (liver flapping tremor) – coarse tremor characterized by rapid, nonrhythmic extension and flexion of the wrists and fingers
    - Fetor hepaticus (liver breath) – fruity or musty odor
  - Laboratory Tests
    - Serum liver enzymes: elevated initially
      - Alanine aminotransferase (ALT) (expected reference range – 8 to 20 units/L; 3 to 35 IU/L).
      - Aspartate aminotransferase (AST) (expected reference range – 5 to 40 units/L).
      - Alkaline phosphatase (ALP) (expected reference range – 30 to 120 units/L).
      - ALT and AST are elevated initially due to hepatic inflammation, and return to normal when liver cells are no longer able to create an inflammatory response. ALP increases in cirrhosis due to intrahepatic biliary obstruction.
    - Serum bilirubin: elevated
      - Bilirubin – indirect (unconjugated): elevated (expected reference range – 0.2 to 0.8 mg/dL).
      - Bilirubin – total: elevated (expected reference range – 0.1 to 1.0 mg/dL).
      - Bilirubin levels are elevated in cirrhosis due to the inability of the liver to excrete bilirubin.
    - Serum protein: decreased (expected reference range – 6 to 8 g/dL) are lowered due to the lack of hepatic synthesis.
    - Serum albumin: decreased (expected reference range – 3.5 to 5 g/dL) are lowered due to the lack of hepatic synthesis.

- Hematological Tests

  □ RBC: decreased (expected reference range for female 4.2 to 5.4 million/uL; male 4.7 to 6.1 million/uL).

  □ Hemoglobin: decreased (expected reference range for female 12 to 16 g/dL; male 14 to 18 g/dL).

  □ Hematocrit: decreased (expected reference range for female 37 to 47%; male 42 to 52%).

  □ Platelet count: decreased (expected reference range 150,000 to 400,000 mm³).

- PT/INR is prolonged due to decreased synthesis of prothrombin (expected reference range PT 11 to 12.5 sec; INR 0.7 to 1.8).

- Ammonia levels (expected reference range 11 to 32 µmol/L [15 to 45 mcg/dL]) rise when hepatocellular injury (cirrhosis) prevents the conversion of ammonia to urea for excretion.

- Serum creatinine levels (expected reference range for female 0.5 to 1.1 mg/dL; male: 0.6 to 1.2 mg/dL) may increase due to deteriorating kidney function, which may occur as a result of advanced liver disease.

○ Diagnostic Procedures

- Ultrasound

  □ This is used to detect ascites, hepatomegaly, splenomegaly, biliary stones, or biliary obstruction.

- Abdominal x-rays and CT scan

  □ Used to visualize possible hepatomegaly, ascites, and splenomegaly.

- MRI

  □ Used to visualize mass lesions and determine whether the liver is malignant or benign.

- Liver biopsy (most definitive)

  □ A liver biopsy identifies the progression and extent of the cirrhosis.

  □ To minimize the risk of hemorrhage, a radiologist may perform the biopsy through the jugular vein, which is threaded to the hepatic vein to obtain tissue for a microscopic evaluation.

  □ This is done under fluoroscopy for safety because this procedure can be problematic for cirrhosis clients due to an increased risk for bleeding complications.

- Esophagogastroduodenoscopy (EGD)

  □ This is performed under moderate (conscious) sedation to detect the presence of esophageal varices, ulcerations in the stomach, or duodenal ulcers and bleeding.

- Endoscopic retrograde cholangiopancreatography (ERCP)

  □ Used to view the biliary tract to assist in removing stones, to collect specimens for biopsy, and for placement of a stent.

Patient-Centered Care

- Nursing Care
  - Assess/Monitor
    - Respiratory status – Monitor oxygen saturation levels and distress. Provide comfort measures by positioning the client to ease respiratory effort (may be compromised by plasma volume excess and ascites). Have the client sit in a chair or elevate the head of the bed to 30° with feet elevated.
    - Skin integrity – Monitor the client closely for skin breakdown. Implement measures to prevent pressure ulcers. Pruritus, which is associated with jaundice, will cause the client to scratch. Encourage washing with cold water and applying lotion to decrease the itching.
    - Fluid balance – Monitor the client for signs of fluid volume excess. Keep strict intake and output, obtain daily weights, and assess ascites and peripheral edema. Restrict fluids and sodium if prescribed.
    - Vital signs – Monitor vital signs and pain level as prescribed.
    - Neurological status – Monitor the client for deteriorating mental status and dementia consistent with hepatic encephalopathy. Lactulose may need to be given to aid in excretion of ammonia.
    - Nutritional status – High-carbohydrate, high-protein, moderate-fat, and low-sodium diet with vitamin supplements such as thiamine, folate, and multivitamins.
    - Gastrointestinal status – In the presence of ascites, measure abdominal girth daily over the largest part of the abdomen. Mark the location of tape for consistency. Observe the client for potential bleeding complications.
    - Pain status – Assess the client's pain and administer analgesics and gastrointestinal antispasmodics as needed.
- Medications
  - Because the metabolism of most medications is dependent upon a functioning liver, general medications are administered sparingly, especially opioids, sedatives, and barbiturates.
  - Diuretics: Decrease excessive fluid in the body.
  - Beta-blocking agent: Used for clients who have varices to prevent bleeding.
  - Lactulose (Cephulac): Used to promote excretion of ammonia from the body through the stool.
  - Nonabsorbable antibiotic: Can be used in place of lactulose.
- Teamwork and Collaboration
  - A dietary consult to assist with special diet needs.
  - Initiate appropriate referrals (social services, Alcoholics Anonymous, Al-Anon).
- Therapeutic Procedures
  - Paracentesis
    - Used to relieve ascites.
    - Nursing Care
      - Prior to the procedure
        - Explain the procedure.
        - Witness informed consent.

- ▸ Obtain vital signs and weight.
- ▸ Assist the client to void.
  - ▫ During the procedure
    - ▸ Position the client supine with head of bed elevated.
    - ▸ Assist the client with relaxation techniques.
    - ▸ Apply dressing over puncture site.
  - ▫ After the procedure
    - ▸ Monitor vital signs as prescribed.
    - ▸ Maintain bed rest as prescribed.
    - ▸ Measure the fluid and document amount, color.
    - ▸ Send specimen to the laboratory.
    - ▸ Access puncture site dressing for drainage.
    - ▸ Weigh client.
  - ○ Endoscopic variceal ligation (EVL)/endoscopic sclerotherapy (EST)
    - ▪ The varices are either sclerosed or banded endoscopically.
    - ▪ There is a decreased risk of hemorrhage with banding.
  - ○ Transjugular intrahepatic portosystemic shunt (TIPS)
    - ▪ Performed in interventional radiology for clients who require further intervention with ascites or hemorrhage.
- Surgical Interventions
  - ○ Surgical bypass shunting procedures
    - ▪ This is a last resort for clients who have portal hypertension and esophageal varices. The ascites is shunted from the abdominal cavity to the superior vena cava.
  - ○ Liver transplantation
    - ▪ Portions of healthy livers from trauma victims or living donors may be used for transplant.
    - ▪ The transplanted liver portion will regenerate and grow in size based on the needs of the body.
    - ▪ The client must meet the transplant criteria to be eligible.
    - ▪ Clients who have severe cardiac and respiratory disease, metastatic malignant liver cancer, and a continued history of alcohol/substance abuse are not candidates for liver transplantation.
    - ▪ Nursing Actions
      - ▫ Prior to surgery
        - ▸ Multidisciplinary approach.
        - ▸ Witness informed consent.
      - ▫ After surgery
        - ▸ Intensive unit care.
        - ▸ Monitor vital signs frequently.
        - ▸ Monitor neurological status.
        - ▸ Monitor for acute graft rejection: tachycardia, fever, right upper quadrant pain, change in bile color or increased jaundice, increased ALT and AST levels.

- ▸ Monitor for infection: fever or excessive, foul-smelling drainage.
- ▸ Monitor for clotting problems: blood in drainage tubes, petechiae.
- ▸ Monitor for hepatic complications: decreased bile drainage, increased right upper quadrant pain with distention, nausea and vomiting, increased jaundice.
- ▸ Monitor for acute renal failure: change in urine output, increased BUN and creatinine levels and electrolyte imbalance.
- ▸ Administer immunosuppressant agents.
- ▸ Administer antibiotic prophylaxis.
- ▸ Obtain blood cultures as prescribed.
- ▸ Keep T-tube in dependant position, and empty frequently, documenting amount and description.

- ○ Client Education
  - ▪ Encourage the client abstain from alcohol and engage in alcohol recovery program.
    - ▫ Helps prevent further scarring and fibrosis of liver.
    - ▫ Allows healing and regeneration of liver tissue.
    - ▫ Prevents irritation of the stomach and esophagus lining.
    - ▫ Helps decrease the risk of bleeding.
    - ▫ Helps to prevent other life-threatening complications.
  - ▪ Consult with provider prior to taking any over-the-counter medications or herbal supplements.
  - ▪ Follow diet guidelines
    - ▫ High-calorie, moderate-fat diet
    - ▫ Low-sodium diet (if the client has excessive fluid in the peritoneal cavity)
    - ▫ Low-protein (if encephalopathy, elevated ammonia)
    - ▫ Small, frequent, well-balanced nutritional meals
    - ▫ Supplemental vitamin-enriched liquids (Ensure, Boost)
    - ▫ Replacement and administration of vitamins due to the inability of the liver to store them
    - ▫ Fluid intake restrictions if serum sodium is low

Complications

- Portal systemic encephalopathy (PSE) — ammonia [handwritten]
  - ○ Clients who have a poorly functioning liver are unable to convert ammonia and other waste products to a less toxic form. These products are carried to the brain and cause neurological symptoms. Clients are treated with medications such as lactulose to reduce the ammonia levels in the body via intestinal excretion. Reductions in dietary protein are indicated as ammonia is formed when protein is broken down by intestinal flora.
  - ○ Nursing Actions
    - ▪ Administer lactulose as prescribed.
    - ▪ Monitor laboratory findings, including potassium, because clients can become hypokalemic with increased stools from the lactulose therapy.

- Assess for changes in the level of consciousness and orientation.
- Report asterixis (flapping of the hands) and fetor hepaticus (liver breath) immediately to the provider. These are clinical signs that the client's encephalopathy is worsening.
  - ○ Client Education
    - Instruct client on prescribed diet.
- Esophageal varices
  - ○ Causes
    - Portal hypertension (elevated blood pressure in veins that carry blood from the intestines to the liver) is caused by impaired circulation of blood through the liver. Collateral circulation is subsequently developed, creating varices in the upper stomach and esophagus. Varices are fragile and can bleed easily.
  - ○ Nursing Actions
    - Assist with saline lavage (vasoconstriction), esophagogastric balloon tamponade, blood transfusions, ligation and sclerotherapy, and shunts to stop bleeding and reduce the risk for hypovolemic shock.
    - Monitor the client's hemoglobin level and vital signs.
    - Monitor for any bleeding.
- Acute graft rejection post liver transplantation
  - ○ This typically occurs between 4 and 10 days after surgery.
  - ○ Symptoms of rejection
    - Tachycardia
    - Upper right flank pain
    - Jaundice
    - Laboratory findings indicative of liver failure
  - ○ Causes
    - Graft versus host disease (GVHD) – recipient's bone marrow creates T-cells to attack the new organ.
  - ○ Nursing Actions
    - Early diagnosis of graft rejection is necessary to successfully prevent total rejection of the liver.
    - Administer immunosuppressants as prescribed by the provider.
    - Monitor laboratory findings.
  - ○ Client Education
    - Inform the client of the importance of taking immunosuppressants and monitoring white blood cell count.
    - Instruct the client to report signs of rejection to the provider immediately.

APPLICATION EXERCISES

1. A nurse on a medical-surgical unit is admitting a client who has hepatitis B with ascites. Which of the following actions should the nurse include in the plan of care?

    A. Initiate contact precautions.

    B. Weigh client weekly.

    C. Measure abdominal girth 7.5 cm (3 in) above the umbilicus.

    (D.) Provide a high-calorie, high-carbohydrate diet.

2. A nurse is caring for a client who has a new diagnosis of hepatitis C. Which of the following is an expected laboratory finding?

    A. Presence of immunoglobin G antibodies (IgG)

    (B.) Presence of enzyme immunoassay (EIA)

    C. Aspartate aminotransferase (AST) 35 units/L

    D. Alanine aminotransferase (ALT) 15 IU/L

-ammonia

3. A nurse is caring for a client who has advanced cirrhosis with worsening hepatic encephalopahy. Which of the following is an expected assessment finding? (Select all that apply.)

    _____ A. Anorexia

    ✗_____ B. Change in orientation

    ✗_____ C. Asterixis

    _____ D. Ascites

    ✗_____ E. Fetor hepaticus

4. A nurse is caring for a client who has cirrhosis. Which of the following medications can the nurse expect to administer to this client? (Select all that apply.)

    ✗_____ A. Diuretic

    ✗_____ B. Beta-blocking agent

    _____ C. Opioid analgesic

    ✗_____ D. Lactulose (Cephulac)

    _____ E. Sedative

5. A nurse is teaching a client who has hepatitis B about home care. Which of the following should the nurse include in the teaching? (Select all that apply.)

_____ A. Limit physical activity.

_____ B. Avoid alcohol.

_____ C. Take acetaminophen for comfort.

_____ D. Wear a mask when in public places.

_____ E. Eat small frequent meals.

6. A nurse is caring for a client who has hepatitis C and has been prescribed a liver biopsy. Use the ATI Active Learning Template: Diagnostic Procedure to complete the following:

A. Description of the procedure.

B. One preprocedure nursing action, one intraprocedure, and one postprocedure nursing action.

C. Identify one potential complication of the procedure.

APPLICATION EXERCISES KEY

1. A. INCORRECT: Hepatitis B is transmitted via blood; therefore standard precautions are adequate.

    B. INCORRECT: Daily weights are obtained to monitor fluid status.

    C. INCORRECT: Abdominal girth is measured over the largest part of the abdomen, which will vary from client to client.

    D. **CORRECT:** A high-calorie, high-carbohydrate diet is recommended for clients who have hepatitis B.

    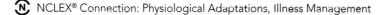 NCLEX® Connection: Physiological Adaptations, Illness Management

2. A. INCORRECT: The presence of immunoglobulin G antibodies (IgG) is an expected laboratory finding in a client who has hepatitis A infection.

    B. **CORRECT:** The presence of enzyme immunoassay is an expected laboratory finding in a client who has a new diagnosis of hepatitis C.

    C. INCORRECT: The aspartate aminotransferase (AST) is elevated in clients with hepatitis C infection; 35 units/L is within the expected reference range.

    D. INCORRECT: The alanine aminotransferase (ALT) is elevated in clients with hepatitis C infection; 15 IU/L is within the expected reference range.

    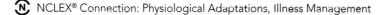 NCLEX® Connection: Reduction of Risk Potential, Laboratory Values

3. A. INCORRECT: Anorexia is present in a client who has liver dysfunction, but it is not a sign of worsening hepatic encephalopathy.

    B. **CORRECT:** A change in orientation indicates worsening hepatic encephalopathy in a client who has advanced cirrhosis.

    C. **CORRECT:** Asterixis, a coarse tremor of the wrists and fingers, is observed as a late complication in a client who has cirrhosis and hepatic encephalopathy.

    D. INCORRECT: Ascites may be present in a client who has liver dysfunction, but it is not a sign of worsening hepatic encephalopathy.

    E. **CORRECT:** Fetor hepaticus, a fruity breath odor, is a clinical finding of worsening hepatic encephalopathy in the client who has advanced cirrhosis.

    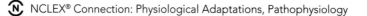 NCLEX® Connection: Physiological Adaptations, Pathophysiology

4. A. **CORRECT:** Diuretics facilitate excretion of excess fluid from the body in a client who has cirrhosis.

   B. **CORRECT:** Beta-blocking agents are prescribed for a client who has cirrhosis to prevent bleeding from varices.

   C. INCORRECT: Opioid analgesics are metabolized in the liver. Therefore, they should not be administered to a client who has cirrhosis.

   D. **CORRECT:** Lactulose (Cephulac) is prescribed for a client who has cirrhosis to aid in the elimination of ammonia in the stool.

   E. INCORRECT: Sedatives are metabolized in the liver. Therefore, they should not be administered to a client who has cirrhosis.

   Ⓝ NCLEX® Connection: Pharmacological and Parenteral Therapies, Medication Administration

5. A. **CORRECT:** Limiting physical activity and taking frequent rest breaks conserves energy and assists in the recovery process for a client who has hepatitis B.

   B. **CORRECT:** Alcohol is metabolized in the liver and should be avoided by the client who has hepatitis B.

   C. INCORRECT: Acetaminophen is metabolized in the liver and should be avoided by the client who has hepatitis B.

   D. INCORRECT: Hepatitis B is a blood-borne disease. Therefore, wearing a mask is not appropriate for this client.

   E. **CORRECT:** A client who has hepatitis B should eat small frequent meals to promote improved nutrition due to the presence of anorexia.

   Ⓝ NCLEX® Connection: Physiological Adaptations, Illness Management

6. *Using the ATI Active Learning Template: Diagnostic Procedure*

   A. Description of the procedure
      - A liver biopsy is a procedure to collect a sample of liver tissue for diagnostic testing. A needle is inserted in the intercostal space between the two right lower ribs and into the liver. An aspirate of liver tissue is then collected.

   B. One preprocedure nursing action, one intraprocedure, and one postprocedure nursing action
      - Preprocedure
        ○ Explain the procedure to the client/family.
        ○ Witness informed consent.
        ○ Ensure the client has been fasting for at least 2 hr.
        ○ Administer preprocedure medication as prescribed.
      - Intraprocedure
        ○ Assist the client into the supine position with the upper right quadrant of the abdomen exposed.
        ○ Assist client with relaxation techniques.
        ○ Instruct client to exhale breath and hold for at least 10 seconds while the needle is inserted.
        ○ Instruct client to resume breathing once the needle is withdrawn.
        ○ Apply pressure to the puncture site.
      - Postprocedure
        ○ Assist client to a right side-lying position and maintain for several hours.
        ○ Monitor client's vital signs.
        ○ Assess for abdominal pain.
        ○ Assess for bleeding from puncture site.

   C. Identify one potential complication of the procedure
      - Bleeding.
      - Bile peritonitis.

   Ⓝ NCLEX® Connection: Reduction of Risk Potential, Diagnostic Tests

UNIT 8 — Nursing Care of Clients with Renal Disorders

SECTIONS

› Diagnostic and Therapeutic Procedures
› Renal System Disorders

NCLEX® CONNECTIONS

When reviewing the chapters in this unit, keep in mind the relevant sections of the NCLEX® outline, in particular:

Client Needs: Basic Care and Comfort	Client Needs: Reduction of Risk Potential	Client Needs: Physiological Adaptation

› Relevant topics/tasks include:
» Elimination
  › Use alternative methods to promote voiding.
» Nonpharmacological Comfort Interventions
  › Assess the client's need for pain management and intervene as needed using non-pharmacological comfort measures.
» Nutrition and Oral Hydration
  › Provide/maintain special diets based on the client's diagnosis/nutritional needs and cultural considerations.
	› Relevant topics/tasks include:
	» Diagnostic Tests
	  › Apply knowledge of related nursing procedures and psychomotor skills when caring for clients undergoing diagnostic testing.
	» Laboratory Values
	  › Educate the client about the purpose and procedure of prescribed laboratory tests.
	» Potential for Complications of Diagnostic Tests/Treatments/Procedures
	  › Intervene to manage potential circulatory complications.
		› Relevant topics/tasks include:
		» Alterations in Body Systems
		  › Perform and manage care of the client receiving peritoneal dialysis.
		» Hemodynamics
		  › Manage the care of a client receiving hemodialysis.
		» Unexpected Response to Therapies
		  › Promote the recovery of the client from unexpected responses to therapy.

chapter 56

Overview

- Renal diagnostic procedures and laboratory assessments are used to evaluate kidney function. By testing the kidney function, diagnosis of disease and efficacy of treatment can be determined.

- Renal diagnostic procedures that nurses should be knowledgeable about include the following:

  - Radiography (x-ray)

  - Excretory urography

  - Computer tomography (CT scan)

  - Magnetic resonance imaging (MRI)

  - Cystography

  - Cystourethrography

  - Voiding cystourethrogram (VCUG)

  - Kidney biopsy

  - Cystoscopy

  - Cystourethroscopy

  - Retrograde pyelogram, cystogram, urethrogram

  - Renography (kidney scan)

  - Ultrasound

- Laboratory assessments that nurses should be knowledgeable about include the following:

  - Serum creatinine – produced due to protein and muscle breakdown.

    - Kidney disease is the only condition that increases serum creatinine level.

    - Kidney function loss of at least 50% will cause an elevation of serum creatinine values.

    - Serum creatinine values remain constant in older adults unless kidney disease is present.

  - Blood urea nitrogen (BUN) – results from breakdown of protein in the liver, creating the by-product urea nitrogen excreted by the kidneys.

    - Factors affecting BUN are dehydration, infection, chemotherapy, steroid therapy, and reabsorption of blood in the liver from damaged tissue.

    - Elevated BUN is highly suggestive of kidney disease.

  - Urinalysis – evaluates waste products from the kidney and detects urologic disorders.

    - Collection of an early-morning specimen provides a more concentrated sample.

    - Urine is analyzed for color; clarity; concentration or dilution; specific gravity; acidity or alkalinity; and presence of drug metabolites, glucose, ketone bodies, and protein.

- Glucose, ketone bodies, and protein, including leukoesterase and nitrites, are not normally present in urine. These abnormal findings may indicate the client has diabetes mellitus, fat metabolism, infection, or if a cytology analysis is performed, cancer.
- Urine for culture and sensitivity is collected when bacteria is found in the urine to determine the type of antibiotic most sensitive for the treatment of possible infection.
- Urine collected for 24 hr is used to measure urine levels of creatinine or urea nitrogen, sodium, chloride, calcium, catecholamines, and proteins.
- Urine creatinine clearance 24-hr collection measures glomerular filtration rate for clients who have suspected renal dysfunction.

RADIOGRAPHY (X-RAY)	
Purpose	› An x-ray of the kidneys, ureters, and bladder (KUB) (may also be prescribed as a "flat plate")
	› Allows for visualization of structures and to detection of renal calculi, strictures, calcium deposits, or obstructions.
Nursing Interventions	› Ask female client if pregnant. Inform client that clothes over the area will need to be removed as well as all jewelry and metal objects.
Complications	› No known complications
CT SCAN	
Purpose	› Provides three-dimensional imaging of renal/urinary system to assess for kidney size and obstruction, cysts, or masses.
	› IV contrast dye (iodine-based) may be used to enhance images.
Nursing Interventions	› Same as KUB without contrast dye.
	› Same as excretory urography with contrast dye (exclude bowel preparation).
Complications	› Dye can cause acute kidney injury.
MRI	
Purpose	› Useful in staging cancer, similar to CT
Nursing Interventions	› Client will lie down and have to remain still for test.
Complications	› Poor imaging if client is unable to lie still.
ULTRASOUND	
Purpose	› Used to assess size of kidney, image the ureters, bladder, masses, cysts, calculi, and obstructions of the lower urinary tract.
Nursing Interventions	› Provide skin care by removing gel on completion of the procedure.
	› Good option if not able to do excretory urography.
Complications	› Minimal risk for the client.

CYSTOGRAPHY; CYSTOURETHROGRAPHY; VCUG	
Purpose	› Detects urethral or bladder injury when contrast dye is instilled through a urinary catheter to provide an image of the bladder (cystography), and image of the ureters (cystourethrography). VCUG detects whether urine refluxes into the ureters as an x-ray is taken while the client is voiding.
Nursing Interventions	› Monitor client for infection for the first 72 hr after the procedure. › Encourage increased fluid intake to dilute urine and minimize burning on urination. › Monitor urine output (less than 30 mL/hr) if suspected pelvic or urethral trauma.
Complications	› Contrast dye does not reach the kidneys and is not nephrotoxic. Dye is not absorbed into the bloodstream. › Urinary tract infection due to catheter placement. » Cloudy, foul-smelling urine » Urgency » Urine positive for leukoesterase and nitrites, sediment, and RBCs
KIDNEY BIOPSY	
Purpose	› Removal of sample of tissue by excision or needle aspiration for cytological (histological) examination.
Nursing Interventions	› Client receives sedation and is monitored for procedure. › Preprocedure » Review coagulation studies. » Nothing by mouth for 4 to 6 hr. › Postprocedure » Monitor vital signs following sedation. » Assess dressings and urinary output (hematuria). » Review Hgb and Hct values. » Administer PRN pain medication.
Complications	› Hemorrhage › Infection » Cloudy, foul-smelling urine » Urgency » Urine positive for leukoesterase and nitrites, sediment, and RBCs

CYSTOGRAPHY; CYSTOURETHROGRAPHY

Purpose	› Used to discover abnormalities of bladder wall (cystoscopy) and/or occlusions of ureter or urethra (cystourethroscopy).
Nursing Interventions	› Client is given anesthesia for the procedure.
	› Check for signs of bleeding and infection. Monitor client for infection for the first 72 hr after the procedure.
	› Preprocedure
	» NPO after midnight.
	» Administer laxative or enemas for bowel preparation the night before the procedure.
	› During the procedure
	» Monitor vital signs if local anesthetic is administered.
	» General anesthesia is an option.
	» Place in lithotomy position.
	› Postprocedure
	» Monitor vital signs and urine output.
	» Document color of urine; may be pink-tinged.
	» Irrigate urinary catheter with 0.9% normal saline if blood clots are present or urine output is decreased or absent.
	» Encourage oral fluids to increase urine output and reduce burning sensation with voiding.
Complications	› Possible urinary tract infection from instrumentation.
	» Cloudy, foul-smelling urine
	» Urgency
	» Urine positive for leukoesterase, nitrites, sediment, and RBCs

RETROGRADE PYELOGRAM, CYSTOGRAM, URETHROGRAM

Purpose	› Used to identify obstruction or structural disorders of the ureters and renal pelvis of the kidneys (pyelogram) by instilling contrast dye during a cystoscopy.
	› Fistulas, diverticula, and tumors are identified in the bladder (cystogram) and urethra (urethrogram) by instilling contrast dye during a cystoscopy.
Nursing Interventions	› Same as a cystoscopy.
Complications	› Same as a cystoscopy.

RENOGRAPHY (KIDNEY SCAN)	
Purpose	› Used to assess renal blood flow and estimates glomerular filtration rate (GFR) after IV injection of radioactive material to produce a scanned image of the kidneys.
Nursing Interventions	› Postprocedure » Assess BP frequently during and after procedure if captopril (Capoten) is given during the procedure to change blood flow to the kidneys. » Alert client about possible orthostatic hypotension following the procedure if captopril is used. » Increase fluid intake if hypotension occurs. » Implement standard precautions when handling urine after procedure.
Complications	› Radioactive material does not cause nephrotoxicity. › Client is not at risk from radioactive material excreted in the urine and then voided.
EXCRETORY UROGRAPHY	
Purpose	› Used to detect obstruction, assess for a parenchymal mass, and assess size of the kidney. IV contrast dye (iodine-based) is used to enhance images.
Nursing Interventions	› Same as KUB › Preprocedure » Encourage increased fluids the day before procedure. » Bowel cleansing with laxative or enema to remove fecal contents, fluid, and gas from the colon for a more clear visualization. » NPO after midnight. » Determine client allergy to iodine, seafood, eggs, milk, chocolate; or if client has asthma. » Check the client's creatinine and BUN levels. » Hold metformin (Glucophage) for 24 hr before procedure (risk for lactic acidosis from contrast dye with iodine). › Postprocedure » Administer parenteral fluid, or encourage oral fluids to flush dye through the renal system and prevent complications. » Diuretics may be administered to increase dye excretion. » Follow-up creatinine and BUN serum levels before metformin is resumed.
Complications	› Dye can cause acute renal injury.

Ⓖ • Gerontological Considerations

  ○ Kidney size and function decrease with aging.

  ○ Blood flow adaptability decreases, especially during a hypotensive or hypertensive crisis.

  ○ Glomerular filtration rate (GFR) decreases by half the rate of a young adult.

  ○ Medical conditions – diabetes, hypertension, and heart failure can affect GFR.

  ○ Kidney injury can occur more easily from contrast dyes and medication due to decreased renal size, blood flow, and GFR.

  ○ Tubular changes can cause urgency and nocturnal polyuria.

  ○ Weak urinary sphincter muscle and shorter urethra in women can cause incontinence and urinary tract infections.

  ○ Enlarged prostate in men can cause urinary retention and infection.

APPLICATION EXERCISES

1. A nurse is providing teaching to a client who is to have an x-ray of the kidneys, ureters, and bladder (KUB). Which of the following statements should the nurse include in the teaching?

    A. "Contrast dye is given during the procedure."

    B. "An enema is necessary before the procedure."

    C. "You will need to lie in a prone position during the procedure."

    D. "The procedure determines whether a kidney stone is present."

2. A nurse is monitoring for postoperative complications in a client who had a kidney biopsy. Which of the following complications causes the most immediate risk to the client?

    A. Infection

    B. Hemorrhage

    C. Hematuria

    D. Kidney failure

3. A nurse is reviewing a client's laboratory findings for urinalysis. The findings indicate the urine is positive for leukoesterase and nitrites. Which of the following is an appropriate nursing action?

    A. Repeat the test early the next morning.

    B. Start a 24-hr urine collection for creatinine clearance.

    C. Obtain a clean-catch urine specimen for culture and sensitivity.

    D. Insert a urinary catheter to collect a urine specimen.

4. A nurse is caring for a client who has type 2 diabetes mellitus and is to undergo excretory urography. Which of the following are appropriate nursing actions prior to this procedure? (Select all that apply.)

    _____ A. Identify client allergy to seafood.

    _____ B. Hold metformin (Glucophage) for 24 hr.

    _____ C. Administer an enema.

    _____ D. Obtain client's serum coagulation profile.

    _____ E. Assess client for history of asthma.

5. A nurse administered captopril (Capoten) to a client during renography (kidney scan). Which of the following is an appropriate action by the nurse?

    A. Assess the client for hypertension.

    B. Limit the client's fluid intake.

    C. Monitor for orthostatic hypotension.

    D. Encourage early ambulation.

6. A nurse is developing a plan of care for a client who is to have a cystoscopy with retrograde pyelogram. Which of the following should the nurse include in the plan of care? Use the ATI Active Learning Template: Diagnostic Procedure to complete this item to include the following:

    A. Procedure Name: Define the procedure.

    B. Indications: Identify one indication for cystoscopy and two for retrograde pyelogram.

    C. Nursing Actions: Describe two nursing actions for preprocedure and two for postprocedure.

APPLICATION EXERCISES KEY

1. A. INCORRECT: No contrast dye is injected for this procedure.

   B. INCORRECT: An enema is not administered before this procedure.

   C. INCORRECT: The client will be asked to lie supine, not prone.

   D. **CORRECT:** A KUB can identify renal calculi, strictures, calcium deposits, or obstructions.

   Ⓝ NCLEX® Connection: Reduction of Risk Potential, Diagnostic Tests

2. A. INCORRECT: Infection is not the most immediate risk following a kidney biopsy. However, if a hematoma develops, the kidney may become infected.

   B. **CORRECT:** Hemorrhage is the most immediate client risk following a kidney biopsy if clotting does not occur at the puncture site.

   C. INCORRECT: Hematuria is not the most immediate risk following a kidney biopsy, but it is a common complication the first 48 to 72 hr after the biopsy.

   D. INCORRECT: Kidney failure is not the most immediate risk following a kidney biopsy. However, the client should be monitored for hemorrhage, which can lead to kidney failure.

   Ⓝ NCLEX® Connection: Reduction of Risk Potential, Diagnostic Tests

3. A. INCORRECT: Repeating the test early the next morning is not an appropriate nursing action because leukoesterase and nitrites in the urine indicate the client has a urinary tract infection.

   B. INCORRECT: Starting a 24-hr urine collection for creatinine clearance is not an appropriate nursing action because leukoesterase and nitrites in the urine indicate the client has a urinary tract infection.

   C. **CORRECT:** Obtaining a clean-catch urine specimen for culture and sensitivity is an appropriate nursing action because this determines the antibiotic that will be most effective for treatment of the urinary tract infection.

   D. INCORRECT: Inserting a urinary catheter to collect a urine specimen is not an appropriate nursing action because leukoesterase and nitrites in the urine indicate the client has a urinary tract infection.

   Ⓝ NCLEX® Connection: Reduction of Risk Potential, Diagnostic Tests

4. A. **CORRECT:** The client who has an allergy to seafood is at higher risk for an allergic reaction to the contrast dye used in the procedure.

    B. **CORRECT:** The client who takes metformin is at risk for lactic acidosis from the contrast dye with iodine used during the procedure.

    C. **CORRECT:** The client should receive an enema to remove fecal contents, fluid, and gas from the colon for a more clear visualization.

    D. INCORRECT: A serum coagulation profile should be obtained for a client prior to a kidney biopsy.

    E. **CORRECT:** A client who has a history of asthma has a higher risk of having an asthma attack as an allergic response to the contrast dye used during the procedure.

    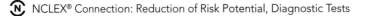 NCLEX® Connection: Reduction of Risk Potential, Diagnostic Tests

5. A. INCORRECT: This is not an appropriate action by the nurse because captopril is an antihypertensive medication, and the client should be assessed for hypotensive effects.

    B. INCORRECT: This is not an appropriate action by the nurse. Increasing the client's fluids can help to resolve any hypotensive effects following the administration of captopril, an antihypertensive medication.

    C. **CORRECT:** The appropriate action by the nurse is to monitor for orthostatic hypotension because the antihypertensive effect of captopril results in a change in blood flow to the kidneys when an initial dose is administered.

    D. INCORRECT: This is not an appropriate action by the nurse because the client may be at risk for a fall when ambulating due to the hypotensive effects of captopril, an antihypertensive medication.

    NCLEX® Connection: Pharmacological and Parenteral Therapies, Medication Administration

6. *Using ATI Active Learning Template: Diagnostic Procedure*

A. Procedure Name

- Cystoscopy is instrumentation into the urinary tract to inspect the bladder wall.

- Retrograde pyelogram is the injection of dye up the ureters to inspect the ureters and pelvis of the kidney.

B. Indications

- Cystoscopy discovers abnormalities of the bladder wall (cysts, tumors, stones).

- Retrograde pyelogram discovers obstructions or structural disorders of the ureters and kidney pelvis (strictures, stones, mass).

C. Nursing Actions

- Preprocedure nursing actions: Client to be NPO after midnight, and administer a laxative the night before the procedure.

- Postprocedure nursing actions: Monitor vital signs; encourage increase in oral fluid intake to reduce burning sensation when voiding; document color of urine; if client has a urinary catheter, irrigate with 0.9% sodium chloride solution when active bleeding or clots are noted, or there is decreased or absent urine output.

Ⓝ NCLEX® Connection: Pharmacological and Parenteral Therapies, Medication Administration

chapter 57

Overview

- Functions of dialysis
  - Rids the body of excess fluid and electrolytes
  - Achieves acid-base balance
  - Eliminates waste products
  - Restores internal homeostasis by osmosis, diffusion, and ultrafiltration
- Dialysis can sustain life for clients who have both acute and chronic renal failure.
- Dialysis does not replace the hormonal functions of the kidneys.
- Two types of dialysis are hemodialysis and peritoneal dialysis.

Hemodialysis

- Hemodialysis shunts the client's blood from the body through a dialyzer and back into circulation. Vascular access is needed for hemodialysis.
- Indications
  - Diagnoses
    - Renal insufficiency
    - Acute kidney injury
    - Chronic kidney disease
    - Drug overdose
    - Persistent hyperkalemia
    - Hypervolemia unresponsive to diuretics
  - Client Manifestations
    - Related to fluid volume changes, electrolyte and pH imbalances, and nitrogenous wastes.
    - Hemodialysis is based on symptoms, not glomerular filtration rate (GRF).
    - Client symptoms include fluid overload, neurological changes, bleeding, or signs of uremia.
- Preprocedure
  - Nursing Actions
    - Check for an informed consent.
    - Use the temporary hemodialysis dual- or triple-lumen catheter, or subcutaneous device until a long-term device is inserted and available for access.

- Assess patency of a long-term device – arteriovenous (AV) fistula, or arteriovenous graft (presence of bruit, palpable thrill, distal pulses, and circulation).

- Avoid taking blood pressure, administering injections, performing venipunctures or inserting IV lines on an arm with an access site. Elevate the extremity following surgical development of AV fistula to reduce swelling.

- **Assess** vital signs, laboratory values (BUN, serum creatinine, electrolytes, Hct), and weight.

- Discuss with the provider medications that need to be withheld until after dialysis. Dialyzable medications and medications that lower blood pressure are withheld.

  ○ Client Education

  - Advise the client that hemodialysis is usually done three times per week, for 3- to 5-hr sessions. Two needles are inserted, one into an artery and the other into a vein.

- Intraprocedure

 View Animation: Hemodialysis

  ○ Nursing Actions

  - Monitor for complications during dialysis.

    □ Dialysis circuit clotting, air bubbles in blood tubing, temperature of the dialysate (37.8° C [100° F]), regulation of the ultrafiltration.

    □ Hypotension, cramping, vomiting, bleeding at the access site, contamination of equipment.

  - Monitor vital signs and coagulation studies during dialysis. Monitor for bleeding, such as oozing from insertion site.

    □ Administer anticoagulants as prescribed.

    □ Heparin is used to prevent clotting of the blood with foreign surfaces.

    □ Monitor the aPTT for risk of hemorrhage.

  - Have protamine sulfate ready to reverse heparin if needed.

  - Provide emotional support. Offer activities, such as books, magazines, music, cards, or television, to occupy the client.

  ○ Client Education

  - Advise the client to notify the nurse of headache, nausea, or dizziness during dialysis. Advise the client not to eat during dialysis.

- Postprocedure

  ○ Nursing Actions

  - Monitor vital signs and laboratory values (BUN, serum creatinine, electrolytes, Hct). Decreases in blood pressure and laboratory values are expected following dialysis.

  - Compare the client's preprocedure weight with the postprocedure weight as a way to estimate the amount of fluid removed (1 liter of fluid is equal to 1 kg or 2.2 lb).

- Assess for the following:
    - Complications (hypotension, clotting of vascular access, headache, muscle cramps, bleeding)
    - Indications of bleeding, and/or infection at the access site
    - Signs of disequilibrium syndrome
    - Signs of hypovolemia (hypotension, dizziness, tachycardia)
- Avoid invasive procedures for 4 to 6 hr after dialysis due to the risk of bleeding related to an anticoagulant.
- Client Education
    - Reinforce AV fistula or AV graft precautions.
    - Teach the client to perform the following:
        - Alert the nurse of early signs of disequilibrium syndrome, such as nausea and headache.
        - Check the access site at intervals following dialysis. Apply light pressure if bleeding.
        - Check the graft for patency by checking for thrill or bruit.
        - Monitor the access site for signs of an infection such as fever, redness, drainage or swelling.
        - Contact the provider if bleeding from the insertion site lasts longer than 30 min following dialysis, for absence of thrill/bruit, or signs of infection.
        - Take medications and supplements as prescribed to replace folate loss.
        - Eat well-balanced meals to include foods high in folate (beans, green vegetables), and take supplements. Protein is lost with each exchange during dialysis and also requires the client to increase protein intake.
        - Avoid lifting heavy objects with access-site arm.
        - Avoid carrying objects that compress or constrict the extremity.
        - Avoid sleeping on top of the extremity with the access device.
        - Perform hand exercises that promote fistula maturation.
- Complications
    - Clotting/infection of access site
        - Anticoagulants are often given to prevent blood clots from forming. Monitor for hemorrhage at the insertion site.
        - Infections of the access site are likely introduced during cannulation.
            - Immunosuppressive disorders increase the risk for infection.
            - Advanced age is a risk factor for dialysis-induced hypotension and access site complications related to chronic illnesses and/or fragile veins.
        - Nursing Actions
            - Use surgical aseptic technique during cannulation.
            - Avoid compression of access site, and venipuncture or blood pressure measurements on extremity with access site.

□ Administer anticoagulants as prescribed.

□ Assess graft site for palpable thrill or audible bruit indicating vascular flow.

□ Assess the access site for redness, swelling, or drainage. Monitor for fever.

○ Disequilibrium syndrome

▪ Disequilibrium syndrome is caused by too rapid a decrease of BUN and circulating fluid volume. It may result in cerebral edema and increased intracranial pressure.

□ Early recognition of disequilibrium syndrome is essential. Signs include nausea, vomiting, change in level of consciousness, seizures, and agitation.

□ Advanced age is a risk factor for dialysis disequilibrium and hypotension due to rapid changes in fluid and electrolyte status.

▪ Nursing Actions

□ Use a slow dialysis exchange rate, especially for older adult clients and those being treated with hemodialysis for the first time.

□ Administer anticonvulsants/barbiturates if needed.

○ Hypotension

▪ Rapid fluid depletion during dialysis may cause hypotension. Other causes include antihypertensives and splanchnic vasodilation due to food ingestion during dialysis.

▪ Nursing Actions

□ Carefully replace fluid volume with transfusion of intravenous fluids or colloid as prescribed. Slow the dialysis exchange rate.

□ Lower the head of the client's bed.

□ For severe hypotension that is unresponsive to fluid replacement, discontinue the dialysis.

○ Anemia

▪ Blood loss and removal of folate during dialysis may contribute to an existing anemia that often occurs with chronic kidney disease (caused by decreased RBC production due to decreased erythropoietin secretion).

▪ Nursing Actions

□ Administer prescribed medication therapy (erythropoietin) to stimulate the production of red blood cells.

□ Monitor Hgb and RBC level.

□ Monitor for hypotension and tachycardia.

□ Transfuse blood products if prescribed.

○ Infectious Diseases

▪ Blood transfusions and frequent blood access due to hemodialysis pose a risk for transmission of blood-borne diseases such as HIV and hepatitis B and C.

▪ Nursing Actions

□ Maintain sterility of equipment.

□ Use standard precautions.

□ Administer medications as prescribed.

Peritoneal Dialysis

- Peritoneal dialysis involves instillation of hypertonic dialysate solution into the peritoneal cavity. Allow the hypertonic dialysate solution to dwell in the peritoneal cavity as ordered by the provider. Drain the dialysate solution that includes the waste products. The peritoneum serves as the filtration membrane.

  ○ The client should have an intact peritoneal membrane, without adhesions from infection or multiple surgeries.

- Indications

  ○ Peritoneal dialysis is the treatment of choice for the older adult.

  ○ Peritoneal dialysis is indicated for clients requiring dialysis who

    ▪ Are unable to tolerate anticoagulation.

    ▪ Have difficulty with vascular access.

    ▪ Have chronic infections or are unstable.

- Preprocedure

  ○ Nursing Actions

    ▪ Assess dry weight (obtained when dialysate is drained), serum electrolytes, creatinine, BUN, and blood glucose.

    ▪ Determine the client's ability to perform self-peritoneal dialysis and follow sterile technique.

      ▫ Level of alertness

      ▫ Past experience with dialysis

      ▫ Understanding of procedure

  ○ Client Education

    ▪ The client should be instructed about the procedure. The client may feel fullness when the dialysate is dwelling. There may be discomfort initially with dialysate infusion.

    ▪ Continuous ambulatory peritoneal dialysis (CAPD) is usually done 7 days a week for 4 to 8 hr. Clients may continue normal activities during CAPD.

    ▪ Continuous-cycle peritoneal dialysis (CCPD) is a 24-hr dialysis. The exchange occurs at night while the client is sleeping. The final exchange is left in to dwell during the day.

    ▪ Automated peritoneal dialysis (APD) is a 30-min exchange repeated over 8 to 10 hr while the client is sleeping.

- Intraprocedure

 View Animation: Peritoneal Dialysis

  ○ Nursing Actions

    ▪ Monitor the client's vital signs frequently during initial dialysis of clients in a hospital setting.

    ▪ Monitor the client's serum glucose level (dialysate contains glucose, a hypertonic solution).

    ▪ Record the amount of inflow compared to outflow of dialysate.

- Monitor the color (clear, light yellow is expected) and amount (expected to equal or exceed amount of dialysate inflow) of outflow.
- Monitor for signs of infection (fever; bloody, cloudy, or frothy dialysate return; drainage at access site) and for complications (respiratory distress, abdominal pain, insufficient outflow, discolored outflow).
- Check the access site dressing for wetness (risk of dialysate leakage) and exit site infections.
- Warm the dialysate prior to instilling. Avoid the use of microwaves, which cause uneven heating.
- Follow prescribed times for infusion, dwell, and outflow.
- Maintain surgical asepsis of the catheter insertion site and when accessing the catheter.
- Keep the outflow bag lower than the client's abdomen (drain by gravity, prevent reflux).
- Reposition the client if inflow or outflow is inadequate.
- Carefully milk peritoneal dialysis catheter if fibrin clot has formed.
- Provide emotional support to the client and family.

- Postprocedure
  - Nursing Actions
    - Monitor weight, serum electrolytes, creatinine, BUN, and blood glucose.
  - Client Education
    - Teach the client home care of the access site.
      - Instruct the client and family how to perform peritoneal dialysis exchanges at home. Provide support for home peritoneal dialysis with home visits.
      - Seek additional information from the National Kidney Foundation for local support groups.
      - Instruct the client to follow instructions carefully and to take all medications as directed.
      - Instruct the client to take prescribed essential minerals and vitamins with supplements of phosphorus, calcium, sodium, potassium.

      - Older adult clients may be unable to care for a peritoneal access site due to cognitive or physical deficits.
      - Body image changes from bloating may be a concern for clients.

- Complications
  - Peritonitis
    - Peritoneal dialysis can allow micro-organisms into the peritoneum and cause peritonitis.
    - Nursing Actions
      - Maintain surgical asepsis during the procedure.
      - Monitor for infection, such as fever, purulent drainage, redness or swelling, and cloudy or discolored drained dialysate.
    - Client Education
      - Educate the client to use strict sterile technique during exchanges.
      - Instruct the client to notify the provider about any sign of infection.

○ Infection at the access site

▪ Infection at the access site may be related to leakage of dialysate. Access site infections may cause peritonitis.

□ Advanced age is a risk factor for access site complications related to chronic illnesses and/or fragile veins.

▪ Nursing Actions

□ Maintain surgical asepsis of access site.

□ Assess site for wetness from a leaking catheter.

□ Monitor for infection, such as fever, purulent drainage, redness, or swelling.

▪ Client Education

□ Educate the client to use strict sterile technique during exchanges.

□ Instruct the client to notify the provider with any sign of infection.

□ Advise the client to assess the site for leaks, and prevent tugging or twisting of tubing.

○ Protein Loss

▪ Peritoneal dialysis may remove needed protein from the blood as well as excess fluid, wastes, and electrolytes.

▪ Nursing Actions

□ Increase dietary intake of protein.

□ Monitor serum albumin level.

▪ Client Education

□ Instruct the client to follow recommended renal diet with an increase in dietary protein.

○ Hyperglycemia and Hyperlipidemia

▪ Hyperglycemia can result due to the hyperosmolarity of the dialysate.

□ Glucose may be absorbed from the dialysate into the blood.

□ Hyperlipidemia may also occur from long-term therapy and lead to hypertension.

▪ Nursing Actions

□ Monitor serum glucose.

□ Administer insulin for glycemic control.

□ Administer antilipemic medication for triglyceride control.

▪ Client Education

□ Instruct the client to check serum glucose.

□ Instruct the client to follow a recommended diet.

□ Instruct the client to take prescribed antihypertensive medication for elevated blood pressure.

○ Poor dialysate inflow or outflow

▪ The tubing may become obstructed or twisted, causing a decrease in flow.

▪ Constipation is a common cause of poor inflow or outflow.

- Nursing Actions
  - □ Reposition the client if inflow or outflow is inadequate.
  - □ Milk tubing to break up fibrin clot.
  - □ Check tubing for kinks or closed clamps.
  - □ Tell the client to avoid constipation by using stool softeners and consuming a diet high in fiber.
- Client Education
  - □ Advise the client to check the tubing for kinks, and teach the client how to remove a fibrin clot.
  - □ Remind the client to monitor the inflow and outflow, and to change position or lower or raise the dialysate bag as needed to improve flow.
  - □ Advise the client to prevent constipation with diet and stool softeners if needed.
  - □ Encourage the client to lie supine with head slightly elevated during CCPD and APD treatment.

APPLICATION EXERCISES

1. A nurse is providing teaching to a client who has chronic kidney disease and is to start hemodialysis. Which of the following information should the nurse include in the teaching?

    A. Hemodialysis restores renal function.

    B. Hemodialysis replaces hormonal function of the renal system.

    C. Hemodialysis allows an unrestricted diet.

    (D.) Hemodialysis returns a balance to serum electrolytes.

2. A nurse is preparing to initiate hemodialysis for a client who has acute kidney injury and has been hospitalized. Which of the following are appropriate nursing actions? (Select all that apply.)

    X   A. Review the client's current medication history.

    X   B. Assess the client's arteriovenous fistula for a bruit.

    _____   C. Calculate the client's total urine output during the shift.

    X   D. Obtain the client's weight.

    X   E. Check the client's serum electrolytes.

    _____   F. Use the client's access site area for venipuncture.

3. A nurse is planning postprocedure care for a client who received hemodialysis. Which of the following should the nurse include in the plan of care? (Select all that apply.)

    X   A. Check BUN and serum creatinine.

    X   B. Administer medications held prior to dialysis

    X   C. Observe for signs of hypovolemia

    X   D. Assess the access site for bleeding.

    _____   E. Evaluate blood pressure on side of AV access.

4. A nurse is caring for a client who is receiving hemodialysis and develops disequilibrium syndrome. Which of the following is an appropriate action by the nurse?

    A. Administer an opioid medication.

    B. Monitor for hypertension.

    (C.) Assess level of consciousness.

    D. Increase the dialysis exchange rate.

5. A nurse is planning care for a client who is having peritoneal dialysis. Which of the following are appropriate nursing actions? (Select all that apply.)

_____X_____ A. Monitor serum glucose levels.

_____X_____ B. Report cloudy dialysate return.

_____ C. Warm the dialysate in a microwave.

_____X_____ D. Assess for shortness of breath.

_____ E. Check the access site dressing for wetness.

_____ F. Maintain medical asepsis when accessing the catheter insertion site.

6. A nurse is reviewing possible complications that a client can experience when receiving peritoneal dialysis. Which of the following complications and actions should the nurse consider in the review? Use the ATI Active Learning Template: Diagnostic Procedure to complete this item. Include the following:

A. Procedure Name: Write out the name, and define the diagnostic test.

B. Potential Complications: List three.

C. Nursing Actions: List two nursing actions for each of the three complications listed.

APPLICATION EXERCISES KEY

1. A. INCORRECT: Hemodialysis does not restore kidney function, but it sustains the life of a client who has kidney disease.

    B. INCORRECT: Hemodialysis does not replace hormonal function of the renal system because of tissue damage causing dysfunction of the renin-angiotensin-aldosterone system.

    C. INCORRECT: Hemodialysis does not allow an unrestricted diet. It requires a diet high in folate and protein, and low in sodium, potassium, and phosphorus.

    D. **CORRECT:** Hemodialysis returns a balance to serum electrolytes by removing excess sodium, potassium, fluids, and waste products; and restores acid-base balance.

     NCLEX® Connection: Physiological Adaptations, Hemodynamics

2. A. **CORRECT:** Reviewing the client's current medication history will determine what medications to hold until after dialysis.

    B. **CORRECT:** Assessing the client's AV fistula for a bruit determines the patency of the fistula for dialysis.

    C. INCORRECT: The client's total urine output over the shift may vary according to the remaining kidney function and does not determine the need for dialysis.

    D. **CORRECT:** Obtaining the client's weight before dialysis is needed to compare with the client's weight after dialysis.

    E. **CORRECT:** Checking the client's serum electrolytes determines the need for dialysis.

    F. INCORRECT: The client's access site area should never be used for venipuncture because it can cause loss of the vascular access.

     NCLEX® Connection: Physiological Adaptations, Alterations in Body Systems

3. A. **CORRECT:** The nurse should check the BUN and serum creatinine to determine the presence and degree of uremia or waste products that remain following dialysis.

    B. **CORRECT:** Medications that can be partially dialysed during the treatment should be withheld. After the treatment, the nurse should administer the medications.

    C. **CORRECT:** A client who is post-dialysis is at risk for hypovolemia due to a rapid decease in fluid volume.

    D. **CORRECT:** The nurse should assess the access site for bleeding because heparin is administered during the procedure to prevent clotting of blood with the dialyzing surfaces.

    E. INCORRECT: The blood pressure should never be taken on the extremity that has the AV access site because it can cause collapse of the AV fistula or graft.

     NCLEX® Connection: Physiological Adaptations, Hemodynamics

4. A. INCORRECT: An altered level of consciousness is a clinical manifestation of disequilibrium syndrome. The nurse should not administer an opioid medication. The provider may prescribe medication to decrease seizure activity.

    B. INCORRECT: The nurse should not monitor for hypertension but for hypotension due to rapid change in fluids and electrolytes causing disequilibrium syndrome.

    C. **CORRECT:** The nurse should assess the client's level of consciousness. A change in urea levels can cause increased intracranial pressure, and subsequently, the client's level of consciousness is decreased.

    D. INCORRECT: The nurse should decrease the dialysis exchange rate to slow the rapid changes in fluid and electrolyte status when a client develops disequilibrium syndrome.

     NCLEX® Connection: Physiological Adaptations, Unexpected Response to Therapies

5. A. **CORRECT:** The nurse should monitor serum glucose levels because the dialysate solution contains glucose.

    B. **CORRECT:** The nurse should monitor for cloudy dialysate return, which indicates an infection. Clear, light yellow solution is expected during the outflow process.

    C. INCORRECT: The nurse should avoid warming the dialysate in a microwave, which causes uneven heating of the solution.

    D. **CORRECT:** The nurse should assess for shortness of breath, which may indicate the client's inability to tolerate a large volume of dialysate.

    E. **CORRECT:** The nurse should check the access site dressing for wetness and determine whether the tubing is kinked, pulled, clamped, or twisted, which can increase the risk for exit site infections.

    F. INCORRECT: The nurse should maintain surgical, not medical, asepsis when accessing the catheter insertion site to prevent infection caused from contamination.

     NCLEX® Connection: Physiological Adaptations, Alterations in Body Systems

6. *Using ATI Active Learning Template: Diagnostic Procedure*

A. Procedure Name

- Peritoneal dialysis – to instill a hypertonic dialysate solution into the peritoneal cavity, allow the solution to dwell for prescribed amount of time, and drain the solution that includes the waste products.

B. Potential Complications

- Peritonitis

- Protein loss from protein wasting

- Hyperglycemia

- Poor dialysate inflow or outflow

C. Nursing Actions

- Peritonitis

  ○ Maintain surgical asepsis.

  ○ Monitor color of outflow solution, pain, fever.

- Protein loss

  ○ Increase dietary intake of protein.

  ○ Monitor albumin level.

- Hyperglycemia

  ○ Monitor serum glucose level.

  ○ Administer insulin.

- Poor dialysate inflow or outflow

  ○ Reposition the client.

  ○ Milk the tubing to break up fibrin clots.

  ○ Check the tubing for kinks or closed clamps.

  ○ Encourage stool softeners and high-fiber diet to prevent constipation.

Ⓝ NCLEX® Connection: Physiological Adaptations, Alterations in Body Systems

chapter 58

Overview

- End-stage kidney disease, when the kidneys can no longer function, may be treated with a kidney transplant as another life-sustaining treatment option other than dialysis. Transplantation may greatly improve the quality of life for a person who is otherwise dependent on dialysis.

- The recipient's tissue must be matched with a donor's.

  ○ Donors for kidney transplantation may be living, non heart-beating, or cadaver donors.

  ○ In-depth tissue typing includes assessment of blood type (ABO) compatibility and histocompatibility, including human leukocytic antigen (HLA) and other minor antigens.

  ○ Clients receiving a donor kidney from a living, related donor – with matching tissue type – have the greatest chance of graft survival.

- The donated kidney is surgically implanted in the client.

Transplantation Procedure

- Indications

  ○ Diagnoses

    ▪ Client indications of end-stage kidney disease necessitating kidney transplantation:

      ▫ Anuria

      ▫ Proteinuria

      ▫ Marked azotemia (elevated BUN and serum creatinine)

      ▫ Severe electrolyte imbalance (hyperkalemia, hypernatremia)

      ▫ Fluid volume excess conditions (heart failure, pulmonary edema)

      ▫ Uremic lung

  ○ Risks

    ▪ Conditions that increase the risks involved in kidney transplantation surgery, lifelong immunosuppression, and organ rejection:

      ▫ Age younger than 2 years

      ▫ Age older than 70 years

        ▸ Older adult clients are more likely to have advanced heart disease and malignancies, which make them less than ideal candidates for kidney transplantation surgery.

      ▫ Advanced, untreatable cardiac disease

      ▫ Active cancer

      ▫ Chemical dependency

- □ Chronic infections or systemic diseases (HIV, hepatitis B or C)
- □ Coagulopathies and certain immune disorders
- □ Morbid obesity
- □ Diabetes
- ○ Client Presentation
  - ▪ Signs and symptoms of end-stage kidney disease may include:
    - □ Subjective Data
      - ▸ Anorexia, fatigue, numbness and tingling of extremities, shortness of breath, dry itchy skin, metallic taste in the mouth, muscle cramping
    - □ Objective Data
      - ▸ Decreased attention span, seizures, tremor, heart failure, edema of hands and feet, dyspnea, distended jugular veins, anemia, vomiting, pulmonary edema, hypertension, cardiac dysrhythmias, pallor, dry itchy skin, bruising, halitosis, and diminished or dark-colored urine
  - ▪ Laboratory Data
    - □ Proteinuria
    - □ Hematuria
    - □ Elevated blood urea nitrogen (BUN) levels
    - □ Elevated serum creatinine
    - □ Decreased glomerular filtration rate (GRF), either estimated from serum or urine creatinine 24 hr values
    - □ Decreased hemoglobin and hematocrit
    - □ Elevated potassium and phosphorus levels
    - □ Sodium normal, increased, or decreased
- • Preprocedure
  - ○ Nursing Actions
    - ▪ Schedule preoperative laboratory assessments, including blood chemistry studies, CBC and differential, bleeding times, urine culture, blood type, and crossmatch.
    - ▪ Administer preoperative medications as prescribed.
      - □ Prophylactic antibiotics
      - □ Immunosuppressant therapy

        - ▸ Methylprednisolone sodium succinate (Solu-Medrol) an anti-inflammatory and immunosuppressant to decrease the immune system response of inflammation and rejection of the donor kidney.
        - ▸ Cyclosporine (Neoral) an immunosuppressant medication to prevent rejection of the donor kidney.
      - □ Monoclonal antibodies
        - ▸ Basiliximab (Simulect) or daclizumab (Zenapax) antibodies that bind to reduce T-cell growth and activation at the receptor site to prevent rejection of the donor kidney
    - ▪ The client is usually dialyzed within 24 hr of surgery.

- ○ Client Education
  - ▪ Prepare the client mentally and emotionally for the procedure.
  - ▪ Inform the client of the interprofessional transplant team involved in the procedure.
    - ▫ Includes nurses, provider, transplant surgeon, anesthesiologists and nephrologists, and clinical nurse specialist and other interprofessional health care workers.
  - ▪ Advise the client that compliance with the posttransplant interventions (lifelong immunosuppression) and risk factor reduction (smoking cessation, blood pressure and blood glucose control) are crucial to the success of the transplantation.
- • Intraprocedure
  - ○ Nursing Actions
    - ▪ Provide padding to the client's bony prominences to provide comfort and prevent skin breakdown.
    - ▪ Communicate surgical progress to the client's family members, if appropriate.
    - ▪ Assist in monitoring urine output and blood loss.
    - ▪ Document appropriate surgical events.
    - ▪ Assist in arranging postoperative unit placement and communicate postoperative needs of the client.
- • Postprocedure
  - ○ Nursing Actions
    - ▪ Assess/monitor
      - ▫ Vital signs every 15 min initially and advance to every hour (follow institutional protocol)
        - ‣ Maintain the client's blood pressure within prescribed parameters.
      - ▫ Intake and output at least hourly
        - ‣ Urine output should be greater than 30 mL/hr. Notify the provider of oliguria as evidenced by urine output of 100 to 400 mL in 24 hr.
        - ‣ Monitor for abrupt decrease in urine output, indicating rejection, tissue injury, thrombosis of the renal artery, or obstruction in the renal system.
      - ▫ Urine appearance and odor hourly (initially pink and bloody, gradually returning to normal in a few days to several weeks)
      - ▫ Daily urinalysis to check for protein, WBCs, RBCs, ketones, glucose, specific gravity, and pH
      - ▫ Daily weight assists in monitoring fluid status
      - ▫ For fluid and electrolyte imbalances, such as hypervolemia, hypovolemia, hypokalemia, and hyponatremia
      - ▫ For signs of infection, such as dyspnea, fever, incisional drainage, and redness
      - ▫ For early signs of organ rejection (fever, hypertension, pain at the transplant site)
      - ▫ Surgical dressing for bloody drainage, which can indicate hemorrhage or hematoma formation.
    - ▪ Administer intravenous fluids as prescribed, usually calculated to replace hourly urine output.
    - ▪ Administer oral fluids and discontinue IV fluid once bowel function returns and fluids are tolerated.

- Encourage the client to turn, cough, and deep breathe to prevent atelectasis and pneumonia.
- Provide urinary catheter care
  - Attach the large indwelling urinary catheter to dependent bedside drainage.
  - Maintain continuous bladder irrigation as prescribed to prevent obstruction from blood clot formation, which can cause damage to the transplanted kidney.
  - Remove the urinary catheter as soon as possible to decrease the risk of infection.
- Intervene for oliguria as prescribed. Diuretics and/or dialysis may be necessary until kidney function is satisfactory.
  - Mannitol, an osmotic diuretic, preserves urine flow and reduces the risk of acute kidney injury. Filtered mannitol draws water into the nephrons of the kidney and promotes diuresis.
  - Thiazides and loop diuretics are less effective when filtration rate is lower causing less diuresis.
- Administer immunosuppressive medications to prevent rejection (prednisone [deltasone], cyclosporines [Neoral], or other medication prescribed by the provider and Monoclonal antibodies, Basiliximab [Simulect] or daclizumab [Zenapax])
  - Monitor for side effects, such as infection and fluid retention.
- Immediately notify the surgeon if any signs of organ rejection appear.
- Administer stool softeners to prevent straining and constipation (risk associated with bowel manipulation during abdominal surgery and the effects of general anesthetics and analgesics).
- Arrange for counseling for the client and family if necessary.
- Arrange for posttransplant follow-up appointments and interventions.
- Client Education
  - Instruct the client to monitor and report signs of infection, such as fever, incisional drainage, and redness.
  - Instruct the client to adhere to the pharmacological regimen (corticosteroids, antilymphocyte preparations, cyclosporine, monoclonal antibodies).
  - Instruct the client and family about prescribed diet and activity level.
    - Diet recommendations:
      - Low fat to decrease cholesterol, high fiber to avoid constipation, increased protein to promote healing, rebuild and maintain muscle mass.
      - Normal intake of potassium, calcium, and phosphorus.
      - Restrict sodium intake to prevent fluid retention and hypertension especially when taking prednisone.
      - Avoid concentrated sugars or carbohydrates to control glycemic factors when on prednisone.
      - Magnesium supplements because cyclosporine (Neoral) can reduce magnesium levels.
      - Avoid grapefruit when taking cyclosporine, which causes increased cyclosporine blood levels.
    - Activity recommendations:
      - Avoid contact sports that may cause an injury to the transplanted kidney.
      - Increase activity as tolerated.

- Complications
    - Organ rejection
        - Clients undergoing kidney transplant face the possibility of organ rejection.
        - Nursing Actions
            - Monitor for and report signs of rejection immediately.
                - Hyperacute – occurs within 48 hr after surgery.
                    - Etiology – An antibody-mediated response causing small blood clots to form in the transplanted kidney that occlude vessels and result in massive cellular destruction. The process can not be reversed.
                    - Findings – fever, hypertension, pain at the transplant site.
                    - Treatment – immediate removal of the donor kidney.
                - Acute – occurs 1 week to 2 years after surgery.
                    - Etiology – An antibody mediated response causing vasculitis in the donor kidney, and cellular destruction starts with inflammation that causes lysis of the donor kidney.
                    - Findings – Oliguria, anuria, low-grade fever, hypertension, tenderness over the transplanted kidney, lethargy, azotemia, and fluid retention.
                    - Treatment – Involves increased doses of immunosuppressive medications.
                - Chronic – occurs gradually over months to years.
                    - Etiology – Blood vessel injury from over-growth of the smooth muscles of the blood vessels causing fibrotic tissue to replace normal tissue resulting in a nonfunctioning donor kidney.
                    - Findings – Findings include gradual return of azotemia, fluid retention, electrolyte imbalance, and fatigue.
                    - Treatment – Conservative (monitor kidney status, continue immunosuppressive therapy) until dialysis is required.
        - Client Education
            - Teach the client to monitor for signs of rejection and to contact the primary care provider immediately.
                - Instruct the client that rejection is diagnosed through a kidney scan and kidney biopsies.
            - Instruct the client to adhere to the pharmacological regimen.
    - Acute tubular necrosis (ATN)
        - A delay in transplanting the donor kidney after harvesting may result in hypoxic injury of the donor kidney.
        - Nursing Actions
            - Monitor the client's urine output, serum creatinine, and BUN levels to detect failure of the transplanted kidney.
            - Report hourly output volumes of less than 30 mL/hr.
            - Assist the client with dialysis as indicated.
            - Prepare the client for a kidney biopsy to distinguish ATN from organ rejection.
        - Client Education
            - Advise the client that dialysis may be needed until the donor kidney heals.

- ○ Renal Artery Stenosis

  - ▪ Renal artery stenosis is due to scarring of surgical anastomosis.

  - ▪ Nursing Actions

    - ▫ Monitor for and report hypertension, bruit over artery anastomosis site, and decreased kidney function, such as oliguria and elevated BUN and creatinine.

    - ▫ Prepare the client for a kidney scan to verify the status of renal blood flow.

    - ▫ Angioplasty and/or surgical intervention may be necessary.

  - ▪ Client Education

    - ▫ Advise the client to monitor for peripheral edema and have blood pressure checked often.

- ○ Thrombosis

  - ▪ A blood clot may form in a major vessel of the transplanted kidney.

  - ▪ Nursing Actions

    - ▫ Monitor the client for and report a sudden decrease in urine output.

    - ▫ Prepare the client for emergency surgery requiring an emergency transplant nephrectomy (removal of the transplant kidney).

  - ▪ Client Education

    - ▫ Keep the client informed about the risk of a blood clot.

    - ▫ Advise the client to inform the provider of a sudden decrease in urine output.

- ○ Infection

  - ▪ Infection is the most common cause of first-transplant-year morbidity and mortality.

  - ▪ Detection of early sign of infection is difficult when the client is prescribed immunosuppressive therapy.

    - ▫ Vague symptoms include low-grade fevers, mild reports of discomfort, and mental status changes.

  - ▪ Nursing Actions

    - ▫ Give high priority to infection control measures, such as frequent hand hygiene.

    - ▫ Monitor for and report signs of a localized (wound) or systemic infection (pneumonia, sepsis).

  - ▪ Client Education

    - ▫ Instruct the client to monitor and report signs of infection, such as fever, incisional drainage, and redness. Later signs of infection may include fatigue and discomfort. Report any signs of infection to the primary care provider.

    - ▫ Educate the client and family about the increased risk for infection during immunosuppressant therapy and infection control measures, such as frequent hand hygiene and avoiding crowds and people who have a communicable disease. The client may need to wear a facemask when out in public.

    - ▫ Instruct the client to adhere to the pharmacological regimen.

APPLICATION EXERCISES

1. A nurse who is a member of the transplant team is assessing information on a client who has end-stage kidney disease. Which of the following client indications should the nurse expect to find?

___✗___ A. Anuria

___✗___ B. Marked azotemia — elevated BUN + creatine

___✗___ C. Crackles in the lungs

_____ D. Increased calcium level

___✗___ E. Proteinuria

2. A nurse is planning postoperative care for a client who had kidney transplant surgery. Which of the following should the nurse include in the plan of care? (Select all that apply.)

___✗___ A. Obtain daily weights

___✗___ B. Assess dressings for bloody drainage

___✗___ C. Replace hourly urine output with IV fluids

_____ D. Position in semi-Fowler's

___✗___ E. Monitor serum electrolytes

3. A nurse is teaching diet recommendations to a client who had a kidney transplant and is taking cyclosporine (Neoral). Which of the following recommendations should the nurse include in the teaching?

A. Decrease protein rich foods

B. Drink grapefruit juice

(C.) Take a magnesium supplement

D. Restrict intake of bananas and raisins

4. A nurse is providing information to a client who has chronic rejection of a transplanted kidney. Which of the following statements should the nurse include?

_____ A. "Immediate removal of the donor kidney is planned."

___✗___ B. "Monitoring electrolytes frequently determines kidney status."

___✗___ C. "Scheduled kidney biopsies determine kidney status."

___✗___ D. "Restarting dialysis depends on marked azotemia."

___✗___ E. "Plan to have the immunosuppressive medication increased."

5. A client who is scheduled for kidney transplantation surgery is assessed by the nurse for risk factors of surgery. Which of the following findings increase the client's risk of surgery?

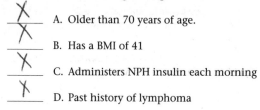

_____ A. Older than 70 years of age.

_____ B. Has a BMI of 41

_____ C. Administers NPH insulin each morning

_____ D. Past history of lymphoma

_____ E. Blood pressure averages 120/70 mm Hg

6. A nurse is planning catheter care for a client who had kidney transplantation surgery. To maintain indwelling urinary catheter patency and avoid complication, which of the following are appropriate nursing actions? Use the ATI Active Learning Template: Nursing Skill to complete this item. Include the following:

A. Indications: List two reasons for an indwelling urinary catheter.

B. Potential Complications: Indicate three risk factors.

C. Nursing Actions: List three postoperative actions.

APPLICATION EXERCISES KEY

1. A. **CORRECT:** Anuria indicates the client has end-stage kidney disease, necessitating kidney transplantation as a treatment.

   B. **CORRECT:** Marked azotemia is elevated BUN and serum creatinine, indicates the client has end-stage kidney disease, necessitating kidney transplantation as a treatment.

   C. **CORRECT:** Crackles in the lungs can indicate the client has pulmonary edema, caused from end-stage kidney disease necessitating kidney transplantation as a treatment.

   D. INCORRECT: Calcium levels are decreased due to increase in serum phosphate levels when the client has end-stage kidney disease.

   E. **CORRECT:** Proteinuria indicates the client has end-stage kidney disease, necessitating kidney transplantation as a treatment.

   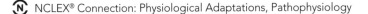 NCLEX® Connection: Physiological Adaptations, Pathophysiology

2. A. **CORRECT:** Daily weights should be obtained by the nurse to assess the client's fluid status.

   B. **CORRECT:** Bloody drainage should be assessed by the nurse, which can indicate hemorrhage or hematoma.

   C. **CORRECT:** Hourly urine output with IV fluid replacement should be monitored by the nurse to detect abrupt decrease in urine output, which may indicate rejection or other serious conditions of the transplant kidney.

   D. INCORRECT: A semi-Fowler's position is not indicated for a client until the client is not at risk for hypotension postoperative.

   E. **CORRECT:** Serum electrolytes should be monitored by the nurse, because electrolytes loss may occur with postoperative diuresis.

   NCLEX® Connection: Physiological Adaptations, Illness Management

3. A. INCORRECT: A client should not decrease protein rich foods in the diet. There are no restrictions of protein intake following a kidney transplant, which promotes healing and rebuilds muscle.

    B. INCORRECT: The client should not drink grapefruit juice, which causes increased cyclosporine serum levels.

    C. **CORRECT:** The client should take a magnesium supplement, because magnesium is lost when taking cyclosporine.

    D. INCORRECT: The client should not restrict intake of bananas and raisins, which are high in potassium and can be consumed in normal amounts.

     NCLEX® Connection: Basic Care and Comfort, Nutrition and Oral Hydration

4. A. INCORRECT: Immediate removal of the donor kidney is treatment for hyperacute rejection.

    B. **CORRECT:** Frequent monitoring of electrolyte studies determines the progression of kidney failure and the need for dialysis.

    C. **CORRECT:** Kidney biopsies do determine the progression of kidney failure and the need for dialysis.

    D. **CORRECT:** Marked azotemia does determine the progression of kidney failure and the need to restart this treatment.

    E. **CORRECT:** Increasing immunosuppressive medication may suppress the progression of kidney failure and the need to restart this dialysis.

     NCLEX® Connection: Reduction of Risk Potential, System Specific Assessments

5.   A. **CORRECT:** A client older than 70 years of age is placed at a greater risk from complication of surgery, lifelong immunosuppression, and organ rejection.

     B. **CORRECT:** A client with a BMI of 41 is morbidly obese and is placed at a greater risk for complication of surgery, lifelong immunosuppression, and organ rejection.

     C. **CORRECT:** A client who requires NPH insulin for Type 1 diabetes mellitus is placed at a greater risk from complication of surgery, lifelong immunosuppression, and organ rejection.

     D. **CORRECT:** A client with a past history of cancer such as lymphoma is placed at a greater risk for complication of surgery, lifelong immunosuppression, and organ rejection.

     E. INCORRECT: Blood pressure averaging 120/70 mm Hg is within normal limits and does not place the client at a greater risk for complication of surgery, lifelong immunosuppression, and organ rejection.

   ⓝ NCLEX® Connection: Health Promotion and Maintenance, Health Promotion/Disease Prevention

6.   *Using the ATI Active Learning Template: Nursing Skill*

     A. Indications for a catheter
     - Monitor hourly urinary output.
     - Monitor color of urine and clots.

     B. Potential Complications
     - Risk for oliguria
     - Risk for infection from an indwelling urinary catheter
     - Risk for blood clot formation

     C. Nursing Actions
     - Regulate IV fluids is accordance to urinary output, as the provider prescribes.
     - Connect the indwelling urinary catheter to the bed lower than the client to promote gravity drainage.
     - Remove the indwelling urinary catheter within a few days postprocedure.
     - Implement continuous bladder irrigation as prescribed to remove blood clots that can obstruct the indwelling urinary catheter and and cause damage to the donor kidney.

   ⓝ NCLEX® Connection: Reduction of Risk Potential, Potential for Complications of Diagnostic Tests/ Treatments/Procedures

chapter 59

Overview

- Glomerulonephritis is an inflammation of the glomerular capillaries, usually following a streptococcal infection. It is an immune complex disease, not an infection of the kidney.
- Glomerulonephritis exists as an acute, latent, and chronic disease.
- Acute glomerulonephritis (AGN)
  - Insoluble immune complexes develop and become trapped in the glomerular tissue producing swelling and capillary cell death.
  - Prognosis varies depending upon the specific cause, but spontaneous recovery generally occurs after the acute illness.
- Chronic glomerulonephritis (CGN)
  - CGN can occur without a previous history or known onset.
  - This involves the progressive destruction of glomeruli and eventual hardening (sclerosis).
  - CGN is the third leading cause of end-stage kidney disease (ESKD), with the prognosis varying depending on the specific cause.

M⬧ View Image: Glomerulonephritis

Health Promotion and Disease Prevention

- Consume a diet low in sodium and restrict fluid intake. Consult a health care provider regarding diet restrictions.

Assessment

- Risk Factors
  - Immunological reactions
    - Primary infection with group A beta-hemolytic streptococcal infection (most common)
    - Systemic lupus erythematosus
  - Vascular injury (hypertension)
  - Metabolic disease (diabetes mellitus)
  - Excessively high protein and high sodium diets

  - Older adult clients may report vague symptoms (nausea, fatigue, joint aches) which may mask glomerular disease.
  - Older adult clients tend to have decreased working nephrons and are at increased risk for chronic kidney failure.

- Clinical Manifestations
  - Renal symptoms
    - Decreased urine output
    - Smoky or coffee-colored urine (hematuria)
    - Proteinuria
  - Fluid volume excess symptoms
    - Pitting edema in lower extremities
    - Weight gain
    - Shortness of breath
    - Orthopnea
    - Bibasilar rales
    - Periorbital edema
    - Mild to severe hypertension, greater than 140/90 mm Hg
  - Older adult fluid volume excess symptoms
    - Shortness of breath, distended neck veins, cardiomegaly, and pulmonary edema
    - Rare symptoms of the older adult are confusion, sleepiness, and possible seizures
  - Changes in the level of consciousness
  - Anorexia/nausea
  - Headache
  - Back pain
  - Fever (AGN)
  - Pruritus (CGN)
  - Laboratory Tests
    - Throat culture to identify possible streptococcus infection
    - Serum BUN (elevated: 100 to 200 mg/dL; expected reference range: 10 to 20 mg/dL) and creatinine (elevated: greater than 6 mg/dL; expected reference range: males: 0.6 to 1.2 mg/dL, and females: 0.5 to 1.1 mg/L)
    - Creatinine clearance 24 hr urine collection (decreased: 50 mL/min/m²; expected reference range: males: 90 to 139 mL/min/m², females: 80 to 125 mL/min/m²)
      - Glomerular filtration rate (GFR): filtration rate of kidneys, best indicator of kidney function is decreased to 50 mL/min (expected reference range greater than 90 mL/min).
    - Urinalysis: proteinuria, hematuria, cell debris (red cells and casts), increased urine specific gravity
    - Electrolytes: hyperkalemia, hypoalbuminemia, and hyperphosphatemia
    - Antistreptolysin-O (ASO) titer (positive indicating the presence of strep antibodies)
    - Erythrocyte sedimentation rate (ESR) (elevated indicating active inflammatory response)
    - White blood cell count (elevated indicating inflammation and presence of active strep infection)

○ Diagnostic Procedures

▪ X-ray of kidney, ureter, bladder (KUB), and renal ultrasound (to detect structural abnormalities [atrophy])

▪ Kidney biopsy (to confirm or rule out diagnosis)

▪ Dialysis can be an intervention to treat end-stage kidney failure with severe uremia (large amounts of urea and other nitrogenous waste found in the blood)

Patient-Centered Care

- Nursing Care
  - ○ Monitor the client's daily weight and note any recent weight gain.
  - ○ Monitor intake and output.
  - ○ Observe the client for changes in urinary pattern.
  - ○ Monitor serum electrolytes, BUN, and creatinine.
  - ○ Observe the client's skin for pruritus.
  - ○ Maintain bed rest to decrease metabolic demands.
  - ○ Maintain prescribed dietary restrictions.
    - ▪ Fluid restriction (24 hr output + 500 to 600 mL)
    - ▪ Sodium restriction (1 to 3 g/day) begins when fluid retention occurs
    - ▪ Protein restriction (if azotemia is present = increased BUN)
      - ▫ Protein restricted to 0.6 to 0.75 g/kg/day reduces nitrogen waste and can slow the progression of renal failure.
- Medications
  - ○ Administer antibiotics, such as penicillin G potassium (Megacillin), erythromycin (Erythrocin), or azithromycin (zithromax), on time to maintain blood levels for an effective elimination of the strep infection.
  - ○ Administer diuretics (thiazide diuretic, loop diuretic, and/or potassium-sparing diuretic) to reduce edema.
  - ○ Use vasodilators to decrease blood pressure.
  - ○ Administer corticosteroids to decrease the inflammatory response.
- Interprofessional Care
  - ○ Nephrology services may be consulted to manage renal function.
    - ▪ Nephrologist
      - ▫ Provides medical care of the client who has kidney disease
      - ▫ Provides medical care for related conditions, diabetes, hypertension, and long-term follow-up care
    - ▪ Nephrology Nurse
      - ▫ Registered nurse specializing in chronic kidney failure
      - ▫ Coordinates client care to include dialysis and transplant treatment

- ▪ Renal Nutritionist (Dietitian)
  - ▫ Provides a comprehensive diet plan and education for the client
  - ▫ May be consulted for diet modifications and fluid restriction
- ▪ Nephrology Social Worker
  - ▫ Assists the client and family to cope with changes related to the kidney disease (job, family, community)
  - ▫ Provides services with community, state, and federal agencies to improve the client's quality of life
- ▪ Renal Technologist
  - ▫ Assists the RN and orders supplies
- ▪ Financial Counselor
  - ▫ Assists in answering billing questions and payment plans
- • Therapeutic Procedures
  - ○ Plasmapheresis (filters antibodies out of circulating blood volume by removing the plasma)
    - ▪ Nursing Actions
      - ▫ Monitor the client carefully during and following the procedure.
        - ‣ Weigh the client before and after the procedure to determine fluid deficit.
        - ‣ Monitor for hypovolemia (hypotension, tachycardia, dizziness, diaphoresis).
        - ‣ Administer replacement fluids with a colloid such as albumin as needed.
        - ‣ Monitor for signs of tetany if too much calcium is removed with the plasma.
        - ‣ Administer calcium chloride or calcium gluconate if prescribed.
        - ‣ Monitor for signs of infection at the access site.
    - ▪ Client Education
      - ▫ Encourage the client to rest, report dizziness, muscle twitching, nausea, vomiting, paresthesias of the extremities, and signs of infection.
- • Care after Discharge
  - ○ Home care services may be indicated if the client is homebound or living in a nursing facility.
  - ○ Outpatient services are routinely set up to follow the client's medications and status.
  - ○ Laboratory services are routinely set up to follow the client's renal function.
  - ○ Client Education
    - ▪ Instruct the client to take medications as prescribed.
    - ▪ Instruct the client to weigh daily, at the same time, and to notify the provider for a weight gain of 2 lb in 24 hr or 5 lb in 1 week.
    - ▪ Educate the client on methods of detecting fluid retention.

- Advise the client to maintain fluid and sodium restriction – a dietary consult may be necessary to create a modified diet.

- Educate the client and family regarding the illness and encourage the expression feelings.

  □ Encourage the client to balance activity and rest.

  □ Promote a plan to decrease stress with diversional activities and relaxation techniques.

  □ Instruct the client to report early signs of infection to the provider.

Complications

- Uremia

  ○ Nursing Actions

    - Monitor the client for muscle cramps, fatigue, pruritus, anorexia, and a metallic taste in mouth.

    - Intervene to maintain skin integrity.

    - Offer a variety of high-carbohydrate foods. Encourage mouth rinses, chewing gum, or hard candy.

    - Prepare the client for prescribed hemodialysis or peritoneal dialysis.

- Pulmonary edema, congestive heart failure, pericarditis

  ○ Nursing Actions

    - Monitor the client for dyspnea, crackles, edema, tachycardia, hypotension, and decreased urine output.

      □ Treat dyspnea with oxygen; crackles and edema with diuretics if blood pressure stable; improve tachycardia with inotropic medications; monitor ECG.

      □ Intervene with dialysis if client fails to respond.

- Anemia

  ○ Nursing Actions

    - Monitor the client's hemoglobin.

    - Assess the client for fatigue, pallor, and weakness.

    - Administer iron and erythropoietin and other blood products, such as packed RBCs, plasma, and fresh frozen platelets, as prescribed.

    - Implement fall risk precautions.

APPLICATION EXERCISES

1. A nurse is presenting information to a client who has a new diagnosis of chronic glomerulonephritis. Which of the following nursing statements is appropriate?

    A. "A high-sodium diet is recommended."

    B. "The destruction of the glomeruli occurs rapidly."

    C. "The cause of the disease is not known."

    D. "To compensate, the number of functioning nephrons is increased."

2. A nurse is assessing laboratory values for a client who may have acute glomerulonephritis. Which of the following findings should the nurse report to the provider?

    A. Urine specific gravity of 1.022

    B. BUN of 16 mg/dL

    C. Creatinine clearance of 48 mL/min/m²

    D. Potassium level of 4.2 mEq/L

3. A nurse is assessing a client who has a diagnosis of acute glomerulonephritis. Which of the following is an expected finding? (Select all that apply.)

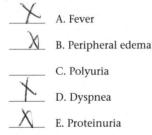

    ___ A. Fever

    ___ B. Peripheral edema

    ___ C. Polyuria

    ___ D. Dyspnea

    ___ E. Proteinuria

4. A nurse is monitoring a client who is receiving plasmapheresis. Which of the following should indicate to the nurse that the client is experiencing side effects from the procedure? (Select all that apply.)

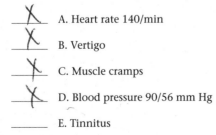

    ___ A. Heart rate 140/min

    ___ B. Vertigo

    ___ C. Muscle cramps

    ___ D. Blood pressure 90/56 mm Hg

    ___ E. Tinnitus

5. A nurse is providing teaching on the manifestation of complications to a client who has acute glomerulonephritis. Which of the following complications should the client report to the provider?

    A. Dry cough

    B. Pitting edema

    C. Weight gain of 2 lb in 1 week

    D. Temperature of 36.8° C (98.4° F)

6. A nurse is planning care for complications experienced by a client who has chronic glomerulonephritis. Which actions should the nurse include in the plan of care? Use ATI Active Learning Template: Basic Concept to complete this item. Include the following:

    A. Related Content: List three complications.

    B. Underlying Principles: List three principles to monitor for each complication.

    C. Nursing Interventions: List two intervention for each complication monitored.

APPLICATION EXERCISES KEY

1. A. INCORRECT: With chronic glomerulonephritis, a low-sodium diet is recommended to slow fluid retention.

    B. INCORRECT: With chronic glomerulonephritis, destruction of the glomeruli is progressive over a long period of time.

    C. **CORRECT:** With chronic glomerulonephritis, the kidney atrophies, and tissue is not available for biopsy and diagnosis, making it difficult to determine the cause.

    D. INCORRECT: With chronic glomerulonephritis, the number of functioning nephrons decrease over time, leading to end-stage kidney failure.

    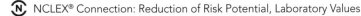 NCLEX® Connection: Physiological Adaptations, Illness Management

2. A. INCORRECT: The urine specific gravity value is within the expected reference range and does not need to be reported to the provider.

    B. INCORRECT: The BUN is within the expected reference range and does not need to be reported to the provider.

    C. **CORRECT:** The creatinine clearance 24 hr urine is not within the expected reference range, indicating possible renal failure, and needs to be reported to the provider.

    D. INCORRECT: The potassium level is within the expected reference range and does not need to be reported to the provider.

    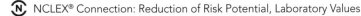 NCLEX® Connection: Reduction of Risk Potential, Laboratory Values

3. A. **CORRECT:** A client who has acute glomerulonephritis may have a low-grade fever because of the possible streptococcus infection.

    B. **CORRECT:** Peripheral edema indicates fluid retention caused by fluid and sodium retention with acute glomerulonephritis.

    C. INCORRECT: Polyuria is not a finding of acute glomerulonephritis; however, fluid retention occurs, causing dilution of the urine.

    D. **CORRECT:** A client who has acute glomerulonephritis may display dyspnea because of fluid retention, causing pulmonary edema or congestive heart failure.

    E. **CORRECT:** A client who has acute glomerulonephritis will have protein loss in the urine because of glomeruli involvement.

    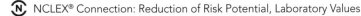 NCLEX® Connection: Physiological Adaptations, Pathophysiology

4. A. **CORRECT:** The client's heart rate of 140/min indicates tachycardia, which is a sign of hypovolemia caused by the removal of blood plasma, which decreases fluid volume.

    B. **CORRECT:** Vertigo is a sign of hypovolemia caused by the removal of blood plasma, which decreases fluid volume.

    C. **CORRECT:** Muscle cramping is a sign of tetany caused by the removal of calcium with the blood plasma.

    D. **CORRECT:** The client's blood pressure of 90/56 mm Hg is a sign of hypovolemia caused by the removal of blood plasma, which decreases fluid volume.

    E. INCORRECT: Tinnitus is not related to plasmapheresis, which can cause hypovolemia.

    (N) NCLEX® Connection: Reduction of Risk Potential, Potential for Complications of Diagnostic Tests/ Treatments/Procedures

5. A. INCORRECT: A dry cough does not indicate fluid overload. Fluid overload manifests with a wet cough and crackles as a complication of acute glomerulonephritis.

    B. **CORRECT:** Pitting edema is an indication of fluid overload, a manifestation of a complication of acute glomerulonephritis.

    C. INCORRECT: A weight gain of 2 lb in 1 week is not a complication. However, a weight gain of 5 lb in 1 week is a sign of fluid overload, a complication of acute glomerulonephritis.

    D. INCORRECT: A temperature of 36.8° C (98.4° F) is not a complication of acute glomerulonephritis. However, a low-grade fever may indicate an infection.

    (N) NCLEX® Connection: Physiological Adaptations, Medical Emergencies

6. *Using ATI Active Learning Template: Basic Concept*

    A. Related Content
        - Uremia
        - Pulmonary edema, congestive heart failure, pericarditis
        - Anemia

    B. Underlying Principles
        - Uremia
          o   Monitor for muscle cramps, anorexia, and metallic taste in mouth.
        - Pulmonary edema, congestive heart failure, pericarditis
          o   Monitor for dyspnea, crackles, edema, hypotension, tachycardia, low urine output.
        - Anemia
          o   Monitor hemoglobin, and monitor for fatigue, pallor, and weakness.

    C. Nursing Interventions
        - Uremia
          o   Maintain skin integrity.
          o   Offer a variety of high-carbohydrate foods.
          o   Encourage mouth rinses, chewing gum, or hard candy.
        - Pulmonary edema, congestive heart failure, pericarditis
          o   Apply oxygen, administer diuretics, dialysis, monitor ECG.
        - Anemia
          o   Administer iron, erythropoietin, packed RBCs, plasma, fresh frozen platelets as prescribed.

    (N) NCLEX® Connection: Physiological Adaptations, Unexpected Response to Therapies

chapter 60

Overview

- There are several disorders that affect the renal system and its ability to function.

- Some of these disorders include acute kidney injury and chronic kidney disease.

- The kidneys regulate fluid, acid-base, and electrolyte balance while also eliminating wastes from the body.

- Kidney failure may be diagnosed as acute kidney injury or chronic kidney disease. Acute kidney injury can result in chronic kidney disease without aggressive treatment, or when complicating preexisting conditions exist.

ACUTE KIDNEY INJURY

- Acute kidney injury (AKI) is the sudden cessation of renal function that occurs when blood flow to the kidneys is significantly compromised. Clinical manifestations occur abruptly with AKI.

  ○ AKI is comprised of four phases:

    ▪ Onset – Begins with the onset of the event, ends when oliguria develops, and lasts for hours to days.

    ▪ Oliguria – Begins with the kidney insult, urine output is 100 to 400 mL/24 hr with or without diuretics, and lasts for 1 to 3 weeks.

    ▪ Diuresis – Begins when the kidneys start to recover, diuresis of a large amount of fluid occurs, and can last for 2 to 6 weeks.

    ▪ Recovery – Continues until kidney function is fully restored and can take up to 12 months.

- Types of Acute Kidney Injury

  ○ Prerenal acute kidney injury – occurs as a result of volume depletion and prolonged reduction of blood flow to the kidneys, which leads to ischemia of the nephrons. Occurs before damage to the kidney. Early intervention restoring fluid volume deficit can reverse AKI and prevent chronic kidney disease (CKD).

    ▪ Causes

      □ Renal vascular obstruction

      □ Shock

      □ Decreased cardiac output causing decreased renal profusion

      □ Sepsis

      □ Hypovolemia

      □ Peripheral vascular resistance

- Nursing Care

  □ Monitor central venous pressure (CVP) and for hypotension, tachycardia, and decreased cardiac output.

  □ Prevent prolonged episodes of hypotension and hypovolemia.

  □ Monitor fluid intake and output (oliguria).

  □ Prepare for fluid challenge and diuretics with signs of azotemia and fluid volume deficit.

    ▸ Administer IV fluid challenge if no fluid restrictions.

    ▸ Administer diuretic to promote increased filtration of blood by kidney.

  □ Administer calcium channel blocker to prevent the movement of calcium into the kidney cells, maintain cell integrity, and increase glomerular filtration rate (GFR).

  □ Review laboratory values (BUN, creatinine, electrolytes, hematocrit).

  □ Assess for lethargy.

  □ Avoid using nephrotoxic medications or combining two or more, which may increase nephron destruction.

- Intrarenal acute kidney injury – Occurs as a result of direct damage to the kidney from lack of oxygen (acute tubular necrosis).

  - Causes

    □ Physical injury – trauma

    □ Hypoxic injury – renal artery or vein stenosis or thrombosis

    □ Chemical injury – acute nephrotoxins (e.g. antibiotics, NSAIDs, contrast dye, heavy metal, blood transfusion reaction)

    □ Immunologic injury – infection, vasculitis, acute glomerulonephritis

  - Nursing Care

    □ Assess for oliguria or anuria.

    □ Assess for edema and manifestations of heart failure or pulmonary edema.

    □ Restrict fluid intake as prescribed.

    □ Review laboratory values for elevated potassium, low calcium levels.

    □ Monitor for ECG dysrhythmias and changes (tall T waves).

    □ Assess for flank pain, nausea, and vomiting.

    □ Assess for lethargy, tremors, and confusion.

    □ Monitor daily weights.

- Postrenal acute kidney injury – Occurs as a result of bilateral obstruction of structures leaving the kidney.

  - Causes

    □ Stone, tumor, bladder atony

    □ Prostate hyperplasia, urethral stricture

    □ Spinal cord disease or injury

**Q
PCC**

- Nursing Care

  □ Monitor for oliguria or intermittent anuria.

  □ Assess for lethargy and other symptoms of uremia.

  □ Assess for changes in urination stream or difficulty starting the stream of urine.

  □ Assess the urine for blood or particles.

  □ Monitor for pain.

- Laboratory Values

  □ Serum creatinine gradually increases 1 to 2 mg/dL every 24 to 48 hr, or 1 to 6 mg/dL in 1 week or less.

  □ Blood urea nitrogen (BUN) can increase to 80 to 100 mg/dL within 1 week with AKI.

  □ Urine specific gravity greater than 1.000 to 1.010 in postrenal type (1.030 in prerenal type, 1.010 in intrarenal type).

- Diagnostic Assessment

  □ X-ray to detect calculi and determine size of kidneys.

  □ Ultrasound to detect an obstruction in the urinary tract.

  □ CT scan without contrast dye to identify obstruction or tumors.

  □ Kidney biopsy to detect immunological disease or determine kidney dysfunction reversibility and need for dialysis therapy.

- Nutrition

  □ Restrict dietary intake of potassium, phosphate, and magnesium during oliguric phase (restriction is for the client not requiring dialysis).

  □ Potassium and sodium is regulated according to the stage of kidney injury.

  □ High-protein diet to replace the high rate of protein breakdown due to stress from the illness. Possible total parenteral nutrition (TPN).

  □ Identify and assist with correcting the underlying cause.

- Health Promotion and Disease Prevention of Acute Kidney Injury

  ○ Encourage clients to drink at least 2 to 3 L daily. Consult with the provider regarding prescribed fluid restriction if needed.

  ○ Promote smoking cessation, weight loss, cautious use of NSAIDs, and control of diabetes and hypertension with prescribed medication.

  ○ Insruct clients to take all antibiotics prescribed for infections.

CHRONIC KIDNEY DISEASE

- Chronic kidney disease (CKD) is a progressive, irreversible kidney disease.
  - A client who has a diagnosis of CKD may be asymptomatic except during periods of stress (infection, surgery, trauma). As kidney dysfunction progresses, clinical manifestations become apparent.
  - Older adult clients are at an increased risk for chronic kidney disease related to the normal aging process (decreased number of functioning nephrons, decreased GFR).
  - Older adults clients who are on bed rest, confused, have a lack of thirst, and do not have easy access to water are at a higher risk for dehydration leading to chronic kidney disease.
  - Risk Factors and Causes of Chronic Kidney Disease
    - Acute kidney injury
    - Diabetes mellitus
    - Chronic glomerulonephritis
    - Nephrotoxic medications (gentamicin, NSAIDs) or chemicals
    - Hypertension, especially if African American
    - Autoimmune disorders (systemic lupus erythematosus)
    - Polycystic kidney
    - Pyelonephrosis
    - Renal artery stenosis
    - Recurrent severe infections
  - CKD is comprised of five stages:
    - Stage 1: Minimal kidney damage with normal GFR (greater than 90 mL/min)
    - Stage 2: Mild kidney damage with mildly decreased GFR (60 to 89 mL/min)
    - Stage 3: Moderate kidney damage with moderate decrease in GFR (30 to 59 mL/min)
    - Stage 4: Severe kidney damage with severe decrease in GFR (15 to 29 mL/min)
    - Stage 5: Kidney failure and end-stage kidney disease with little or no glomerular filtration (less than 15 mL/min)
  - End-stage kidney disease exists when 90% of the functioning nephrons have been destroyed and are no longer able to maintain fluid, electrolyte, and acid-base homeostasis.
  - Dialysis or kidney transplantation can maintain life, but neither is a cure for CKD.

Health Promotion and Disease Prevention of Chronic Kidney Disease

- Encourage clients to drink at least 3 L of water daily. Consult with the provider regarding any restrictions.
- Promote smoking cessation.
- Encourage diet and activities to control or prevent diabetes and hypertension.
- Teach the client the importance of adherence to a medication regimen when prescribed.
- Encourage yearly testing for albumin in the urine if the client has diabetes or hypertension.

- Instruct the client to take all antibiotics until completed.
- Limit over-the-counter NSAIDs.
- Subjective Data
  - ○ Fatigue, lethargy, involuntary movement of legs, depression, intractable hiccups
- Objective Data
  - ○ In most cases, findings of chronic kidney disease are related to fluid volume overload and include the following:
    - Neurologic – lethargy, decreased attention span, slurred speech, tremors or jerky movements, ataxia, seizures, coma
    - Cardiovascular – fluid overload (jugular distention; sacrum, ocular or peripheral edema), hypertension, dysrhythmias, heart failure, orthostatic hypotension
    - Respiratory – uremic halitosis with deep sighing, yawning, shortness of breath, tachypnea, hyperpnea, Kussmaul respirations, crackles, pleural friction rub, frothy pink sputum
    - Hematologic – anemia (pallor, weakness, dizziness), ecchymoses, petechiae, melena
    - Gastrointestinal – ulcers in mouth and throat, foul breath, blood in stools, nausea, vomiting
    - Musculoskeletal – osteodystrophy (thin fragile bones)
    - Renal – urine contains protein, blood, particles; change in the amount, color, concentration
    - Skin – decreased skin turgor, yellow cast to skin, dry, pruritus, urea crystal on skin (uremic frost)
    - Reproductive – erectile dysfunction
  - ○ Laboratory Tests
    - Urinalysis
      - □ Hematuria, proteinuria, and decrease in specific gravity.
    - Serum creatinine
      - □ Gradual increase over months to years for CKD exceeding 4 mg/dL. May be as high as 15 to 30 mg/dL.
    - BUN
      - □ Gradual increase with elevated serum creatinine over months to years for CKD. May be as high as 180 to 200 mg/dL.
    - Serum electrolytes
      - □ Decreased sodium (dilutional) and calcium; increased potassium, phosphorus, and magnesium.
    - CBC
      - □ Decreased hemoglobin and hematocrit from anemia secondary to the loss of erythropoietin in CKD.
  - ○ Diagnostic Procedures
    - Radiologic procedures to detect disease processes, obstruction, and arterial defects.
      - □ Ultrasound
      - □ Kidneys, ureter, and bladder (KUB)
      - □ Computerized tomography (CT)
      - □ Magnetic resonance imaging (MRI) without contrast dye

□ Aortorenal angiography

□ Cystoscopy

□ Retrograde pyelography

□ Kidney biopsy

- Complications of CKD
  ○ Potential complications of kidney failure include electrolyte imbalance, dysrhythmias, fluid overload, hypertension, metabolic acidosis, secondary infection, and uremia.

Patient-Centered Care

- Nursing Care
  ○ Abnormal findings to be reported and monitored
    ▪ Urinary elimination patterns (amount, color, odor, and consistency)
    ▪ Vital signs (blood pressure may be increased or decreased)
    ▪ Weight – 1 kg (2.2 lb) daily weight increase is approximately 1 L of fluid retained.
  ○ Assess and monitor vascular access or peritoneal dialysis insertion site.
  ○ Obtain a detailed medication and herb history to determine the client's risk for continued kidney injury.
  ○ Control protein intake based on the client's stage of chronic kidney disease and type of dialysis prescribed.
  ○ Restrict the client's dietary sodium, potassium, phosphorous, and magnesium.
  ○ Provide the client a diet that is high in carbohydrates and moderate in fat.
  ○ Restrict the client's intake of fluids (based on urinary output).
  ○ Monitor for weight gain trends.
  ○ Adhere to meticulous cleaning of areas on skin not intact and access sites to control infections.
  ○ Balance the client's activity and rest.
  ○ Prepare the client for hemodialysis, peritoneal dialysis, and hemofiltration if indicated.
  ○ Provide skin care to the client in order to increase comfort and prevent breakdown.
  ○ Protect the client from injury.
  ○ Provide emotional support to the client and family.
  ○ Encourage the client to ask questions and discuss fears.
  ○ Administer medications as prescribed.
- Medications (See the *Pharmacology Review Module* for detailed information on these medications.)
  ○ Avoid administering antimicrobial medications (e.g., aminoglycosides and amphotericin B), NSAIDs, angiotensin-converting enzyme inhibitors and angiotensin-receptor blockers, and IV contrast dye, which are nephrotoxic.
  ○ Digoxin (Lanoxin), a cardiac glycoside, increases contractility of the myocardium and promotes cardiac output.
    ▪ Monitor digoxin laboratory levels due to slow excretion of the medication with CKD.
    ▪ Administer digoxin (Lanoxin) after receiving dialysis.

- ○ Sodium polystyrene (Kayexalate) to increase elimination of life-threatening serum potassium, which may cause dangerous cardiac dysrhythmias and peaked T waves.

  - ▪ Restrict sodium intake. Sodium polystyrene contains sodium and can cause fluid retention and hypertension, a complication of CKD.

- ○ Erythropoietin alfa (Epogen, Procrit) to stimulate production of red blood cells, given for anemia

- ○ Ferrous sulfate (Feosol), an iron supplement to prevent severe iron deficiency.

- ○ Aluminum hydroxide gel (Amphojel)

  - ▪ Taken with meals to bind phosphate in food and stop phosphate absorption.

  - ▪ Take 2 hr before or after digoxin.

- ○ Furosemide (Lasix), a loop-diuretic administered to excrete excess fluids.

  - ▪ Avoid administering to a client who has end-stage kidney disease.

  - ▪ Clients may also receive thiazide diuretics, potassium-sparing diuretics, and osmotic diuretics.

- • Teamwork and Collaboration

  - ○ Nephrology services may be consulted to manage dialysis or kidney failure.

  - ○ Nutritional services may be consulted to manage the nutritional needs of the client.

- • Therapeutic Procedures

  - ○ Hemodialysis

- • Care after Discharge

  - ○ Nephrology services may be indicated if the client is to receive outpatient dialysis.

  - ○ Refer the client to a community support group relating to the disease.

  - ○ Nutritional services may be consulted for the client's dietary needs.

  - ○ Refer the client to a smoking-cessation support group and counseling if needed.

- • Client Education

  - ○ Instruct the client to monitor the daily intake of carbohydrates, proteins, sodium, and potassium, according to the provider.

  - ○ Instruct the client to monitor fluid intake according to fluid restriction prescribed by the provider.

  - ○ Encourage the client who has diabetes mellitus to adhere to strict blood glucose control because uncontrolled diabetes is a major risk factor for chronic kidney disease.

  - ○ Instruct the client to avoid antacids containing magnesium.

  - ○ Encourage the client to take rest periods from activity.

  - ○ Educate the client who is receiving hemodialysis or peritoneal dialysis on an outpatient basis.

  - ○ Educate the client on how to measure blood pressure and weight at home.

  - ○ Encourage the client to ask questions and discuss fears.

  - ○ Encourage the client to diet, exercise, and take medication as prescribed.

  - ○ Advise the client to notify the provider if she observes signs of skin breakdown.

APPLICATION EXERCISES

1. A nurse is planning care for a client who has prerenal acute kidney injury following abdominal aortic aneurysm repair. The client's urinary output is 80 mL in the past 4 hr, and blood pressure is 92/58 mm Hg. Which of the following should be included in the plan of care?

    A. Prepare the client for a CAT scan with contrast dye.

    B. Anticipate urine specific gravity to be 1.010.

    C. Plan to administer a fluid challenge.

    D. Place client in Trendelenburg position.

2. A nurse is planning care for a client who has postrenal acute kidney injury due to metastatic cancer. The client has a serum creatinine of 5 mg/dL. Which of the following are appropriate actions by the nurse? (Select all that apply.)

    _____ A. Provide a high-protein diet.

    _____ B. Assess the urine for blood.

    _____ C. Monitor for intermittent anuria.

    _____ D. Administer diuretic medication.

    _____ E. Provide NSAIDs for pain.

3. A nurse is planning care for a client who has stage 4 chronic kidney disease. Which of the following should the nurse include in the plan of care? (Select all that apply.)

    _____ A. Assess for jugular vein distention.

    _____ B. Provide frequent mouth rinses.

    _____ C. Auscultate for a pleural friction rub.

    _____ D. Assess using the Glasgow Coma Scale.

    _____ E. Monitor for dysrhythmias.

4. A nurse is caring for a client who has stage 4 chronic kidney disease. Which of the following is an expected laboratory finding?

    A. Blood urea nitrogen (BUN) 54 mg/dL

    B. Glomerular filtration rate (GRF) 20 mL/min

    C. Serum creatinine 1.2 mg/dL

    D. Serum potassium 5.0 mEq/L

5. A nurse is assessing a client who has prerenal acute kidney injury (AKI). Which of the following should the nurse include in the assessment? (Select all that apply.)

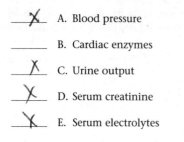

_____X____ A. Blood pressure

_____ B. Cardiac enzymes

_____X____ C. Urine output

_____X____ D. Serum creatinine

_____X____ E. Serum electrolytes

6. A nurse is preparing to administer medication to a client who has chronic kidney disease. What information should the nurse consider when administering medication? Use the ATI Active Learning Template: Medication and the ATI Pharmacology Review Module to complete this item to include the following:

A. Medications: Identify three.

B. Nursing Interventions: Describe two for each medication.

C. Client Education: List two for each medication.

APPLICATION EXERCISES KEY

1. A. INCORRECT: The nurse should not plan for a CAT scan as an intervention in the care of the client. Contrast dye is also contraindicated in a client who has possible acute kidney injury.

    B. INCORRECT: The nurse should expect a specific gravity of 1.030 for a client who has prerenal acute kidney injury.

    C. **CORRECT:** The nurse should plan to administer a fluid challenge for hypovolemia, which is indicated by the client's low urinary output and blood pressure.

    D. INCORRECT: The nurse should position the client in reverse Trendelenburg, with the head down and feet up to treat hypotension.

     NCLEX® Connection: Physiological Adaptations, Fluid and Electrolyte Imbalances

2. A. **CORRECT:** The nurse should provide the client with a high-protein diet because of the high rate of protein breakdown that occurs with acute kidney injury.

    B. **CORRECT:** The nurse should assess the client's urine for blood, stones, and particles indicating an obstruction of the urinary structures that leave the kidney.

    C. **CORRECT:** The nurse should assess the client for intermittent anuria because of possible bilateral obstruction of the urinary structures that leave the kidney.

    D. INCORRECT: The nurse should not administer a diuretic medication because it can increase destruction of the remaining nephrons in the kidney.

    E. INCORRECT: The nurse should not administer NSAIDs, which are nephrotoxic to the nephrons in the kidney, for pain.

     NCLEX® Connection: Physiological Adaptations, Alterations in Body Systems

3.   A. **CORRECT:** The nurse should assess for jugular vein distention, which may indicate fluid overload and congestive heart failure.

     B. **CORRECT:** The nurse should provide frequent mouth rinses due to uremic halitosis caused by urea waste in the blood.

     C. **CORRECT:** The nurse should auscultate for a pleural friction rub related to respiratory failure and pulmonary edema caused by acid base imbalances and fluid retention.

     D. INCORRECT: The Glasgow Coma Scale is used for a client who has a head injury to identify increased intracranial pressure, not for a client who has chronic kidney disease.

     E. **CORRECT:** The nurse should monitor for dysrhythmias related to increased serum potassium, which is not being excreted by the kidneys.

     Ⓝ NCLEX® Connection: Physiological Adaptations, Alterations in Body Systems

4.   A. INCORRECT: A BUN of 180 to 200 mg/dL is indicative of stage 4 chronic kidney disease.

     B. **CORRECT:** The GRF is severely decreased to approximately 20 mL/min, which is indicative of stage 4 chronic kidney disease.

     C. INCORRECT: In stage 4 chronic kidney disease, a creatinine level can be as high as 15 to 30 mg/dL.

     D. INCORRECT: A client in stage 4 chronic kidney disease would have a potassium level greater than 5.0 mEq/L.

     Ⓝ NCLEX® Connection: Reduction of Risk Potential, Laboratory Values

5.   A. **CORRECT:** Assessment of blood pressure for hypotension in a client who has prerenal AKI should assist in determining hypovolemia.

     B. INCORRECT: Assessment of cardiac enzymes is not indicated for a client who has prerenal AKI.

     C. **CORRECT:** Assessment of urine output in a client who has prerenal AKI should assist in determining oliguria.

     D. **CORRECT:** Assessment of serum creatinine should assist in determining the extent of the AKI and the need for intervention.

     E. **CORRECT:** Assessment of serum electrolytes should assist in determining the extent of the AKI and the need for intervention.

     Ⓝ NCLEX® Connection: Physiological Adaptations, Illness Management

6. *Using the ATI Active Learning Template: Medication*

A. Medications
- Digoxin (Lanoxin)
- Sodium polystyrene (Kayexalate)
- Epoetin alfa (Epogen)
- Ferrous sulfate (Feosol)
- Aluminum hydroxide gel (Amphojel)
- Furosemide (Lasix)

B. Nursing Interventions
- Digoxin – Take apical pulse for 1 min, and monitor laboratory levels for signs of toxicity.
- Sodium polystyrene – Monitor for hypokalemia, and restrict sodium intake.
- Epoetin alfa – Administer by subcutaneous route, and monitor for hypertension .
- Ferrous sulfate – Administer following dialysis and with a stool softener.
- Aluminum hydroxide gel – Avoid administering if client has gastrointestinal disorders; administer a stool softener with this medication.
- Furosemide – Monitor intake and output and blood pressure.

C. Client Education
- Digoxin – Instruct the client not to take medication within 2 hr of eating, and teach client how to take an apical pulse for 1 min.
- Sodium polystyrene – Instruct the client to take a mild laxative if constipated, and teach how to take blood pressure.
- Epoetin alfa – Instruct the client about having blood tests twice a week and how to take blood pressure.
- Ferrous sulfate – Instruct the client to take medication with food and that stools will be dark in color.
- Aluminum hydroxide gel – Instruct the client to report constipation to the provider and to take 2 hr before or after receiving digoxin.
- Furosemide – Instruct the client to weigh self each morning and to notify provider of light-headedness, excess thirst, and unusual coughing.

N NCLEX® Connection: Physiological Adaptations, Illness Management

chapter 61

Overview

- There are three components to the urinary system: the ureter, bladder, and urethra. The goal of the urinary system is to promote optimal kidney function. Two infections that affect the renal and urinary system are urinary tract infections, and pyelonephritis.

URINARY TRACT INFECTION

Overview

- A urinary tract infection (UTI) refers to any portion of the lower urinary tract (ureters, bladder, urethra, prostate). This includes the following:
  - Cystitis - Bladder
  - Urethritis - urethra
  - Prostatitis - prostate
- An upper UTI refers to conditions such as pyelonephritis (inflammation of the kidney pelvis).
- UTIs are caused by Enterobacteriaceae micro-organisms (klebsiella, proteus), pseudomonas, *Staphylococcus saprophyticus*, and most commonly, *Escherichia coli*.
- Untreated UTIs may lead to pyelonephritis and urosepsis, which can cause septic shock and death.

Assessment

- Risk Factors
  - Female gender
    - Short urethra predisposes women to UTIs
    - Close proximity of the urethra to the rectum
    - Decreased estrogen in aging women promotes atrophy of the urethral opening toward the rectum (increases the risk of urosepsis in women)
    - Sexual intercourse
    - Frequent use of feminine hygiene sprays, tampons, sanitary napkins, and spermicidal jellies
    - Pregnancy
    - Poorly fitted diaphragm
    - Hormonal influences within the vaginal flora

- Synthetic underwear and pantyhose
- Wet bathing suits
- Frequent submersion into baths or hot tubs
  - ○ Indwelling urinary catheters (significant source of infection in clients who are hospitalized)
  - ○ Stool incontinence
  - ○ Bladder distention
  - ○ Urinary conditions (anomalies, stasis, calculi, residual urine)
  - ○ Possible genetic links
  - ○ Disease (diabetes mellitus)
  - ○ Older adult clients have an increased risk of bacteremia, sepsis, and shock.
    - Incomplete bladder emptying caused by an enlarged prostate or prostatitis in males
    - Bladder prolapse in females
    - Inability to empty bladder (neurogenic bladder) as a result of a stroke or Parkinson's disease
    - Fecal incontinence with poor perineal hygiene
    - Hypoestrogen in females affecting the mucosa of the vagina and urethra, causing bacteria to adhere to the mucosal surface
    - Renal complications increase due to decreased number of functioning nephrons and fluid intake
- Subjective Data
  - ○ Lower back or lower abdominal discomfort and tenderness over the bladder area
  - ○ Nausea
  - ○ Urinary frequency and urgency
  - ○ Dysuria, bladder cramping, spasms
  - ○ Feeling of incomplete bladder emptying or retention of urine
  - ○ Perineal itching
  - ○ Hematuria (red-tinged, smoky, coffee-colored urine)
  - ○ Pyuria (greater than 4 WBC in urine sample)
- Objective Data
  - ○ Fever
  - ○ Vomiting
  - ○ Voiding in small amounts
  - ○ Nocturia
  - ○ Urethral discharge
  - ○ Cloudy or foul-smelling urine

Ⓖ
- ○ Older Adult Clinical Manifestation of UTI
  - Mental confusion
  - Incontinence
  - Loss of appetite
  - Nocturia and dysuria
  - Hypotension, tachycardia, tachypnea, and fever (signs of urosepsis)
- ○ Laboratory Tests
  - Urinalysis and urine culture and sensitivity
    - □ Nursing Actions
      - ‣ Instruct the client regarding proper technique for the collection of a clean-catch urine specimen.
      - ‣ Collect catheterized urine specimens using sterile technique.
    - □ Expected findings include the following:
      - ‣ Bacteria, sediment, white blood cells (WBC), and red blood cells (RBC)
      - ‣ Positive leukocyte esterase and nitrates (68% to 88% positive results indicates UTI)
  - WBC count and differential if urosepsis is suspected
    - □ White blood cell count at or above 10,000/uL with a shift to the left, indicating an increased number of immature cells (neutrophils) in response to infection
  - Rule out sexually transmitted infections, which can cause symptoms of a UTI.
    - □ *Chlamydia trachomatis, Neisseria gonorrhoeae,* and herpes simplex can cause acute urethritis.
    - □ Trichomonas or candida can cause acute vaginal infections.
- ○ Diagnostic Procedures
  - Cystoscopy is used for complicated UTIs.
  - Cystourethroscopy to detect strictures, calculi, tumors, cystitis.
  - Computed tomography (CT) scan to detect pyelonephritis.
  - Ultrasonography to detect cysts, tumors, calculi, and abscesses.
  - Transrectal ultrasonography to detect prostate and bladder conditions in males.

Patient-Centered Care

- Nursing Care
  - ○ Promote fluid intake up to 3 L daily.
  - ○ Consult with the provider regarding prescribed fluid restrictions if needed.
  - ○ Administer antibiotic medications as prescribed.
  - ○ Encourage clients to urinate every 3 to 4 hr instead of waiting until the bladder is completely full.
  - ○ Recommend warm sitz bath two or three times a day to provide comfort.
  - ○ Encourage clients to bathe daily to promote good body hygiene.
  - ○ Avoid the use of indwelling catheters if possible. This reduces the risk for infection.

- Medications
  - Fluoroquinolones (ciprofloxacin, norfloxacin, levofloxacin), nitrofurantoin (Macrodantin, Furadantin, Macrobid), trimethoprim, or sulfonamides (Bactrim or Septra) are antibiotics used to treat urinary infections by directly killing bacteria and inhibiting bacterial reproduction.
    - Penicillins and cephalosporins are administered less frequently because the medication is less effective and tolerated.
    - Nitrofurantoin is an antibacterial medication where therapeutic levels are achieved in the urine only.
    - Nursing Considerations
      - If sulfonamide is prescribed, ask the client about allergy to sulfa.
    - Client Education
      - Educate the client regarding the need to take all of the prescribed antibiotics even if symptoms subside.
      - Encourage the client to take the medication with food.
  - Phenazopyridine (Pyridium, Urogesic) is bladder analgesic used to treat UTIs.
    - Nursing Considerations
      - The medication will not treat the infection, but it will help relieve bladder discomfort.
      - Inform the client that the medication will turn urine orange.
    - Client Education
      - Encourage the client to take the medication with food.
- Teamwork and Collaboration
  - Urology services may be consulted for managing UTIs.
- Care after Discharge
  - Urology services may be consulted for management of long-term antibiotic therapy for chronic UTIs.
- Client Education
  - Instruct the client to drink at least 3 L of fluid daily.
  - Instruct the client to bathe daily to promote good body hygiene.
  - Advise the client to empty bladder every 3 to 4 hr instead of waiting until the bladder is completely full.
  - Advise the client to urinate before and after intercourse.
  - Advise the client to drink cranberry juice to decrease the risk of infection.
    - The compound in cranberries may stop certain bacteria from adhering to the mucosa of the urinary tract.
    - Clients who have chronic cystitis should avoid cranberry juice, which irritates the bladder.

- ○ Advise the client to empty the bladder as soon as there is an urgency to void.
- ○ Instruct female clients to:
  - ▪ Wipe the perineal area from front to back.
  - ▪ Avoid using bubble baths, and feminine products and toilet paper containing perfumes.
  - ▪ Avoid sitting in wet bathing suits.
  - ▪ Avoid wearing pantyhose with slacks or tight clothing.

Complications

- • Urethral obstruction, pyelonephritis, chronic kidney disease, urosepsis, septic shock, and death

---

PYELONEPHRITIS

Overview

- • Pyelonephritis is an infection and inflammation of the kidney pelvis, calyces, and medulla. The infection usually begins in the lower urinary tract with organisms ascending into the kidney pelvis.
- • *Escherichia coli* organisms are the cause of most acute cases of pyelonephritis.
- • Repeated infections create scarring that changes the blood flow to the kidney, glomerulus, and tubular structure.
- • Filtration, reabsorption, and secretion are impaired, which results in a decrease in renal function.
- • Acute pyelonephritis is an active bacterial infection that can cause the following:
  - ○ Interstitial inflammation
  - ○ Tubular cell necrosis
  - ○ Abscess formation in the capsule, cortex, or medulla
  - ○ Temporarily altered kidney function (this rarely progresses to chronic kidney disease)
- • Chronic pyelonephritis is the result of repeated infections that cause progressive inflammation and scarring.
  - ○ This can result in the thickening of the calyces and postinflammatory fibrosis with permanent renal tissue scarring.
  - ○ It is more common with obstructions, urinary anomaly, and vesicoureteral urine reflux.
  - ○ Reflux of urine occurs at the junction where the ureter connects to the bladder.

Assessment

- Risk Factors
  - Ⓖ Men over 65 years of age who have prostatitis and hypertrophy of the prostate
  - Chronic urinary stone disorders (stones harbor bacteria)
  - Spinal cord injury (clients have a higher incidence of reflux)
  - Pregnancy
  - Congenital malformations
  - Bladder tumors
  - Chronic illness (diabetes mellitus, hypertension, chronic cystitis)
  - Urine pH increases, becoming more alkaline, in older adult clients and promotes bacterial growth.
  - Incomplete bladder emptying is more common among older adult clients.
  - Ⓖ Older adult clients may exhibit gastrointestinal or pulmonary symptoms instead of febrile responses because an older adult client's temperature may vary at a lower than normal state.
    - Causes are inadequate diet, loss of adipose tissue, lack of exercise, and reduction in the client's thermoregulator.
- Subjective Data
  - Chills
  - Colicky-type abdominal pain
  - Nausea
  - Malaise, fatigue
  - Burning, urgency, and frequency with urination
  - Costovertebral tenderness
- Objective Data
  - Fever, tachycardia, tachypnea, hypertension
  - Flank and back pain
  - Vomiting
  - Nocturia
  - Inability to concentrate urine or conserve sodium (chronic pyelonephritis)
  - Asymptomatic bacteremia
- Laboratory Tests
  - Urinalysis and urine culture and sensitivity same as for a UTI (positive leukocyte esterase and nitrites, WBCs, and bacteria).
  - WBC count and differential: Same as for a UTI.
  - Blood cultures will be positive for the presence of bacteria if a systemic infection is present.
  - Serum creatinine and blood urea nitrogen (BUN) are elevated during acute episodes and consistently elevated with chronic infection.
  - C-reactive protein is elevated during exacerbating inflammatory processes of the kidneys.
    - Erythrocyte sedimentation rate (ESR) is elevated during acute or chronic inflammation.

- Diagnostic Procedures

  - An x-ray of the kidneys, ureters, and bladder (KUB) may demonstrate calculi or structural abnormalities.

  - Ultrasonography to detect cysts, tumors, calculi, and abscesses.

  - Gallium scan – a nuclear medicine test that uses injectable radioactive dye to visualize organs, glands, bones, and blood vessels that have infection and inflammation.

  - Intravenous pyelogram (IVP) may demonstrate calculi, structural, or vascular abnormalities.

- Surgical Interventions

  - Inform the client of the purpose of the surgery and expected outcomes.

  - Intravenous antibiotics and analgesics are usually administered for each procedure.

  - Pyelolithotomy – This is the removal of a large stone from the kidney that causes infections and blocks the flow of urine from the kidney.

  - Nephrectomy – This is the removal of the kidney when all procedures to clear the client of infection were unsuccessful.

  - Ureteroplasty – This is done to repair or revise the ureter and can involve reimplantation of the ureter in the bladder wall to preserve the function of the kidney and eliminate infection.

Complications of Chronic Pyelonephritis

- Septic shock (hypotension, tachycardia, fever) due to bacterial organism entering the blood stream.

- Chronic kidney disease (elevated BUN, creatinine, electrolytes) from inflammation and infection that causes fibrosis of the kidney pelvis and calyx, scarring, and changes in the blood vessels and the glomerular and tubular filtration system.

- Hypertension (related to fluid and sodium retention) indicating chronic kidney disease caused by destruction of the filtration system of the kidney due to infection.

Patient-Centered Care

- Nursing Care (Nonsurgical)

  - Assess/Monitor

    - Nutritional status

    - Intake and output

    - Fluid and electrolyte balance

    - Pain status

    - Temperature

    - The onset, quality, duration, and severity of the pain

  - Increase fluid intake to 2 to 3 L/day unless contraindicated.

  - Administer antipyretic, such as acetaminophen (Tylenol), as needed for fever and opioid analgesics for pain associated with pyelonephritis and following procedures.

  - Provide emotional support.

  - Assist with personal hygiene.

- Nursing Care (Surgical)
  - Includes all the above information.
  - Assess the dressings and incision.
  - Balance rest and activities.
  - Instruct on monitoring signs of infection.
  - Instruct on the role of nutritious meals and adequate fluid intake.
- Medications (See the *Pharmacology Review Module* for more detailed information.)
  - Opioid analgesics (opioid agonists), morphine sulfate, and morphine for moderate to severe pain
  - Antibiotics
    - Mild to moderate pyelonephritis treated at home for 14 days with the following:
      - Anti-infective – trimethoprim (Primsol), sulfamethoxazole/trimethoprim (Bactrim, Septra)
      - Quinolone antibiotic -- ciprofloxacin (Cipro), levofloxacin (Levaquin)
    - Severe pyelonephritis treated in the hospital for 24 to 48 hr with IV medication:
      - Quinolone antibiotic – ciprofloxacin (Cipro)
      - Cephalosporin antibiotic – ceftriaxone (Cefizox), ceftazidime (Fortaz)
      - Aminopenicillin antibiotic – ampicillin (Principen), ampicillin/sulbactam (Unasyn)
      - Aminoglycoside antibiotic – gentamicin, tobramycin (Tobrex), amikacin (Amikin)
- Teamwork and Collaboration
  - Urology services may be consulted to manage pyelonephritis.
  - Nutritional services may be consulted to promote adequate calories for the client.
- Care After Discharge
  - Home care services may be indicated if the client needs assistance with medications or nutritional therapy.
  - Follow up with the provider as directed.
- Client Education
  - Educate the client regarding adequate nutritional status.
  - Encourage the client to drink at least 3 L of fluids daily unless otherwise indicated by the provider.
  - Instruct the client to take medications as prescribed.
  - Instruct the client to notify the provider if acute onset of pain occurs or a fever is present.
  - Encourage the client and family to express their fears and anxiety related to the disease.
  - Encourage the client to take rest periods as needed from activity.

APPLICATION EXERCISES

1. A nurse is caring for a client who has a urinary tract infection. The client reports pain and a burning sensation upon urination, and cloudy urine with an odor. Which of the following is the priority intervention by the nurse?

    A. Offer a warm sitz bath.

    B. Recommend drinking cranberry juice.

    C. Encourage increased fluids.

    D. Administer an antibiotic.

2. A nurse is preparing educational material to present to a female client who has frequent urinary tract infections (UTIs). Which of the following information should the nurse include? (Select all that apply.)

     A. Avoid sitting in a wet bathing suit.

    B. Wipe the perineal area back to front following elimination.

    C. Empty the bladder when there is an urge to void.

    D. Wear synthetic fabric underwear.

    E. Take a tub bath daily.

3. A nurse is reviewing the laboratory findings for urinalysis (UA) of a client who reports urgency and nocturia. Which of the following findings should the nurse report to the provider?

    A. Positive for casts

    B. Positive leukocyte esterase

    C. Positive for epithelial cells

    D. Positive for crystals

4. A nurse on a medical unit is caring for several clients. Which of the following clients are at risk for developing pyelonephritis? (Select all that apply.)

    A. A client who is 32 weeks of gestation

    B. A client who has kidney calculi

    C. A client who has a urine pH of 4.2

    D. A client who has a neurogenic bladder

    E. A client who has diabetes mellitus

5. A nurse is planning care for a client who has chronic pyelonephritis. Which of the following are appropriate actions by the nurse? (Select all that apply.)

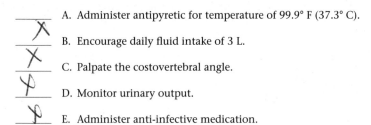

A. Administer antipyretic for temperature of 99.9° F (37.3° C).

B. Encourage daily fluid intake of 3 L.

C. Palpate the costovertebral angle.

D. Monitor urinary output.

E. Administer anti-infective medication.

6. A nurse is educating a client who has chronic pyelonephritis. What information should the nurse include in the teaching? Use the ATI Active Learning Template: Systems Disorder to complete this item. Include the following:

A. Description of Disorder/Disease Process

B. Potential Complications: List three, and explain why these occur.

C. Management of Client Care: Identify three teaching points for the client.

APPLICATION EXERCISES KEY

1. A. INCORRECT: Offering a warm sitz bath will provide temporary relief of the symptoms of a UTI, but it is not the priority intervention by the nurse.

    B. INCORRECT: Recommending that the client drink cranberry juice may help prevent a UTI in the future, but it is not the priority intervention by the nurse.

    C. INCORRECT: Encouraging the client to increase fluid intake will help to relieve temporary symptoms of a UTI, but it is not the priority intervention by the nurse.

    D. **CORRECT:** The greatest risk to the client is injury to the renal system from the UTI. Therefore, the priority intervention is to administer antibiotics.

    (N) NCLEX® Connection: Physiological Adaptations, Unexpected Response to Therapies

2. A. **CORRECT:** The client should avoid sitting in a wet bathing suit, which can increase the risk for a UTI by colonization of bacteria in a moist, warm environment.

    B. INCORRECT: The client should wipe the perineal area from front to back after elimination to prevent contaminating the urethra with bacteria.

    C. **CORRECT:** The client should empty the bladder when there is an urge to void rather than retain urine for an extended period of time, which increases the risk for a UTI.

    D. INCORRECT: The client should wear cotton underwear that absorbs moisture and keeps the perineal area drier, thus decreasing colonization of bacteria that can cause a UTI.

    E. **CORRECT:** The client should take a tub bath or shower daily to promote good body hygiene and decrease colonization of bacteria in the perineal area that can cause a UTI.

    (N) NCLEX® Connection: Health Promotion and Maintenance, Health Promotion/Disease Prevention

3. A. INCORRECT: The client may have a few casts in the UA, which is a normal finding.

    B. **CORRECT:** The client who has positive leukocyte esterase indicates 68% to 88% positive urine for UTI, and the nurse should report this finding to the provider.

    C. INCORRECT: The client may have a few epithelial cells in the UA, indicating contamination of the urine during voiding.

    D. INCORRECT: The client may have a few crystals in the UA, which is a normal finding.

    (N) NCLEX® Connection: Reduction of Risk Potential, Laboratory Values

4.　A. **CORRECT:** A client who is at 32 weeks of gestation is at risk for developing pyelonephritis because of increased pressure on the urinary system during pregnancy causing reflux or retention of urine.

　　B. **CORRECT:** A client who has kidney calculi is at risk for pyelonephritis because stones harbor bacteria.

　　C. INCORRECT: A client who has a urine pH of 4.2 has decreased acidity; therefore, the urine does not promote bacterial growth.

　　D. **CORRECT:** The client who has a neurogenic bladder may retain urine, promoting bacterial growth and causing pyelonephritis.

　　E. **CORRECT:** The client who has diabetes mellitus is at risk of pyelonephritis because glucose that may be in the urine promotes bacterial growth.

　　Ⓝ NCLEX® Connection: Health Promotion and Maintenance, Health Promotion/Disease Prevention

5.　A. INCORRECT: Administering an antipyretic medication for a low-grade fever is not an appropriate nursing action.

　　B. **CORRECT:** The nurse should encourage fluid intake greater than 2 to 3 L daily to maintain dilute urine during the day and night.

　　C. **CORRECT:** The nurse should gently palpate the costovertebral angle for flank tenderness, which may indicate inflammation and infection.

　　D. **CORRECT:** The nurse should monitor urinary output to determine that 1 to 3 L of urine is excreted daily.

　　E. **CORRECT:** The nurse should administer anti-infective medication to treat the bacteriuria and decrease progressive damage to the kidney.

　　Ⓝ NCLEX® Connection: Physiological Adaptations, Illness Management

6. *Using the ATI Active Learning Template: Systems Disorder*

   A. Description of Disorder/Disease Process
      - Chronic pyelonephritis is a repetitive infection and inflammation of the kidney pelvis, calyces, and medulla, which generally begins from bacteria that ascends from a lower urinary tract infection.

   B. Potential Complications
      - Septic shock caused by micro-organisms entering the bloodstream from the infected kidney.
      - Chronic kidney disease caused by inflammation, fibrosis, and scarring of the kidney filtration structure.
      - Hypertension (related to fluid and sodium retention) indicating chronic kidney disease caused by destruction of the filtration system of the kidney from infection.

   C. Management of Client Care – Client Education
      - Encourage at least 3 L of fluids daily.
      - Instruct the client to take all medications prescribed.
      - Instruct the client to notify the provider if having acute, rapid onset of pain.
      - Encourage verbalization of fears and anxiety.
      - Encourage a balance of rest and activity.

   (N) NCLEX® Connection: Physiological Adaptations, Illness Management

chapter 62

Overview

- Urolithiasis is the presence of calculi (stones) in the urinary tract.

- The majority of stones (75%) are composed of calcium phosphate or calcium oxalate, but they may contain other substances (uric acid, struvite, cystine).

- A diet high in calcium is not believed to increase the risk of stone formation unless there is a preexisting metabolic disorder or renal tubular defect.

- Reoccurrence is increased (35% to 50%) in individuals with calcium stones who have a family history or whose first occurrence of urinary calculi is prior to the age of 25.

- Most clients can expel stones without invasive procedures. Factors that influence whether a stone will pass spontaneously or not include the composition, size, and location of the stone.

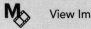   View Image: Renal Calculus

Assessment

- Risk Factors

  ○ The cause of urolithiasis is unknown.

  ○ There is an increased incidence of urolithiasis in males.

  ○ Urolithiasis formation is associated with:

    ▪ Urinary tract lining that is damaged.

    ▪ Urine flow that is decreased, concentrated, and contains particles (calcium).

    ▪ Metabolic defects including:

      □ Increased intestinal absorption or decreased renal excretion of calcium.

      □ Increased oxalate production (genetic) or inability to metabolize oxalate from foods (black tea, spinach, beets, Swiss chard, chocolate, and peanuts).

      □ Increased production or decreased clearance of purines (contributing to increased uric-acid levels).

  ○ Can be attributed to high alkalinity or acidity of the urine.

  ○ Urinary stasis, urinary retention, immobilization, and dehydration contribute to an environment favorable for stone formation.

  ○ Decreased fluid intake or increased incidence of dehydration among older adult clients may increase the risk of stone formation.

- Subjective Data
  - Severe pain (renal colic)
    - Pain intensifies as the stone moves through the ureter.
    - Flank pain suggests stones are located in the kidney or ureter.
    - Flank pain that radiates to the abdomen, scrotum, testes, or vulva is suggestive of stones in the ureter or bladder.
  - Urinary frequency or dysuria (stones in the bladder)
  - Fever
- Objective Data
  - Diaphoresis
  - Pallor
  - Nausea/vomiting
  - Tachycardia, tachypnea, increased or decreased blood pressure with pain
  - Oliguria/anuria (occurs with stones that obstruct urinary flow); urinary tract obstruction is a medical emergency and needs to be treated to preserve kidney function.
  - Hematuria (smoky-looking urine)
  - Laboratory Tests – Urinalysis
    - Altered odor of the urine and increased urine turbidity if infection is present
    - Increased RBCs, WBCs, and bacteria (presence of infection)
    - Crystals noted on microscopic exam
    - Abnormal serum calcium, phosphate, and uric-acid levels in the presence of metabolic disorders/defects
  - Diagnostic Procedures
    - Radiology examination
      - KUB (x-ray of kidney, ureters, bladder), or intravenous pyelogram (IVP) is used to confirm the presence and location of stones. IVP is contraindicated if there is a urinary obstruction.
    - CT or MRI
      - A CT (noncontrast helical scan) or MRI is used to identify cystine or uric-acid stones, which cannot be seen on standard x-rays.
    - A renal ultrasound or cystoscopy may confirm the diagnosis.

Patient-Centered Care

- Nursing Care
  - Report laboratory and diagnostic findings to the provider.
  - Provide preoperative and postoperative care as indicated.
  - Assess/Monitor for:
    - Pain status.
    - Intake and output.
    - Urinary pH.

- ○ Administer prescribed medications.
- ○ Strain all urine to check for passage of the stone and save the stone for laboratory analysis.
- ○ Encourage increased oral intake to 3 L/day unless contraindicated.
- ○ Administer IV fluids as prescribed.
- ○ Encourage ambulation to promote passage of the stone.
- Medications
  - ○ Analgesics
    - ▪ Opioids (morphine sulfate) are used in the first 24 hr with the acute onset of stones.
      - ▫ Opioid agents are used to treat moderate to severe pain. These drugs act on the mu and kappa receptors that help alleviate pain. Activation of these receptors produces analgesia (pain relief), respiratory depression, euphoria, sedation, and a decrease in GI motility.
      - ▫ Use cautiously with clients who have asthma or emphysema due to the risk of respiratory depression.
      - ▫ Nursing Considerations
        - ▸ Assess every 4 hr.
        - ▸ Watch for evidence of respiratory depression, especially in older adult clients. If respirations are 12 or less, stop the medication and notify the provider immediately.
        - ▸ Monitor vital signs for hypotension and decreased respirations.
        - ▸ Assess the client's level of sedation (drowsiness, level of consciousness).
      - ▫ Client Education
        - ▸ Encourage the client to suck on hard candies to alleviate dry mouth.
        - ▸ Encourage the client to drink plenty of fluids to prevent constipation.
    - ▪ NSAIDs (ketorolac) are used to treat mild to moderate pain, fever, and inflammation.
      - ▫ Nursing Considerations – Observe for signs of bleeding.
      - ▫ Client Education
        - ▸ Instruct the client to watch for bleeding (dark stools, blood in stools).
        - ▸ Instruct the client to notify the provider if abdominal pain occurs, which may be due to gastric ulceration.
  - ○ Spasmolytic drugs
    - ▪ Oxybutynin chloride (Ditropan) alleviates pain with a neurogenic or overactive bladder.
    - ▪ Nursing Considerations
      - ▫ Ask the client if there is a history of glaucoma, as this medication increases intraocular pressure.
      - ▫ Monitor for dizziness and tachycardia.
      - ▫ Monitor for urinary retention.
    - ▪ Client Education
      - ▫ Instruct the client to report palpitations and problems with voiding or constipation.
      - ▫ Inform the client that dizziness and dry mouth are common with the medication.

- ○ Antibiotics (gentamicin, cephalexin [Keflex]) are used to treat UTIs.
  - ▪ Nursing Considerations
    - ▫ Administer medication with food to decrease GI distress.
    - ▫ Monitor for nephrotoxicity and ototoxicity for clients taking gentamicin.
  - ▪ Client Education
    - ▫ Inform the client that urine may have foul odor related to the antibiotic.
    - ▫ Instruct the client to report loose stools related to the medication.
- • Teamwork and Collaboration
  - ○ Urology services may be consulted for management of urolithiasis.
  - ○ Nutritional services may be consulted for dietary modifications concerning foods related to stone formation.
- • Therapeutic Procedures
  - ○ Extracorporeal shock wave lithotripsy (ESWL)
    - ▪ Uses sound, laser, or shock-wave energies to break stones into fragments.
    - ▪ Requires moderate (conscious) sedation and ECG monitoring during the procedure.
    - ▪ Nursing Actions
      - ▫ Educate the client regarding ESWL.
      - ▫ Assess for gross hematuria and strain urine following the procedure.
      - ▫ Administer analgesics as prescribed.
    - ▪ Client Education
      - ▫ Inform the client that bruising is normal at the site where waves are applied.
      - ▫ Explain to the client that there will be hematuria postprocedure.
- • Surgical Interventions
  - ○ Stenting is the placement of a small tube in the ureter during a ureteroscopy to dilate the ureter and allow passage of a stone.
  - ○ Retrograde ureteroscopy uses a basket, forceps, or loop on the end of the ureteroscope to grasp and remove the stone.
  - ○ Percutaneous ureterolithotomy/nephrolithotomy is the insertion of an ultrasonic or laser lithotripter into the ureter or kidney to grasp and extract the stone.
  - ○ Open surgery
    - ▪ Open surgery uses a surgical incision to remove the stone. This surgery is used for large or impacted stones (staghorn calculi) or for stones not removed by other approaches.
    - ▪ Ureterolithotomy (into the ureter).
    - ▪ Pyelolithotomy (into the kidney pelvis).
    - ▪ Nephrolithotomy (into the kidney)
- • Care after Discharge
  - ○ Nutritional services may be consulted for dietary modifications concerning foods related to stone formation.

- Client Education
  - Educate the client regarding the role of diet and medications in the treatment and prevention of urinary stones.
    - Calcium phosphate
      - Limit intake of food high in animal protein (reduction of protein intake decreases calcium precipitation).
      - Limit sodium intake.
      - Reduced calcium intake (dairy products) is individualized.
      - Medications
        - Thiazide diuretics (hydrochlorothiazide) are used to increase calcium reabsorption.
        - Orthophosphates are used to decrease urine saturation of calcium oxalate.
        - Sodium cellulose phosphate is used to reduce the intestinal absorption of calcium.
    - Calcium oxalate
      - Avoid oxalate sources: Spinach, black tea, rhubarb, cocoa, beets, pecans, peanuts, okra, chocolate, wheat germ, lime peel, and Swiss chard.
      - Limit sodium intake.
    - Struvite (magnesium ammonium phosphate)
      - Avoid high-phosphate foods (dairy products, red and organ meats, whole grains).
    - Uric acid (urate)
      - Decrease intake of purine sources (organ meats, poultry, fish, gravies, red wine, sardines).
      - Medications
        - Allopurinol (Zyloprim) is used to prevent the formation of uric acid.
        - Potassium or sodium citrate or sodium bicarbonate is used to alkalinize the urine.
    - Cystine
      - Limit animal protein intake.
      - Medications
        - Alpha mercaptopropionylglycine (AMPG) is used to lower urine cystine.
        - Captopril (Capoten) is used to lower urine cystine.

Complications

- Obstruction – A stone may block the passage of urine into the kidney, ureter, or bladder. The client's urinary output may be diminished or absent.
  - Nursing Actions
    - Notify the provider immediately.
    - Prepare the client for removal of the stone.
- Hydronephrosis occurs when a stone has blocked a portion of the urinary tract. The urine backs up and causes distention of the kidney.
  - Nursing Actions
    - Notify the provider immediately.
    - Prepare the client for removal of the stone.

APPLICATION EXERCISES

1. A nurse is completing the admission assessment of a client who has a kidney stone. Which of the following is an expected finding?

    A. Bradycardia

    B. Diaphoresis ~ _sweating_

    C. Nocturia

    D. Bradypnea

2. A nurse is caring for a client who has a left renal calculus and an indwelling urinary catheter. Which of the following assessment findings requires immediate intervention by the nurse?

    A. Flank pain that radiates to the lower abdomen

    B. Client report of nausea

    C. Absent urine output for 2 hr

    D. Client report of feeling sweaty

3. A nurse is reviewing discharge instructions with a client who had spontaneous passage of a calcium phosphate kidney stone. Which of the following should be included in the teaching? (Select all that apply.)

    _____ A. Limit intake of food high in animal protein.

    _____ B. Reduce sodium intake.

    _____ C. Strain urine for 48 hr.

    _____ D. Report burning with urination to the provider.

    _____ E. Increase fluid intake to 3 L/day.

4. A nurse is completing teaching for a client who is scheduled for extracorporeal shock wave lithotripsy (ESWL). Which of the following statements made by the client indicates understanding of the teaching?

    A. "I will be fully awake during the procedure."

    B. "Lithotripsy will reduce my chances of having stones in the future."

    C. "I will report any bruising that occurs to my doctor."

    D. "Straining my urine following the procedure is important."

5. A nurse is completing discharge instructions with a client who has spontaneously passed a calcium oxalate stone. Which of the following foods should the nurse instruct the client to avoid? (Select all that apply.)

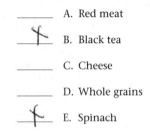

_____ A. Red meat

_____ B. Black tea

_____ C. Cheese

_____ D. Whole grains

_____ E. Spinach

6. A nurse is providing teaching to a client who is scheduled for extracorporeal shock wave lithotripsy (ESWL). What should be included in the teaching? Use the ATI Active Learning Template: Therapeutic Procedure to complete this item to include the following:

A. Description of Procedure

B. Client Education: Describe at least four teaching points.

APPLICATION EXERCISES KEY

1. A. INCORRECT: Tachycardia is a clinical manifestation associated with a client who has a kidney stone.

    B. **CORRECT:** Diaphoresis is a clinical manifestation associated with a client who has a kidney stone.

    C. INCORRECT: Oliguria is a clinical manifestation associated with a client who has a kidney stone.

    D. INCORRECT: Tachypnea is a clinical manifestation associated with a client who has a kidney stone.

     NCLEX® Connection: Physiological Adaptations, Pathophysiology

2. A. INCORRECT: Flank pain radiating to the lower abdomen is a finding associated with renal calculus, but there is another finding that requires immediate intervention by the nurse.

    B. INCORRECT: Client report of nausea is a finding associated with renal calculus, but there is another finding that requires immediate intervention by the nurse.

    C. **CORRECT:** When using the acute vs. chronic approach to care, no urine output for 2 hr requires immediate intervention by the nurse. This indicates kidney dysfunction, and the provider should be notified immediately.

    D. INCORRECT: Diaphoresis is a finding associated with renal calculus, but there is another finding that requires immediate intervention by the nurse.

     NCLEX® Connection: Physiological Adaptations, Unexpected Response to Therapies

3. A. **CORRECT:** The client should limit the intake of food high in animal protein, which contains calcium phosphate.

    B. **CORRECT:** The client should limit intake of sodium, which affects the precipitation of calcium phosphate in the urine.

    C. INCORRECT: Straining urine is not indicated once the stone has passed.

    D. **CORRECT:** The client should report burning with urination to the provider because this can be an indication of infection.

    E. **CORRECT:** The client should increase fluid intake to 3 L/day. A decrease in fluid intake can cause dehydration, which increases the risk of stone formation.

     NCLEX® Connection: Reduction of Risk Potential, Therapeutic Procedures

4.   A. INCORRECT: The client receives moderate (conscious) sedation for this procedure. The client is not fully awake.

   B. INCORRECT: Lithotripsy does not decrease the recurrence rate of kidney stones. The procedure breaks the stone into fragments so they will pass into urine.

   C. INCORRECT: Bruising is an expected finding following lithotripsy and does not need to be reported to the provider.

   D. **CORRECT:** A client is instructed to strain urine following lithotripsy to verify that the stone has been passed.

    NCLEX® Connection: Basic Care and Comfort, Nutrition and Oral Hydration

5.   A. INCORRECT: Red meat contains struvite (magnesium ammonium phosphate) and does not need to be avoided.

   B. **CORRECT:** Black tea contains calcium oxalate and should be avoided.

   C. INCORRECT: Cheese contains struvite (magnesium ammonium phosphate) and does not need to be avoided.

   D. INCORRECT: Whole grains contains struvite (magnesium ammonium phosphate) and do not need to be avoided.

   E. **CORRECT:** Spinach contains calcium oxalate and should be avoided.

    NCLEX® Connection: Reduction of Risk Potential, Therapeutic Procedures

6.   *Using the ATI Active Learning Template: Therapeutic Procedure*

   A. Description of Procedure
   - Use of sound, laser, or shock-wave energy to break urinary calculi into fragments.

   B. Client Education
   - Moderate (conscious) sedation is used, and the client is not fully awake.
   - The client will have cardiac monitoring during the procedure.
   - Hematuria will occur postprocedure.
   - Analgesics will be administered following the procedure.
   - The client will be instructed to strain urine following the procedure.
   - Bruising at the site where waves were applied is an expected finding.

    NCLEX® Connection: Reduction of Risk Potential, Therapeutic Procedures

UNIT 9   Nursing Care of Clients with Reproductive Disorders

SECTIONS

› Female Reproductive Disorders
› Male Reproductive Disorders

NCLEX® CONNECTIONS

When reviewing the chapters in this unit, keep in mind the relevant sections of the NCLEX® outline, in particular:

Client Needs: Basic Care and Comfort	Client Needs: Reduction of Risk Potential	Client Needs: Physiological Adaptation

› Relevant topics/tasks include:
» Elimination
  › Perform irrigations.
  › Evaluate whether the client's elimination is restored/maintained.
	› Relevant topics/tasks include:
	» Diagnostic Tests
	  › Compare the client's diagnostic findings with pretest results.
	» Laboratory Values
	  › Educate the client about the purpose and procedure of prescribed laboratory tests.
	» Potential for Alterations in Body Systems
	  › Monitor the client's output for changes from baseline.
		› Relevant topics/tasks include:
		» Alterations in Body Systems
		  › Assess the client for signs and symptoms of adverse effects of radiation therapy.
		» Illness Management
		  › Identify client data that needs to be reported immediately.
		» Pathophysiology
		  › Understand general principles of pathophysiology.

chapter 63

Overview

- Diagnostic procedures used to evaluate the structure, condition, and function of a female client's reproductive tissues and organs:
  - Pelvic exam with Papanicolaou (Pap) and human papilloma virus (HPV) tests
  - Colposcopy and cervical biopsy
  - Cone biopsy
  - Endometrial biopsy
  - Screening studies
  - Mammography
  - Hysterectomy
- Biopsies can also serve as therapeutic purposes in removing abnormal tissue. Another therapeutic procedure that nurses should be knowledgeable about is a hysterectomy.

Pelvic Exam with Papanicolaou (Pap) and Human Papilloma Virus (HPV) Tests

- Bimanual examination of the cervix, uterus, fallopian tubes, and ovaries is performed by the provider. The provider inserts two gloved fingers into the vagina and traps the reproductive structures between the fingers of the one hand and the fingers of the opposite hand that is on the abdomen. Palpation of the structures is done during this time.
- Two tests are used for cervical cancer screening, the Pap test and the test for HPV. Both can be performed prior to the pelvic examination.
  - The Pap test is use to identify precancerous and cancerous cells of the cervix.
  - The HPV test is used to identify HPV infections that can lead to cervical cancer.
- Screening Guidelines
  - The American Cancer Society provides guidelines for the prevention and early detection of cervical cancer. See www.cancer.org.

AGE	TESTING RECOMMENDATIONS
21	› All women begin screening for cervical cancer
21-29	› Pap test every 3 years › HPV unnecessary unless needed following an abnormal Pap test
30-65	› Pap and HPV every 5 years
Older than 65	› May discontinue testing if regular screenings have been negative › If diagnosed with cervical precancer, continue to screen

- ○ Screening is unnecessary for women who have had a hysterectomy with removal of the cervix and have a negative history of cervical cancer.
- ○ Women who are at high risk for cervical cancer need to be screened more frequently based on the advice of her provider.
- Preprocedure
  - ○ Nursing Actions
    - ■ Advise the client that she should schedule the test when she is not menstruating.
    - ■ Inform the client that use of vaginal medications, douching, or sexual intercourse within the past 24 hr may alter test results.
    - ■ Have the client empty her bladder.
    - ■ Place the client in the lithotomy position and drape appropriately.
    - ■ Explain to the client how the procedure will be carried out.
    - ■ Have all necessary equipment available (cervical scraping tools, glass slides, fixative, perineal pad).
- Intraprocedure
  - ○ Nursing Actions
    - ■ Remain with the client and provide support.
    - ■ Have ready the necessary equipment for the provider during procedure.
    - ■ Transfer specimens to slides and apply fixative to slides.
- Postprocedure
  - ○ Nursing Actions
    - ■ Provide the client with perineal pad and tissues.
  - ○ Client Education
    - ■ Inform the client that minimal bleeding may occur from the cervix.
    - ■ Inform the client of the time frame for results to be available.
    - ■ Educate the client about the importance of following up with provider if results are abnormal.

Colposcopy and Cervical Biopsy

- A colposcopy is the examination of the tissues of the vagina and cervix using an electric microscope. Typically, the provider also performs a biopsy. Several options are available.
  - ○ The provider may perform an endocervical curettage if a lesion is visible.
  - ○ A cone biopsy is an extensive surgical biopsy. The provider excises a cone-shaped sample of tissue to remove potentially harmful cells. In some cases, anesthesia is used for the procedure. Margins of the excised tissue are examined to ensure removal of all harmful cells. The surgeon may destroy the cells using a scalpel, cryosurgery (extreme cold, which freezes the tissue), lasers, or a procedure known as loop electorsurgical excision (LEEP). LEEP uses an electric current, and the laser procedure uses a laser beam that vaporizes the abnormal tissue.
  - ○ The best time to perform the procedure is in the early phase of the menstrual cycle because the cervix is less vascular then.

- Indications
  - Pap tests that demonstrate atypical or abnormal cells must be followed up with a colposcopy and cervical biopsy.
- Preprocedure
  - Nursing Actions
    - Provide psychological support.
    - Explain the procedure to the client and inform her that when the specimen is obtained, she can expect to experience temporary discomfort and cramping.
    - Preprocedure care is the same as that for a Pap test, except a sterile biopsy cup will be needed instead of the other equipment.
- Postprocedure
  - Nursing Actions
    - Postprocedure care is the same as that for a Pap test.
    - Provide client with perineal pad and tissues.
  - Client Education
    - Instruct the client to rest for the first 24 hr after the procedure.
    - Instruct the client to abstain from sexual intercourse and avoid using a douche, vaginal creams, or tampons until all discharge has stopped (usually about 2 weeks).
    - Instruct the client to avoid lifting heavy objects for approximately 2 weeks (to allow time for the cervix to heal).
    - Instruct the client to report excessive bleeding, fever, or foul-smelling drainage to the provider.
- Complications
  - Bleeding
    - Heavy bleeding can result from the excision of tissue.
    - Nursing Actions
      - Assess the client for heavy bleeding.
    - Client Education
      - Instruct the client to notify the provider for abnormal vaginal bleeding.
  - Infection
    - Infection can result from this invasive procedure.
    - Nursing Actions
      - Assess the client for fever, chills, severe pain, foul odor, or purulent vaginal discharge.
    - Client Education
      - Instruct the client to notify the provider regarding symptoms.

Endometrial Biopsy

- A thin, hollow tube is inserted through the cervix, and a curette or suction equipment is used to obtain the endometrial tissue sample.
- Indications
  - Potential Diagnoses
    - Endometrial biopsies are done to assess for uterine cancer as well as evaluate for menstrual irregularities and potential causes of infertility.
  - Client Presentation
    - Abnormal or postmenopausal bleeding
- Preprocedure
  - Nursing Actions
    - Obtain the client's menstrual history.
    - Administer an analgesic prior to the procedure.
    - Prepare the client using same procedure as pelvic examination.
    - Witness consent.
  - Client Education
    - Educate the client about the procedure.
      - Biopsies are done with the client awake.
      - Some discomfort and cramping will be felt by the client.
      - Instruct the client on use of relaxation techniques.
    - Have the client empty her bladder.
- Postprocedure
  - Nursing Actions
    - Postprocedure care is the same as that for a Pap test.
    - Encourage the client to rest on the examination table until cramping has diminished.
  - Client Education
    - Inform the client that spotting may be present for 1 to 2 days.
    - Tell the client that results will be available in approximately 72 hr.
    - Instruct the client to abstain from sexual intercourse and avoid using a douche, vaginal creams, or tampons until all discharge has stopped (usually about 1 to 2 days).
    - Have the client notify the provider of heavy vaginal bleeding, fever, severe pain, and/or foul discharge.
- Complications
  - Bleeding
    - Heavy vaginal bleeding is a potential complication of an endometrial biopsy.
    - Nursing Actions
      - Assess the client for heavy bleeding.
    - Client Education
      - Instruct the client to notify the provider of abnormal vaginal bleeding.

- ○ Infection

  - ▪ Infection can result from this invasive procedure.

  - ▪ Nursing Actions

    - □ Assess the client for fever, chills, severe pain, foul odor, and purulent vaginal discharge.

  - ▪ Client Education

    - □ Instruct the client to notify the provider regarding these symptoms.

Screening for Reproductive Disorders

- Syphilis

  - ○ There are two serologic (blood) studies used to screen for syphilis.

    - ▪ Venereal disease research laboratory (VDRL) – the oldest test for syphilis that is still performed

    - ▪ Rapid plasma regain (RPR) – a newer test for syphilis and has replaced the VDRL test in many institutions

  - ○ Interpretation of Findings

    - ▪ Both tests are done using a sample of blood and reported as nonreactive (negative for syphilis) or reactive (positive for syphilis).

    - ▪ False positives may occur secondary to infection, pregnancy, malignancies, and autoimmune disorders.

    - ▪ If either test is reactive, diagnosis should be confirmed using one of the following tests:

      - □ Fluorescent treponemal antibody absorbed (FTA-ABS)

      - □ Treponema pallidum particle agglutination assay (TPPA)

- Human Immune Deficiency Virus (HIV)

  - ○ The enzyme immunoassay (EIA) test and Western blot assay are used to detect the presence of HIV

  - ○ Interpretation of Findings

    - ▪ The enzyme immunoassay (EIA) test, formerly the enzyme-linked immunosorbent assay (ELISA) is an antibody test used to measure the client's response to HIV. The test is typically positive 3 weeks to 3 months after the infection occurs, but it can be delayed for as long as 36 months. False positive results can occur; therefore further testing is needed.

      - □ If the EIA is positive, the Western blot assay is used to confirm the diagnosis of HIV.

- Genital Herpes

  - ○ Although a diagnosis of genital herpes can be based on the client's history and physical, the diagnosis can be confirmed with laboratory testing, which include the following:

    - ▪ Herpes viral culture – Fluid from a lesion is obtained using a swab and placed in a cup for culture.

    - ▪ Polymerase chain reaction (PRC) test – Identifies genetic material of the virus. Cells from a lesion, blood, or other body fluids can be tested. Identifies type of virus (herpes simplex 1 [HSV 1] or herpes simplex 2 [HSV 2]).

    - ▪ Antibody test – Blood is tested for antibodies to the virus. Some tests can identify the type of virus. The HerpeSelect Immnoblot, HerpeSelect ELISA and the Western Blot can be used to differentiate between HSV 1 and HSV 2.

Mammography

- During a mammogram, a woman's breast is mechanically compressed both vertically and horizontally by the x-ray machine while radiologic pictures are taken of each breast.

- Indications

  - Screening mammograms detect breast cancer lesions in women who do not have symptoms. Screening mammograms decrease cancer death rates because the treatment options and outcomes are best when the cancer is detected early.

  - A number of organizations provide guidelines for screening mammograms, including the American Cancer Society and the U.S. Preventive Services Task Force (USPSTF). For current guidelines, see www.cancer.org and www.uspreventiveservicestaskforce.org, respectively.

  - Diagnostic mammograms are used when a screening mammograms reveals abnormal findings or when breast cancer symptoms are present. The diagnostic mammogram provides a more detailed picture and is more accurate than the screening mammogram.

  - There are two types of mammography screening tools. Traditional mammography images are stored on film. Digital mammography takes an electronic image, which can be stored electronically. Both types are effective diagnostic tools; however, the digital mammogram can be more useful in women who have dense breast tissue. It is also more costly.

  - A breast ultrasound can be used to determine whether a mass is fluid filled (cyst) or a solid mass, which could be a cancerous lesion. A wire needle biopsy can be used if the abnormal area is too small to be palpated. Ultrasound is used to identify the area of concern. Then a small wire is placed into the area. Subsequently the surgeon performs a biopsy using the wire to locate the area.

- Preprocedure

  - Client Education

    - Instruct the client to avoid the use of deodorant, lotion, or powders in the axillary region or on the breasts prior to the exam.

    - Tell the client she should not have a mammogram if she is pregnant.

- Intraprocedure

  - Nursing Actions

    - Radiologic technicians are often the members of the health care team who perform mammograms.

- Postprocedure

  - Client Education

    - Inform the client that she will be contacted about results of diagnostic examination.

    - Reinforce education about self-breast examinations.

    - Encourage the client to follow the advice of her provider regarding when to return for a follow-up mammogram.

Hysterectomy

- A hysterectomy is the removal of the uterus.
- A bilateral salpingo oophrectomy is the removal of the ovaries and fallopian tubes.
- There are three methods of performing a hysterectomy
  - Abdominal approach, also known as a total abdominal hysterectomy
  - Vaginal approach (TVA)
  - Laparoscopy-assisted vaginal hysterectomy (LAVH)
- There are a number of options available for a woman who requires a hysterectomy or other reproductive procedure. In some cases, the decision regarding which procedure is based on the client's preference in conjunction with the surgeon's recommendation.

NAME OF PROCEDURE	EXTENT OF PROCEDURE
Total hysterectomy	› Uterus and cervix are removed.
Subtotal hysterectomy	› Uterus is removed; cervix is not.
Bilateral salpingo oophorectomy	› Ovaries and fallopian tubes are removed.
Panhysterectomy	› Uterus, cervix, ovaries, and fallopian tubes are removed.
Radical hysterectomy	› Uterus, cervix, upper part of the vagina, adjacent tissue, including lymph nodes, are removed.

- To treat leiomyomas (benign fibroid tumors), uterine-sparing procedures are available.
- Indications
  - Diagnoses
    - Uterine cancer
    - Noncancerous conditions – fibroids, endometriosis (inflammation of the endometrium), and genital prolapse – that cause pain, bleeding, or emotional stress
  - Client Presentation
    - Painful intercourse
    - Hypermenorrhea
    - Pelvic pressure
    - Urinary urgency or frequency
    - Constipation
- Preprocedure
  - Nursing Actions
    - Ensure that clients who have been taking anitcoagulant medications, aspirin, nonsterodial anti-inflammatory drugs (NSAIDs), or vitamin E have discontinued their use.
    - Rule out pregnancy.
    - Administer preoperative antibiotics.
    - Place antiembolism stockings.

- Complete psychological assessment.

- Maintain NPO status.

- Ensure that informed consent has been obtained.

- ○ Client Education

  - Teach the client how to turn, cough, and deep breathe, and the importance of early ambulation.

  - Instruct the client how to use an incentive spirometer.

  - Teach the client about preoperative and postoperative medications.

- Postprocedure

  - ○ Nursing Actions

    - Postoperatively, the nurse must monitor the client for vaginal bleeding. Excess bleeding is more than one saturated pad in 4 hr.

    - An indwelling urinary catheter is generally inserted intraoperatively and in place for the first 24 hr postoperatively.

    - Priority assessments and interventions following a total abdominal hysterectomy:

      - □ Monitor the client's vital signs (fever, hypotension).

      - □ Monitor the client's breath sounds (risk of atelectasis; turn, cough, and deep breathe; use of incentive spirometry; ambulation).

      - □ Monitor the client's bowel sounds (risk of paralytic ileus).

      - □ Monitor the client's urine output (call the provider if less than 30 mL/hr).

      - □ Provide IV fluid and electrolyte replacement (until bowel sounds return).

      - □ Monitor the client's incision (infection, integrity, risk of dehiscence).

      - □ Monitor the client for signs of thrombophlebitis (warmth, tenderness, edema).

      - □ Take thromboembolism precautions (sequential compression devices, ambulation).

      - □ Monitor the client's blood loss (Hgb and Hct).

  - ○ Client Education

    - Instruct the client about a well-balanced diet that is high in protein and vitamin C for wound healing, and high in iron if the client is anemic.

    - If the client's ovaries have been removed, she can develop menopausal symptoms. Discuss issues related to hormone therapy with the client.

    - Instruct the client to restrict activity (heavy lifting, strenuous activity, driving, stairs, sexual activity) for as long as 6 weeks depending on the procedure that was performed.

    - Remind the client to avoid the use of tampons.

    - Tell the client to notify the surgeon of temperatures over 37.8° C (100° F), foul-smelling drainage from incision, pain, redness, swelling in calf, or burning on urination.

- Complications
  - ○ Complications for clients following a hysterectomy are similar to that of clients who are postoperative following other abdominal surgeries. Monitor the client for complications including the following:
    - Hypovolemic shock
      - □ Hypovolemic shock due to blood loss is a potential complication following a hysterectomy.
      - □ Nursing Actions
        - ‣ Monitor the client's vital signs, Hgb, and Hct.
        - ‣ Check for excessive vaginal bleeding (more than one saturated perineal pad in 4 hr).
        - ‣ Provide fluid replacement therapy and/or blood transfusions as indicated.
    - Infection, which can be indicated by foul-smelling vaginal drainage, temperatures greater than 37.8° C (100° F), and redness, swelling, or drainage at the site of the incision.
    - Psychological reactions
      - □ Psychological reactions can occur months to years after surgery.
      - □ Nursing Actions
        - ‣ Encourage the client to discuss the positive aspects of life.
        - ‣ Understand that occasional sadness in the client is normal, but persistent sadness or depression indicates a need for counseling assistance.
  - ○ Client Education
    - Encourage the client to attend a support group.

APPLICATION EXERCISES

1. A nurse is preparing a client for her first Papanicolaou (Pap) test. Which of the following statements is appropriate for the nurse to make?

    A. "You should urinate immediately after the procedure is over."

    B. "You will not feel any discomfort."

    C. "You may experience some bleeding after the procedure."

    D. "You will need to hold your breath during the procedure."

2. A nurse in a provider's office is reviewing a client's laboratory results. The client's rapid plasma regain (RPR) is positive. Which of the following tests confirm the diagnosis of syphilis?

    A. Venereal Disease Research Laboratory (VDRL)

    B. D-dimer

    C. Treponema pallidum particle agglutination assay

    D. Sickledex

3. A nurse in a clinic is reviewing the facility's testing process and procedures for human immune deficiency virus (HIV) with a new employee. Which of the following information should the nurse include in the review?

    A. In the presence of HIV, the enzyme immunoassay (EIA) test is typically reactive within 72 hr after the client is infected.

    B. The Western blot assay is used to confirm the diagnosis of HIV.

    C. The polymerase chain reaction (PRC) test is used to confirm the diagnosis of HIV.

    D. In the presence of HIV the enzyme immunoassay (EIA) test is typically reactive within 48 hr after the client is infected.

4. A nurse is providing instructions to a client before a mammogram. Which of the following should the nurse instruct the client to avoid prior to the procedure?

    A. Multivitamin

    B. Deodorant

    C. Sexual intercourse

    D. Exercise

5. A nurse is providing instructions for a client who is scheduled for a cervical biopsy. Which of the following should the nurse include in the instructions? (Select all that apply.)

_____ A. "The procedure is painless."

_____ B. "Avoid heavy lifting for approximately 2 weeks after the procedure."

_____ C. "Heavy bleeding is common during the first 12 hours after the procedure."

_____ D. "Plan to rest for the first 72 hours after the procedure."

_____ E. "Avoid the use of tampons for 2 weeks after the procedure."

6. A nurse is planning care for a client who is to have a total abdominal hysterectomy. Use the ATI Active Learning Template: Therapeutic Procedure to complete this item to include the following sections: Identify nursing actions the nurse should include both preprocedure and postprocedure. List at least two nursing actions the nurse should include preprocedure and at least four actions the nurse should include postprocedure.

APPLICATION EXERCISES KEY

1. A. INCORRECT: The client is instructed to urinate immediately before the procedure.

    B. INCORRECT: The client may experience discomfort when the provider obtains the cervical sample.

    C. **CORRECT:** The client may experience a small amount of vaginal bleeding due to scraping of the cervix.

    D. INCORRECT: The client should use relaxation techniques such as taking deep breaths during the procedure.

    Ⓝ NCLEX® Connection: Reduction of Risk Potential, Therapeutic Procedures

2. A. INCORRECT: The VDRL is another screening test for syphilis.

    B. INCORRECT: The D-dimer is a test used measure fibrin and is used to diagnose disseminated intravascular coagulation.

    C. **CORRECT:** The treponema pallidum particle agglutination assay is used to confirm the diagnosis of syphilis.

    D. INCORRECT: The sickledex is used to diagnose sickle cell anemia.

    Ⓝ NCLEX® Connection: Reduction of Risk Potential, Laboratory Values

3. A. INCORRECT: The EIA test is typically reactive 3 weeks to 3 months after the infection occurs, but it can be delayed for as long as 36 months.

    B. **CORRECT:** Confirming HIV is a two-step process. If the EIA is positive, a second test, the Western blot assay, is done.

    C. INCORRECT: The PRC test is used to confirm the diagnosis of genital herpes.

    D. INCORRECT: The EIA test is typically reactive 3 weeks to 3 months after the infection occurs, but it can be delayed for as long as 36 months.

    Ⓝ NCLEX® Connection: Reduction of Risk Potential, Laboratory Values

4. A. INCORRECT: Taking a multivitamin does not alter the accuracy of a mammogram.

    B. **CORRECT:** Applying deodorant or powder can alter the accuracy of a mammogram by causing a shadow to appear.

    C. INCORRECT: Having sexual intercourse does not alter the accuracy of a mammogram.

    D. INCORRECT: Exercising does not alter the accuracy of a mammogram.

    Ⓝ NCLEX® Connection: Reduction of Risk Potential, Therapeutic Procedures

5.   A. INCORRECT: Typically the client will experience temporary discomfort and cramping when the specimen is obtained.

     B. **CORRECT:** The client should avoid heavy lifting until the cervix has healed, which is approximately 2 weeks.

     C. INCORRECT: Some bleeding is common after a cervical biopsy, but excessive bleeding is a complication and should be reported to the provider.

     D. INCORRECT: The client should plan to rest for the first 24 hr after the procedure.

     E. **CORRECT:** The client should not use tampons until the cervix has healed, which is approximately 2 weeks.

    (**N**) NCLEX® Connection: Reduction of Risk Potential, Therapeutic Procedures

6.   *Using the ATI Active Learning Template: Therapeutic Procedure*
   - Preprocedure
     - Maintain NPO status.
     - Ensure that informed consent has been obtained.
     - Teach the client to turn, cough, deep breathe, to use the incentive spirometer, and the importance of early ambulation
     - Teach the client about preoperative and postoperative medications.
     - Rule out pregnancy.
     - Ensure that clients who have been taking anticoagulant medications, aspirin, nonsteroidal anti-inflammatory drugs (NSAIDs), or vitamin E have discontinued their use.
     - Administer preoperative antibiotics.
     - Place antiembolism stockings
     - Complete psychological assessment.
   - Postprocedure
     - Monitor vaginal bleeding. The client should have no more than one saturated perineal pad in 4 hr.
     - Maintain indwelling urinary catheter and monitor urine output. The client should have at least 30 mL/hr.
     - Monitor vital signs.
     - Monitor breath sounds and use of incentive spirometer.
     - Assist with ambulation.
     - Monitor bowel sounds.
     - Provide IV fluid and electrolyte replacement.
     - Monitor the client's incision.
     - Monitor the client's Hgb and Hct.
     - Monitor for signs of thrombosis and take thromboembolism precautions.
     - Instruct the client about diets that promote wound healing (high protein and vitamin C).
     - Instruct the client to restrict activity.
     - If ovaries have been removed, discuss issues related to hormone therapy.
     - Remind the client to avoid the use of tampons.
     - Tell the client to notify the surgeon of temperature over 37.8° C (100° F), foul-smelling drainage from incision, pain, redness, swelling in calf, and burning on urination.
     - Assess psychological status.

    (**N**) NCLEX® Connection: Reduction of Risk Potential, Therapeutic Procedures

chapter 64

Overview

- The average age of menarche (first menses) in the United States is 13 years of age. If an adolescent has not begun having periods by 15 years of age, possible causes should be investigated.

- Menstrual cycles are typically 28 days long, with a range from 21 to 42 days. The first day of menstruation is day 1 of a menstrual cycle. Ovulation typically occurs around day 14. Menstruation begins 14 days after ovulation and typically lasts 4 to 5 days, but it can continue for up to 7 days.

- Menstrual cycles continue until menopause or surgical removal of the uterus. Menopause is the time when ovulation ceases and menstrual cycles become irregular and eventually stop. The median age of onset of menopause is 51 years of age.

MENSTRUAL DISORDERS

Overview

- Painful menstruation, or dysmenorrhea, is common in adolescents and young women. In many women, this pain is significantly decreased after the birth of a child or as a woman becomes older.

- Dysfunctional uterine bleeding (DUB) is believed to be due to a hormonal imbalance and may include menorrhagia and metrorrhagia. Menorrhagia is excessive bleeding (in amount and duration), possibly with clots and for longer than 7 days. Metrorrhagia is bleeding between menstrual periods more frequently than every 21 days. It is more common in women who are entering menopause and adolescent females who have begun menstruating in the past 1 to 2 years.

- Amenorrhea is the absence of menses. In a woman who has had menstrual cycles, this can be a sign of a medical disorder, such as thyroid disorder or structural disorders of the reproductive system. A common cause is low percentage of body fat in women who are involved in sports or women who overexercise. Anorexia nervosa also can result in amenorrhea due to a decrease in body fat.

- Premenstrual syndrome (PMS) is thought to be caused by an imbalance between estrogen and progesterone. Symptoms can vary among women and can vary for an individual woman from one cycle to the next. Common symptoms include irritability, impaired memory, depression, poor concentration, mood swings, binge eating, breast tenderness, bloating, weight gain, headache, and back pain. Premenstrual dystrophic disorder (PMDD) is a severe form of PMS seen in only a small number of women, and it interferes with a woman's ability to carry out her daily activities. With either condition, symptoms begin a few days before the menstrual period and end a few days after the onset of the menstrual period.

- Endometriosis is characterized by an overgrowth of endometrial tissue that extends outside the uterus into the fallopian tubes, onto the ovaries, and into the pelvis. Blockage of the fallopian tubes by endometrial tissue is a common cause of infertility.

Assessment

- Subjective data
  - Menstrual history (age of first menses, monthly cycle)
  - Sexual history
  - Nutritional history
  - Report of premenstrual depression, irritability, changes in appetite, abdominal bloating, fatigue, emotional lability, or fluid retention
  - Characteristics of flow
  - Characteristics and location of pain during menstrual cycle
- Objective data
  - Pelvic tenderness during palpation of the lower abdomen and the pelvic examination
  - Metabolic disorders (thyroid disorders)
  - Laboratory tests
    - Hemoglobin and hematocrit
      - May be below expected reference range due to excessive blood loss.
    - CA-125 is an immunodiagnostic test in which findings are elevated in ovarian cancer. Endometriosis and other conditions may also cause CA-125 to be elevated above the expected reference range.
  - Diagnostic procedures
    - Endometrial biopsy
      - Determines the relationship between menstrual flow and the hormone cycle, as well as possible pathologic reasons for bleeding, such as uterine cancer.
    - Transvaginal ultrasound
      - Can identify the presence of uterine fibroids, endometrial abnormalities, or leiomyomas.

Patient-Centered Care

- Medications
  - Hormonal contraceptives
    - May be used to decrease symptoms of PMS, PMDD, dysmenorrhea and DUB
    - May be the initial treatment for endometriosis
  - Diuretic – Aldosterone antagonist – spironolactone (Aldactone)
    - May be used to treat bloating and weight gain associated with PMS and PMDD
  - Leuprolide (Lupron) – synthetic luteinizing hormone
    - Reduces the follicle-stimulating and luteinizing hormone levels in DUB
    - Suppresses estrogen and testosterone production in the body, making it an effective treatment for endometriosis (promotes atrophy of ectopic tissue)
    - Can cause birth defects, so a reliable form of contraception should be used
    - May cause decreased libido and increased risk of osteoporosis

- ○ NSAIDs – ibuprofen (Motrin)
  - ■ May be given for endometriosis to inhibit production of prostaglandins
  - ■ Aids in treatment of pain and discomfort related to PMS and PMDD
- ○ Oral iron supplements
  - ■ Used to treat anemia associated with DUB
- ○ SSRIs – fluoxetine (Prozac), sertraline (Zoloft)
  - ■ Are used to treat both the emotional and physical symptoms of PMS and PMDD
- • Surgical Interventions
  - ○ DUB
    - ■ Dilatation and curettage
      - □ Used to diagnosis and treat DUB. The cervix is dilated, and the wall of the uterus is scraped with a curette. Endometrium scraped from the uterine wall is sent to the laboratory for examination.
    - ■ Endometrial ablation
      - □ Used to remove endometrial tissue in the uterus.
      - □ The tissue may be removed by laser, heat, electricity, or cryotherapy.
    - ■ Hysterectomy if other treatments are unsuccessful
  - ○ Endometriosis
    - ■ Laparoscopic removal of ectopic tissue and adhesions
      - □ A laser may be used to remove tissue.

MENOPAUSE

Overview

- • Menopause is the cessation of menses. Menses will appear on an infrequent cycle for a period of time that does not exceed 2 years. Menopause is considered complete when no menses have occurred for 12 months.
- • Menopause may be natural or surgically induced.

Assessment

- • Subjective and Objective Data
  - ○ Vasomotor symptoms – Hot flashes and irregular menses
  - ○ Genitourinary – Atrophic vaginitis, shrinking of labia, decreased vaginal secretions, dyspareunia, increased vaginal pH, vaginal dryness, incontinence
  - ○ Psychologic – Mood swings, changes in sleep patterns, and decreased REM sleep
  - ○ Skeletal – Decreased bone density

- ○ Cardiovascular – Decreased HDL and increased LDL

- ○ Dermatologic – Decreased skin elasticity and loss of hair on head and in the pubic area

- ○ Reproductive – Breast tissue changes

- ○ Laboratory Tests

  - ▪ Follicle stimulating hormone (FSH) – Increased during menopause

  - ▪ Blood, urine, and saliva hormone levels (estrogens, progesterone, dehydroepiandrosterone sulfate [DHEA-S], testosterone)

- ○ Diagnostic Procedures

  - ▪ Pelvic examination with Papanicolaou (PAP) smear to rule out cancer in cases of abnormal bleeding

  - ▪ Breast examination with mammogram to rule out cancer in cases of a palpable change from predominantly glandular tissue to fatty tissue

  - ▪ Biopsy of uterine lining in cases of undiagnosed abnormal uterine bleeding in a woman over 40 years of age or in a woman whose menses has stopped for a year and bleeding has begun again

  - ▪ Bone mineral density measurement using dual-energy x-ray absorptiometry (DXA) to determine the client's risk for osteoporosis

Patient-Centered Care

- • Medications

  - ○ Menopausal hormone therapy (HT)

    - ▪ Estrogen deficiency symptoms occur naturally as part of the aging process during menopause. Menopausal hormone therapy is prescribed to suppress hot flashes associated with menopause, to prevent atrophy of vaginal tissue, and to reduce the risk of fractures due to osteoporosis. For a woman who has a uterus, HT will include estrogen and progestin. For a woman who no longer has a uterus (following a hysterectomy), estrogen alone is prescribed.

    - ▪ Many preparations of HT are available (oral, transdermal, intravaginal, intramuscular). HT may be prescribed as a continuous, combined estrogen-progesterone therapy or a variety of cyclic patterns.

    - ▪ Based on their individual risk factors and health care needs, women should discuss the risks and benefits of using HT with their providers. The risk associated with the use of HT depends on many factors (the age of the woman, her personal/family history, the regimen prescribed). HT places women at risk for a number of adverse conditions, including coronary heart disease, myocardial infarction, deep-vein thrombosis, stroke, and breast cancer.

    - ▪ If the use of HT is required for management of menopausal symptoms, the best recommendation is to use HT on a short-term basis, generally less than 5 years.

    - ▪ Client Education

      - □ Reinforce to the client the advantages and disadvantages of HT.

      - □ Instruct the client in self-administration of HT.

      - □ Advise the client to quit smoking immediately if applicable.

- □ Teach the client how to prevent and assess the development of venous thrombosis.
  - ▸ Avoid wearing knee-high stockings and clothing or socks that are restrictive.
  - ▸ Note and report symptoms of unilateral leg pain, edema, warmth, and redness.
  - ▸ Avoid sitting for long periods of time.
  - ▸ Take short walks throughout the day to promote circulation.
  - ▸ Perform frequent ankle pumps, and move and stretch legs.
- □ Instruct the client about atypical clinical manifestations of myocardial infarction (abdominal pain, vague chest symptoms, arm pain, pain between the shoulders), and instruct the client to seek assistance immediately.
- □ If oral therapy causes nausea, taking medication with food may help.
- □ If the client is using vaginal creams or suppositories of estrogen compounds, be sure to refrain from inserting them prior to intercourse, or the client's partner may absorb some of the product.
- Alternative therapies
  - □ Ask the client about her use of complementary and alternative therapies such as black cohosh, ginseng, and red clover to relieve the effects of menopause. Research regarding their usefulness has been inconsistent.
  - □ Phytoestrogens interact with estrogen receptors in the body. Vegetables such as dandelion greens, alfalfa sprouts, black beans, and soy beans contain phytoestrogens.
  - □ Vitamins E and B_6 have been reported to decrease hot flashes in some women.
  - ○ Client Education
    - HT is beneficial in the prevention of age-related problems.
      - □ Osteoporosis
      - □ Atrophic vaginitis, which is characterized by vaginal burning and bleeding, pruritus, and painful intercourse, may improve with HT. Vaginal instillations of estrogen may be the best option because systemic absorption is reduced.
      - □ Older adult clients also may decrease the risk of osteoporosis by performing regular weight-bearing exercises; increasing intake of high-protein and high-calcium foods; avoiding alcohol, caffeine, and tobacco; and taking calcium with vitamin D supplements.

Complications

- Embolic complications (risk increased by concurrent smoking)
  - ○ Myocardial infarction, especially during the first year of therapy
  - ○ Stroke
  - ○ Venous thrombosis – Thrombophlebitis, especially during the first year of therapy
- Cancer
  - ○ In some studies, long-term use of HT has been found to increase the risk for breast cancer.
  - ○ Also some studies indicate that, long-term use of estrogen-only HT increases the risk for ovarian and endometrial cancer.

APPLICATION EXERCISES

1. A school nurse is providing an education session about menstruation with a group of adolescent female students. Which of the following statements should the nurse include? (Select all that apply.)

_____ A. "The average age of onset of menstruation for girls in the U.S. is 11."

_____ B. "The range for a typical menstrual cycle is between 21 and 42 days."

_____ C. "The first day of the menstrual cycle begins with the last day of the menstrual period."

_____ D. "Ovulation typically occurs around the 14th day of the menstrual cycle."

_____ E. "It is not unusual for a menstrual period to last as long as 7 days."

2. A nurse in a provider's office is providing information to a client who has dysfunctional uterine bleeding (DUB). Which of the following statements by the client indicate understanding of the information? (Select all that apply.)

_____ A. "My heavy bleeding may be due to a hormonal imbalance."

_____ B. "If I do not ovulate, my menstrual flow will be lighter."

_____ C. "Oral contraceptives are contraindicated for women who heavy uterine bleeding like mine."

_____ D. "My doctor may perform a D&C to find out what's causing my abnormal bleeding."

_____ E. "My condition is more common in women who are in their 30s."

3. A nurse is reviewing the medical record of a client who has premenstrual syndrome (PMS). Which of the following medications are used to treat premenstrual syndrome? (Select all that apply.)

_____ A. Fluoxetine (Prozac)

_____ B. Spironolactone (Aldactone)

_____ C. Ethinyl estradiol/drospirenone (Yasmin)

_____ D. Ferrous sulfate (Feosol)

_____ E. Methylergonovine (Methergine)

4. A nurse is providing support to a client who has a recent diagnosis of endometriosis. The nurse should reinforce with the client that which of the following conditions is a complication of endometriosis?

    A. Insulin resistance

    B. Infertility

    C. Vaginitis

    D. Pelvic inflammatory disease

5. A client who is menopausal asks the nurse about use of herbal therapy to treat hot flashes. Which of the following herbal supplements should the nurse recommend?

    A. Ginger root

    B. Black cohosh

    C. Saw palmetto

    D. Kava

6. A nurse is instructing a client who is being evaluated for premenstrual syndrome (PMS) to journal her symptoms to aid in the diagnosis. Use the ATI Active Learning Template: Systems Disorder to complete this item to include the following section: Client Education: Identify six symptoms of PMS.

APPLICATION EXERCISES KEY

1. A. INCORRECT: Although some females experience the onset of menstruation as early as age 11, the average age is 13.

   B. **CORRECT:** Although a typical menstrual cycle is 28 days, a range of 21 to 42 days is considered a regular menstrual cycle.

   C. INCORRECT: The first day of the menstrual cycle begins with the first day of the menstrual period.

   D. **CORRECT:** The first half of the menstrual cycle is the follicular phase, and the second half of the menstrual cycle is the luteal phase. Ovulation typically occurs around the middle of the cycle, or day 14 in a 28-day menstrual cycle.

   E. **CORRECT:** A menstrual period typically lasts from 4 to 7 days.

   Ⓝ NCLEX® Connection: Physiological Adaptations, Pathophysiology

2. A. **CORRECT:** DUB can be caused by a progesterone deficiency.

   B. INCORRECT: Anovulation is associated with a deficiency in estrogen and progesterone, which contributes to DUB.

   C. INCORRECT: DUB occurs when progesterone levels are low. Contraceptives that contain progestin can be used to treat the condition.

   D. **CORRECT:** When the provider performs a dilatation and curettage, endometrium scraped from the uterine wall is sent to the laboratory for evaluation.

   E. INCORRECT: DUB is more common in young women who are just starting to menstruate and in women who are nearing menopause.

   Ⓝ NCLEX® Connection: Physiological Adaptations, Pathophysiology

3. A. **CORRECT:** Fluoxetine, an SSRI, is used to treat the emotional symptoms of PMS, such as irritability and mood swings, and has an added effect of treating physical symptoms.

   B. **CORRECT:** Spironolactone is a diuretic and can reduce bloating and weight gain associated with PMS.

   C. **CORRECT:** Oral contraceptives that contain drospirenone reduce the symptoms of PMS.

   D. INCORRECT: Oral iron supplements, such as ferrous sulfate, are used to treat anemia associated with dysfunctional uterine bleeding.

   E. INCORRECT: Methylergonovine is used to treat postpartum hemorrhage.

   Ⓝ NCLEX® Connection: Pharmacological and Parenteral Therapies, Medication Administration

4. A. INCORRECT: Insulin resistance is a complication of polycystic ovary syndrome.

    B. **CORRECT:** Infertility is a complication of endometriosis because endometrial tissue overgrowth can block the fallopian tubes.

    C. INCORRECT: Vaginitis is typically caused by an infection.

    D. INCORRECT: Pelvic inflammatory disease is caused by an infection of the pelvic organs.

    Ⓝ NCLEX® Connection: Reduction of Risk Potential, Potential for Complications from Surgical Procedures and Health Alterations

5. A. INCORRECT: Ginger root is used to treat nausea and vomiting.

    B. **CORRECT:** The action of black cohosh is unknown. However, research studies indicate it is useful in the treatment of menopausal symptoms, including hot flashes.

    C. INCORRECT: Saw Palmetto is used to treat benign prostate hyperplasia.

    D. INCORRECT: Kava is used to treat anxiety. However, it can cause severe liver damage, and its use is not recommended.

    Ⓝ NCLEX® Connection: Basic Care and Comfort, Nutrition and Oral Hydration

6. *Using the ATI Active Learning Template: Systems Disorder*
    - Client Education
        - Irritability
        - Impaired memory
        - Depression
        - Poor concentration
        - Mood swings
        - Binge eating
        - Breast tenderness
        - Bloating
        - Weight gain
        - Headache
        - Back pain

    Ⓝ NCLEX® Connection: Physiological Adaptations, Pathophysiology

chapter 65

Overview

- A cystocele is a protrusion of the posterior bladder through the anterior vaginal wall. It is caused by weakened pelvic muscles and/or structures.
    - For a cystocele with mild signs and symptoms, medical treatment may be attempted. If this is not successful, surgery may be indicated.
- A rectocele is a protrusion of the anterior rectal wall through the posterior vaginal wall. It is caused by a defect of the pelvic structures, a difficult delivery, or a forceps delivery.
    - For a rectocele with mild clinical manifestations, medical treatment may be attempted. If this is not successful, surgery may be indicated.

Health Promotion and Disease Prevention

- Inform the client of measures to prevent atrophic vaginitis and the advantages of prevention.
- Advise clients who are at risk to lose weight if obese.
- Instruct clients to eat high-fiber diets and drink adequate fluids to prevent constipation.
- Administer estrogen therapy to prevent uterine atrophy and atrophic vaginitis if the client is not at risk for complications from hormone therapy (cardiovascular or embolic history).

Assessment

- Risk Factors
    - Cystocele
        - Obesity
        - Advanced age (loss of estrogen)
        - Chronic constipation
        - Family history
        - Vaginal childbirth
        - Multiparity
        - Increased abdominal pressure
        - Hysterectomy (can contribute to weakening of the floor of the pelvis)
    - Rectocele
        - Pelvic structure defects
        - Obesity
        - Aging

- Family history
- Difficult vaginal childbirth necessitating repair of a tear
- Forceps delivery
- Previous hysterectomy
  - ○ Cystocele and rectocele develop in older adult females, usually following menopause.
  - ○ Older adult clients are more susceptible to constipation and chronic bearing down during elimination, which can displace weakened structures.
- Subjective Data
  - ○ Cystocele
    - Urinary frequency and/or urgency
    - Stress incontinence
    - History of frequent urinary tract infections
    - Sense of vaginal fullness
    - Dyspareunia
    - Fatigue
    - Back and pelvic pain
  - ○ Rectocele
    - Constipation and/or the need to place fingers in the vagina to elevate the rectocele to complete evacuation of feces
    - Sensation of a mass in the vagina
    - Pelvic/rectal pressure or pain
    - Dyspareunia
    - Fecal incontinence
    - Uncontrollable flatus
    - Hemorrhoids
- Objective Data
  - ○ Diagnostic Procedures
    - Cystocele
      - □ A pelvic examination reveals a bulging of the anterior vaginal wall when the client is instructed to bear down.
      - □ Bladder ultrasound measures residual voiding.
      - □ Urine culture and sensitivity is used to diagnosis urinary tract infection associated with urinary stasis.
      - □ A voiding cystourethrography is performed to identify the degree of bladder protrusion and the amount of urine residual.
    - Rectocele
      - □ A pelvic examination reveals a bulging of the posterior wall when the client is instructed to bear down.
      - □ A rectal examination and/or barium enema reveals the presence of a rectocele.

Patient-Centered Care

- Therapeutic Procedures
  - ○ Intravaginal estrogen
    - ▪ Intravaginal estrogen is used to prevent atrophy of the pelvic muscles in postmenopausal women.
  - ○ Bladder training contributes to urinary continence.
  - ○ Vaginal pessary
    - ▪ A removable rubber, plastic, or silicone device inserted into the vagina to provide support and block protrusion of other organs into the vagina. The provider selects the type of pessary and ensures that it fits correctly.

 View Image: Pessary

    - ▪ Nursing Actions
      - □ Teach the client how to insert, remove, and clean the device.
      - □ Monitor for possible bleeding or fistula formation.
  - ○ Kegel exercises
    - ▪ Exercises done to strengthen the pelvic floor
    - ▪ Client Education
      - □ Teach the client how to perform the exercises.
        - ▸ Contract the circumvaginal and perirectal muscles.
        - ▸ Tightening pelvic muscles.
        - ▸ Gradually increase the contraction period to 10 seconds.
        - ▸ Follow each contraction period with a relaxation period of 10 to 15 seconds.
        - ▸ Perform while lying down, sitting, and standing.
        - ▸ Perform a set of exercises at least 4 times daily.
        - ▸ Keep abdominal muscles relaxed during contractions.
- Surgical Interventions
  - ○ Transvaginal repair
    - ▪ A transvaginal repair is performed to treat prolapse of pelvic organs. Vaginal mesh is used to create a sling that supports the pelvic floor.
  - ○ Cystocele
    - ▪ Anterior colporrhaphy
      - □ Using a vaginal or laproscopic approach, the pelvic muscles are shortened and tightened.
  - ○ Rectocele
    - ▪ Posterior colporrhaphy
      - □ Using a vaginal/perineal approach, the pelvic muscles are shortened and tightened.

- ○ Anterior-posterior repair
  - In some cases, surgery for both a cystocele and a rectocele is needed; this is called an anterior-posterior repair.
  - A hysterectomy may be performed at the same time as any of the procedures listed above.
  - Nursing Actions
    - □ Postoperative
      - ▸ Provide routine postoperative care to prevent complications.
      - ▸ Administer analgesics, antimicrobials, and stool softeners/laxatives as prescribed.
      - ▸ Provide perineal care at least twice daily following surgery and after every urination or bowel movement.
      - ▸ Apply an ice pack to the perineal area to relieve pain and swelling.
      - ▸ Suggest that the client take frequent sitz baths to soothe the perineal area.
      - ▸ Provide a liquid diet immediately following surgery followed by a low-residue diet until normal bowel function returns.
      - ▸ Recommend that the client drink at least 2 L of fluid daily, unless contraindicated.
      - ▸ Following removal of the catheter, instruct the client to void every 2 to 3 hr to prevent a full bladder and stress on stitches.
      - ▸ The client may be discharged with either a suprapubic or an indwelling urinary catheter.

- **Care After Discharge**
  - ○ Client Education
    - Instruct the client on how to care for the urinary catheter at home if applicable. Instruct the client to notify the provider about signs of infection (elevated temperature, pulse, respirations, foul smelling drainage).
    - Caution the client to avoid straining at defecation; sneezing; coughing; lifting; and sitting, walking, or standing for prolonged periods following surgery.
    - Instruct the client to tighten and support pelvic muscles when coughing or sneezing.
    - Advise the client of postoperative restrictions, including avoidance of strenuous activity, lifting anything weighing greater than 5 lb, and sexual intercourse for 6 weeks.
    - Inform the client that if the provider did not schedule her for removal of stitches, they will be absorbed by the body, negating the need for removal.

Complications

- Complications are similar to those associated with a vaginal hysterectomy.
- Vaginal erosion and serious infection has led to the recall of some surgical mesh implants used to repair pelvic organ prolapse. For more information, see www.fda.gov.
- Dyspareunia (painful sexual intercourse) is a possible surgical complication due to surgical alteration of the vaginal orifice.

FIBROCYSTIC BREAST CONDITION

Overview

- Fibrocystic breast condition is a noncancerous breast condition.
- It is most common in younger women. It occurs less frequently in postmenopausal women.
- The condition is thought to occur due to cyclic hormonal changes.
- Fibrosis (of connective tissue) and cysts (fluid-filled sacs) develop.
- Risk Factors
  - Premenopausal status
  - Hormone therapy
  - Caffeine consumption
- Subjective Data
  - Breast pain
  - Tender lumps, commonly in upper, outer quadrant
- Objective Data
  - Physical Assessment Findings
    - Palpable rubberlike lumps, usually in the upper, outer quadrant
  - Diagnostic/Therapeutic Procedures
    - Breast ultrasound is used to confirm the diagnosis.
    - Fine needle aspiration is also used to confirm the diagnosis or to reduce pain due to fluid build-up.

Patient-Centered Care

- Medications
  - Over-the-counter analgesics such as acetaminophen (Tylenol) or ibuprofen (Motrin)
  - Oral contraceptives to suppress estrogen/progesterone secretion.
  - Diuretics to decrease breast engorgement.
  - Danazol and androgen/anabolic steroid to suppress ovarian function. Use of this medication is limited to clients who have severe fibrocystic breast condition due to its many adverse effects.
  - Vitamin E to reduce pain.
- Nursing Actions
  - Suggest that the client reduce the intake of salt before menses, wear a supportive bra, and use apply either local heat or cold to temporarily reduce pain.
  - Encourage the client to follow the provider's recommendations and to journal the effectiveness of the treatment plan.

APPLICATION EXERCISES

1. A nurse is instructing a client how to perform Kegel exercises. Which of the following instructions should the nurse include? (Select all that apply.)

_____ A. Perform a set of exercises four times a daily.

_____ B. Contract the circumvaginal and/or perirectal muscles.

_____ C. Gradually increase the contraction period to 10 seconds.

_____ D. Follow each contraction with at least a 10-second relaxation period.

_____ E. Perform while sitting, lying, and standing.

_____ F. Tighten abdominal muscles during contractions.

2. A client is admitted to the gynecology unit for an anterior colporrhaphy. Which of the following client statements is consistent with the physiological alteration that necessitates this type of surgery?

A. "I have to push the feces out of a pouch in my vagina with my fingers."

B. "I have pain and bleeding when I have a bowel movement."

C. "I have had frequent urinary tract infections."

D. "I am embarrassed by uncontrollable flatus."

3. A nurse is preparing to discharge a client who has had an anterior and posterior colporrhaphy. Which of the following instructions should the nurse provide?

A. "Do not bend over for at least 6 weeks."

B. "You can lift objects as heavy as 10 pounds."

C. "Do not engage in intercourse for at least 6 weeks."

D. "You may have foul-smelling draining within the first week after surgery."

4. A nurse in a provider's office is reviewing the medical record of a client who has fibrocystic breast condition. Which of the following is an expected finding?

A. Palpable rubberlike lump in the upper outer quadrant

B. BRCA1 gene mutation

C. An elevated CA-125

D. *Peau d'orange* dimpling of the breast

5. A nurse is preparing an educational session for a group of women on medications used to treat fibrocystic breast condition. Use the ATI Active Learning Template: Medication to complete this item. Include the following section: Therapeutic Uses – Identify three classes of medications that are used to treat the condition, and provide a brief description of the purpose of the medications in treating fibrocystic breast condition.

APPLICATION EXERCISES KEY

1. A. **CORRECT:** The client should perform a set of exercises at least four times a day.

    B. **CORRECT:** The client should contract her circumvaginal and perirectal muscles as if trying to stop the flow of urine or passing flatus.

    C. **CORRECT:** The client should hold the contraction for 10 seconds. She may need to gradually increase the contraction period to reach this goal.

    D. **CORRECT:** The client should follow each contraction with a period of relaxation of 10 to 15 seconds.

    E. **CORRECT:** The client should perform the exercises in all three positions.

    F. INCORRECT: The client should relax her other muscles, such as those in her abdomen and her thighs.

    Ⓝ NCLEX® Connection: Health Promotion and Maintenance, Health Promotion/Disease Prevention

2. A. INCORRECT: Pouching of feces is a physiological alteration associated with a rectocele. The surgical procedure for a rectocele is posterior colporrhaphy.

    B. INCORRECT: Pain and bleeding with a bowel movement is a physiological alteration associated with a rectocele. The surgery for a rectocele is a posterior colporrhaphy.

    C. **CORRECT:** Due to urinary stasis associated with a cystocele, this finding is consistent with a cystocele. The surgery for a cystocele is an anterior colporrhaphy.

    D. INCORRECT: Uncontrollable flatus is a physiological alteration associated with a rectocele. The surgery for a rectocele is a posterior colporrhaphy.

    Ⓝ NCLEX® Connection: Physiological Adaptations, Alterations in Body Systems

3. A. INCORRECT: The client does not have a restriction regarding bending over.

    B. INCORRECT: The client should not lift an object that weighs more than 5 lb.

    C. **CORRECT:** The client should refrain from intercourse to allow time for the surgical site to heal, which is typically about 6 weeks.

    D. INCORRECT: Foul-smelling draining is a sign of infection, which should be reported to the provider.

    Ⓝ NCLEX® Connection: Reduction of Risk Potential, Therapeutic Procedures

4. A. **CORRECT:** Clients who have fibrocystic breast condition typically have breast pain and rubbery lumps in the upper outer quadrant of the breasts.

    B. INCORRECT: BRCA1 gene mutation is a risk factor for breast cancer.

    C. INCORRECT: An elevated CA-125 is a finding associated with ovarian cancer.

    D. INCORRECT: *Peau d'orange* dimpling of the breast is a finding associated with breast cancer.

    Ⓝ NCLEX® Connection: Physiological Adaptations, Pathophysiology

5. *Using ATI Active Learning Template: Medication*
    - Therapeutic Uses
      ○ Analgesics, such as acetaminophen (Tylenol) or ibuprofen (Motrin), are used to relieve pain.
      ○ Oral contraceptives to suppress estrogen/progesterone secretion.
      ○ Diuretics to decrease breast engorgement.
      ○ Androgen/anabolic steroid danazol (Danocrine) to suppress ovarian function.
      ○ Vitamin E to reduce pain.

    Ⓝ NCLEX® Connection: Physiological Adaptations, Pathophysiology

chapter 66

Overview

- Changes to the prostate gland are common as men age, and routine diagnostic procedures should be performed to evaluate these changes.

  ○ Enlargement of the prostate gland is usually benign and is called benign prostatic hyperplasia.

  ○ Prostate cancer is one of the most common forms of cancer in men.

- Diagnostic procedures for male reproductive disorders include the following:

  ○ Prostate-specific antigen

  ○ Digital rectal exam

  ○ Transrectal ultrasound

Prostate-Specific Antigen (PSA) and Digital Rectal Exam (DRE)

- The PSA measures the amount of a protein produced by the prostate gland in the bloodstream. It is performed prior to the DRE because a rise in the PSA may occur due to the irritation that occurs upon palpation of the gland.

  ○ A sample of blood is used to determine the PSA level.

  ○ A client who has an elevated PSA should undergo a DRE by a provider to validate the findings.

- The DRE is done in an office or clinic.

  ○ With the client leaning over the examination table, the provider places a gloved, lubricated finger in the client's anus and palpates the posterior portion of the prostate gland through the rectal wall. The client also can be placed on his side or in the lithotomy position for the exam.

  ○ If the DRE reveals an abnormality, the location of the potentially cancerous prostate lesion is determined by ultrasonography and confirmed by a biopsy.

- Indications

  ○ Many providers recommend an annual PSA and DRE on men over 50 years old to better ensure early detection of prostate cancer. African American men and men who have a family history of prostate cancer should begin screening at an earlier age.

  ○ For additional information regarding screening for and treatment of prostate cancer, see www.cdc.gov.

  ○ Client Presentation

    ▪ As the prostate gland enlarges, it encroaches on the urethra and causes diminished flow and retention of urine. Blood may also be found in the urine. These symptoms can indicate BPH (benign prostatic hyperplasia) or prostate cancer.

- Interpretation of Findings
  - ○ PSA
    - An increase in PSA may indicate that a client has prostatic cancer.
      - □ PSA levels increase with age. For a man younger than 50 years of age, a PSA level of 2.5 ng/mL is within the expected range.
      - □ A PSA value over 4 ng/mL requires further evaluation. An elevated PSA is an indication of a number of conditions, including prostate cancer, BPH, and acute prostatitis.
  - ○ DRE
    - Abnormal findings during the DRE include an abnormally large and hard prostate with an irregular shape or lumps.

Transrectal Ultrasound (TRUS)

- With the client in a left, side-lying position, a probe is inserted into the client's rectum, and sound waves are bounced off the surface of the prostate gland to provide an image.
- Indications
  - ○ A TRUS is done if a client's PSA and/or DRE reveal a possible abnormality.
- Interpretation of Findings
  - ○ If an irregularity is found, the image will be used to guide a needle biopsy.

APPLICATION EXERCISES

1. An older adult client is having an annual physical exam at a provider's office. Which of the following client findings indicates additional follow-up is needed in regard to the prostate gland? (Select all that apply.)

_____ A. Prostate-specific antigen (PSA) is 7.1 ng/mL.

_____ B. A digital rectal exam (DRE) reveals an enlarged prostate that is smooth and firm.

_____ C. The client reports a weak urine stream.

_____ D. The client reports urinating once during the night.

_____ E. Smegma is present below the glands of the penis.

2. A nurse is providing information to a client who is scheduled for a transrectal ultrasound (TRUS). Which of the following information should the nurse include?

A. "This procedure will determine whether you have prostate cancer."

B. "The provider will insert a finger into your anus during the procedure."

C. "Sound waves will be used to create a picture of your prostate."

D. "An anesthetic will be used during the procedure."

3. A nurse in a provider's office is providing information to an older adult client who is to have prostate-specific antigen (PSA) and a digital rectal exam (DRE). Use the ATI Active Learning Template: Diagnostic Procedure to complete this item to include the following:

A. Description of the procedures and the order in which they are performed.

B. Nursing Actions: Identify two factors that place the client at risk for prostate cancer.

APPLICATION EXERCISES KEY

1. A. **CORRECT:** Although the PSA level is typically elevated in an older adult male, a PSA level of greater than 4 ng/mL warrants additional follow-up.

    B. INCORRECT: A prostate that is enlarged and smooth is an expected finding in an older adult male.

    C. **CORRECT:** A weak urine stream is a clinical manifestation of benign prostatic hyperplasia and warrants follow-up.

    D. INCORRECT: Urinating once during the night is an expected finding for an older adult male.

    E. INCORRECT: Smegma is a normal secretion that can accumulate beneath the glans penis.

    Ⓝ NCLEX® Connection: Health Promotion and Maintenance, Health Screening

2. A. INCORRECT: A biopsy is used to make the diagnosis of prostate cancer.

    B. INCORRECT: A rectal probe transducer is inserted into the client's rectum when a TRUS is performed.

    C. **CORRECT:** A transrectal ultrasound creates an image of the prostate using sound waves.

    D. INCORRECT: Anesthesia is not used for this procedure.

    Ⓝ NCLEX® Connection: Reduction of Risk Potential, Diagnostic Tests

3. *Using ATI Active Learning Template: Diagnostic Procedure*

    A. Description of the procedures and the order in which they are performed
    * PSA: A blood sample is taken to measure a specific protein produced by the prostate gland that is present in the bloodstream. The PSA is performed first because examination of the prostate (DRE) irritates the prostate and can cause the PSA to rise.
    * DRE: With the client leaning over the exam table, or placed on his side, or in the lithotomy position, the examiner uses a gloved, lubricated finger to palpate the prostate through the rectal wall to identify any abnormalities in size, shape, and consistency.

    B. Nursing Actions
    * African American descent
    * Family history of prostate cancer

    Ⓝ NCLEX® Connection: Reduction of Risk Potential, Diagnostic Tests

chapter 67

Overview

- As an adult male ages, the prostate gland enlarges. When the enlargement of the gland begins to cause urinary dysfunction, it is called benign prostatic hyperplasia (BPH).
- Disorders of the male reproductive system include testicular and prostate cancer and benign prostatic hyperplasia (BPH). Content on male reproductive cancer is included in the *Cancer Disorders* chapter.
- Benign prostatic hyperplasia is a very common condition of the older adult male.

BENIGN PROSTATIC HYPERPLASIA (BPH)

Overview

- BPH can significantly impair the outflow of urine from the bladder, making a client susceptible to infection and retention. Excessive amounts of urine retained can cause reflux of urine into the kidney, dilating the ureter and causing kidney infections.

Assessment

- Risk Factors
  - Age
  - Family history
- Clinical Manifestations
  - The International Prostate Symptom Score (I-PSS) is an assessment tool used to determine the severity of symptoms and their effect on the client's quality of life. The client rates the severity of lower urinary tract symptoms using a 0 to 5 scale and also rates his quality of life as affected by urinary tract symptoms.
  - Clients who have BPH typically report urinary frequency, urgency, incomplete emptying of the bladder, urinary hesitancy, urinary incontinence, dribbling post-voiding, nocturia, diminished force of urinary stream, straining with urination, and painless hematuria.
  - Urinary stasis and persistant urinary retention leads to frequent urinary tract infections.
  - If BPH persists, back flow of urine into the ureters and kidney can lead to kidney damage.
- Laboratory Tests
  - Urinalysis and culture (WBCs elevated and bacterial present with urinary tract infection)
  - Elevated BUN and creatinine (indicates kidney damage)
  - Prostate-specific antigen (PSA) to rule out prostate cancer

- Diagnostic Procedures

  ○ A digital rectal exam (DRE) will reveal an enlarged, smooth prostate.

  ○ A transrectal ultrasound (TRUS) and needle or aspiration biopsy is performed to rule out prostate cancer in the presence of an enlarged prostate.

Patient-Centered Care

- Nursing Care

  ○ Client Teaching

    ▪ Frequent ejaculation has been found to release prostatic fluids, thereby decreasing the size of the prostate.

    ▪ Tell the client to avoid drinking large amounts of fluids at one time, and to urinate when the urge is initially felt.

    ▪ Tell the client to avoid bladder stimulants, such as alcohol and caffeine.

    ▪ Tell the client to avoid medications that cause decreased bladder tone, such as anticholinergics, decongestants, and antihistamines.

    ▪ BPH may initially be treated conservatively with medication.

  ○ Medications

    ▪ The goal of medication for BPH is to re-establish an uninhibited urine flow out of the bladder.

      □ Dihydrotestosterone (DHT)-lowering medications – 5-alpha reductase inhibitor (5-ARI), such as finasteride (Proscar)

        ▸ DHT-lowering medications decrease the production of testosterone in the prostate gland.

        ▸ Decreasing a male client's DHT often causes a decrease in the size of the prostate.

        ▸ Client Education

          ▷ Reinforce that it may take 6 months to 1 year before effects of the medication are evident.

          ▷ Inform the client that impotence and a decrease in libido are possible side effects.

          ▷ Report breast enlargement to the provider.

          ▷ Finasteride is teratogenic to a male fetus. The medication can be absorbed through the skin. Pregnant women should not be in contact with tablets that are crushed or broken.

      □ Alpha-blocking agents – tamsulosin (Flomax)

        ▸ Alpha-adrenergic receptor antagonists cause relaxation of the bladder outlet and prostate gland.

        ▸ These agents decrease pressure on the urethra, thereby re-establishing a stronger urine flow.

        ▸ Client Education

          ▷ Warn the client that postural hypotension may occur, and that changes in position must be made slowly.

          ▷ Warn the client that concurrent use with cimetidine (Tagamet) can potentiate the hypotensive effect.

- Therapeutic Procedures
  - ○ Transurethral needle ablation (TUNA) – Low-level radiation is used to shrink the prostate.
  - ○ Transurethral microwave therapy (TUMT) – Heat is applied to the prostate to decease its size.
  - ○ Prostatic stent – Can be placed to keep the urethra patent, especially if client is a poor candidate for surgery.
- Surgical Interventions
  - ○ Surgical resection is an option for clients who do not receive adequate relief from conservative measures.
    - ▪ Transurethral incision of the prostate (TUIP) involves incisions into the prostate to relieve constriction of the urethra. Tissue is not removed with this procedure. It is minimally invasive and typically performed in an outpatient setting.
    - ▪ Transurethral resection of the prostate (TURP) is the most common surgical procedure for BPH.
    - ▪ TURP is performed using a resectoscope (similar to a cystoscope) that is inserted through the urethra and trims away excess prostatic tissue, enlarging the passageway of the urethra through the prostate gland.
    - ▪ Typically, epidural and spinal anesthesia are used.
    - ▪ Nursing Actions
      - □ Preoperative
        - ▸ Cardiovascular, respiratory, and renal systems should be carefully assessed prior to surgery.
        - ▸ Ensure that the client fully understands the procedure and what to expect postoperatively.
      - □ Postoperative
        - ▸ Postoperative treatment usually includes placement of an indwelling three-way catheter.
          - ▷ The urinary catheter drains urine and allows for instillation of a continuous bladder irrigation (CBI) of normal saline (isotonic) or another prescribed irrigating solution to keep the catheter free of obstruction.

 View Animation: Continuous Bladder Irrigation

          - ▷ The rate of the CBI is adjusted to keep the irrigation return pink or lighter. For example, if bright-red or ketchup-appearing (arterial) bleeding with clots is observed, the nurse should increase the CBI rate.
          - ▷ If the catheter becomes obstructed (bladder spasms, reduced irrigation outflow), turn off the CBI and irrigate with 50 mL of irrigation solution using a large piston syringe. Contact the surgeon if unable to dislodge the clot.
          - ▷ Record the amount of irrigating solution instilled (generally very large volumes) and the amount of return. The difference equals urine output.
          - ▷ The catheter has a large balloon (30 to 45 mL) that is taped tightly to the leg, creating traction so that the balloon will apply firm pressure to the prostatic fossa to prevent bleeding. This makes the client feel a continuous need to urinate. Instruct the client to not void around the catheter as this causes bladder spasms. Avoid kinks in the tubing.

- ▸ Monitor the client's vital signs and urinary output.

- ▸ Administer/provide increased fluids to the client.

- ▸ Monitor the client for bleeding (persistent bright-red bleeding unresponsive to increase in CBI and traction on the catheter or reduced Hgb levels) and report to the provider.

- ▸ Assist the client to ambulate as soon as possible to reduce the risk of deep-vein thrombosis and other complications that occur due to immobility.

- ▸ Administer medications to the client.

    - ▹ Analgesics (surgical manipulation or incisional discomfort)

    - ▹ Antispasmodics (bladder spasms)

    - ▹ Antibiotics (prophylaxis)

    - ▹ Stool softeners (avoid straining)

- ▸ When the catheter is removed, monitor the client's urinary output. The initial voiding following removal may be uncomfortable, red in color, and contain clots. The color of the urine should progress toward amber in 2 to 3 days. Instruct the client that expected output is 150 to 200 mL every 3 to 4 hr. The client should contact the provider if unable to void.

- Client Education

    - □ Tell the client to avoid heavy lifting, strenuous exercise, straining, and sexual intercourse for the prescribed length of time (usually 2 to 6 weeks).

    - □ Tell the client to drink 12 or more 8-oz glasses of water each day.

    - □ Tell the client that nonsteroidal anti-inflammatory medications promote bleeding and should be avoided.

    - □ Tell the client to avoid bladder stimulants, such as caffeine and alcohol.

    - □ Tell the client that if urine becomes bloody, stop activity, rest, and increase fluid intake.

    - □ Tell the client to contact the surgeon for persistent bleeding or obstruction (less than expected output or distention).

Complications

- TURP Complications

    - ○ Urethral trauma, urinary retention, bleeding, and infection are complications associated with TURP.

    - ○ Other complications include regrowth of prostate tissue and reoccurrence of bladder neck obstruction.

    - ○ Nursing Actions

        - Monitor the client and intervene for bleeding.

        - Provide antibiotic prophylaxis to the client.

APPLICATION EXERCISES

1. A nurse in a provider's office is obtaining a history from a client who is being evaluated for benign prostatic hyperplasia (BPH). Which of the following findings are indicative of this condition? (Select all that apply.)

_____ A. Backache

_____ B. Frequent urinary tract infections

_____ C. Weight loss

_____ D. Hematuria

_____ E. Urinary incontinence

2. A nurse is caring for a client who has a new diagnosis of benign prostatic hyperplasia (BPH). The nurse should anticipate a prescription for which of the following medications?

A. Oxybutynin (Ditropan)

B. Diphenhydramine (Benadryl)

C. Ipratropium (Atrovent)

D. Tamsulosin (Flomax)

3. A nurse is instructing a client who is scheduled for a transurethral resection of the prostate (TURP) about his postoperative care. Which of the following information should the nurse include in the teaching?

A. "You may have a continuous sensation of needing to void even though you have a catheter."

B. "You will be on bed rest for the first 2 days after the procedure."

C. "You will be instructed to limit your fluid intake after the procedure."

D. "Your urine should be clear yellow the evening after the surgery."

4. A nurse is providing discharge instructions to a client who is postoperative from a TURP. Which of the following instructions should the nurse include? (Select all that apply.)

_____ A. Avoid sexual intercourse for 3 months after the surgery.

_____ B. If urine appears bloody, stop activity and rest.

_____ C. Avoid drinking caffeinated beverages.

_____ D. Take a stool softener once a day.

_____ E. Treat pain with ibuprofen (Motrin).

5. A nurse is teaching a client who has a new prescription for finasteride (Proscar) about the medication. Use the ATI Active Learning Template: Medication to complete this item to include the following sections:

A. Therapeutic Uses: Identify the therapeutic use of this medication for this client.

B. Client Education: Identify four instructions the nurse should include.

APPLICATION EXERCISES KEY

1. A. INCORRECT: Backache occurs in the presence of prostate cancer that has spread to other areas of the body.

    B. **CORRECT:** In the presence of BPH, pressure on urinary structures leads to urinary stasis, which in turn promotes the occurrence of urinary tract infections.

    C. INCORRECT: Weight loss occurs in the presence of prostate cancer.

    D. **CORRECT:** Painless hematuria occurs in the presence of BPH.

    E. **CORRECT:** Overflow incontinence occurs in the presence of BPH due to an increased volume of residual urine.

    Ⓝ NCLEX® Connection: Physiological Adaptations, Pathophysiology

2. A. INCORRECT: Oxybutynin is an anticholinergic medication that is used to treat overactive bladder. Anticholinergic medications are contraindicated for a client who has BPH. Oxybutynin causes urinary retention.

    B. INCORRECT: Diphenhydramine is an antihistamine and is contraindicated for a client who has BPH. Diphenhydramine causes urinary retention.

    C. INCORRECT: Ipratropium is an anticholinergic used to treat asthma and other respiratory conditions. Anticholinergic medications are contraindicated for a client who has BPH. Ipratropium causes urinary retention.

    D. **CORRECT:** Tamsulosin is an alpha-adrenergic receptor antagonist that relaxes the bladder outlet and the prostate gland, which improves urinary flow.

    Ⓝ NCLEX® Connection: Pharmacological and Parenteral Therapies, Medication Administration

3. A. **CORRECT:** To reduce the risk of postoperative bleeding, the client will have a catheter with a large balloon that places pressure on the internal sphincter of the bladder. Pressure on the sphincter causes a continuous sensation of needing to void.

    B. INCORRECT: The client is ambulated early in the postoperative period to reduce the risk of deep-vein thrombosis and other complications that occur due to immobility

    C. INCORRECT: The client is encouraged to increase his fluid intake unless contraindicated by another condition. A liberal fluid intake reduces the risks of urinary tract infection and dysuria.

    D. INCORRECT: The client's urine is expected to be pink the first 24 hr after surgery.

    Ⓝ NCLEX® Connection: Reduction of Risk Potential, Therapeutic Procedures

4. A. INCORRECT: The client should follow the provider's instructions, which typically includes avoidance of sexual intercourse for 2 to 6 weeks after the surgery.

    B. **CORRECT:** Excessive activity may cause recurrence of bleeding. The client should rest to promote reclotting at the incisional site.

    C. **CORRECT:** Caffeine is a bladder stimulant and should be avoided.

    D. **CORRECT:** The client should take a stool softener to keep the stool soft and thus prevent the complication of bleeding at the time of a bowel movement.

    E. INCORRECT: The client should avoid taking nonsteroidal anti-inflammatory medications because they can cause bleeding.

    Ⓝ NCLEX® Connection: Reduction of Risk Potential, Therapeutic Procedures

5. *Using the ATI Active Learning Template: Medication*

    A. Therapeutic Uses
    - Finasteride inhibits 5-alpha reductase and enzyme, which converts testosterone to dihydrotesterone. Production of testosterone in the prostate gland is reduced, which in turn reduces the size of prostate tissue.

    B. Client Education
    - The medication must be taken on a long-term basis. It may take as long as a year before the effects of the medication are evident.
    - Impotence and a decreased libido are possible adverse effects.
    - Report breast enlargement to the provider.
    - Finasteride is teratogenic to the male fetus. The medication can be absorbed through the skin. Pregnant women should not be in contact with tablets.

    Ⓝ NCLEX® Connection: Pharmacological and Parenteral Therapies, Medication Administration

UNIT 10   Nursing Care of Clients with Musculoskeletal Disorders

SECTIONS
› Diagnostic and Therapeutic Procedures
› Musculoskeletal Disorders

NCLEX® CONNECTIONS

When reviewing the chapters in this unit, keep in mind the relevant sections of the NCLEX® outline, in particular:

Client Needs: Basic Care and Comfort	Client Needs: Reduction of Risk Potential	Client Needs: Physiological Adaptation

› Relevant topics/tasks include:
» Assistive Devices
  › Assess the client's use of assistive devices.
» Mobility/Immobility
  › Apply and maintain devices used to promote venous return.
	› Relevant topics/tasks include:
	» Potential for Alterations in Body Systems
	  › Identify the client with an increased risk for insufficient vascular perfusion.
	» Potential for Complications of Diagnostic Tests/ Treatments/Procedures
	  › Intervene to prevent potential neurological complications.
	» System Specific Assessment
	  › Assess the client for peripheral edema.
		› Relevant topics/tasks include:
		» Alterations in Body Systems
		  › Provide wound care and/or assist with dressing change.
		» Illness Management
		  › Promote and provide continuity of care in illness management activities.
		» Medical Emergencies
		  › Notify the provider about the client's unexpected response/emergency situation.

chapter 68

Overview

- Imaging studies are the primary diagnostic procedures used for musculoskeletal disorders.

- Evaluation of the conduction of electrical impulses in muscles may also be assessed in the presence of muscle weakness.

- Arthroscopy is performed to assess the condition of a joint and may simultaneously be used to repair tears and other joint defects.

- Musculoskeletal diagnostic procedures that nurses should be knowledgeable about include the following:

  - Arthroscopy

  - Nuclear scans (bone scan, gallium scan, and thallium scan)

  - Dual x-ray absorptiometry scans (DXA)

  - Electromyography (EMG) and nerve conduction studies

- Other diagnostic procedures used to detect joint conditions and musculoskeletal structures are x-ray studies, ultrasound, computed tomography (CT) scans, and magnetic resonance imaging (MRI).

Arthroscopy

- Arthroscopy is done to visualize the internal structures of a joint, most commonly the knee or shoulder joints.

- Number and placement of incisions depend on the area of the joint needing to be visualized and the extent of the needed repair.

- Arthroscopy cannot be done if infection is present in the joint or if the client is unable to bend the joint at least 40°.

- Indications

  - Potential Diagnoses

    - A client who has sustained injuries to his joints may undergo arthroscopy to ascertain the extent of damage, during which time repair may also be done using the arthroscope (torn ligament, meniscus, or synovial biopsy).

  - Client Presentation

    - Joint swelling, pain, and crepitus

    - Joint instability

- Preprocedure
  - Nursing Actions
    - Teach the client postprocedure exercises or refer him to a physical therapist (straight leg raising, quadriceps setting isometrics).
    - Ensure that the client has signed the informed consent form.
  - Client Education
    - Provide postoperative joint exercises.
    - Reinforce explanation of the procedure.
- Postprocedure
  - Nursing Actions
    - The client's postprocedure care for an arthroscopy, which was performed under sterile technique, is done on an outpatient basis.
    - Assess neurovascular status and dressings of the client's limb every hour or per hospital protocol.
  - Client Education
    - Ice and elevate the extremity for 24 hr.
    - Instruct the client to take a prescribed analgesic for pain.
    - Apply a splint or sling if prescribed.
    - Maintain activity restrictions as prescribed.
    - Have the client use crutches if limited weight bearing is prescribed.
    - Monitor the color and temperature of the extremity as well as pain and sensation.
    - Notify the provider of any changes, such as swelling, increased joint pain, thrombophlebitis, and infection.
- Complications
  - Infection
    - Complications are uncommon after this procedure, but infection may occur as with any procedure that disrupts the integrity of the skin.
    - Client Education
      - Notify the provider immediately of swelling, redness, or fever.

Nuclear Scans

- Bone scans are done when a client's entire skeletal system is to be evaluated.
  - A radionuclide test involves radioactive material injected 2 to 3 hr before scanning.
  - Bone scans can most commonly detect hairline bone fractures. They detect tumors, fractures, and diseases of the bone (osteomyelitis, osteoporosis, vertebral compression fractures).
- Gallium and thallium scans are more sensitive to detecting bone problems than a bone scan.
  - The radioisotope migrates to tissues of the brain, liver, and breast and is used to detect disease of these organs also.
  - Radionuclide is injected 4 to 6 hr before scanning.

- ○ The scan takes 30 to 60 min and may require sedation in order for the client to lay still during that time. Repeat scanning occurs at 24, 48, and 72 hr.
- ○ Indications for gallium and thallium scans
  - ▪ Potential Diagnoses
    - ▫ Arthritis
    - ▫ Osteomyelitis
    - ▫ Fractures
    - ▫ Osteoporosis
    - ▫ Primary or metastatic bone cancer
    - ▫ Bone pain of unknown origin
  - ▪ Client Presentation
    - ▫ Bone pain
- Preprocedure

  - ○ Nursing Actions
    - ▪ Inform the client about how the procedure will be done.
    - ▪ Assess for allergy to radioisotope or conditions that would prevent performing the procedure (pregnancy, kidney disease).
  - ○ Client Education
    - ▪ Explain to the client the need to lie still during the length of the procedure.
    - ▪ Instruct client to empty bladder before the procedure.
- Postprocedure
  - ○ Client Education
    - ▪ Following the procedure, the client does not need to take any radioactive precautions.
    - ▪ Encourage the client to drink fluids to increase excretion of radioisotope in the urine and feces.

Dual X-ray Absorptiometry (DXA)

- DXA scans are done to estimate the density of a client's bone mass – usually in the hip or spine – and the presence/extent of osteoporosis.
- A DXA scan uses two beams of radiation and findings are analyzed by a computer and interpreted by a radiologist. No contrast material is used. Clients receive a score that relates their amount of bone density to that of other people in their age group and gender.
- The client will lie on an x-ray table while a scan of a selected area is done.
- Indications
  - ○ Potential Diagnoses
    - ▪ Osteoporosis
    - ▪ Postmenopausal state (baseline may be done at age 40)
  - ○ Client Presentation
    - ▪ Loss of height
    - ▪ Bone pain
    - ▪ Fractures

- Preprocedure
  - ○ Nursing Actions/Client Education
    - ▪ Inform the client about how the procedure will be done.
    - ▪ Instruct the client to stay dressed but remove metallic objects.
- Postprocedure
  - ○ Client Education
    - ▪ Follow up with the provider regarding supplements and medications that may be needed if bone loss is present.

Electromyography and Nerve Conduction Studies

- Electromyography (EMG) and nerve conduction studies are done to determine the presence and cause of muscle weakness.
- EMG
  - ○ EMG is performed at the bedside or in a EMG laboratory.
  - ○ Thin needles are placed in the muscle under study and attached to an electrode, which is attached to an oscilloscope. Electrical activity is recorded during a muscle contraction.
- Nerve conduction study
  - ○ Flat electrodes are taped on the skin.
  - ○ Low electrical currents are sent through the electrodes and muscle response to the stimulus is recorded.
- Indications
  - ○ Potential Diagnoses
    - ▪ Neuromuscular disorders
    - ▪ Motor neuron disease (amyotrophic lateral sclerosis, myasthenia gravis, Guillain Barré)
    - ▪ Peripheral nerve disorders (carpal tunnel)
- Preprocedure
  - ○ Nursing Actions
    - ▪ Inform the client about what to expect.
    - ▪ Ask whether the client is taking an anticoagulant or muscle relaxants (contraindicated for this procedure).
    - ▪ Have the client sign the consent form.
  - ○ Client Education
    - ▪ Inform the client that when both EMG and nerve conduction are ordered, the nerve conduction is completed first.
    - ▪ Discomfort may be felt during needle insertion and when electrical current is sent through electrodes.
    - ▪ The client may be asked to flex her muscle while the needle is inserted.
- Postprocedure
  - ○ Client Education
    - ▪ Inform the client that some bruising may occur at needle insertion sites.
    - ▪ Have the client report swelling or tenderness at any of the sites to the provider.
    - ▪ Instruct the client to apply ice to prevent hematoma formation at the needle insertion sites and to reduce swelling and pain.

APPLICATION EXERCISES

1. A nurse is completing preoperative teaching for a client who is to undergo an arthroscopy to repair injury to a shoulder. Which of the following statements by the nurse is appropriate? (Select all that apply.)

_____ A. "Avoid damage or moisture to the cast on your arm."

___X___ B. "Inspect your incision daily for signs of infection."

_____ C. "Resume normal activity within 12 hr."

_____ D. "Position your affected extremity in a dependent position."

___X___ E. "Perform isometric exercises as directed."

2. A nurse is planning care for a client who is postoperative following an arthroscopy of the knee. Which of the following is an appropriate action by the nurse? (Select all that apply.)

___X___ A. Assess color and temperature of the extremity.

_____ B. Apply warm compresses to incision sites.

___X___ C. Elevate the extremity.

___X___ D. Administer opioid medication.

___X___ E. Assess pulse and sensation in the foot.

3. A nurse is providing teaching to a client who is scheduled for a bone scan. Which of the following statements by the nurse is appropriate?

A. "The procedure will take about 1 hour."

B. "You will be placed in a tubelike structure during the procedure."

C. "You will need to take precautions with your urine for 24 hours after the procedure."

(D.) "A radioactive substance will be injected before the procedure."

4. A nurse is educating clients at a health fair about dual x-ray absorptiometry (DXA) scans. Which of the following should the nurse include in the teaching? (Select all that apply.)

_____ A. The test requires the use of contrast material.

___X___ B. The hip and spine are the usual areas to be scanned.

___X___ C. The scan is used to detect osteoarthritis. osteoporosis

___X___ D. Bone pain may indicate a need for a scan.

___X___ E. At age 40 years, a baseline scan is recommended.

5. A nurse is planning care for a client who is to have an electromyography (EMG). Which of the following should the nurse include in the plan of care? (Select all that apply.)

_____ A. Assess the client for bruising.

_____ B. Apply ice to insertion sites.

_____ C. Determine whether the client takes a muscle relaxant.

_____ D. Instruct the client to flex muscles while the needle is inserted.

_____ E. Expect swelling, redness, and tenderness at the insertion sites.

6. A nurse is providing teaching to a client who is having a gallium scan. What should the nurse include in the teaching? Use the ATI Active Learning Template: Diagnostic Procedure to complete this item to include the following:

A. Procedure Name: Define.

B. Indications: List three.

C. Nursing Actions: List two preprocedure and one postprocedure.

APPLICATION EXERCISES KEY

1. A. INCORRECT: A sling is applied to immobilize the arm of the affected shoulder to limit activity and promote healing.

    B. **CORRECT:** The incision should be inspected daily for evidence of infection, such as redness, swelling, or purulent drainage.

    C. INCORRECT: Normal activity will resume as prescribed by the provider.

    D. INCORRECT: The affected extremity should be placed across the chest in a nondependent position to reduce swelling.

    E. **CORRECT:** Isometric exercises are recommended by the provider and directed by the physical therapist.

    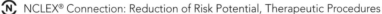 NCLEX® Connection: Reduction of Risk Potential, Therapeutic Procedures

2. A. **CORRECT:** Assessing color and temperature of the affected extremity identifies alterations in circulation.

    B. INCORRECT: Cold compresses are applied the first 24 hr to the incisional site to decrease swelling and pain.

    C. **CORRECT:** Elevating the leg will help decrease swelling and pain in the affected extremity.

    D. **CORRECT:** Administering prescribed opioid medication will help to relieve joint pain in the affected extremity.

    E. **CORRECT:** Assessing pulse and sensation of the affected extremity identifies alterations in circulation.

    (N) NCLEX® Connection: Physiological Adaptations, Alterations in Body Systems

3. A. INCORRECT: The entire procedure will take several hours. The radionuclide substance is injected and must be absorbed by the bone prior to the procedure. The client must wait several hours after the injection before the scan can be completed.

    B. INCORRECT: The client is placed in a tubelike structure during an MRI.

    C. INCORRECT: Radioactive precautions related to the client's urine are not necessary following the procedure.

    D. **CORRECT:** A radioactive substance is injected 2 to 3 hr before the procedure to allow for visualization of tumors, fractures, or diseases of the bone.

    (N) NCLEX® Connection: Reduction of Risk Potential, Therapeutic Procedures

4. A. INCORRECT: Contrast material is not used for a DXA scan.

   B. **CORRECT:** The most common areas for a DXA scan is the hip and spine for more clear visualization of a large area of bone.

   C. INCORRECT: Osteoporosis, not osteoarthritis, is detected by a DXA scan.

   D. **CORRECT:** Bone pain, loss of height, and fractures are findings that may indicate the need for a DXA scan.

   E. **CORRECT:** A baseline scan at age 40 is recommended to compare with a scan done during the postmenopausal period.

   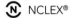 NCLEX® Connection: Reduction of Risk Potential, Therapeutic Procedures

5. A. **CORRECT:** The nurse should inform the client that some bruising might occur at the needle insertion sites.

   B. **CORRECT:** The nurse should apply ice to the insertion sites to prevent hematoma from developing.

   C. **CORRECT:** The nurse should assess the client's prescribed medications to determine whether the client takes a muscle relaxant, which may create a false reading.

   D. **CORRECT:** The nurse should ask the client to flex muscles for an easier insertion of the needle into the muscle.

   E. INCORRECT: The nurse should instruct the client to report swelling, redness, and tenderness at the insertion sites to the provider because this may indicate an infection.

   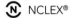 NCLEX® Connection: Reduction of Risk Potential, Diagnostic Tests

6. *Using ATI Active Learning Template: Diagnostic Procedure*

   A. Procedure Name: A gallium scan involves a radioisotope called radionuclide that is injected into the client 4 to 6 hr before the scan to view the client's bones. The radionuclide also migrates to the tissues of the brain, liver, and breast and is used to detect disease of these organs.

   B. Indications: Detect fractures, osteoporosis, bone lesions, osteomyelitis, and arthritis.

   C. Nursing Actions

   - Preprocedure nursing actions
     - Assess the client for allergy to radioisotopes.
     - Assess for existing conditions such as pregnancy or kidney disease.
     - Have the client empty his bladder before the procedure.
   - Postprocedure nursing actions – Inform the client to increase fluid intake to promote the excretion of the radioisotope in the urine and feces.

   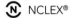 NCLEX® Connection: Reduction of Risk Potential, Therapeutic Procedures

UNIT 10   **NURSING CARE OF CLIENTS WITH MUSCULOSKELETAL DISORDERS**
SECTION: DIAGNOSTIC AND THERAPEUTIC PROCEDURES

CHAPTER 69   Arthroplasty

Overview

- Most musculoskeletal surgical procedures are performed to repair damaged joints, in particular the knees and the hips.
- Arthroplasty refers to the surgical removal of a diseased joint due to osteoarthritis, osteonecrosis, rheumatoid arthritis, trauma, or congenital anomalies, and replacing it with prosthetics or artificial components made of metal and/or plastic.
- Total joint arthroplasty, which can also be called total joint replacement, involves replacement of all components of an articulating joint.
- Musculoskeletal surgical procedures that nurses should be knowledgeable about
  - Knee arthroplasty
  - Hip arthroplasty

Knee and Hip Arthroplasty

- Total knee arthroplasty involves the replacement of the distal femoral component, the tibia plate, and the patellar button. Total knee arthroplasty is a surgical option when conservative measures fail.

 View Image: Artificial Knee Joint

- Unicondylar knee replacements are done when a client's joint may be diseased in one compartment of the joint.
- Total hip arthroplasty involves the replacement of the acetabular cup, the femoral head, and the femoral stem.

 View Image: Artificial Hip Joint

- Hemiarthroplasty refers to half of a joint replacement. Fractures of the femoral neck can be treated only with the replacement of the femoral component.
- Indications
  - Diagnoses
    - Knee and hip arthroplasty treats degenerative disease (osteoarthritis, rheumatoid arthritis).
  - Client Presentation
    - Pain when bearing weight on the joint (walking, running)
    - Joint crepitus and stiffness
    - Joint swelling (primarily occurs in the knees)

- Desired Therapeutic Outcome
  - The goal of both hip and knee arthroplasty is to eliminate pain, restore joint motions, and improve a client's functional status and quality of life.
- Preprocedure
  - Nursing Actions
    - Review diagnostic test results.
      - □ CBC, urinalysis, electrolytes, BUN, creatinine – Assess a client's surgical readiness, and rule out anemia, infection, or organ failure. Epoetin alfa may be prescribed preoperatively to increase Hgb.
      - □ Chest x-ray – Rule out pulmonary surgical contraindications (infection, tumor).
      - □ ECG – Gather a baseline rhythm to identify cardiovascular surgical contraindications (dysrhythmia).
    - Contraindications
      - □ Recent or active infection (urinary tract infection) can cause micro-organisms to migrate to the surgical area and cause the prosthesis to fail
      - □ Arterial impairment to the affected extremity
      - □ The client's inability to follow the postsurgery regimen
      - □ A comorbid condition (uncontrolled diabetes mellitus or hypertension, osteoporosis, progressive inflammatory condition, unstable cardiac or respiratory conditions)
  - Client Education
    - Postoperative care (incentive spirometry, transfusion, surgical drains, dressing, pain control, transfer, exercises, activity limits)
    - Autologous blood donation (client donates blood prior to procedure to be used postoperatively)
    - Scrubbing of the surgical site with a prescribed antiseptic soap the night before and on the morning of surgery decreases bacterial count on skin, which helps lower the chance of infection
    - Wearing clean clothes and sleeping on clean linens the night before surgery
    - May take antihypertensive medication, as well as other medications that the surgeon allows with a sip of water the morning of surgery
- Intraprocedure
  - May use general or spinal anesthesia
  - Removal and replacement of joint components with artificial components
  - Components may or may not be cemented in place. Components that do not use cement allow the bone to grow into the prosthesis to stabilize it. Weight bearing is delayed several weeks until the femoral shaft has grown into the prosthesis.
- Postprocedure
  - Nursing Actions
    - Knee arthroplasty
      - □ Provide postoperative care, and prevent postoperative complications (deep vein thrombosis, anemia, infection).
      - □ Older adult clients are at a higher risk for medical complications related to chronic conditions, including hypertension, diabetes mellitus, coronary artery disease, and obstructive pulmonary disease.

- □ A continuous passive motion (CPM) machine may be prescribed to promote motion in the knee and prevent scar tissue formation. CPM is usually placed and initiated immediately after surgery. CPM provides passive range of motion from full extension to the prescribed amount of flexion. The prescribed duration of its use should be followed, but it should be turned off during meals.

- □ Positions of flexion of the knee are limited to avoid flexion contractures. Avoid knee gatch and pillows placed behind the knee.

- □ To prevent pressure ulcers from developing on the heels, place a small blanket or pillow slightly above the ankle area to keep heels off the bed.

- □ Provide medications as prescribed. Focus needs to be about pain medications. This promotes client participation in early ambulation.

  - ▸ Analgesics – opioids (epidural, PCA, IV, oral), NSAIDs

  - ▸ A continuous peripheral nerve block – continuous infusion of local anesthetic directly into sciatic or femoral nerve

    - ▷ A continuous peripheral nerve block provides localized pain relief.

    - ▷ Monitor the client for systemic effects of local anesthetic, such as hypotension, bradycardia, restlessness, or seizure.

  - ▸ Antibiotics – prophylaxis and postoperatively

  - ▸ Anticoagulant – low-molecular weight heparin, such as enoxaparin (Lovenox); warfarin (Coumadin)

- □ Ice or cold therapy may be applied to reduce postoperative swelling.

- □ Monitor a client's neurovascular status of surgical extremity every 2 to 4 hr (movement, sensation, color, pulse, capillary refill, and compare with contralateral extremity).

- □ Assess a client frequently for overt bleeding and signs of hypovolemia, such as hypotension and tachycardia.

  - ▸ Monitor compression bandage and wound suction drain for excessive drainage.

  - ▸ Monitor the autotransfusion drainage system, if used, and reinfuse blood as prescribed by the provider.

- ▪ Hip arthroplasty

  - □ Provide postoperative care, and prevent postoperative complications.

    - ▸ Deep vein thrombosis may develop and result in a pulmonary embolism, a life-threatening complication after total hip arthroplasty.

      - ▷ Monitor a client for symptoms of pulmonary embolism, including acute dyspnea, tachycardia, and pleuritic chest pain.

      - ▷ Follow deep vein thrombosis prophylaxis to include pharmacological management, antiembolic stockings, and sequential compression devices while in bed.

      - ▷ Encourage plantar flexion, dorsiflexion, and circumduction exercises to prevent clot formation.

      - ▷ Encourage early ambulation with physical and occupational therapy.

    - ▸ Other complications include hip dislocation, infection, anemia, and neurovascular compromise.

Ⓖ
- □ The older adult client is at a higher risk for medical complications related to chronic conditions, including hypertension, diabetes mellitus, coronary artery disease, and obstructive pulmonary disease.

- □ The older adult client is at greatest risk for a potentially life-threatening complication (deep vein thrombosis, pulmonary emboli) because of age and compromised circulation before surgery.

- □ Clients who are obese, and those with a history of deep vein thrombosis, are also at a greater risk for developing deep vein thrombosis or pulmonary emboli.

- □ Monitor a client for bleeding.
  - ▶ Check the dressing site frequently, noting any evidence of bleeding. Monitor and record drainage from surgical drains.
  - ▶ Monitor daily laboratory values, including Hgb and Hct levels. The client's Hgb and Hct may continue to drop 24 to 48 hr after surgery. Autologous blood from presurgery donation or blood salvaged intraoperatively or postoperatively using special collection devices may be used for postoperative blood replacement. Blood transfusions are relatively common for Hgb levels less than 9 g/dL.

- □ Monitor the neurovascular status of the surgical extremity every 2 to 4 hr (movement, sensation, color, pulse, capillary refill, and compare with contralateral extremity).

- □ Provide medications as prescribed.
  - ▶ Analgesics – opioids (epidural, PCA, IV, oral), NSAIDs
  - ▶ Antibiotics – prophylaxis and postoperatively
  - ▶ Anticoagulant – low-molecular weight heparin, such as enoxaparin (Lovenox); warfarin (Coumadin), dalteparin (Fragmin), fondaparinux (Arixtra)

- □ Early Ambulation
  - ▶ Transfer the client out of bed from his unaffected side into a chair or wheelchair.
  - ▶ The client's weight-bearing status is determined by the orthopedic surgeon and by choice of cemented (usually partial/full weight-bearing as tolerated) versus noncemented prostheses (usually only partial weight-bearing until after a few weeks of bone growth).

Ⓠ
Ⓢ
  - ▶ Use assistive devices (walker) and adaptive devices (raised toilet seat) when caring for the client.
  - ▶ Apply ice to the surgical site following ambulation as a nonpharmacological measure to decrease pain and discomfort.

- □ Client position – Place the client supine with the head slightly elevated and the affected leg in a neutral position. Place a pillow or abduction device between the legs when turning to the unaffected side. The client should not be turned to the operative side, which could cause hip dislocation.

- □ Use total hip precautions to prevent dislocation of the new joint.

- □ Monitor the client for new joint dislocation: acute onset of pain, reports hearing "a pop," internal rotation of the affected extremity, and shortened affected extremity.

AFTER ARTHROPLASTY	
DOS	**DON'TS**
› Use elevated seating/raised toilet set.	› Avoid flexion of hip greater than 90°.
› Use straight chairs with arms.	› Avoid low chairs.
› Use an abduction pillow, or a pillow, if prescribed, between the client's legs while in bed (and with turning, if restless, or is in an altered mental state).	› Do not cross a client's legs.
› Externally rotate a client's toes.	› Do not internally rotate a client's toes.

- ○ Client Education
  - ▪ Knee and hip arthroplasty
    - □ The client requires extensive physical therapy to regain mobility. The client may be discharged home or to an acute rehabilitation facility. If discharged home, outpatient or in-home therapy must be provided. Home care should be available for 4 to 6 weeks.
    - □ Monitor for evidence of incisional infection (fever, increased redness, swelling, purulent drainage), and care for the incision (clean daily with soap and water).
    - □ Monitor for deep vein thrombosis (swelling, redness, pain in calf), pulmonary embolism (shortness of breath, chest pain), and bleeding if the client is taking an anticoagulant.
    - □ Hip arthroplasty – Follow position restrictions to avoid dislocation (see table above). Arrange for and instruct the client about the use of raised toilet seats, and care items (long-handled shoehorn, dressing sticks).
    - □ Knee arthroplasty – Dislocation is not common following total knee arthroplasty. Kneeling and deep-knee bends are, however, limited indefinitely.

APPLICATION EXERCISES

1. A nurse is reviewing the health record of a client who is to undergo total joint arthroplasty. The nurse should recognize which of the following findings as a contraindication to this procedure?

    A. Age of 78

    B. History of cancer

    C. Previous joint replacement

    D. Bronchitis 2 weeks ago

2. A nurse is admitting a client to the orthopedic unit following a total knee arthroplasty. Which of the following actions by the nurse are appropriate? (Select all that apply.)

    _X_ A. Maintain continuous passive motion device.

    _X_ B. Palpate dorsopedal pulses.

    _____ C. Place pillow behind the knee.

    _X_ D. Elevate heels off bed.

    _____ E. Apply heat therapy to incision.

3. A nurse is planning discharge teaching for a client who had a total hip arthroplasty. Which of the following should the nurse include in the teaching? (Select all that apply.)

    _X_ A. Clean the incision daily with soap and water.

    _____ B. Turn the toes inward when sitting or lying.

    _X_ C. Sit in a straight-backed armchair.

    _____ D. Bend at the waist when putting on socks.

    _X_ E. Use a raised toilet seat.

4. A nurse is assessing a client who is to undergo a right knee arthroplasty. Which of the following are expected findings? (Select all that apply.)

    _____ A. Skin reddened over the joint

    _X_ B. Pain when bearing weight

    _X_ C. Joint crepitus

    _X_ D. Swelling of the affected joint

    _X_ E. Limited joint motion

5. A nurse is completing a preoperative teaching plan for a client who is to have a total hip arthroplasty. Which of the following should the nurse include in the teaching plan? (Select all that apply.)

_____X_____ A. Encouraging complete autologous blood donation

_____ B. Sitting in a low reclining chair

_____ C. Having the client roll onto the operative hip

_____X_____ D. Using an abductor pillow when turning

_____X_____ E. Performing isometric exercises

6. A nurse is preparing to administer enoxaparin (Lovenox) to a client who had a total knee arthroplasty. Which of the following should the nurse consider before administering the medication? Use the ATI Active Learning Template: Medication and the Pharmacology Review Module to complete this item. Include the following:

A. Expected Pharmacological Action: Define.

B. Nursing Interventions: List two nursing interventions.

C. Client Education: List three client teaching points.

7. A nurse is preparing to administer enoxaparin (Lovenox) 60 mg subcutaneous to a client who had a total knee arthroplasty. Available is enoxaparin injection 100 mg/1 mL. How many mL should the nurse plan to administer? (Round the answer to the nearest tenth.)

$$\frac{100}{1} \qquad \frac{60}{X}$$

$$100X = 60$$

$$X = 0.6 \ mL$$

APPLICATION EXERCISES KEY

1. A. INCORRECT: Age greater than 70 is not a contraindication for a total joint arthroplasty unless there are comorbidity factors.

    B. INCORRECT: History of cancer is not a contraindication for a total joint arthroplasty unless there are comorbidity factors.

    C. INCORRECT: Previous joint arthroplasty surgery is not contraindicated for total joint arthroplasty unless there are comorbidity factors.

    D. **CORRECT:** A recent infection can cause micro-organisms to migrate to the surgical area and cause the prosthesis to fail.

    Ⓝ NCLEX® Connection: Physiological Adaptations, Pathophysiology

2. A. **CORRECT:** A continuous passive motion device promotes motion in the knee and prevents scar tissue formation.

    B. **CORRECT:** The nurse should assess the strength of the pulses of both lower extremities to help determine adequate circulation.

    C. INCORRECT: A pillow should not be placed behind the knee to avoid flexion contractures.

    D. **CORRECT:** The nurse should prevent pressure ulcers on the client's heels by elevating the heels off the bed with a pillow.

    E. INCORRECT: The nurse should apply cold therapy, not heat therapy, to reduce postoperative swelling.

    Ⓝ NCLEX® Connection: Reduction of Risk Potential, Therapeutic Procedures

3. A. **CORRECT:** Washing the surgical incision daily with soap and water decreases the risk of infection.

    B. INCORRECT: Toes should be externally rotated. This prevents dislocation of the hip prosthesis.

    C. **CORRECT:** The client who uses a straight-backed armchair decreases the chance of bending at a greater than 90° angle, which may cause dislocation of the hip prosthesis.

    D. INCORRECT: The client who bends at the waist places the hip in a position greater than a 90° angle, which may cause dislocation of the hip prosthesis.

    E. **CORRECT:** The client who uses a toilet riser decreases the chance of bending greater than 90° degrees, which may cause dislocation of the hip prosthesis.

    Ⓝ NCLEX® Connection: Reduction of Risk Potential, Potential for Complications of Diagnostic Tests/ Treatments/Procedures

4. A. INCORRECT: Skin over the knee that's red may indicate infection and is not an expected finding.

    B. **CORRECT:** Pain when bearing weight due to degeneration of the joint tissue is an expected finding.

    C. **CORRECT:** Joint crepitus due to degeneration of the joint tissue is an expected finding.

    D. **CORRECT:** Swelling of the affected joint due to degeneration of the joint tissue is an expected finding.

    E. **CORRECT:** Limited joint motion is due to degeneration of the joint tissue and is an expected finding.

    Ⓝ NCLEX® Connection: Physiological Adaptations, Alterations in Body Systems

5. A. **CORRECT:** The client should be encouraged to donate blood that can be used postoperatively.

    B. INCORRECT: The client should anticipate sitting in a high chair to keep the hip at a 90° angle. This prevents dislocation.

    C. INCORRECT: The client should not turn to the operative side.

    D. **CORRECT:** The client should use an abductor device or pillow between the legs when turning. This helps avoid dislocation of the affected hip.

    E. **CORRECT:** The client should perform isometric exercises to prevent blood clots and maintain muscle tone.

    Ⓝ NCLEX® Connection: Reduction of Risk Potential, Therapeutic Procedures

6. *Using ATI Active Learning Template: Medication*

    A. Expected Pharmacological Action
       • Enoxaparin is an anticoagulant.
       • Use low molecular-weight heparin after abdominal and orthopedic surgery to prevent deep vein thrombosis that may lead to pulmonary embolism.

    B. Nursing Interventions
       • Do not expel the air bubble from the syringe before injection. It's nitrous oxide and allows the client to receive all the medication during the injection.
       • Rotate injection sites.
       • Monitor for manifestations of unexplained bleeding.

    C. Client Education
       • Encourage the use of a soft toothbrush and shaving with an electric razor to prevent bleeding.
       • Avoid over-the-counter medication unless prescribed by a provider.
       • Don't take enoxaparin with garlic, ginger, ginkgo, or feverfew. These supplements may increase the risk of bleeding.

    Ⓝ NCLEX® Connection: Pharmacological and Parenteral Therapies, Expected Actions/Outcomes

7. **0.6** mL

Using Ratio and Proportion

STEP 1: *What is the unit of measurement to calculate?*
mL

STEP 2: *What is the dose needed? Dose needed = Desired*
60 mg

STEP 3: *What is the dose available? Dose available = Have*
100 mg

STEP 4: *Should the nurse convert the units of measurement?*
No

STEP 5: *What is the quantity of the dose available?*
1 mL

STEP 6: *Set up an equation, and solve for X.*

$$\frac{Have}{Quantity} = \frac{Desired}{X}$$

$$\frac{100\ mg}{1\ mL} = \frac{60\ mg}{X\ mL}$$

X = 0.6

STEP 7: *Round if necessary.*

STEP 8: *Reassess to determine whether the amount to give makes sense.*
If there is 100 mg/mL and the prescribed amount is 60 mg, it makes sense to give 0.6 mL. The nurse should administer enoxaparin injection 0.6 mL subcutaneous.

Using Desired Over Have

STEP 1: *What is the unit of measurement to calculate?*
mL

STEP 2: *What is the dose needed? Dose needed = Desired*
60 mg

STEP 3: *What is the dose available? Dose available = Have*
100 mg

STEP 4: *Should the nurse convert the units of measurement?*
No

STEP 5: *What is the quantity of the dose available?*
1 mL

STEP 6: *Set up an equation, and solve for X.*

$$\frac{Desired \times Quantity}{Have} = X$$

$$\frac{60\ mg \times 1\ mL}{100\ mg} = X\ mL$$

0.6 = X

STEP 7: *Round if necessary.*

STEP 8: *Reassess to determine whether the amount to give makes sense.*
If there is 100 mg/mL and the prescribed amount is 60 mg, it makes sense to give 0.6 mL. The nurse should administer enoxaparin injection 0.6 mL subcutaneous.

Using Dimensional Analysis

STEP 1: *What is the unit of measurement to calculate?*
mL

STEP 2: *What quantity of the dose is available?*
1 mL

STEP 3: *What is the dose available? Dose available = Have*
100 mg

STEP 4: *What is the dose needed? Dose needed = Desired*
60 mg

STEP 5: *Should the nurse convert the units of measurement?*
No

STEP 6: *Set up an equation of factors, and solve for X.*

$$X = \frac{Quantity}{Have} \times \frac{Conversion\ (Have)}{Conversion\ (Desired)} \times \frac{Desired}{}$$

$$X\ mL = \frac{1\ mL}{100\ mg} \times \frac{60\ mg}{}$$

X = 0.6

STEP 7: *Round if necessary.*

STEP 8: *Reassess to determine whether the amount to give makes sense.*
If there is 100 mg/mL and the prescribed amount is 60 mg, it makes sense to give 0.6 mL. The nurse should administer enoxaparin injection 0.6 mL subcutaneous.

Ⓝ NCLEX® Connection: Pharmacological and Parenteral Therapies, Dosage Calculation

chapter 70

Overview

- Amputation is the removal of a body part, most commonly an extremity.

- Amputations can be elective due to complications of peripheral vascular disease and arteriosclerosis, or traumatic due to an accident.

- Amputations are described in regard to the extremity and whether they are located above or below the designated joint.

- The term disarticulation describes an amputation performed through a joint.

- Upper extremity amputations include above- and below-the-elbow amputations, wrist and shoulder disarticulations, and finger amputations. Traumatic amputation is the primary cause of upper extremity amputations.

- Lower extremity amputations include above- and below-the-knee amputations, hip and knee disarticulations, Syme amputation (removal of foot with ankle saved), midfoot and toe amputations.

- Lower extremity amputations are usually done due to peripheral vascular disease as a result of arteriosclerosis, and every effort is made to save as much of the extremity as possible. Even loss of the big toe can significantly affect balance and ambulation. Salvage of the knee with a below-the-knee amputation (BKA) also improves function over an above-the-knee amputation (AKA).

- The higher the level of amputation, the greater the amount of effort that will be required to use a prosthesis.

- The level of the amputation is determined by the presence of adequate blood flow needed for healing.

- Older adult clients are poor candidates for prosthetic training due to the amount of energy required for ambulation.

- Significant changes to a client's body image occur after an amputation and should be addressed during the client's perioperative and rehabilitative phases.

Health Promotion and Disease Prevention

- Clients who have diabetes mellitus should monitor blood glucose and maintain within the expected reference range.

- Use safety measures when working with heavy machinery or in areas where there is a risk of electrocution or burns.

- Encourage clients to quit or not start smoking, maintain a healthy weight, and exercise regularly.

- Tell clients to maintain good foot care and seek early medical attention for nonhealing wounds.

Assessment

- Risk Factors
  - Traumatic injury (motor vehicle crashes, industrial equipment, and combat/war injuries)
  - Thermal injury (frostbite, electrocution, burns)
  - Peripheral vascular disease
  - Malignancy
  - Chronic disease processes
    - Peripheral vascular disease resulting in ischemia/gangrene
    - Diabetes mellitus resulting in peripheral neuropathy and peripheral vascular disease
    - Infection (osteomyelitis)
  - Older adult clients have a higher risk of peripheral vascular disease and diabetes mellitus resulting in decreased tissue perfusion and peripheral neuropathy. Both conditions place older adult clients at risk for lower extremity amputation.
- Clinical manifestations of decreased tissue perfusion
  - Clients may or may not report pain.
  - History of injury or disease process precipitating amputation
  - Altered peripheral pulses (may need to use Doppler)

M◈   View Video: Doppler Assessment of Pulses

  - Differences in temperature of extremities (level of leg at which temperature becomes cool)
  - Altered color of extremities (black indicates gangrene, cyanosis indicates vascular compromise)
  - Presence of infection and open wounds
  - Lack of sensation in the affected extremity
- Nursing Actions
  - Monitor capillary refill by comparing the extremities. In older adult clients, capillary refill may be difficult to monitor due to thickened and opaque nails.
  - Observe for edema, necrosis, and lack of hair distribution of the extremity due to inadequate peripheral circulation.
- Diagnostic procedures to determine blood flow at various levels of an extremity
  - Angiography – Allows visualization of peripheral vasculature and areas of impaired circulation
  - Doppler laser and ultrasonography studies – Measure speed of blood flow in an extremity
  - Transcutaneous oxygen pressure (TcPO$_2$) – Measures oxygen pressures in an extremity to indicate blood flow in the extremity, which is a reliable indicator for healing
  - Ankle-brachial index – Measures difference between ankle and brachial systolic pressures

Patient-Centered Care

- Management of Traumatic Amputation
  - Implement medical emergency system.
  - Apply direct pressure using gauze, if available, or clean cloth to prevent life-threatening hemorrhage.
  - Elevate the extremity above the heart to decrease blood loss.
  - Wrap the severed extremity in dry sterile gauze (if available) or in a clean cloth, and place in a sealed plastic bag.
  - Submerge the bag in ice water, and send with the client.
- Surgical Interventions – Surgical Amputation Techniques
  - Closed amputation
    - This is the most common technique used. Skin flap is sutured over end of residual limb, closing site.
  - Open amputation
    - This technique is used when an active infection is present. Skin flap is not sutured over end of residual limb allowing for drainage of infection. Skin flap is closed at a later date.
- Nursing Actions (pre, post)
  - Prevent postoperative complications (hypovolemia, pain, infection).
  - Assess surgical site for bleeding. Monitor vital signs frequently.
  - Monitor tissue perfusion of end of residual limb.
    - Palpate residual limb for warmth. Heat may indicate infection.
    - Compare pulse most proximal to incision with pulse in other extremity.
  - Monitor and treat pain.
    - Differentiate between phantom limb and incisional pain.
      - Phantom limb pain is the sensation of pain in the location of the extremity following the amputation.
      - Phantom limb pain is related to severed nerve pathways and is a frequent complication in clients who experienced chronic limb pain before the amputation. This pain or sensation may be experienced immediately after surgery, up to several weeks, or indefinitely.
      - Phantom limb pain occurs less frequently following traumatic amputation.
      - Clients often describe the pain as deep and burning, cramping, shooting, or aching.
    - Incisional pain is treated with analgesics.
    - Phantom limb pain is treated much differently from incisional pain.
      - Administering beta blockers such as propranolol (Inderal) may relieve the continual dull, burning sensation associated with the amputated limb.
      - Administering antiepileptics such as gabapentin (Neurontin) or carbamazepine (Tegretol) may relieve sharp, stabbing, and burning phantom limb pain.
      - Some clients may have relief from antispasmodics and antidepressant medication.
      - The nurse should recognize the pain is real and manage it accordingly.
      - Alternative treatment for phantom limb pain may include nonpharmacological methods such as massage, heat, biofeedback, or relaxation therapy.
      - Teach the client how to push the residual limb down toward the bed while supported on a soft pillow; it helps to reduce phantom limb pain and prepare the limb for a prosthesis.

- ○ Monitor for signs of infection and/or nonhealing of incision. Infection can lead to osteomyelitis.
  - Amputation may not heal if performed below the level of adequate tissue perfusion.
  - Position the affected extremity in dependent position to promote blood flow/oxygenation.
  - Administer antibiotics and change dressings as prescribed if open amputation was performed.
  - Record characteristics of drainage, such as amount, color, and odor.
- ○ Client's perception and feelings regarding amputation of body part
  - Allow for the client/family to grieve for the loss of the body part and change in body image.
  - Feelings may include depression, anger, withdrawal, and grief.
  - The nurse should assess the psychosocial well-being of the client. Assess for feelings of altered self-concept and self-esteem, and willingness and motivation for rehabilitation.
  - The nurse should facilitate a supportive environment for both the client and family so grief can be processed. Refer the client to religious/spiritual adviser, social worker, or counselor.
  - Rehabilitation should include adaptation to new body image and integration of prosthetic and adaptive devices into self image.
- ○ Residual limb preparation and prosthesis fitting
  - Residual limb must be shaped and shrunk in preparation for prosthetic training.
  - Shrinkage interventions
    - □ Wrapping the stump, using elastic bandages (figure-eight wrap) to prevent restriction of blood flow and decrease edema.
    - □ Using a stump shrinker sock (easier for the client to apply).
    - □ Using an air splint (plastic inflatable device) inflated to protect and shape the residual limb and for easy access to inspect the wound.
- ○ Client Education
  - Explain to the client how to care for and wrap the residual limb and perform limb-strengthening exercises.
  - Reinforce the proper application and care of the prosthesis to the client.
  - Explain to the client how to safely transfer and use mobility devices and adaptive aids.
  - Explain to the client how to manage phantom limb pain.
- Teamwork and Collaboration (consultations, referrals)
  - ○ Intensive efforts by the interprofessional team will be necessary to facilitate successful rehabilitation.
  - ○ A certified prosthetic orthotist will fit client with prosthesis after wound is healed and stump has shrunk.
  - ○ A physical therapist will train client in the application and care of prosthesis and mobility aids.
  - ○ A psychologist may be needed to help with adjustment to loss of extremity.
  - ○ A social worker assist the client with financial issues and can refer the client to resources and a support group or organization for those who had an amputation.

- Flexion Contractures
  - Flexion contractures are more likely with the hip or knee joint following amputation due to improper positioning.
  - Nursing Actions
    - Prevention includes range-of-motion (ROM) exercises and proper positioning immediately after surgery.
    - Avoid elevating the stump on a pillow after the first 24 hr following surgery.
    - Have the client lie prone for 20 to 30 min several times a day.
    - Discourage prolonged sitting in a chair.
  - Client Education
    - Have physical therapist teach client some exercises that will prevent contractures.
    - Have the client stand using good posture with residual limb in extension. This also will aid in balance.

APPLICATION EXERCISES

1. A nurse is presenting information to clients at a health fair on measures to reduce the risk of amputation. Which of the follow information should the nurse provide? (Select all that apply.)

_____ A. Encourage clients who smoke to consider smoking cessation programs.

_____ B. Encourage clients who have diabetes mellitus to maintain blood glucose within the reference range.

_____ C. Instruct clients to unplug electrical equipment when performing repairs.

_____ D. Encourage clients who have vascular disease to maintain good foot care.

_____ E. Advise clients to wait 2 hr after taking pain medication before driving.

2. A nurse is assessing an older adult client who has arteriosclerosis and is scheduled for a possible right lower extremity amputation. Which of the following are expected findings in the affected extremity? (Select all that apply.)

_____ A. Skin cool to touch from mid-calf to the toes

_____ B. Lower leg appears dusky when client is sitting

_____ C. Palpable pounding pedal pulse

_____ D. Lack of hair on lower leg

_____ E. Blackened areas on several toes

3. A nurse is caring for a client following a below-the-elbow amputation. Which of the following are appropriate actions by the nurse? (Select all that apply.)

_____ A. Encourage dependent positioning of the residual limb.

_____ B. Inspect for presence and amount of drainage.

_____ C. Implement shrinkage intervention of the residual limb.

_____ D. Wrap the residual limb in a circular manner using gauze.

_____ E. Assess for feelings of body image changes.

4. A client who had an above-the-knee amputation reports having sharp, stabbing type of phantom pain. Which of the following is an appropriate action by the nurse?

A. Facilitate counseling services.

B. Encourage use of cold therapy.

C. Question whether the pain is real.

D. Administer an antiepileptic medication.

5. A nurse is preparing a plan of care to prevent a client from developing flexion contractions following a below-the-knee amputation 24 hr ago. Which of the following should the nurse include in the plan of care?

    A. Elevate the residual limb on a pillow.

    B. Position the client prone several times each day.

    C. Wrap the stump in a figure-eight pattern.

    D. Encourage sitting in a chair during the day.

6. A nurse is completing discharge planning for a client who had an amputation. What members of an interprofessional team will the nurse include in the discharge planning process? Use the ATI Active Learning Template: Basic Concept to complete this item to include the following:

    A. Related Content: List three members of the interprofessional team.

    B. Underlying Principles: Describe the principal purpose of each member.

APPLICATION EXERCISES KEY

1. A. **CORRECT:** Smoking cessation can decrease the development of arteriosclerosis and possible amputation of a lower extremity.

    B. **CORRECT:** Regulation of blood glucose within a normal reference range may decrease the development of arteriosclerosis and possible amputation of a lower extremity.

    C. **CORRECT:** Unplugging electrical equipment when performing repairs prevents electrocution and injury to an extremity, which may lead to amputation.

    D. **CORRECT:** Maintaining good foot care may prevent a possible infection which can result in amputation.

    E. INCORRECT: Driving under the influence of pain medication may lead to an accident and injury to an extremity requiring amputation.

     NCLEX® Connection: Health Promotion and Maintenance, Health Promotion/Disease Prevention

2. A. **CORRECT:** The client may have coolness of the affected extremity where decreased vascularization starts.

    B. **CORRECT:** The client's affected extremity may become dusky when sitting due to decreased vascularization of the extremity.

    C. INCORRECT: The client will have a lack of or diminished pedal pulse of the affected extremity due to decreased vascularization.

    D. **CORRECT:** The client may have decreased hair growth on areas of the affected extremity due to decreased vascularization.

    E. **CORRECT:** The client may have blackened areas on several toes suggestive of gangrene due to decreased vascularization to the affected extremity.

     NCLEX® Connection: Physiological Adaptations, Pathophysiology

3. A. **CORRECT:** Dependent positioning of the residual limb can improve circulation to the end of the stump and promote healing.

    B. **CORRECT:** Inspecting for the presence and amount of drainage can assist in determining early manifestations of infection.

    C. **CORRECT:** Residual limb preparation includes shrinkage interventions before fitting of the prosthesis.

    D. INCORRECT: Wrap the residual limb with an elastic bandage in a figure-eight manner to prevent restriction of blood flow before fitting for the prosthesis.

    E. **CORRECT:** The client may have feelings of depression, anger, withdrawal, and grief due to body image changes, and the nurse should assess for these feelings.

     NCLEX® Connection: Physiological Adaptations, Alterations in Body Systems

4.   A. INCORRECT: Counseling services can assist clients to cope with body image changes and is not prescribed for treatment of phantom pain.

   B. INCORRECT: Heat therapy, not cold therapy, to the residual limb is an alternative therapy that may relieve phantom pain.

   C. INCORRECT: Phantom pain is related to the severed nerve pathways following the amputation, and the nurse should not question whether the pain is real.

   D. **CORRECT:** Antiepileptic medication may relieve the client's phantom pain.

   Ⓝ NCLEX® Connection: Pharmacological and Parenteral Therapies, Pharmacological Pain Management

5.   A. INCORRECT: To avoid flexion contractures, the residual limb should not be elevated with a pillow after 24 hr of the amputation.

   B. **CORRECT:** The client should lie prone several times each day for 20 to 30 min to prevent flexion contractures developing.

   C. INCORRECT: The client may have the residual limb wrapped in a figure eight to prepare for the prosthesis, but this action does not prevent flexion contractures.

   D. INCORRECT: The client may develop flexion contractures by allowing the residual stump to hang in a bent position when sitting for an extended period following the amputation.

   Ⓝ NCLEX® Connection: Reduction of Risk Potential, Potential for Complications of Diagnostic Tests/ Treatments/Procedures

6.   *Using the ATI Active Learning Template: Basic Concept*

   A. Related Content
   - Certified prosthetic orthotist
   - Physical therapist
   - Psychologist
   - Social worker

   B. Underlying Principles
   - Certified prosthetic orthotist fits the client with the prosthesis following healing and shrinking of the stump.
   - Physical therapist provides training for applying the prosthesis, assists in mobility training, and reviews mobility aids.
   - Psychologist assists the client/family in adjusting to the loss of an extremity.
   - Social worker provides referral information for financial assistance, resources and support groups, or organizations to help adjust to life-changing physical conditions.

   Ⓝ NCLEX® Connection: Health Promotion and Maintenance, Aging Process

chapter 71

Overview

- Osteoporosis is a common chronic metabolic bone disorder resulting in low bone density. Osteoporosis occurs when the rate of bone resorption (osteoclast cells) exceeds the rate of bone formation (osteoblast cells) resulting in fragile bone tissue and subsequent fractures.

- Osteopenia, the precursor to osteoporosis, refers to low bone mineral density relative to the client's age and sex.

- Bone mineral density peaks between the ages of 18 to 30. After peak years, bone density decreases, with a significant increase in the rate of loss in postmenopausal women due to estrogen loss.

Health Promotion and Disease Prevention

- Ensure the client's diet includes adequate amounts of calcium and vitamin D, especially before age 35.
  - Foods rich in vitamin D are most fish, egg yolks, fortified milk, and cereal.
  - Foods rich in calcium are milk products, green vegetables, fortified orange juice and cereals, red and white beans, and figs.
- Encourage the client to take a calcium supplement with vitamin D if dietary intake is inadequate (lactose intolerant).
- Encourage the client to limit the amount of carbonated beverages, which may cause calcium loss.
- Encourage the client to expose areas of skin to sun 5 to 30 min twice a week. Exposure to the sun for any length of time should include wearing sunscreen to avoid getting a sunburn.
- Encourage the client to discuss the pros and cons of hormone replacement therapy postmenopausally with her provider.
- Encourage the client to engage in weight-bearing exercises (e.g. walking, lifting weights).

Assessment

- Risk Factors
  - Female gender, family history, and thin, lean body build are precursors to low bone density.
  - If the client is over age 60, is a female who has postmenopausal estrogen deficiency, has low levels of calcitonin, or is male with low testosterone, increased bone loss may occur.
  - History of low calcium intake with suboptimal levels of vitamin D decreases bone formation.
  - History of smoking and high alcohol intake (three or more drinks per day) causes decreased bone formation and increased bone absorption.

- ○ Excess caffeine consumption causes excretion of calcium in the urine.

- ○ Inadequate intake of calcium and vitamin D in the diet stimulates the parathyroid hormone to be released and triggers calcium to be pulled from the bone.

- ○ Lack of physical activity/prolonged immobility places the client at risk for osteoporosis because bones need the stress of weight-bearing activity for bone rebuilding and maintenance.

- ○ Secondary osteoporosis results from medical conditions including:

  - Hyperparathyroidism.

  - Long-term corticosteroid use (asthma, systemic lupus erythematosus).

  - Long-term anticonvulsant medication use (phenytoin [Dilantin] and phenobarbital affect the absorption and metabolism of calcium).

  - Long-term lack of weight-bearing (spinal cord injury).

- ○ Older adult clients have an increased risk of falls related to impaired balance, generalized weakness, gait changes, and impaired vision and hearing. Medication side effects can cause orthostatic hypotension, urinary frequency, or confusion, which can also raise the client's risk for falls.

- • Clinical Manifestations

  - ○ Reduced height (postmenopausal)

  - ○ Acute back pain after lifting or bending (worse with activity, relieved by rest)

  - ○ Restriction in movement and spinal deformity

  - ○ History of fractures (wrist, femur, thoracic spine)

  - ○ Thoracic (kyphosis) of the dorsal spine

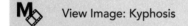
View Image: Kyphosis

  - ○ Pain upon palpation over affected area

  - ○ Laboratory Tests

    - Serum calcium, vitamin D, phosphorus, and alkaline phosphatase levels are drawn to rule out other metabolic bone diseases (Paget's disease or osteomalacia).

    - Thyroid tests and serum protein levels also are checked to rule out hyperthyroidism.

  - ○ Diagnostic Procedures

    - Radiographs

      □ Radiographs of the spine and long bones reveal low bone density and fractures.

    - Dual x-ray absorptiometry (DXA)

      □ A DXA scan is used to screen for early changes in bone density and is usually done on the hip or spine.

      □ A peripheral DXA scan is used to assess the bone density of the heel, forearm, or finger.

      □ DXA uses two beams of radiation. Findings are analyzed by a computer and interpreted by a radiologist. Clients receives a score that relates their amount of bone density to other people in their age group and gender.

      □ The client will lie on an x-ray table while a scan of a selected area is done.

- Peripheral quantitative ultrasound (pQUS)
  - □ An ultrasound, usually of the heel, tibia, and patella. pQUS is an inexpensive, portable, and low-risk method to determine osteoporosis and assessing for risk of fracture, especially in men over age 70 years.
- Quantitative Computed Tomography (QCT)
  - □ QCT is used to measure bone density, especially in the vertebral column.

Patient-Centered Care

- Nursing Care
  - ○ Administer medications as prescribed.
  - ○ Instruct the client and family regarding dietary calcium food sources and to limit excess caffeine, alcohol, and carbonated beverage consumption, all of which increase bone loss.
  - ○ Provide information regarding calcium and vitamin D supplementation (take with food).
  - ○ Instruct the client on the need for adequate amounts of protein, magnesium, vitamin K, and other trace minerals needed for bone formation.
  - ○ Reinforce the need for exposure to vitamin D (moderate sun exposure using sunscreen, fortified milk).
  - ○ Encourage weight-bearing exercises (at least 30 min, three to five times a week) to improve strength and reduce bone loss.
  - ○ Assess the home environment for safety (remove throw rugs, provide adequate lighting, clear walkways) to prevent falls, which may result in fractures.
    - Reinforce the use of safety equipment and assistive devices.
    - Instruct the client to avoid inclement weather (ice, slippery surfaces).
    - Clearly mark thresholds, doorways, and steps.
- Medications
  - ○ Medications such as calcium and vitamin D can slow or prevent osteoporosis. A combination of several of these medications may be used in place of just one.

OSTEOPOROSIS CLASSIFICATIONS/MEDICATIONS	
THERAPEUTIC INTENT	**NURSING CONSIDERATIONS**
Thyroid Hormone – calcitonin human, calcitonin salmon (Miacalcin, Fortical)	
› Decreases bone resorption by inhibiting osteoclast activity for prevention and treatment of osteoporosis, hypercalcemia, and Paget's disease of the bone	› Calcitonin human can only be administered subcutaneously. › Calcitonin salmon can be administered subcutaneously, intramuscularly, and intranasally.
Teriparatide (Forteo)	
› A parathyroid hormone that stimulates osteoblasts to increase new bone formation to increase bone mass › Stimulates calcium absorption	› Administered only subcutaneously. › Contraindicated if hypercalcemic. › Report leg cramps or bone pain to the provider.

| OSTEOPOROSIS CLASSIFICATIONS/MEDICATIONS | |
THERAPEUTIC INTENT	NURSING CONSIDERATIONS
Estrogen Hormone Supplements – estrogen (Premarin), estrogen and medroxyprogesterone (Prempro)	
› Replaces estrogen lost due to menopause or surgical removal of ovaries	› Instruct client on potential complications, including breast and endometrial cancers and deep-vein thrombosis (DVT). › Reinforce monthly breast self-examinations. Estrogen should be given along with progesterone in women who still have their uterus.
Estrogen Agonist/Antagonists – raloxifene hydrochloride (Evista)	
› Decreases osteoclast activity, subsequently decreasing bone resorption and increasing bone mineral density › Treats postmenopausal osteoporosis as well as breast cancer	› Avoid for clients with a history of DVT. › Monitor liver function tests. › Instruct client on need for calcium and vitamin D supplements. › Monitor and instruct client to report unusual calf pain or tenderness to the provider.
Calcium Supplement – calcium-carbonate (Os-Cal, Caltrate 600), calcium-citrate (Citracal)	
› Supplements calcium that is consumed in food products to promote healthy bones (not to slow osteoporosis)	› Give with food in divided doses with 6 to 8 oz of water. › Calcium supplements may cause GI upset. › Monitor for kidney stones.
Vitamin D Supplement	
› Increases absorption of calcium from the intestinal tract and availability of calcium in the serum needed for remineralization of bone › Needed by individuals who are not exposed to adequate amounts of sunlight or who do not meet its daily requirements	› Vitamin D is a fat-soluble vitamin, so toxicity can occur. Symptoms of toxicity include weakness, fatigue, nausea, constipation, and kidney stones.
Bisphosphonates (inhibit bone resorption) – alendronate (Fosamax), ibandronate (Boniva), risedronate (Actonel)	
› Decreases number and actions of osteoclasts, subsequently inhibiting bone resorption for prevention and treatment of osteoporosis, hypercalcemia, and Paget's disease of the bone	› Risk for esophagitis and esophageal ulcers. Report early signs of indigestion, chest pain, difficulty swallowing, or bloody emesis to provider immediately. › Take with 8 oz of water in the early morning before eating. › Remain upright for 30 min after taking medication.

- Teamwork and Collaboration (consultations, referrals)
  - Physical therapy may be used to establish an exercise regimen: 20 to 30 min of aerobic exercise (e.g. walking) at least three times per week with addition of weight lifting.
  - Clients may need rehabilitation if fractures cause immobilization or disability.
  - Most hip fractures are due to osteoporosis. Joint repair or joint arthroplasty requires physical therapy for a full recovery.
- Therapeutic Procedures
  - Orthotic devices are available for immobilization of the spine immediately after a compression fracture of the spine.
    - The device provides support and decreases pain.
    - A physical therapist fits the device for the client and teaches him how to apply it.
    - Nursing Actions
      - Teach the client how to check for skin breakdown under the orthotic device.
      - Instruct the client on the importance of good posture and body mechanics.
      - Teach the client to log roll when getting out of bed.
      - Instruct the client to use heat and back rubs to promote muscle relaxation.
- Surgical Interventions
  - Joint repair or joint arthroplasty may be necessary to repair or replace a joint weakened by osteoporosis. This is most often the hip joint.
  - Vertebroplasty or kyphoplasty are minimally invasive procedures performed by a radiologist. Bone cement is injected into the fractured space of the vertebral column with or without balloon inflation. Balloon inflation of the fracture is to contain the cement and add height to the fractured vertebra.
    - Mild sedation is used.
    - Client lies in a supine position for 1 to 2 hr following procedure.
    - Monitor vital signs for shortness of breath and the puncture site for bleeding.
    - Complete a neurological assessment.
    - Apply cold therapy to the injection site.

Complications

- Fractures are the leading complication of osteoporosis. Early recognition and treatment is essential.
  - Nursing Actions
    - Review risk factors for osteoporosis and falls, assess the client's dietary intake of calcium, reinforce daily exercise including weight-bearing activities, and ensure proper screening with a DXA scan.

APPLICATION EXERCISES

1. A nurse is admitting an older adult client who has suspected osteoporosis. Which of following is an expected clinical finding? (Select all that apply.)

_____ A. History of consuming one glass of wine daily

__X__ B. Loss in height of 2 in (5.1 cm)

__X__ C. Body mass index (BMI) of 21

__X__ D. Kyphotic curve at upper thoracic spine

__X__ E. History of lactose intolerance

2. A nurse is performing health screenings of clients at a health fair. Which of the following clients are at risk for osteoporosis? (Select all that apply.)

__X__ A. A 40-year-old client who takes prednisone (Deltasone) for asthma

_____ B. A 30-year-old client who jogs 3 miles daily

__X__ C. A 45-year-old client who takes phenytoin (Dilantin) for seizures

__X__ D. A 65-year-old client who has a sedentary lifestyle

__X__ E. A 70-year-old client who has smoked for 50 years

3. A nurse is planning discharge teaching on home safety for an older adult client who has osteoporosis. Which of the following information should the nurse include in the teaching? (Select all that apply.)

__X__ A. Remove throw rugs in walkways.

__X__ B. Use prescribed assistive devices.

__X__ C. Remove clutter from the environment.

_____ D. Walk with caution on icy surfaces.

__X__ E. Maintain lighting of doorway areas.

4. A nurse is providing dietary teaching about calcium-rich foods to a client who has osteoporosis. Which of the following foods should the nurse include in the instructions?

A. White bread

(B.) White beans

C. White meat of chicken

D. White rice

5. A nurse is providing care for a client who had a vertebroplasty of the thoracic spine. Which of the following is an appropriate action by the nurse?

    A. Apply heat to the client's puncture site.

    B. Place the client in a supine position.

    C. Turn the client every 4 hr.

    D. Ambulate the client within the first hour post-procedure.

6. A nurse is administering raloxifene hydrochloride (Evista) to a client who has osteoporosis. What should the nurse consider before administering the medication? Use the ATI Active Learning Template: Medication to complete this item to include the following:

    A. Therapeutic Uses: List two.

    B. Nursing Interventions: Describe two.

    C. Evaluation of Medication Effectiveness: Describe one.

APPLICATION EXERCISES KEY

1.   A. **INCORRECT:** A client who consumes more than three glasses of alcohol each day is at risk for developing osteoporosis because alcohol can increase bone loss.

     B. **CORRECT:** The loss of 2 inches of height is suggestive of having osteoporosis due to fractures of the vertebral column.

     C. **CORRECT:** A client who has a BMI of 21 is at risk of developing osteoporosis due to low body weight and thin body build, suggesting decreased bone mass.

     D. **CORRECT:** Kyphosis curve is highly suggestive of having osteoporosis due to fractures of the vertebrae causing the curve.

     E. **CORRECT:** Lactose intolerance is highly suggestive of having osteoporosis due to possible lack of calcium intake.

      NCLEX® Connection: Physiological Adaptations, Pathophysiology

2.   A. **CORRECT:** Prednisone affects the absorption and metabolism of calcium and places the client at risk for osteoporosis.

     B. **INCORRECT:** Weight-bearing activities decrease the risk for osteoporosis due to placing stress on bones, which promotes bone rebuilding and maintenance.

     C. **CORRECT:** Phenytoin affects the absorption and metabolism of calcium and places the client at risk for osteoporosis.

     D. **CORRECT:** A sedentary lifestyle places the client at risk for osteoporosis because bones need the stress of weight bearing activity for bone rebuilding and maintenance.

     E. **CORRECT:** Smoking increases the risk for osteoporosis because it decreases osteogenesis.

      NCLEX® Connection: Health Promotion and Maintenance, Health Promotion/Disease Prevention

3.   A. **CORRECT:** Removing throw rugs in walkways may help to prevent a fall and bone fracture.

     B. **CORRECT:** Using prescribed assistive devices may help to prevent a fall and bone fracture.

     C. **CORRECT:** Removing clutter from the environment may help to prevent tripping, falling, and a bone fracture.

     D. **INCORRECT:** The client should avoid walking on icy surfaces during inclement weather to help prevent a fall and bone fracture.

     E. **CORRECT:** Good lighting in doorway areas may prevent a fall and bone fracture.

      NCLEX® Connection: Basic Care and Comfort, Nutrition and Oral Hydration

4.   A. INCORRECT: White bread is not a calcium-rich food, but it is a good source of carbohydrates.

   B. **CORRECT:** White beans should be included in the teaching because they are a good source of calcium.

   C. INCORRECT: White meat of chicken is not a calcium-rich food, but it is a good source of protein.

   D. INCORRECT: White rice is not a calcium-rich food, but it is a good source of carbohydrates.

    NCLEX® Connection: Safety and Infection Control, Home Safety

5.   A. INCORRECT: The client should have cold therapy applied to the puncture site to decrease bleeding and swelling following the procedure.

   B. **CORRECT:** The client should remain in a supine position with bed flat for the first 1 to 2 hr following the procedure to allow for hardening of the cement.

   C. INCORRECT: The client should not turn frequently but remain in a supine position with bed flat for 1 to 2 hr following the procedure.

   D. INCORRECT: The client should not ambulate but lay in a supine position with bed flat for 1 to 2 hr following the procedure.

    NCLEX® Connection: Reduction of Risk Potential, Diagnostic Tests

6.   *Using the ATI Active Learning Template: Medication*

   A. Therapeutic Uses

   • Estrogen agonist/antagonist

   • Decreases bone resorption and increases bone density

   • Treatment of postmenopausal osteoporosis

   • Treatment of breast cancer by reducing the risk of cancer metastasis

   B. Nursing Interventions

   • Avoid administering to a client who has a history of DVT.

   • Instruct the client to report unusual calf pain or tenderness, a sign of DVT.

   • Assess liver function tests periodically.

   • Review need for calcium and vitamin D supplements when taking the medication.

   C. Evaluation of Medication Effectiveness

   • Improved bone mineral density

   • No further loss in height

   • No metastasis of the cancer

    NCLEX® Connection: Pharmacological and Parenteral Therapies, Medication Administration

chapter 72

Overview

- A fracture is a break in a bone secondary to trauma or a pathological condition.

- Fractures caused by trauma are the most common type of bone fracture.

- Pathological fractures may be caused by metastatic cancer, osteoporosis, or Paget's disease.

- Bone is continually going through a process of remodeling as osteoclasts release calcium from the bone and osteoblasts build up the bone.

- Remodeling of bone occurs at equal rates until an individual reaches their thirties. From this age on, the activity of the osteoclasts outpace the osteoblasts, increasing an individual's risk of osteoporosis. In women, this process significantly increases following menopause. Subsequently, women experience fractures secondary to osteoporosis a decade or so earlier than men.

Health Promotion and Disease Prevention

- Ensure recommended intake of calcium for developmental stage in life.

- Ensure adequate intake of vitamin D and/or exposure to sunlight.

- Monitor for development of osteoporosis, especially in postmenopausal clients and clients who have a thyroid disorder.

- Engage in weight-bearing exercise on a regular basis.

- Take a bisphosphonate if prescribed by the provider to slow bone resorption and treat osteoporosis.

- Use caution to prevent falls or accidents.

- Prevent injury with the use of seat belts and helmets.

FRACTURES

Overview

- A closed, or simple, fracture does not break through the skin surface.

- An open, or compound, fracture disrupts the skin integrity, causing an open wound and tissue injury with a risk of infection.

- Open fractures are graded based upon the extent of tissue injury.

  - Grade I – minimal skin damage

  - Grade II – damage includes skin and muscle contusions but without extensive soft tissue injury

  - Grade III – damage is excessive to skin, muscles, nerves, and blood vessels

- A complete fracture goes through the entire bone, dividing it into two distinct parts. An incomplete fracture goes through part of the bone.

- A simple fracture has one fracture line, while a comminuted fracture has multiple fracture lines splitting the bone into multiple pieces.

- A displaced fracture has bone fragments that are not in alignment, and a non-displaced fracture has bone fragments that remain in alignment.

- A fatigue (stress) fracture results when excess strain occurs from recreational and athletic activities.

- Compression fracture occurs from a loading force pressing on callus bone. This condition is common in the older adult client who has osteoporosis.

- Common Types of Fractures

  - Comminuted: Bone is fragmented.

  - Oblique: Fracture occurs at oblique angle and across bone.

  - Spiral: Fracture occurs from twisting motion (common with physical abuse).

  - Impacted: Fractured bone is wedged inside opposite fractured fragment.

  - Greenstick: Fracture occurs on one side (cortex) but does not extend completely through the bone (most often in children).

- Hip fractures are the most common injury in older adults and are usually associated with falls.

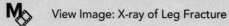

M View Image: X-ray of Leg Fracture

Assessment

- Risk Factors

  - Osteoporosis

    - Excessive exercising and weight loss from dieting and malnutrition can lead to osteoporosis.

    - Women who do not use estrogen replacement therapy after menopause lose estrogen and are unable to form strong new bone.

    - Clients on long-term corticosteroid therapy lose calcium from their bones due to direct inhibition of osteoblast function, inhibition of gastrointestinal calcium absorption, and enhancement of bone resorption.

  - Falls

  - Motor vehicle crashes

  - Substance use disorder

  - Diseases (bone cancer, Paget's disease)

  - Contact sports and hazardous recreational activities (football, skiing)

  - Physical abuse

  - Lactose intolerance

  - Age, as bone becomes less dense with advancing age

- Clinical Manifestations
  - History of trauma, metabolic bone disorders, chronic conditions, and possible use of corticosteroid therapy
  - Pain and/or reduced movement manifests at the area of fracture or the area distal to the fracture.
  - Physical Assessment Findings
    - Crepitus: A grating sound created by the rubbing of bone fragments
    - Deformity: Internal rotation of extremity, shortened extremity, visible bone with open fracture
    - Muscle spasms: Due to the pulling forces of the bone when not aligned
    - Edema: Swelling from trauma
    - Ecchymosis: Bleeding into underlying soft tissues from trauma
  - Diagnostic Procedures
    - Standard radiographs, computed tomography (CT) imaging scan used to detect fractures of the hip and pelvis, and/or magnetic resonance imagery (MRI)
      - Identify the type of fracture and location.
      - Indicate pathological fracture resulting from tumor or mass.
      - Determine soft tissue damage around fracture (MRI).
    - A bone scan using radioactive material determines hairline fractures and complications/ delayed healing.

Patient-Centered Care

- Nursing Care
  - Provide emergency care at time of injury.
  - Maintain ABCs.
  - Monitor the client's vital signs and neurological status because injury to vital organs may occur due to bone fragments (fractures of pelvis, ribs).
  - Stabilize the injured area, including the joints above and below the fracture, by using a splint and avoiding unnecessary movement.
  - Maintain proper alignment of the affected extremity.
  - Elevate the limb above the heart and apply ice.
  - Assess for bleeding and apply pressure, if needed.
  - Cover open wounds with a sterile dressing.
  - Remove clothing and jewelry near the injury or on the affected extremity.
  - Keep the client warm.
  - Assess pain frequently and follow pain management protocols, both pharmacologic and nonpharmacologic.
  - Initiate and continue neurovascular checks at least every hour. Immediately report any change in status to the provider.
  - Prepare the client for any immobilization procedure appropriate for the fracture.

IMMOBILIZING INTERVENTIONS: CASTS, SPLINTS, AND TRACTION

Overview

- Immobilization secures the injured extremity in order to:
  - Prevent further injury.
  - Promote healing/circulation.
  - Reduce pain.
  - Correct a deformity.
- Types of Immobilization Devices
  - Casts
  - Splints/immobilizers
  - Traction
  - External fixation
  - Internal fixation
- Closed reduction is when a pulling force (traction) is applied manually to realign the displaced fractured bone fragments. Once the fracture is reduced, immobilization is used to allow the bone to heal.
- Open reduction is when a surgical incision is made and the bone is manually aligned and kept in place with plates and screws. This is known as an open reduction and internal fixation (ORIF) procedure.

Patient-Centered Care

- Nursing Care
  - Neurovascular assessment is essential throughout immobilization. Assessments are performed every hour for the first 24 hr and every 1 to 4 hr thereafter following initial trauma to monitor neurovascular compromise related to edema and/or the immobilization device. Neurovascular assessment includes the assessment of:
    - Pain – Assess the client's pain level, location, and frequency. Assess pain using a 0 to 10 pain rating scale and have the client describe the pain. Immobilization, ice, and elevation of the extremity with the use of analgesics should relieve most of the pain.
    - Sensation – Assess the client for numbness or tingling sensation of extremity. Loss of sensation may indicate nerve damage.
    - Skin temperature – Check the temperature of the affected extremity. The extremity should be warm, not cool, to touch. Cool skin may indicate decreased arterial perfusion.
    - Capillary refill – Press nail beds of affected extremity until blanching occurs. Blood return should be within 3 seconds. Prolonged refill indicates decreased arterial perfusion. Nail beds that are cyanotic may indicate venous congestion.
    - Pulses – Pulses should be palpable and strong. Pulses should be equal to unaffected extremity. Edema can make it difficult to palpate pulses so Doppler ultrasonography may be required.
    - Movement – Client should be able to move affected extremity in passive motion.

- Casts
    - Casts are more effective than splints or immobilizers because they cannot be removed by the client.
    - Types of Casts
        - Short and long arm and leg casts
        - Walking cast (a rubber walking pad on the sole of the cast assists the client in ambulating when weight bearing is allowed)
        - Spica casts (a portion of the trunk and one or two extremities; typically used on children with congenital hip dysplasia)
        - Body casts (encircle the trunk of the body)
    - Casting Materials
        - Plaster of Paris casts are heavy, not water resistant, and can take 24 to 72 hr to dry.
        - Synthetic fiberglass casts are light, stronger, water resistant, and dry very quickly (in 30 min).
    - Casts, as circumferential immobilizers, are applied once the swelling has subsided (to avoid compartment syndrome). If the swelling continues after cast application and causes unrelieved pain, the cast can be split on one side (univalve) or on both sides (bivalved).
    - A window can be placed in an area of the cast to allow for skin inspection (e.g., if the client has a wound under the cast).
    - Moleskin is used over any rough area of the cast that may rub against the client's skin.
    - Nursing Actions
        - Monitor neurovascular status and assess pain.
        - Apply ice for 24 to 48 hr.
        - Handle a plaster cast with the palms, not fingertips, until the cast is dry to prevent denting the cast.
        - Avoid setting the cast on hard surfaces or sharp edges.
        - Prior to casting, the area is cleaned and dried. Tubular cotton web roll is placed over the affected area to maintain skin integrity. The casting material is then applied.
        - After cast application, position the client so that warm, dry air circulates around and under the cast (support the casted area without pressure under or directly on the cast) for faster drying and to prevent pressure from changing the shape of the cast. Use gloves to touch the cast until it is completely dry.
        - Elevate the cast above the level of the heart during the first 24 to 48 hr to prevent edema of the affected extremity.
        - If any drainage is seen on the cast, it should be outlined, dated, and timed, so it can be monitored for any additional drainage.
        - Older adult clients have an increased risk for impaired skin integrity due to the loss of elasticity of the skin and decreased sensation (comorbidities).
    - Client Education
        - Clients are instructed not to place any foreign objects under the cast to avoid trauma to the skin. Itching under the cast can be relieved by blowing cool air from a hair dryer under the cast.
        - Plastic coverings over the cast can be used to avoid soiling from urine or feces.

□ Demonstrate how plastic bags can be used during baths and showers to keep the cast dry.

□ Report any areas under the cast that become painful, have a "hot spot," have increased drainage, are warm to the touch, or have odor, which may indicate infection.

□ Instruct the client to report immobility and complications such as shortness of breath, skin breakdown, and constipation.

○ Traction

■ Traction uses a pulling force to promote and maintain alignment of the injured area.

■ Goals of traction include:

□ Prevent soft tissue injury.

□ Realign of bone fragments.

□ Decrease muscle spasms and pain.

□ Correct or prevent further deformities.

■ Traction prescriptions should include the type of traction, amount of weight, and whether traction can be removed for nursing care.

■ Classification of Traction

□ Straight or running: The countertraction is provided by the client's body by applying a pulling force in a straight line. Movement of the client's body can alter the traction provided.

□ Balanced suspension: The countertraction is produced by devices such as slings or splints to support the fractured extremity while pulling with ropes and weights. The client's body can be moved without altering the traction.

■ Types of Traction

□ Manual: A pulling force is applied by the hands of the provider for temporary immobilization, usually with sedation or anesthesia, in conjunction with the application of an immobilizing device.

□ Skin: Primary purpose is to decrease muscle spasms and immobilize the extremity prior to surgery. The pulling force is applied by weights that are attached by rope to the client's skin with tape, straps, boots, or cuffs. Examples include Bryant's traction (used for congenital hip dislocation in children) and Buck's traction (used preoperatively for hip fractures for immobilization in adult clients).

 View Image: Buck's Traction

□ Skeletal: The pulling force is applied directly to the bone by weights attached by rope directly to a rod/screw placed through the bone to promote bone alignment. Examples include skeletal tongs (Gardner-Wells) and femoral or tibial pins (Steinmann pin). Weights 15 to 30 lb can be applied as needed.

 View Image: Balanced Suspension Skeletal Traction

□ Halo: Screws are placed through a halo-type bar that encircles the head into the outer table of the bone of the skull. This halo is attached to rods that are secured to a vest worn by the client. Ensure that the wrench to release the rods is attached to the vest when using halo traction in the event CPR is necessary.

- Nursing Actions
  - Assess neurovascular status of the affected body part every hour for 24 hr and every 4 hr after that.
  - Maintain body alignment and realign if the client seems uncomfortable or reports pain.
  - Avoid lifting or removing weights.
  - Ensure that weights hang freely and are not resting on the floor.
  - If the weights are accidentally displaced, replace the weights. If the problem is not corrected, notify the provider.
  - Ensure that pulley ropes are free of knots, fraying, loosening, and improper positioning at least every 8 to 12 hr.
  - Notify the provider if the client experiences severe pain from muscle spasms unrelieved with medications and/or repositioning. Move the client in halo traction as a unit, without applying pressure to the rods. This will prevent loosening of the pins and pain.
  - Routinely monitor skin integrity and document.
  - Use heat/massage, as prescribed, to treat muscle spasms.
  - Use therapeutic touch and relaxation techniques.
  - Pin Site Care
    - Pin care is done frequently throughout immobilization (skeletal traction and external fixation methods) to prevent and to monitor for signs of infection including:
      - Drainage and redness (color, amount, odor).
      - Loosening of pins.
      - Tenting of skin at pin site (skin rising up pin).
    - Pin care protocols (chlorhexidine) are based on provider preference and facility policy. A primary concept of pin care is that one cotton-tip swab is designated for each pin to avoid cross-contamination.
    - Pin care is provided usually once a shift, 1 to 2 times a day, or per facility protocol.
    - Crusting at the pin site should not be removed as this provides a natural barrier to bacteria.
- Medications
  - Prophylactic antibiotics prevent infection when fracture immobilization is achieved. Typically, a broad-spectrum intravenous antibiotic such as cefazolin (Ancef) is administered for 24 to 48 hr post-injury.
  - Analgesics
    - Opioid and nonopioid analgesics may be used as needed to control pain.
    - NSAIDs decrease associated tissue inflammation.
  - Muscle relaxants relieve muscle spasms.
- Splints and immobilizers provide support, control movement, and prevent additional injury.
  - Splints are removable and allow for monitoring of skin swelling or integrity.
  - Splints can be used to support fractured/injured areas until casting occurs and swelling is decreased. Casting is then done or used for post-paralysis injuries to avoid joint contracture.
  - Immobilizers are prefabricated and typically fasten with Velcro straps.
  - Client Education
    - Ensure the client is aware of application protocol regarding full-time or part-time use.
    - Instruct the client to observe for skin breakdown at pressure points.

- Surgical Interventions
  - External Fixation
    - External fixation involves fracture immobilization using percutaneous pins and wires that are attached to a rigid external frame.
    - Used to treat:
      - Comminuted fracture or nonunion fractures with extensive soft tissue damage.
      - Leg length discrepancies from congenital defects.
      - Bone loss related to tumors or osteomyelitis.
    - Advantages include:
      - Immediate fracture stabilization.
      - Minimal blood loss occurring in comparison with internal fixation.
      - Allowing for early mobilization and ambulation.
      - Maintaining alignment of closed fractures that could not be maintained in cast or splint.
      - Permitting wound care with open fractures.
    - Disadvantages include:
      - Risk of pin site infection leading to osteomyelitis.
      - Potential overwhelming appearance to client.
      - Noncompliance issues.
    - Nursing Actions
      - Elevate extremity.
      - Monitor neurovascular status and skin integrity.
      - Assess body image.
      - Pin care every 8 to 12 hr. Monitor site for drainage, color, odor, redness.
      - Observe for signs of fat and pulmonary embolism.
      - Provide antiembolism stockings and sequential compression device to prevent deep-vein thrombosis (DVT).
    - Client Education
      - Teach the client pin care.
      - Discuss clothing and other materials that can be used to cover the device.
      - If activity is restricted, advise the client to perform deep breathing and leg exercises and other techniques to prevent complications to immobilization, such as pneumonia or thrombus formation.
  - Open Reduction and Internal Fixation (ORIF)
    - Open reduction refers to visualization of a fracture through an incision in the skin, and internal fixation with plates, screws, pins, rods, and prosthetics as needed.
    - After the bone heals, the hardware may be removed, depending on the location and type of hardware.
    - Nursing Actions
      - Prevent dislocation, especially of hip.
      - Monitor skin integrity.

- Ensure heels are off bed at all times and inspect bony prominence every shift.

- Perform a neurovascular assessment.

- Observe the cast or dressing for postoperative drainage. The cast may have a window cut in it through which the incision can be viewed. An elastic wrap is used to keep the window block cover in place to decrease localized edema.

- Observe for signs of fat and pulmonary embolism.

- Provide antiembolism stockings and a sequential compression device to prevent DVT and administer prescribed anticoagulants.

- Monitor the client's pain level.

  ▸ Administer analgesics, antispasmodics, and/or anti-inflammatory medication (NSAIDS) and assess relief.

  ▸ Position for comfort and with ice on the surgical site.

- Monitor for signs of infection.

  ▸ Monitor the client's vital signs, observing for fever, tachycardia, incisional drainage, redness, and odor.

  ▸ Monitor laboratory values (WBC, ESR).

  ▸ Provide surgical aseptic wound care.

- Increase physical mobility as appropriate.

  ▸ Consult physical and occupational therapy for ambulation and activities of daily living (ADLs).

  ▸ Monitor orthostatic blood pressure when the client gets out of bed for the first time.

  ▸ Turn and reposition the client every 2 hr.

  ▸ Have the client get out of bed from the unaffected side.

  ▸ Position the client for comfort (within restrictions).

- Support nutrition.

  ▸ Encourage increased calorie intake.

  ▸ Ensure use of calcium supplements.

  ▸ Encourage small, frequent meals with snacks.

  ▸ Monitor for constipation.

Complications

- Compartment syndrome

  ○ Compartment syndrome usually affects extremities and occurs when pressure within one or more of the muscle compartments (an area covered with an elastic tissue called fascia) of the extremity compromises circulation, resulting in an ischemia-edema cycle.

  ○ Capillaries dilate in an attempt to pull oxygen into the tissue. Increased capillary permeability from the release of histamine leads to edema from plasma proteins leaking into the interstitial fluid space.

  ○ Increased edema causes pressure on the nerve endings, resulting in pain. Blood flow is further reduced and ischemia persists, resulting in compromised neurovascular status.

- ○ Pressure can result from external sources, such as a tight cast or a constrictive bulky dressing.
- ○ Internal sources, such as an accumulation of blood or fluid within the muscle compartment, can cause pressure as well.
- ○ Clinical Manifestations
  - Compartment syndrome (ACS) is assessed by using the five P's (pain, paralysis, paresthesia, pallor, and pulselessness).
  - Increased pain unrelieved with elevation or by pain medication.
    - □ Intense pain when passively moved.
  - Paresthesia or numbness, burning, and tingling are early signs.
  - Paralysis, motor weakness, or inability to move the extremity indicate major nerve damage and are late signs.
  - Color of tissue is pale (pallor), and nail beds are cyanotic.
  - Pulselessness is a late sign of compartment syndrome.
  - Palpated muscles are hard and swollen from edema.
- ○ If untreated, tissue necrosis can result. Neuromuscular damage occurs within 4 to 6 hr.
- ○ Surgical treatment is a fasciotomy.
  - A surgical incision is made through the subcutaneous tissue and fascia of the affected compartment to relieve the pressure and restore circulation.
  - After the fasciotomy, the open wounds require sterile packings and dressings until secondary closure occurs. Skin grafts may be necessary.
- ○ Nursing Actions
  - Prevention includes:
    - □ Notifying the provider when compartment syndrome is suspected.
    - □ The provider will cut the cast on one side (univalve) or both sides (bivalve).
    - □ Loosening the constrictive dressing or cutting the bandage or tape.
- ○ Client Education
  - Instruct the client to report pain not relieved by analgesics or pain that continues to increase in intensity.
  - The client should also be instructed to report numbness, tingling, or a change in color of the extremity.

- Fat embolism
  - ○ Adults between age 70 and 80 are at the greatest risk of developing a fat embolism. Hip and pelvis fractures are most common.
  - ○ Fat embolism can occur after the injury, usually within 48 hr following long bone fractures or with total joint arthroplasty.
  - ○ Fat globules from the bone marrow are released into the vasculature and travel to the small blood vessels, including those in the lungs, resulting in acute respiratory insufficiency and organ perfusion. Careful diagnosis should differentiate between fat embolism and pulmonary embolism.

- ○ Clinical manifestations include:
  - Dyspnea, chest pain, decreased oxygen saturation
  - Decreased mental acuity related to low arterial oxygen level (earliest sign)
  - Respiratory distress
  - Tachycardia
  - Tachypnea
  - Fever
  - Cutaneous petechiae – pinpoint-sized subdermal hemorrhages that occur on the neck, chest, upper arms, and abdomen (from the blockage of the capillaries by the fat globules). This is a discriminating finding from pulmonary embolism and is a late sign.
- ○ Nursing Actions
  - Maintain the client on bed rest.
  - Prevention includes immobilization of fractures of the long bones and minimal manipulation during turning if immobilization procedure has not yet been performed.
  - Treatment includes oxygen for respiratory compromise, corticosteroids for cerebral edema, vasopressors, and fluid replacement for shock, as well as pain and antianxiety medications as needed.
- Deep-vein thrombosis (DVT)
  - ○ Deep-vein thrombosis is the most common complication following trauma, surgery, or disability related to immobility.
  - ○ Nursing Actions
    - Encourage early ambulation.
    - Apply antiembolism stockings, sequential compression device (SCD).
    - Administer anticoagulants as prescribed.
    - Encourage intake of fluids to prevent hemoconcentration.
    - Instruct the client to rotate feet at the ankles and perform other lower extremity exercises as permitted by the particular immobilization device.
- Osteomyelitis
  - ○ Osteomyelitis is an infection of the bone that begins as an inflammation within the bone secondary to penetration by infectious organisms (virus, bacteria, or fungi) following trauma or surgery.
  - ○ Clinical Manifestations
    - Bone pain that is constant, pulsating, localized, and worse with movement
    - Erythema and edema at the site of the infection
    - Fever
      - □ Older adults may not have an elevated temperature.
    - Leukocytosis and possible elevated sedimentation rate
    - Many of these manifestations will disappear if the infection becomes chronic.

- ○ Diagnostic procedures

  - ▪ Bone scan using radioactive material to diagnose osteomyelitis and MRI may also facilitate a diagnosis.

  - ▪ Cultures are performed for detection of possible aerobic and anaerobic organisms.

  - ▪ If septicemia develops, blood cultures will be positive for offending microbes.

- ○ Treatment

  - ▪ Long course (3 months) of IV and oral antibiotic therapy.

  - ▪ Surgical debridement may also be indicated. If a significant amount of the bone requires removal, a bone graft may be necessary.

  - ▪ Hyperbaric oxygen treatments may be needed to promote healing in chronic cases of osteomyelitis.

  - ▪ Surgically implanted antibiotic beads in bone cement are packed into the wound as a form of antibiotic therapy.

  - ▪ Unsuccessful treatment can result in amputation.

- ○ Nursing Actions

  - ▪ Administer antibiotics as prescribed to maintain a constant blood level.

  - ▪ Administer analgesics as needed.

  - ▪ Conduct neurovascular assessments if debridement is done.

  - ▪ If the wound is left open to heal, standard precautions are adequate, and clean technique can be used during dressing changes.

- • Avascular necrosis

  - ○ Avascular necrosis results from the circulatory compromise that occurs after a fracture. Blood flow is disrupted to the fracture site and the resulting ischemia leads to tissue (bone) necrosis.

  - ○ Commonly found in hip fractures or in fractures with displacement of a bone.

  - ○ Clients receiving long-term corticosteroid therapy are at greater risk for developing avascular necrosis.

  - ○ Replacement of damaged bone with a bone graft or prosthetic replacement may be necessary.

- • Failure of fracture to heal

  - ○ A fracture that has not healed within 6 months of injury is considered to be experiencing "delayed union."

  - ○ Malunion: Fracture heals incorrectly

  - ○ Nonunion: Fracture that never heals

    - ▪ Electrical bone stimulation and bone grafting can be used to treat nonunion.

    - ▪ May occur more frequently in older adult clients due to impaired healing process.

  - ○ Malunion or nonunion may cause immobilizing deformity of the bone involved.

APPLICATION EXERCISES

1. A nurse is teaching a client how to manage an external fixation device upon discharge. Which of the following statements by the client indicates an understanding of safe management? (Select all that apply.)

_____X_____ A. "I will clean the pins twice a day."

_____X_____ B. "I will use a separate cotton swab for each pin."

_____X_____ C. "I will report loosening of the pins to my doctor."

_____ D. "I will move my leg by lifting the device in the middle."

_____ E. "I will remove any crusting that forms at the pin site."

2. A nurse is assessing a client who has a casted compound fracture of the right forearm. Which of the following findings is an early indication of neurovascular compromise?

A. Paresthesia

B. Pulselessness

C. Paralysis

D. Pallor

3. A nurse is completing an assessment of a client who had an external fixation device applied 2 hr ago for a fracture of the left tibia and fibula. Which of the following findings indicate compartment syndrome? (Select all that apply.)

_____X_____ A. Intense pain when the left foot is passively moved

_____ B. Edematous left toes compared to the right

_____X_____ C. Hard, swollen muscle in the left leg

_____X_____ D. Burning and tingling of the distal left foot

_____X_____ E. Minimal pain relief following a second dose of opioid medication

4. A nurse is completing discharge teaching to a client who had a wound debridement for osteomyelitis. Which of the following information should the nurse include in the teaching?

A. Antibiotic therapy should continue for 3 months.

B. Relief of pain indicates the infection is eradicated.

C. Contact precautions are used during wound care.

D. Dressing changes are performed using aseptic technique.

5. A nurse in the emergency department is planning care for a client who has a right hip fracture. Which of the following immobilization devices should the nurse anticipate in the plan of care?

    A. Skeletal traction

    B. Buck's traction

    C. Halo traction

    D. Gardner-Wells traction

6. A nurse is performing a neurovascular assessment on a client who has a cast applied following a right arm fracture. What are appropriate interventions by the nurse? Use the ATI Active Learning Template: Basic Concept to complete this item to include the following:

    A. Related Content: Identify the purpose of neurovascular assessment.

    B. Underlying Principles: Identify the six components of a neurovascular assessment.

    C. Nursing Interventions: Describe a nursing intervention related to each of the six components.

APPLICATION EXERCISES KEY

1. A. **CORRECT:** Clean the external fixation pins one to two times each day to remove exudate that may harbor bacteria.

   B. **CORRECT:** Using a separate cotton swab on each pin will decrease the risk of cross-contamination, which could cause pin site infection.

   C. **CORRECT:** Notify the provider if a pin is loose because the provider will know how much to tighten the pin and prevent damage to the tissue and bone.

   D. INCORRECT: The external fixation device should never be used to lift or move the affected leg, due to the risk of injuring and dislocating the fractured bone.

   E. INCORRECT: Crusting at the pin site provides a natural barrier from bacteria and should not be removed.

    NCLEX® Connection: Basic Care and Comfort, Mobility/Immobility

2. A. **CORRECT:** Paresthesia is an early sign of neurovascular compromise, which is suggestive of compartment syndrome.

   B. INCORRECT: Pulselessness is a late sign of neurovascular compromise, which is suggestive of compartment syndrome.

   C. INCORRECT: Paralysis is a late sign of neurovascular compromise, which is suggestive of compartment syndrome.

   D. INCORRECT: Pallor is a late sign of neurovascular compromise due to inadequate profusion to the distal extremity, which is suggestive of compartment syndrome.

    NCLEX® Connection: Basic Care and Comfort, Mobility/Immobility

3. A. **CORRECT:** Intense pain of the left foot when passively moved may indicate pressure from edema on nerve endings and is a neurological sign of compartment syndrome.

   B. INCORRECT: Edema of the left toes is an expected finding in a client who has a fracture of the left tibia and fibula.

   C. **CORRECT:** A hard, swollen muscle on the affected extremity indicates edema build-up in the area of injury and is a sign of compartment syndrome.

   D. **CORRECT:** Burning and tingling of the left foot indicates pressure from edema on nerve endings and is an early neurological sign of compartment syndrome.

   E. **CORRECT:** Minimal pain relief after receiving opioid medication may indicate pressure from edema on nerve endings and is an early neurological sign of compartment syndrome.

    NCLEX® Connection: Reduction of Risk Potential, Potential for Complications from Surgical Procedures and Health Alterations

4. A. **CORRECT:** Treatment of osteomyelitis includes continuing antibiotic therapy for 3 months.

    B. INCORRECT: Relief of pain does not indicate that osteomyelitis is resolved, and the client should continue antibiotic therapy as prescribed.

    C. INCORRECT: When performing wound care, standard precautions are implemented, because a wound due to osteomyelitis is classified as a dirty wound and is usually left open for healing.

    D. INCORRECT: Clean technique is used when performing a dressing change of a wound due to osteomyelitis, because the wound is classified as a dirty wound and is usually left open for healing.

     NCLEX® Connection: Reduction of Risk Potential, Potential for Complications from Surgical Procedures and Health Alterations

5. A. INCORRECT: Skeletal traction is an immobilization device applied surgically to a long bone fracture.

    B. **CORRECT:** Buck's traction is a temporary immobilization device applied to diminish muscle spasms and immobilize the affected extremity until surgery is performed.

    C. INCORRECT: Halo traction immobilizes the cervical spine when a cervical fracture occurs.

    D. INCORRECT: Gardner-Wells traction uses tongs to immobilize and realign the cervical spine when a cervical fracture occurs.

    NCLEX® Connection: Reduction of Risk Potential, Therapeutic Procedures

6. *Using the ATI Active Learning Template: Basic Concept*

    A. Related Content

    - Neurovascular assessment is performed to monitor for any compromise in the affected extremity caused by edema and or immobilization device.

    B. Underlying Principles

    - Assess for pain level, location, and type and frequency.
    - Assess sensation of the distal extremity.
    - Assess skin temperature for warmth.
    - Assess capillary refill.
    - Assess the pulses distal to the fracture.
    - Assess finger movement.

    C. Nursing Interventions

    - Pain – Administer pain medication, elevate the extremity, and apply ice.
    - Sensation – Notify the provider of numbness, tingling, or loss of sensation.
    - Skin temperature – Notify the provider if the affected extremity is cool compared to the unaffected extremity.
    - Capillary refill – Notify the provider if nail beds are cyanotic.
    - Pulses – Notify the provider if pulse is absent.
    - Finger movement – Notify the provider if the client is unable to perform passive or active movement of the fingers.

    NCLEX® Connection: Reduction of Risk Potential, Therapeutic Procedures

chapter 73

Overview

- Osteoarthritis (OA) or degenerative joint disease (DJD) is a disorder characterized by progressive deterioration of the articular cartilage. It is a noninflammatory (unless localized), nonsystemic disease.

- It is no longer thought to be only a wear-and-tear disease associated with aging, but rather a process in which new tissue is produced as a result of cartilage destruction within the joint. The destruction outweighs the production. The cartilage and bone beneath the cartilage erode and osteophytes (bone spurs) form, resulting in narrowed joint spaces. The changes within the joint lead to pain, immobility, muscle spasms, and potential inflammation.

- Early in the disease process of OA, it may be difficult to distinguish from rheumatoid arthritis (RA).

CHARACTERISTIC	OSTEOARTHRITIS	RHEUMATOID ARTHRITIS
Disease process	› Cartilage destruction with bone spur growth at joint ends; degenerative	› Synovial membrane inflammation resulting in cartilage destruction and bone erosion; inflammatory
Symptoms	› Pain with activity that improves at rest	› Swelling, redness, warmth, pain at rest or after immobility (morning stiffness)
Effusions	› Localized inflammatory response	› All joints
Body size	› Usually overweight	› Usually underweight
Nodes	› Heberden's and Bouchard's nodes	› Swan neck and boutonnière deformities of hands
Systemic involvement	› No – articular	› Yes – lungs, heart, skin, and extra-articular
Symmetrical	› No	› Yes
Diagnostic tests	› X-rays	› X-rays and positive rheumatoid factor

    View Images: Heberden's and Bouchard's Nodes

Health Promotion and Disease Prevention

- Encourage the client to use joint-saving measures (good body mechanics, labor-saving devices).
- Encourage the client to maintain a healthy weight to decrease joint degeneration of the hips and knees.
- Recommend that the client stop smoking to reduce cartilage loss, especially if there is a family history of OA.
- Encourage the client to avoid or limit repetitive strain on joints (jogging, contact sports, risk-taking activities).
- Recommend wearing well-fitted shoes with supports to prevent falls.

Assessment

- Risk Factors
  - Age (majority of adults over age 60 have joint changes on x-ray)
  - Women have higher incidence of OA than men
  - Obesity
  - Smoking
  - Possible genetic link
  - History of repetitive stress on joints (manual laborers, professional athletes, marathon runners)
- Clinical Manifestations
  - Joint pain and stiffness that resolves with rest or inactivity
  - Pain with joint palpation or range of motion (observe for muscle atrophy, loss of function, limp when walking, and restricted activity due to pain)
  - Crepitus in one or more of the affected joints
  - Enlarged joint related to bone hypertrophy
  - Heberden's nodes enlarged at the distal interphalangeal (DIP) joints
  - Bouchard's nodes located at the proximal interphalangeal (PIP) joints (OA is not a symmetrical disease, but these nodes can occur bilaterally)
  - Inflammation resulting from secondary synovitis, indicating advanced disease
  - Joint effusion (excess joint fluid) that is easily moved from one area of the joint to another area
  - Vertebral radiating pain affected by cervical or lumbar compression of nerve roots
- Laboratory Tests
  - Erythrocyte sedimentation rate (ESR) and high-sensitivity C-reactive protein may be increased slightly related to secondary synovitis. Osteoarthritis without synovitis is not an inflammatory disorder.
- Diagnostic Procedures
  - Radiographs and magnetic resonance imaging (MRI) can determine structural changes within the joint (decreased joint space, bone spurs).

Patient-Centered Care

- Nursing Care
  - Assess/Monitor
    - Pain – location, characteristics, quality, severity
    - Degree of functional limitation
    - Levels of fatigue and pain after activity
    - Range of motion
    - Proper functional/joint alignment
    - Home barriers
    - Ability to perform ADLs
  - Instruct the client about the use of analgesics and NSAIDs prior to activity and around the clock as needed.

○ Balance rest with activity.

○ Instruct the client on proper body mechanics.

○ Encourage the use of thermal applications: heat to alleviate pain and ice for acute inflammation.

○ Encourage the use of complementary and alternative therapies, including acupuncture, tai chi, hypnosis, magnets, and music therapy.

○ Encourage the use of splinting for joint protection, and the use of larger joints.

○ Encourage the use of assistive devices to promote safety and independence, including an elevated toilet seat, shower bench, long-handled reacher, and shoe horn.

○ Encourage the use of a daily schedule of activities that will promote independence (high-energy activities in the morning).

○ Encourage a well-balanced diet and ideal body weight. Consult a dietitian to provide meal planning for balanced nutrition.

- Medications

  ○ Analgesic therapy

    ▪ Acetaminophen (Tylenol)

      □ Does not provide anti-inflammatory benefits, which may not be needed if synovitis is not present

      □ Nursing Actions

        ▸ Limit administration of acetaminophen to a maximum of 4,000 mg/24 hr.

        ▸ Monitor liver function tests.

    ▪ Nonsteroidal Anti-Inflammatory Drugs (NSAIDs)

      □ Analgesics and anti-inflammatories (celecoxib [Celebrex], naproxen [Naprosyn], ibuprofen [Motrin, Advil]) that are used to relieve pain and synovitis if present

      □ May replace acetaminophen with an NSAID if adequate relief is not obtained

      □ Nursing Actions

        ▸ Monitor kidney function (BUN and creatinine).

        ▸ Educate the client that NSAIDs are nephrotoxic and should be taken as prescribed.

        ▸ Teach the client to report evidence of black tarry stool, indigestion, and shortness of breath.

    ▪ Topical analgesics

      □ Trolamine salicylate (Aspercreme) may provide varying amounts of temporary pain relief, depending on client response. Apply topically over the area of involvement. It contains salicylate.

      □ Capsaicin (Axsain, Capsin) may provide varying amounts of temporary pain relief depending on client response. Apply topically over an area of involvement. It is made from alkaloid that is derived from hot peppers. It is thought to prevent transmission of pain sensations from peripheral neural transmitters.

- Client Education
  - ▸ Instruct the client to wear gloves during application.
  - ▸ Advise the client to wear nitrile gloves when applying capsaicin patch.
  - ▸ Instruct the client to avoid applying tight dressings to area where capsaicin cream was applied to prevent skin irritation.
  - ▸ Tell the client to wash hands immediately after applying capsaicin and avoid touching eyes or applying over broken skin areas, which can cause painful burning.
  - ▸ Explain to the client that a burning sensation of the skin after application is normal and should subside.
  - ▸ Instruct the client to apply frequently (up to 4 times a day) for maximum benefit.
- Glucosamine (rebuilds cartilage)
  - Glucosamine is a naturally occurring chemical involved in the makeup of cartilage. Glucosamine sulfate is believed to aid in the synthesis of synovial fluid and rebuild cartilage.
  - Glucosamine may decrease the cells that cause joint inflammation and degradation of cartilage.
  - Glucosamine is often taken in combination with chondroitin and may or may not have a pain reduction effect.
  - Client Education
    - ▸ Consult the provider regarding dosage.
    - ▸ May cause mild GI upset (nausea, heartburn).
    - ▸ Use with caution with shellfish allergy.
    - ▸ Question clients about concurrent use of chondroitin, NSAIDs, heparin, and warfarin.
- Intra-articular injections
  - Glucocorticoids are used to treat localized inflammation.
  - Hyaluronic acid (Hyalgan, Synvisc) is used to replace the body's natural hyaluronic acid, which is destroyed by joint inflammation. It is currently only approved for treatment of hip and knee joints.
  - Client Education
    - ▸ Hyaluronic acid – Instruct the client to notify the provider if allergic to birds, feathers, or eggs because this medication is made from combs of chickens.
- Teamwork and Collaboration
  - ○ Physical therapy services can teach muscle strengthening exercises, application of heat, diathermy (treatment with electrical currents), ultrasonography (treatment with sound waves), or stretching and strengthening exercises.
  - ○ A transcutaneous electrical nerve stimulation (TENS) unit may be prescribed by the provider and applied by the physical therapist with client instruction on how to use it.
  - ○ A nutritionist may assist the client in diet for weight loss or control in relation to reduced activity level.
- Therapeutic Procedures
  - ○ Conservative therapy includes balancing rest with activity, using bracing or splints, cane, and applying thermal therapies (heat or cold).
- Surgical Interventions
  - ○ Total joint arthroplasty – When all other conservative measures fail, the client may choose to undergo total joint arthroplasty to relieve the pain and improve mobility and quality of life.

APPLICATION EXERCISES

1. A nurse is assessing a client who has osteoarthritis of the knees and fingers. Which of the following clinical manifestations should the nurse expect to find? (Select all that apply.)

_____ A. Heberden's nodes

_____ B. Swelling of all joints

_____ C. Small body frame

_____ D. Enlarged joint size

_____ E. Limp when walking

2. A nurse is providing information to a client who has osteoarthritis of the hip and knee. Which of the following information should the nurse include in the information? (Select all that apply.)

_____ A. Apply heat to joints to alleviate pain.

_____ B. Ice inflamed joints following activity.

_____ C. Install an elevated toilet seat.

_____ D. Take tub baths.

_____ E. Complete high-energy activities in the morning.

3. A nurse is providing information about capsaicin (Capsin) cream to a client who reports continuous knee pain from osteoarthritis. Which of the following information should the nurse include in the discussion?

A. Continuous pain relief is provided.

B. Inspect for skin irritation and cuts prior to application.

C. Cover the area with tight bandages after application.

D. Apply the medication every 2 hr during the day.

4. A nurse is preparing a client who is to receive hyaluronic acid (Synvisc) injection for osteoarthritis. Which of the following statements by the nurse is appropriate?

A. "Hyaluronic acid is currently approved for shoulder joint inflammation."

B. "Report an allergy to shellfish before receiving hyaluronic acid."

C. "Hyaluronic acid is a natural joint replacement fluid."

D. "Hyaluronic acid is made from the combs of chickens."

5. A nurse is providing educational information on glucosamine to a group of clients at a health fair. Which of the following should the nurse include in the teaching?

    A. It decreases the amount of synovial fluid produced in the joints.

    B. The medication aids in the rebuilding of cartilage.

    C. A prescription is required for this medication.

    D. This medication is injected into the joint to decrease joint pain.

6. A nurse is providing information on alternative therapies for a client who is having continual joint pain from osteoarthritis. What information should the nurse include? Use the ATI Active Learning Template: Basic Concept to complete this item to include the following:

    A. Related Content:

- List three alternative therapies to treat osteoarthritis.
  - Underlying Principles: Describe two activities involved with each alternative therapy.

APPLICATION EXERCISES KEY

1. A. **CORRECT:** Heberden's nodes are enlarged nodules on the distal interphalangeal joints of the hands and feet of a client who has osteoarthritis.

    B. INCORRECT: Swelling and pain of all joints is a manifestation of rheumatoid arthritis. A local inflammation of a joint is related to osteoarthritis.

    C. INCORRECT: A small body frame is a risk factor for rheumatoid arthritis. Obesity is a risk factor for osteoarthritis.

    D. **CORRECT:** A client may manifest enlarged joints due to bone hypertrophy.

    E. **CORRECT:** A client may manifest a limp when walking due to pain from inflammation in the localized joint.

    Ⓝ NCLEX® Connection: Reduction of Risk Potential, Diagnostic Tests

2. A. **CORRECT:** Applying heat to joints can provide temporary relief of pain.

    B. **CORRECT:** Applying ice to inflamed joints following activity can decrease edema.

    C. **CORRECT:** Installing an elevated toilet seat can help decrease strain and pain of the affected joints.

    D. INCORRECT: Taking a tub bath places the client at risk for increased strain and pain on the affected joints when getting in and out of the tub and increases the risk for falls.

    E. **CORRECT:** Encouraging high-energy activity in the morning is recommended as part of a daily routine to promote independence.

    Ⓝ NCLEX® Connection: Reduction of Risk Potential, Diagnostic Tests

3. A. INCORRECT: Capsaicin cream provides temporary relief of pain when applied up to four times a day.

    B. **CORRECT:** Inspect the skin for irritation and cuts before applying capsaicin cream, because hot peppers in the cream can cause a painful burning sensation in areas of skin breakdown.

    C. INCORRECT: After capsaicin cream is applied, avoid covering the area with a tight bandage, which may cause increased skin irritation.

    D. INCORRECT: For maximum pain relief benefit, apply capsaicin cream up to four times a day.

    Ⓝ NCLEX® Connection: Reduction of Risk Potential, Therapeutic Procedures

4. A. INCORRECT: Hyaluronic acid is currently approved for hip and knee joint inflammation only.

   B. INCORRECT: Allergies to birds, feathers, or eggs should be reported to the provider before hyaluronic acid is injected, because the synthetic fluid is made from the combs of chickens.

   C. INCORRECT: Hyaluronic acid is a synthetic fluid used to replace the natural hyaluronic acid produced in joints.

   D. **CORRECT:** Hyaluronic acid is made from the combs of chickens to replace the natural hyaluronic acid produced in joints.

   Ⓝ NCLEX® Connection: Reduction of Risk Potential, Therapeutic Procedures

5. A. INCORRECT: Glucosamine may increase the amount of synovial fluid produced in the joint and decrease inflammation.

   B. **CORRECT:** Glucosamine can aid in the rebuilding of cartilage and decrease joint pain.

   C. INCORRECT: Glucosamine is an over-the-counter dietary supplement used to decrease pain and build damaged cartilage.

   D. INCORRECT: Glucosamine is administered orally or topically to relieve joint pain.

   Ⓝ NCLEX® Connection: Health Promotion and Maintenance, Health Promotion/Disease Prevention

6. *Using the ATI Active Learning Template: Basic Concept*

   A. Related Content/Underlying Principles
   - Physical Therapy
     - Apply heat, diathermy, and ultrasound.
     - Perform stretching and strengthening exercises.
     - Use transcutaneous electrical nerve stimulation (TENS).
   - Conservative Therapy
     - Balance rest with activity.
     - Use braces, splints, and cane.
     - Apply thermal therapies (heat or cold).
   - Nutritional Therapy
     - Provide nutritional information on weight loss.
     - Provide nutritional information on a balanced diet.

   Ⓝ NCLEX® Connection: Health Promotion and Maintenance, Health Promotion/Disease Prevention

UNIT 11   Nursing Care of Clients with Integumentary Disorders

SECTIONS

› Diagnostic and Therapeutic Procedures
› Integumentary Disorders

Client Needs: Basic Care and Comfort	Client Needs: Reduction of Risk Potential	Client Needs: Physiological Adaptation

› Relevant topics/tasks include:
» Mobility/Immobility
  › Promote circulation.
» Nutrition and Oral Hydration
  › Evaluate the impact of disease/illness on the nutritional status of the client.
	› Relevant topics/tasks include:
	» Laboratory Values
	  › Obtain specimens other than blood for diagnostic testing.
	» Potential for Alterations in Body Systems
	  › Identify the client's potential for skin breakdown.
	» System Specific Assessment
	  › Identify factors that result in delayed wound healing.
		› Relevant topics/tasks include:
		» Alterations in Body Systems
		  › Assess the client for signs and symptoms of adverse effects of radiation therapy.
		» Fluid and Electrolyte Imbalances
		  › Identify signs and symptoms of the client's fluid and/or electrolyte imbalance.
		» Medical Emergencies
		  › Provide emergency care for wound disruption.

chapter 74

Overview

- Integumentary diagnostic procedures involve identification of pathogenic micro-organisms. The most accurate and definitive way to identify micro-organisms and cell characteristics is by examining blood, body fluids, and tissue samples under a microscope.

- Skin lesions or changes in the skin may need confirmation by microscope to determine if the cause is viral, fungal, or bacterial.

- Integumentary diagnostic procedures that nurses should be knowledgeable about
  - Wood's light examination
  - Skin culture and sensitivity
  - Tzanck smear
  - Potassium hydroxide (KOH)
  - Biopsy

Skin Diagnostic Studies

- Wood's light examination
  - Ultraviolet light is used to produce specific colors to reveal a skin infection.
  - Examination is performed in a dark room to evaluate pigment changes in a light-skinned client.

- Skin culture and sensitivity
  - Culture refers to isolation of the pathogen on culture media.
  - Sensitivity refers to the effect that antimicrobial agents have on the micro-organism.
    - If the micro-organism is killed by the antimicrobial, the microbe is considered to be sensitive to that medication.
    - If tolerable levels of the medication are unable to kill the microbe, the microbe is considered to be resistant to that medication.
  - A culture and sensitivity can be done on a sample of purulent drainage from a skin lesion.
  - Cultures should be done prior to initiating antimicrobial therapy.
  - Results of a culture and sensitivity test usually are available preliminarily within 24 to 48 hr, and final results in 72 hr.

- Indications
  - Skin lesions, which may be infectious, may appear raised, reddened, edematous, and/or warm. There may be purulent drainage and/or fever.

- Interpretation of findings for bacterial infection
  - The microbe responsible for the infection is identified in the culture, and the antimicrobials that are sensitive to that microbe are listed.
  - Heavy growth of greater than 100,000 colonies definitively diagnoses an infection. Negative results are less than 10,000 colonies.
  - Indeterminate results are 10,000 to 100,000 colonies.
  - Appropriate medications are those with three to four degrees of sensitivity.
- Tzanck smear confirms a viral skin lesion
  - A microscopic cytology examination is completed after extracting cells from the base of a lesion. Microscopic examination reveals multinucleated giant cells to confirm the lesion is viral.
- Potassium hydroxide (KOH) test confirms a fungal skin lesion
  - A microscopic examination of the scales scraped off a lesion is mixed with potassium hydroxide (KOH). Specimen is positive for fungus if there is the presence of fungal hyphae (threadlike filaments).
- Preprocedure
  - Nursing Actions
    - Use standard precautions when collecting and handling specimens.
    - Most specimens will be collected by the nurse or provider.
- Intraprocedure
  - Nursing Actions
    - Bacterial or viral specimens
      - Express material from the lesion by lifting or puncturing the crusted or scabbed area over the lesion using a small-gauge sterile needle or 0.9% sodium chloride and a sterile cotton swab.
      - Culturette tubes are specific for specimen collection and contain a sterile cotton-tipped applicator and a fixative that is released after the infectious exudate is applied to the applicator and inserted in the tube.
      - A specimen obtained for a viral culture is immediately placed on ice and sent to the laboratory.
    - Fungal specimen
      - Requires a sufficient quantity of scales collected using a wooden tongue depressor and placing the specimen in a clean container to be sent to the laboratory.
      - If a fungal culture is needed because of inconclusive results due to a deeper fungal infection, a punch biopsy is performed.
      - Specimens must be properly labeled and delivered to the laboratory promptly for appropriate storage and analysis.
- Postprocedure
  - Nursing Actions
    - Teach the client about measures to prevent the spread of an infectious skin disorder.
      - Bacterial infections – Bathe daily using an antibacterial soap.
        - Do not squeeze bacterial lesions but remove the crusted exudate so the antibacterial topical medication can penetrate into the lesion.
        - Apply warm compresses twice daily for comfort to furuncles or areas where cellulitis is present.

▫ Viral lesion – Apply compress of Burow's solution (aluminium acetate in water) for 20 min, three times a day to promote the formation of a crust and healing.

▸ Avoid tight, restrictive clothing that may irritate a lesion.

▸ Allow a lesion to dry between treatments, and avoid lying on the lesion to promote circulation and comfort.

▸ Use good hand hygiene to prevent cross-contamination of the infection.

▸ Avoid sharing personal items (combs, brushes, clothing, footwear).

- Medication therapy for bacterial infections

  ▫ Superficial skin infections are treated with topical antibacterial cream or ointment.

  ▫ Extensive bacterial skin infections involving the lymphatic system, or if cellulitis is present, are treated with systemic antibiotic therapy (cephalosporins or penicillins).

  ▫ If allergic to cephalosporins and penicillins, the provider can prescribe tetracycline (Sumycin), erythromycin (Erythrocin), azithromycin (Zithromax, Zmax), amikacin, or tobramycin (Tobrex).

  ▫ If the skin lesion is cultured as having MRSA, IV vancomycin (Vancocin) or oral linezolid (Zyvox) or clindamycin (Cleocin) is prescribed.

- Medication for viral infections

  ▫ Topical treatment with acyclovir (Zovirax), valacyclovir (Valtrex), or famciclovir (Famvir) decreases the number of active viruses on the surface of the skin and reduces the discomfort associated with a herpetic infection or lesion.

- Medication for fungal infections

  ▫ Yeast infections or dermatophyte infections are treated with topical cream or powder. For example, clotrimazole (Lotrimin, Mycelex) cream is applied to the infected skin twice a day and for 1 to 2 weeks after the lesions are no longer present, or as prescribed by the provider.

  ▫ Skin must be clean and dry before applying topical ointments or creams.

Biopsy

- Biopsy is the removal of a sample of tissue by excision or needle aspiration for cytological (histological) examination.

  ○ Biopsy for skin lesions can be a punch biopsy, shave biopsy, or excisional biopsy.

  ○ Biopsy confirms or rules out malignancy.

  ○ Skin biopsies are performed under local anesthesia.

- Indications

  ○ Evidence of skin lesion may include an area of discoloration that is thickened, thinned, raised, flat, rough, painful, open, dry, and/or itchy.

  ○ A biopsy is commonly performed to establish an exact diagnosis or to rule out diseases such as cancer.

- Interpretation of Findings

  ○ After a biopsy is completed, the tissue sample is sent to pathology for interpretation.

- Preprocedure
  - Nursing Actions
    - Ensure that the client has signed the informed consent form.
    - Explain the procedure to the client.
  - Client Education
    - Inform the client about what to expect in regard to the formation of a scar.
    - Teach the client about what to expect about the test/procedure.
- Intraprocedure
  - Punch biopsy
    - A small plug of tissue approximately 2 to 6 mm is removed with a special cutting instrument, with or without sutures to close the site.
  - Shave biopsy
    - Removal of only the part of the lesion that is raised above the surrounding tissue using a scalpel or razor blade with no suturing.
  - Excisional biopsy
    - A larger and deeper specimen is obtained, and suturing is required.
  - Nursing Actions
    - Explain to the client what to expect according to the type of biopsy.
    - Assist the provider with the test/procedure as needed, and assist with local anesthesia.
    - Establish a sterile field.
    - Place the tissue sample in a container containing appropriate solution, label, and send to the laboratory.
    - As appropriate, apply pressure to the biopsy site to control bleeding.
    - As appropriate, place a sterile dressing over the biopsy site.
- Postprocedure
  - Nursing Actions
    - As appropriate, monitor the biopsy site.
    - Postbiopsy discomfort usually is relieved by mild analgesics.
  - Client Education
    - Teach the client to report excessive bleeding and/or evidence of infection (redness, warmth, drainage, fever) to the provider.
    - Teach the client to check the incision daily. The incision should be clean, dry, and intact.
    - May remove dressings after 8 hr, and may use tap water or 0.9% sterile sodium chloride to clean the biopsy site of dried blood or crusts.
    - If prescribed by the provider, may apply an antibacterial topical medication to prevent infection.
    - If sutures are used, return to the provider for removal in 7 to 10 days.
    - Report excessive bleeding to the provider.

APPLICATION EXERCISES

1. A nurse is caring for a client who has a suspected viral skin lesion. Which of the following laboratory findings should the nurse anticipate reviewing to confirm this diagnosis?

    A. Potassium hydroxide (KOH)

    B. Culture and sensitivity

    C. Tzanck smear report

    D. Biopsy

2. A nurse in a clinic is preparing to obtain a skin specimen from a client who has a suspected herpes infection. Which of the following actions should the nurse take? (Select all that apply.)

   _____ A. Scrape the site with a wooden tongue depressor.

   _____ B. Puncture the crusted area with a sterile needle.

   _____ C. Swab the crusted area with a sterile cotton-tipped applicator.

   _____ D. Place cotton-tipped applicator in culturette tube.

   _____ E. Place culturette tube in ice.

3. A nurse is instructing a client on home care after a culture for a bacterial infection and cellulitis. Which of the following information should the nurse include in the teaching? (Select all that apply.)

   _____ A. Bathe with antibacterial soap.

   _____ B. Apply antibacterial topical medication to the crusted exudate.

   _____ C. Apply warm compresses to the affected area.

   _____ D. Cover affected area with snug fitting clothing.

   _____ E. Allow lesions to dry before applying topical medication.

4. A nurse is providing discharge instructions to a client who had a skin biopsy with sutures. Which of the following client statements indicates a need for further teaching?

    A. "I can expect redness around the site for 3 days."

    B. "I will call my doctor if I have a fever."

    C. "I should apply an antibiotic ointment to the area."

    D. "I will make a return appointment in 7 days for removal of my sutures."

5. A nurse is providing teaching to a client about a new prescription for clotrimazole (Lotrimin). Which of the following should the nurse include in the teaching?

    A. "It reduces the discomfort of a herpetic infection."

    B. "This is a cream to treat a bacterial infection."

    C. "Apply the topical medication for up to 2 weeks."

    D. "Allow the area to remain moist before applying."

6. A nurse is caring for a client who is to have a biopsy of a skin lesion. What should the nurse consider in planning for the procedure? Use the ATI Active Learning Template: Basic Concept to complete this item to include the following:

    A. Related Content/Underlying Principles:
- List the three types of integumentary biopsies.
- Describe the biopsies.

    B. Nursing Interventions: Describe two intraprocedure nursing actions.

APPLICATION EXERCISES KEY

1. A. INCORRECT: Findings of a potassium hydroxide (KOH) test reveal if skin lesions are fungal in origin.

    B. INCORRECT: Findings of a skin culture and sensitivity test reveal if lesions are bacterial or fungal and indicate antimicrobial medication to be used in treatment.

    C. **CORRECT:** A Tzanck smear report confirms if a skin lesion is viral in origin.

    D. INCORRECT: Findings of a biopsy report confirm or rule out if a lesion is malignant.

    (N) NCLEX® Connection: Reduction of Risk Potential, Diagnostic Tests

2. A. INCORRECT: A wooden tongue depressor is used to scrape cells of a skin lesion to test for a fungus.

    B. **CORRECT:** Exudate under the crusted area should be collected. The crust or scab should be punctured or lifted to obtain a reliable specimen.

    C. INCORRECT: Swab the moist lesion bed under the crust with a sterile cotton-tipped applicator to obtain a reliable specimen.

    D. **CORRECT:** The cotton-tipped applicator is placed in liquid fixative within the culturette tube.

    E. **CORRECT:** The culturette tube is immediately placed in ice when obtaining a viral specimen.

    (N) NCLEX® Connection: Reduction of Risk Potential, Diagnostic Tests

3. A. **CORRECT:** The client should use antibacterial soap to reduce the bacteria count on the skin.

    B. INCORRECT: The client should apply topical medication directly to the moist lesion bed. The medication will not penetrate the crusted exudate.

    C. **CORRECT:** The client should apply warm compresses to the affected area to promote comfort.

    D. INCORRECT: The client should wear loose-fitting clothes to avoid irritating the lesion.

    E. **CORRECT:** The client should dry the area well before applying a topical medication to allow for spreading the medication more effectively.

    (N) NCLEX® Connection: Reduction of Risk Potential, Therapeutic Procedures

4. A. **CORRECT:** The client should report redness, pain, drainage, or warmth at the biopsy site to the provider.

   B. INCORRECT: A fever is an indication of an infection, and the provider should be notified.

   C. INCORRECT: Antibiotic ointment is applied as prescribed by the provider to prevent infection.

   D. INCORRECT: Removal of the sutures following a biopsy is done 7 to 10 days postprocedure.

   Ⓝ NCLEX® Connection: Reduction of Risk Potential, Therapeutic Procedures

5. A. INCORRECT: Clotrimazole is not an antiviral medication to treat a herpetic infection. It is used to treat a fungal infection.

   B. INCORRECT: Clotrimazole is not an antibacterial medication. It is used to treat a fungal infection.

   C. **CORRECT:** Clotrimazole is a medication used to treat a fungal infection and is applied for 1 to 2 weeks after the infection is resolved.

   D. INCORRECT: Clotrimazole is an antifungal medication and should be applied to a clean, dry surface.

   Ⓝ NCLEX® Connection: Pharmacological and Parenteral Therapies, Medication Administration

6. *Using the ATI Active Learning Template: Basic Concept*

   A. Related Content/Underlying Principles
   - Punch biopsy – A small, 2 to 6 mm plug of tissue is removed from the skin lesion, followed with or without suturing.
   - Shave biopsy – A scalpel or razor blade removes only the raised area of the lesion, with no suturing.
   - Excisional biopsy – A large, deep specimen of tissue is obtained, followed with suturing.

   B. Nursing Interventions
   - Assist with setting up materials for placement of a local anesthetic.
   - Apply pressure to the biopsy site to control bleeding.
   - Place a sterile dressing over the biopsy site if needed.

   Ⓝ NCLEX® Connection: Reduction of Risk Potential, Therapeutic Procedures

chapter 75

Overview

- Psoriasis is a skin disorder that is characterized by scaly, dermal patches and is caused by an overproduction of keratin. This overproduction can occur at a rate up to seven times the rate of normal cells. It is thought to be an autoimmune disorder and has periods of exacerbations and remissions.

- In some clients, psoriasis can also affect the joints, causing arthritis-type changes and pain.

 View Image: Psoriasis

- Seborrheic dermatitis is a skin disorder caused by inflammation of areas of the skin that contain a high number of sebaceous glands. It is characterized by papulopustules (oily form) or flaky plaques (dry form) that develop on the surface of the skin. Dandruff is a type of seborrheic dermatitis.

- Seborrheic dermatitis has periods of remission and exacerbation.

PSORIASIS

Assessment

- Risk Factors

  - Infections (severe streptococcal throat infection, *Candida* infection, upper respiratory infection)

  - Skin trauma, recent surgery

  - Genetics

  - Stress (related to overstimulation of the immune system)

  - Seasons (warm weather improves symptoms)

  - Hormones (puberty or menopause)

  - Medications (lithium, beta-blocker medication, antimalarials, indocin [Indomethacin])

- Clinical Manifestations

  - Psoriasis vulgaris presents as scaly skin with silvery white colored patches.

  - Exfoliative psoriasis displays as erythema and scaling from a severe inflammatory reaction. The reaction can cause dehydration and hypothermia or hyperthermia.

  - Palmoplantar pustulosis manifests as reddened hyperkeratotic areas (accelerated maturation of epidermal cells) due to an inflammatory disorder. Plaques form and pustules turn brown, peel, and form a crust on the palms of the hands and soles of the feet.

- Exacerbation and remission of pruritic lesions
- Physical Assessment Findings
  - Scaly patches
  - Bleeding stimulated by removal of scales
  - Skin lesions primarily on the scalp, elbows and knees, sacrum, and lateral areas of the extremities (psoriasis vulgaris)
  - Pitting, crumbling nails

Patient-Centered Care

- Medications
  - Topical corticosteroids – triamcinolone acetonide (Kenalog)
    - Reduces secondary inflammatory response of lesions
    - Nursing Actions
      - Observe skin for thinning, striae, or hypopigmentation with high-potency corticosteroids.
    - Client Education
      - Instruct the client to apply high-potency corticosteroids as prescribed to prevent adverse effects. (Avoid use on face or in skin folds, and take periodic medication vacations.)
      - The provider may instruct the client to use warm, moist, occlusive dressings of plastic wrap (gloves, plastic garments, booties) after applying the topical medication. These can be left in place up to 8 hr each day.
  - Tar Preparations – coal tar and anthralin (Drithocreme, Lasan)
    - Used for moderate findings with psoriasis.
    - Exposure to short-wave ultraviolet B light is often done in conjunction with the application of coal tar.
    - Remove the creams from the lesions before the short-wave ultraviolet B is exposed to the affected areas.
    - Up to 30 treatments are administered and can produce 80% client remission rate.
    - Coal tar preparations are limited to inpatient and outpatient care clinics.
    - Represses cell division and decreases inflammation and itching.
    - May stain skin and hair.
    - May stimulate growth of skin cancers.
    - Anthralin cream should remain on no more than 2 hr after application to prevent chemical burns.
    - Anthralin is used alone or in conjunction with coal tar baths and short-wave ultraviolet B exposure.
    - Nursing Actions
      - Instruct the client on proper application.
      - Instruct the client on how to assess for cancerous lesions.
    - Client Education
      - Due to odor and staining, the client should apply this product at night and cover areas of body with old pajamas, gloves, and socks.

○ Topical epidermopoiesis suppressive medications – calcipotriene (Dovonex), a synthetic vitamin D$_3$; tazarotene (Tazorac), a vitamin A derivative

  ☐ Recommended for mild to moderate psoriasis.

  ☐ Reduces accelerated development of epidermal cells.

  ☐ Not recommended for older adults or women who are breastfeeding.

  ☐ Tazarotene (Tazorac) may cause birth defects. Women should be advised to use birth control during use.

- Nursing Actions

  ☐ Calcipotriene (Dovonex) – Monitor for symptoms of hypercalcemia (elevated serum calcium, muscle weakness, fatigue, anorexia).

- Client Education

  ☐ Instruct the client to avoid using the product on the face or in skin folds. May apply to the scalp.

  ☐ Instruct the client that burning and stinging can occur upon application.

  ☐ Instruct the client to report muscle weakness, fatigue, anorexia.

  ☐ Advise the client to use sunscreen and avoid sun exposure.

  ☐ Women should obtain a pregnancy test prior to initiating this medication.

○ Cytotoxic medications (severe, intractable cases) – methotrexate (Trexall), acitretin (Soriatane)

  ☐ Reduces turnover of epidermal cells.

  ☐ Decreases the effects of contraceptives

  ☐ Contraindicated in pregnant women and can cause fetal death or congenital anomalies

- Nursing Actions

  ☐ Monitor liver function tests for liver toxicity if methotrexate or acitretin therapy is being used.

  ☐ Methotrexate can cause bone marrow suppression (leukopenia, thrombocytopenia, anemia).

- Client Education

  ☐ Instruct the client to avoid alcohol while taking this medication.

  ☐ Advise the client to monitor for fever, sore throat, increased bleeding or bruising, and fatigue.

• Therapeutic Procedures

○ Photochemotherapy and ultraviolet light (PUVA therapy)

- A psoralen photosensitizing medication, methoxsalen (Oxsoralen, Uvadex), is administered followed by long-wave ultraviolet A (UVA) to decrease proliferation of epidermal cells.

- Psoralen is given 2 hr before ultraviolet treatments.

- Treatments are given 2 to 3 times per week, avoiding consecutive days.

- Nursing Actions

  ☐ Monitor the skin's response to light (redness, tenderness, tanning).

  ☐ Ensure that the client wears eye protection during treatment and for 24 hr indoors and outside following a treatment.

- Client Education

  ☐ Instruct the client to notify the provider of extreme redness, swelling, and discomfort.

  ☐ Inform the client of the long-term affects of premature skin aging, cataracts, and skin cancer.

- Other Systemic Medication
  - Cyclosporine (Sandimmune, Neoral) and azathioprine (Imuran)
    - Immunosuppressant medications are administered when lesions do not respond to other therapies.
    - Nephrotoxicity occurs and increases the risk of infections.
  - Medications that are becoming first-line treatment for moderate to severe plaque psoriasis include subcutaneous administration of adalimumab (Humira), etanercept (Enbrel), and ustekinumab (Stelara), and IV administration of infliximab (Remicade).
  - Nursing Action
    - Evaluate for latent tuberculosis with TB skin test.
    - Inspect prefilled syringe for particles or discoloration.
    - Rotate injection sites, and do not rub after administration.
    - Protect medication from light.
  - Client Education
    - Inform the client not to take if pregnant or breastfeeding.
    - Teach the client how to administer subcutaneous medication.
    - Instruct the client to report signs of infection.
    - Educate the client about need for lifelong treatment and the increased risk of cancer.
    - Instruct the client to not receive any live vaccines while taking the medication.

SEBORRHEIC DERMATITIS

Health Promotion and Disease Prevention

- Keep skin dry. Avoid overheating and perspiring.
- Do not scratch pruritic lesions.

Assessment

- Risk Factors
  - Genetics
  - Stress
  - Hormones
  - Older adults can develop seborrheic keratoses, which are more plaquelike in appearance, ranging from flesh-tone, brown, or black, rough, greasy, wartlike surfaces. They often are removed for cosmetic purposes.

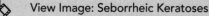
View Image: Seborrheic Keratoses

- Clinical Manifestations
  - ○ Chronic inflammation and scaling of the scalp, face, underarms, chest, and sacral region.
  - ○ Secondary candida infection may develop in body folds and creases and requires treatment with ketoconazole (Kuric, Xolegel).
  - ○ Report of periods of exacerbations and remissions.
  - ○ Pruritic lesions.
  - ○ Physical Assessment Findings
    - ▪ Waxy or flaky-appearing plaques and/or scales
    - ▪ Skin lesions primarily on the oily areas of the body (scalp, forehead, nose, axilla, groin)

Patient-Centered Care

- Medications
  - ○ Topical corticosteroids
    - ▪ Reduce secondary inflammatory response of lesions
    - ▪ Client Education
      - □ Instruct the client to avoid getting medication in the eyes, which can lead to glaucoma or cataracts, or skin folds.
  - ○ Antiseborrheic shampoos
    - ▪ Contain selenium sulfide, sulfur, or salicylic acid
    - ▪ Decrease the growth rate of epithelial cells of the scalp
    - ▪ Client Education
      - □ The client should use at least three times per week.
      - □ The client should leave shampoo on for 2 to 3 min.

APPLICATION EXERCISES

1. A nurse is providing information about a new prescription for corticosteroid cream to a client who has mild psoriasis. Which of the following should the nurse include in the information? (Select all that apply.)

_____ A. Apply an occlusive dressing after application.

_____ B. Apply three to four times per day.

_____ C. Wear gloves after application to lesions on the hands.

_____ D. Avoid applying in skin folds.

_____ E. Use medication continuously over a period of several months.

2. A nurse is teaching a client who has a history of psoriasis about photochemotherapy and ultraviolet light (PUVA) treatments. Which of the following should the nurse include in the teaching?

A. Apply coal tar before each treatment.

B. Administer a psoralen medication before the treatment.

C. Use this treatment every evening.

D. Remove the scales gently following each treatment.

3. A nurse is educating a female client on the use of calcipotriene (Dovonex) topical medication for the treatment of psoriasis. Which of the following information should the nurse include? (Select all that apply.)

_____ A. Recommended for facial lesions.

_____ B. Expect a stinging sensation upon application.

_____ C. Apply to the scalp.

_____ D. Obtain a pregnancy test.

_____ E. Limit application to skin folds.

4. A nurse is providing teaching to a client who has a prescription for methotrexate (Trexall) for severe psoriasis. Which of the following information should the nurse include?

A. Drink a glass of wine daily.

B. Monitor for evidence of infection.

C. Monitor kidney function tests regularly.

D. Expect increased bruising.

5. A nurse is assessing a client who has seborrheic keratosis on the forehead and nose. Which of the following manifestations should the nurse expect to find? (Select all that apply.)

_____ A. Waxy appearance of the lesions

_____ B. Black, rough lesions

_____ C. Pruritus of the lesions

_____ D. Purplish skin stain around the lesion

_____ E. Wartlike surface of the lesions

6. A nurse is providing information to a client who has a prescription for adalimumab (Humira) to treat severe plaque psoriasis. What should the nurse include in the information? Use the ATI Active Learning Template: Medication to complete this item to include the following sections:

A. Therapeutic Uses: List two.

B. Nursing Interventions: Describe three.

C. Client Education: Describe three teaching points.

APPLICATION EXERCISES KEY

1. A. **CORRECT:** An occlusive dressing can enhance the efficacy of the topical corticosteroid on the exposed lesions.

    B. INCORRECT: Corticosteroid cream is applied twice daily to prevent development of local and systemic adverse effects.

    C. **CORRECT:** Gloves worn after the medication can enhance the efficacy of the topical corticosteroid on the exposed lesions of the hands.

    D. **CORRECT:** Corticosteroid cream applied to lesions in skin folds increases the risk of yeast infections.

    E. INCORRECT: Corticosteroid cream used continuously can increase the risk for development of local and systemic adverse effects.

    N NCLEX® Connection: Pharmacological and Parenteral Therapies, Medication Administration

2. A. INCORRECT: PUVA treatment does not involve the use of coal tar.

    B. **CORRECT:** PUVA treatment involves the administration of a medication, such as a psoralen, to enhance photosensitivity.

    C. INCORRECT: PUVA treatments are completed two to three times each week and not on consecutive days.

    D. INCORRECT: Removal of scales may cause bleeding and is not recommended when treating psoriasis.

    N NCLEX® Connection: Reduction of Risk Potential, Therapeutic Procedures

3. A. INCORRECT: Applying calcipotriene to the face is not recommended because it may cause facial dermatitis.

    B. **CORRECT:** Calcipotriene causes stinging and burning sensations when applied to the lesions.

    C. **CORRECT:** Calcipotriene solution is applied to scalp lesions.

    D. **CORRECT:** Calcipotriene can cause birth defects. Female clients should obtain a pregnancy test before using the medication.

    E. **CORRECT:** Applying calcipotriene to skin folds can cause a possible local reaction of itching, irritation, and erythema.

    N NCLEX® Connection: Pharmacological and Parenteral Therapies, Medication Administration

4. A. INCORRECT: The client should not drink alcohol when taking methotrexate because the medication can cause liver damage.

   B. **CORRECT:** The client should monitor for fever and sore throat, which are signs of infection. Methotrexate can cause blood dyscrasias such as leukopenia.

   C. INCORRECT: The client should have liver function levels monitored frequently because the medication can cause liver damage.

   D. INCORRECT: The client should report increased bruising because methotrexate can cause blood dyscrasias such as thrombocytopenia.

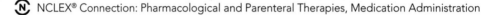 NCLEX® Connection: Pharmacological and Parenteral Therapies, Medication Administration

5. A. **CORRECT:** Seborrheic keratosis lesions appear waxy in texture.

   B. **CORRECT:** Seborrheic keratoses are tan, brown, or black lesions that are rough and become irritated due to friction.

   C. INCORRECT: Seborrheic keratoses may become irritated from friction but are not pruritic lesions.

   D. INCORRECT: Seborrheic keratosis does not cause a purplish skin stain around the lesion.

   E. **CORRECT:** A wartlike surface of the lesions is common for seborrheic keratosis, and the lesions are removed for cosmetic reasons.

NCLEX® Connection: Physiological Adaptations, Pathophysiology

6. *Using the ATI Active Learning Template: Medication*

A. Therapeutic Uses
- Moderate to severe plaque psoriasis and psoriatic arthritis
- Moderate to severe rheumatoid arthritis

B. Nursing Interventions
- Evaluate for latent tuberculosis with a TB skin test.
- Inspect prefilled syringe for particles or discoloration.
- Rotate injection sites and do not rub after medication administration.
- Protect medication from light.

C. Client Education
- Teach client how to administer subcutaneous medication for home use.
- Instruct the client to monitor for evidence of infection.
- Inform the client not to take during pregnancy or when breastfeeding.
- Educate the client that the medication is a lifelong treatment.
- Inform the client of the increased risk of developing cancer.
- Instruct the client to not receive any live vaccines while taking the medication.

NCLEX® Connection: Pharmacological and Parenteral Therapies, Medication Administration

chapter 76

Overview

- Thermal, chemical, electrical, and radioactive agents can cause burns, which result in cellular destruction of the skin layers and underlying tissue. The type of burn and the severity of the burn affect the treatment plan.

  - Thermal burns occur when there is exposure to flames, steam, or hot liquids. This type of burn occurs most frequently, especially in older adults and children.

  - Chemical burns occur when there is exposure to a caustic agent. Cleaning agents used in the home (drain cleaner, bleach) and agents used in the industrial setting (caustic soda, sulfuric acid) cause chemical burns.

  - Electrical burns occur when an electrical current passes through the body and can result in severe damage, including loss of organ function, tissue destruction with subsequent need for amputation of a limb, and cardiac and/or respiratory arrest.

  - Radiation burns most frequently occur as a result of therapeutic treatment for cancer or from sunburn.

- In addition to destruction of body tissue, a burn injury results in the loss of:

  - Temperature regulation

  - Sweat and sebaceous gland function

  - Sensory function

- Metabolism increases to maintain body heat as a result of burn injury and tissue damage.

- The severity of the burn is based on:

  - Percentage of total body surface area (TBSA) – Standardized charts for age groups are used to identify the extent of the injury.

  - Depth of the burn – Burns are classified according to the layers of skin and tissue involved.

  - Body location of the burn – In areas where the skin is thinner, there is more damage to underlying tissue (any part of the face, hand, perineum, feet).

    - Methods to assess burns:

      - Rule of Nines – Quick method to approximate the extent of burn by dividing the body into multiples of nine. The total of the sum is equal to the total body surface area (TBSA). This determines the measurement and the extent of the burn.

      - Lund and Browder Method – A more exact method estimating the extent of burn by the percentage of surface area of anatomic parts, particularly the head and legs of the client injured. Dividing body into smaller parts and providing a TBSA for each body part, an estimate of TBSA can be determined.

      - Palmer Method – Quick method to approximate scattered burns using the palm of the client's hand. The palm of the client's hand (excluding the fingers) is equal to 0.5% TBSA. This method can be used for all age groups.

○ Age of the client – Young clients and older adult clients have less reserve capacity to deal with a burn injury. For the older adult client, the skin is thinner. Thus, more damage to underlying tissue may occur.

○ Causative agent – Thermal, chemical, electrical, or radioactive.

○ Presence of other injuries – The presence of fractures or other injuries increases the risk of complications.

○ Involvement of the respiratory system – Inhalation of deadly fumes, smoke, steam, and heated air can cause respiratory failure or airway edema. Carbon monoxide poisoning also can occur, especially if the injury took place in an enclosed area.

○ Overall health of the client – A client who has a chronic illness has a greater risk of complications and a more serious prognosis.

- Three Phases of Burn Care
  - ○ Emergent (resuscitative phase)
    - ▪ First 24 to 48 hr after the burn occurs
  - ○ Acute
    - ▪ Begins when fluid resuscitation is finished
    - ▪ Ends when the wound is covered by tissue
  - ○ Rehabilitative
    - ▪ Begins when most of the burn area is healed
    - ▪ Ends when reconstructive and corrective procedures are complete (may last for years)

Health Promotion and Disease Prevention

- Ensure that the number and placement of fire extinguishers and smoke alarms in the home is adequate and operable. Family members should know how to use the extinguishers.
- Keep emergency numbers near the phone.
- Have a family exit and meeting plan for fires.
- Review with clients of all ages that in the event that the client's clothing or skin is on fire, the client should "stop, drop, and roll" to extinguish the fire.
- Store matches and lighters out of reach and out of sight of children and adults who lack the ability to protect themselves.
- Reduce setting on water heater to below 140° F (60° C).
- Have an annual professional inspection and cleaning of chimney/fireplace.
- Turn handles of pots/pans to the side or use back burners.
- Don't leave hot cups on the edge of the counter.
- Cover electrical outlets.
- Wear gloves when handling chemicals to prevent injury.
- Teach clients to wear protective clothing during sun exposure and to use sunscreen to avoid sunburn.
- Instruct clients to avoid using tanning beds.
- Avoid smoking in bed and when under the influence of alcohol or sedating medications.

Assessment

- Risk Factors
  - Risk for Death from Burns
    - Age greater than 60 years
    - Burn involves greater than 40% TBSA
    - Inhalation injury
  - Older adults are at higher risk for damage to subcutaneous tissue, muscle, connective tissue, and bone because their skin is thinner.
  - Older adults have a higher risk for complications from burns because of chronic illnesses (e.g., diabetes mellitus, cardiovascular disease).
- Subjective Data
  - Report of burn agent (dry heat, moist heat, chemical, electrical, ionizing radiation)
  - Duration of contact
  - Area of the body in which the burn occurred
- Objective Data
  - Physical Assessment Findings

ASSESS DEPTH OF INJURY		
AREA INVOLVED/APPEARANCE	SENSATION/HEALING	EXAMPLE
Superficial – damage to epidermis		
› Pink to red, tender, no blisters, mild edema, and no eschar	› Painful › Heals within 3 to 6 days › No scarring	› Sunburn
Superficial partial thickness – damage to the entire epidermis and some parts of the dermis		
› Pink to red, blisters, mild to moderate edema, and no eschar	› Painful › Heals within 10 to 21 days › No scarring	› Flame or burn scalds
Deep partial thickness – damage to entire epidermis and deep into the dermis		
› Red to white, with moderate edema, free of blisters, and soft and dry eschar	› Painful and sensitive to touch › Heals within 3 to 6 weeks › Scarring likely › Possible grafting involved	› Flame and burn scalds › Grease, tar, or chemical burns › Exposure to hot objects for prolonged time

ASSESS DEPTH OF INJURY		
AREA INVOLVED/APPEARANCE	SENSATION/HEALING	EXAMPLE
Full thickness – damage to the entire epidermis and dermis, and may extend into the subcutaneous tissue. Nerve damage also occurs.		
› Red to tan, black, brown, or white › Free from blisters, severe edema, and hard and inelastic eschar	› Pain may or may not be present › As burn heals, painful sensations return and severity of pain increases › Heals within weeks to months › Scarring › Grafting required	› Burn scalds › Grease, tar, chemical, or electrical burns › Exposure to hot objects for prolonged time
Deep full thickness – damage to all layers of skin and extends to muscle, tendons and bones		
› Black, no edema	› Heals within weeks to months › Scarring › Grafting required	› Chemical burns

 View Images: Burn Staging

- Levels of Care
  - Inhalation damage findings may include singed nasal hair, eye brows, and eyelashes; a sooty appearance to sputum; hoarseness; and wheezing. Clinical manifestations may not be evident for 24 to 48 hr and are seen as wheezing, hoarseness, and increased respiratory secretions.
  - Carbon monoxide inhalation (suspected if the injury took place in an enclosed area) findings include erythema (pink or cherry red color of skin) and upper airway edema, followed by sloughing of the respiratory tract mucosa.
  - Hypovolemia and shock may result when injury to at least 20% to 30% TBSA occurs. Fluid shifts from the intercellular and intravascular space to the interstitial space. Additional findings include hypotension, tachycardia, and decreased cardiac output.
- Laboratory Tests
  - CBC, serum electrolytes, BUN, ABGs, fasting blood glucose, liver enzymes, urinalysis, and clotting studies.
    - Initial fluid shift (first 24 hr after injury)
      - Hct and Hgb – elevated due to loss of fluid volume and fluid shifts into interstitial space (third spacing)
      - Sodium – decreased due to third spacing (hyponatremia)
      - Potassium – increased due to cell destruction (hyperkalemia)
  - Fluid mobilization (48 to 72 hr after injury)
    - Hgb and Hct – decreased due to fluid shift from interstitial space back into vascular fluid
    - Sodium – remains decreased due to renal and wound loss
    - Potassium – decreased due to renal loss and movement back into cells (hypokalemia)

- WBC count – initial increase then decrease with left shift
- Blood glucose – elevated due to stress response
- ABGs – slight hypoxemia and metabolic acidosis
- Total protein and albumin – low due to fluid loss

Patient-Centered Care

- Nursing Care
  - Minor Burns
    - Stop the burning process.
      - Remove clothing or jewelry that might conduct heat.
      - Apply cool water soaks or run cool water over injury; do not use ice.
      - Flush chemical burns with large volume of water.
      - Cover the burn with clean cloth to prevent contamination and hypothermia.
      - Provide warmth.
      - If necessary, have client go to a health care facility for medical care.
    - Provide analgesics.
    - Cleanse with mild soap and tepid water (avoid excess friction).
    - Use antimicrobial ointment.
    - Apply dressing (nonadherent, hydrocolloid) if the burn area is irritated by clothing.
    - Educate the family to avoid using greasy lotions or butter on burn.
    - Educate family to monitor for evidence of infection.
    - Check immunization status for tetanus and determine need for immunization.
  - Moderate and Major Burns
    - Maintain airway and ventilation. A nasogastric tube may be indicated for clients at risk for aspiration.
    - Assist client to cough and deep breathe every hour.
    - Suction every hour or as needed.
    - Keep head of bed elevated at all times.
    - Provide humidified supplemental oxygen as prescribed.
    - Monitor vital signs.
    - Maintain cardiac output.
      - Initiate intravenous access using a large-bore needle. If a large area of the body is burned, a central venous catheter is inserted.
      - Fluid replacement is important during the first 24 hr.
        - ▸ Rapid fluid replacement is needed during the emergent phase to maintain tissue perfusion and prevent hypovolemic (burn) shock.
        - ▸ Fluid resuscitation is based on individual client needs (evaluation of urine output, cardiac output, blood pressure, status of electrolytes).
        - ▸ Isotonic crystalloid solutions, such as 0.9% sodium chloride or lactated Ringer's solution, are used.

- ▸ Colloid solutions, such as albumin, or synthetic plasma expanders (Hespan, Plasma-Lyte), may be used after the first 24 hr of burn recovery.
- ▸ Maintain urine output of 30 mL/hr (0.5 to 1.0 mL/kg/hr).
- ▸ Be prepared to administer blood products as needed.
  - ▫ Monitor for manifestations of shock.
    - ▸ Alterations in sensorium (confusion)
    - ▸ Increased capillary refill time
    - ▸ Urine output less than 30 mL/hr
    - ▸ Rapid elevations of temperature
    - ▸ Decreased bowel sounds
    - ▸ Blood pressure may remain normotensive, even in hypovolemia.
- ○ Pain Management
  - ▪ Establish ongoing monitoring of pain and effectiveness of pain treatment.
  - ▪ Avoid IM or subcutaneous injections.
  - ▪ Use intravenous opioid analgesics such as morphine sulfate, hydromorphone (Dilaudid), and fentanyl (Sublimaze). Anesthetics such as ketamine (Ketalar), pentobarbital sodium (Nembutal), and nitrous oxide also may be used.
  - ▪ Monitor for respiratory depression when using opioid analgesics.
  - ▪ The use of patient-controlled analgesia is appropriate for some clients. They help decrease pain level, and the client benefits from having a sense of control.
  - ▪ Administer pain medication prior to dressing changes or procedures.
  - ▪ Use nonpharmacologic methods for pain control, such as guided imagery, music therapy, and therapeutic touch, to enhance the effects of analgesic medications and lead to more effective pain management.
- ○ Prevent Infection
  - ▪ Follow standard precautions when performing wound care.
  - ▪ Restrict plants and flowers due to the risk of contact with *Pseudomonas aeruginosa*.
  - ▪ Restrict consumption of fresh fruits and vegetables.
  - ▪ Limit visitors.
  - ▪ Use reverse isolation if prescribed.
  - ▪ Monitor for manifestations of infection and report to provider.
  - ▪ Use client-designated equipment such as BP cuffs, thermometers.
  - ▪ Administer tetanus toxoid if indicated.
  - ▪ Administer antibiotics if infection present.
- ○ Nutritional Support
  - ▪ The client who has a large area of burn injury will be in a hypermetabolic and hypercatabolic state. The client may need 5,000 calories per day.
  - ▪ Increase caloric intake to meet increased metabolic demands and prevent hypoglycemia.
  - ▪ Increase protein intake to prevent tissue breakdown and to promote healing.
  - ▪ Enteral therapy or total parenteral nutrition (TPN) may be necessary due to decreased gastrointestinal motility and increased caloric needs.

- ○ Restoration of Mobility
  - Maintain correct body alignment, splint extremities, and facilitate position changes to prevent contractures.
  - Maintain active and passive range of motion.
  - Assist with ambulation as soon as the client is stable.
  - Apply pressure dressings to prevent contractures and scarring.
  - Monitor areas at high risk for pressure sores (heels, sacrum, back of head).
- ○ Psychological Support of Client and Family
  - Provide emotional support.
  - Assist with coping.
- Medications

TOPICAL AGENTS – ANTIMICROBIAL CREAMS	
USES AND ADVANTAGES	DISADVANTAGES
Silver nitrate 0.5%	
› Used on wounds exposed to air, or with modified or occlusive dressing › May affect joint movement › Reduces fluid evaporation › Bacteriostatic against pseudomonas and staphylococcus › Inexpensive	› Does not penetrate eschar › Stains clothing and linen › Discolors wound, making assessment difficult › Painful on application
Silver sulfadiazine 1% (Silvadene)	
› Used with occlusive dressings › Maintains joint mobility › Effective against gram-negative bacteria, gram-positive bacteria, and yeast	› May cause transient neutropenia › Contraindicated with allergies to sulfa › Does not penetrate eschar › Painful to remove from wound › Decreases granulocyte formation
Mafenide acetate (Sulfamylon)	
› Used on wounds exposed to air › Used as a solution for occlusive dressings to keep the dressing moist › Penetrates eschar and goes into underlying tissues › Effective with electrical and infected wounds › Biostatic against gram-negative and gram-positive bacteria	› Painful to apply and remove › May cause metabolic acidosis or hyperpnea › Inhibits wound healing › Hypersensitivity may develop
Bacitracin	
› Used on wounds exposed to air or with modified dressings › Maintains joint mobility › Bacteriostatic against gram-positive organisms › Painless and easy to apply	› Limited effectiveness on gram-negative organisms

- Teamwork and Collaboration

  ○ Initiate referral to a registered dietitian, social worker, psychological counselor, or occupational/physical therapist if indicated.

  ○ Respiratory therapy to improve pulmonary function also may be needed.

- Therapeutic Procedures

  ○ Wound Care

    ▪ Nonsurgical management, such as hyperbaric oxygen therapy

    ▪ Nursing Actions

      □ Premedicate the client with analgesic as prescribed prior to all wound care.

      □ Remove all previous dressings.

      □ Assess for odors, drainage, and discharge. Assess for evidence of sloughing, eschar, bleeding, and evidence of new skin cell regeneration.

      □ Cleanse the wound as prescribed, removing all previous ointments. (It is important to cleanse the wound thoroughly.)

      □ Assist with debridement.

        ▸ Mechanical – Use scissors and forceps to cut away the dead tissue during the hydrotherapy treatment.

        ▸ Hydrotherapy – Place the client in a warm tub of water or use warm running water, as if to shower, to cleanse the wound.

          ▷ Use mild soap or detergent to gently wash burns and then rinse with room-temperature water.

          ▷ Encourage the client to exercise his joints during the hydrotherapy treatment.

        ▸ Enzymatic – Apply a topical enzyme to break down and remove dead tissue.

      □ Ensure that the client does not become hypothermic during the treatment.

      □ Apply a thin layer of topical antibiotic ointment as prescribed and cover with dressing, using surgical aseptic technique.

  ○ Skin Coverings

    ▪ Biologic skin coverings are temporarily used to promote healing of large burns. Additionally, biologic skin coverings promote the retention of water and protein and provide coverage of nerve endings, thus reducing the amount of pain experienced by the client. The provider stipulates whether skin coverings are to be left open or protected by a dressing.

      □ Allograft (homograft) – Skin is donated from human cadavers and used for partial- and full-thickness burn wounds.

      □ Xenograft (heterograft) – Obtained from animals, such as pigs, for partial-thickness burn wounds.

      □ Amnion – Obtained from human placenta; requires frequent changes.

      □ Synthetic skin coverings – Used for partial-thickness burn wounds.

        ▸ Many of the synthetic skin coverings are made of materials that are clear enough to see through so that the wound can be visualized without removing the dressing.

- Permanent skin coverings may be the treatment of choice for burns covering large areas of the body.
  - □ Autografts – Donor skin from another area of the burn client's body
    - ▸ Sheet graft – Sheet of skin used to cover wound
    - ▸ Mesh graft – Sheet of skin placed in mesher so skin graft has small slits in it; allows graft to be stretched to cover larger areas of the burn wound
  - □ Artificial skin – synthetic product that is used for partial- and full-thickness burn wounds (healing is faster)
  - □ Cultured epithelium – epithelial cells cultured for use when grafting sites are limited
- Nursing Actions
  - □ Maintain immobilization of graft site.
  - □ Elevate extremity.
  - □ Provide wound care to the donor site.
  - □ Administer analgesics.
  - □ Monitor for evidence of infection before and after skin coverings or grafts are applied.
    - ▸ Discoloration of unburned skin surrounding burn wound
    - ▸ Green color to subcutaneous fat
    - ▸ Degeneration of granulation tissue
    - ▸ Development of subeschar hemorrhage
    - ▸ Hyperventilation indicating systemic involvement of infection
    - ▸ Unstable body temperature
- Client Education
  - □ Instruct the client to keep extremity elevated.
  - □ Instruct the client to report signs and symptoms of infection.
  - □ Determine the client's level of pain and provide addition measures to control donor site pain.
  - □ Instruct the client to continue to perform range-of-motion exercises and to work with a physical therapist to prevent contractures.
  - □ Provide client instruction on how to assess the wound for infection and how to perform wound care.
- Care After Discharge
  - ○ Initiate referral for home health nursing care.
  - ○ Initiate referral to occupational therapy for evaluation of the home environment and assistance to relearn how to perform ADLs.
  - ○ Initiate referral to social services for community support services.

Complications

- Airway Injury

  - Thermal injuries to the airway may result from steam or chemical inhalation, aspiration of scalding liquid, and explosion while breathing. If the injury took place in an enclosed space, carbon monoxide poisoning should be suspected.

  - Clinical manifestations may be delayed for 24 to 48 hr.

  - Clinical manifestations include progressive hoarseness, brassy cough, difficulty swallowing, drooling, increased secretions, adventitious breath sounds, and expiratory sounds that include audible wheezes, crowing, and stridor.

  - Nursing Actions – Maintain airway and ventilation, and provide oxygen as prescribed.

  - Client Education – Educate the client and family about airway management, such as deep breathing, coughing, and elevating the head of the bed.

- Fluid and Electrolyte Imbalances

  - Nursing Actions

    - Assess fluid volume status. Weigh daily and maintain strict I&O.

    - Monitor laboratory results and compare to previous data.

    - Administer IV fluids and electrolytes.

  - Client Education – Educate the client and family about signs and symptoms of electrolyte imbalances and the need to alert the provider immediately.

- Wound Infections

  - Nursing Actions

    - Assess for discoloration, edema, odor, and drainage.

    - Assess for fluctuations in temperature and heart rate.

    - Obtain wound culture.

    - Administer antibiotics as prescribed.

    - Monitor laboratory results, observing for anemia and infection.

    - Maintain surgical aseptic technique with dressing changes.

  - Client Education – Educate the client and family on the importance of infection control.

APPLICATION EXERCISES

1. A nurse working in a provider's office is assessing a client who has a severe sunburn. Which of the following is the proper classification of this burn?

    A. Superficial

    B. Superficial partial-thickness

    C. Deep partial-thickness

    D. Full-thickness

2. A nurse is caring for a client who has sustained burns to 35% of his total body surface area. Of this total, 20% are full-thickness burns on the arms, face, neck, and shoulders. The client's voice is hoarse, and he has a brassy cough. These findings are indicative of which of the following?

    A. Pulmonary edema

    B. Bacterial pneumonia

    C. Inhalation injury

    D. Carbon monoxide poisoning

3. A nurse is caring for a client who was admitted 24 hr ago with deep partial-thickness and full-thickness burns to 40% of his body. Which of the following are expected findings in this client? (Select all that apply.)

    _____ A. Hypertension

    _____ B. Bradycardia

    _____ C. Hyperkalemia

    _____ D. Hyponatremia

    _____ E. Decreased hematocrit

4. A nurse is preparing to administer fentanyl (Sublimaze) to a client who was admitted 24 hr ago with deep partial-thickness and full-thickness burns over 60% of his body. The nurse should plan to use which of the following routes to administer the medication?

    A. Subcutaneous

    B. Intramuscular

    C. Intravenous

    D. Transdermal

5. A nurse is planning care for a client who has burn injuries. Which of the following interventions should be included in the plan of care? (Select all that apply.)

_____ A. Use standard precautions when performing wound care.

_____ B. Encourage fresh vegetables in the diet.

_____ C. Increase protein intake.

_____ D. Instruct client to consume 3,000 calories daily.

_____ E. Restrict fresh flowers in room.

6. A nurse is reviewing care of a client who has an autograft skin covering of a burn injury with a nurse who will assume care of the client at the end of the day. What should be included in the review? Use the ATI Active Learning Template: Therapeutic Procedure to complete this item to include the following:

A. Description of Procedure

B. Nursing Actions: Describe at least four interventions.

APPLICATION EXERCISES KEY

1. A. **CORRECT:** A sunburn is a superficial burn. Superficial burns damage the top layer of the skin.

    B. INCORRECT: A superficial partial-thickness burn can be caused by a flame or a burn scald. This damages the entire epidermis layer of the skin.

    C. INCORRECT: A deep partial-thickness burn can be caused by a grease burn. This affects the deep layers of the skin.

    D. INCORRECT: A full-thickness burn can be caused by a tar burn. This affects the dermis and sometimes the subcutaneous fat layer.

     NCLEX® Connection: Physiological Adaptations, Pathophysiology

2. A. INCORRECT: Difficulty breathing and a production of pink frothy sputum are indicative of pulmonary edema.

    B. INCORRECT: Coughing and a fever are indicative of a bacterial infection.

    C. **CORRECT:** Wheezing and hoarseness are indicative of inhalation injury and should be reported to the provider immediately.

    D. INCORRECT: Confusion and headaches are indicative of carbon monoxide poisoning.

     NCLEX® Connection: Physiological Adaptations, Pathophysiology

3. A. INCORRECT: Hypotension occurs when a client is in shock.

    B. INCORRECT: Tachycardia occurs when a client is in shock.

    C. **CORRECT:** Hyperkalemia occurs when a client is in shock as a result of leakage of fluid from the intracellular space.

    D. **CORRECT:** Hyponatremia occurs when a client is in shock as a result in sodium retention in the interstitial space.

    E. INCORRECT: An increased hematocrit occurs when a client is in shock.

     NCLEX® Connection: Physiological Adaptations, Pathophysiology

4. A. INCORRECT: Subcutaneous injections should be avoided due to the risk of infection.

    B. INCORRECT: Intramuscular injections should be avoided due to the risk of infection.

    C. **CORRECT:** The intravenous route is used to administer pain medication to a client who has a major burn during the emergent phase. Once IV access is established, this will provide the most rapid pain relief.

    D. INCORRECT: Transdermal route of administration should not be used due to the risk of tissue damage.

     NCLEX® Connection: Pharmacological and Parenteral Therapies, Pharmacological Pain Management

5. A. **CORRECT:** Standard precautions should be used when performing wound care to decrease the risk of infection.

    B. INCORRECT: The client should restrict consumption of fresh vegetables due to the presence of bacteria on the surface and increased risk for infection.

    C. **CORRECT:** The client should increase protein consumption, which promotes wound healing and prevents tissue breakdown.

    D. INCORRECT: The client should consume 5,000 calories/day.

    E. **CORRECT:** Flowers should not be the client's room due to the bacteria they carry, which increases the risk for infection.

    NCLEX® Connection: Physiological Adaptations, Illness Management

6. *Using the ATI Active Learning Template: Therapeutic Procedure*

    A. Description of Procedure
    - An autograft is donor skin from another area of the burn client's body. This is a permanent skin covering and used for burns on larger areas of the body.

    B. Nursing Actions
    - Maintain immobilization of the graft site.
    - Elevate the extremity.
    - Provide wound care to the donor site.
    - Administer analgesics.
    - Monitor for evidence of infection before and after skin coverings or grafts are applied.
      - Discoloration of unburned skin surrounding burn wound
      - Green color to subcutaneous fat
      - Degeneration of granulation tissue
      - Development of subeschar hemorrhage
      - Hyperventilation indicating systemic involvement of infection
      - Unstable body temperature

    NCLEX® Connection: Physiological Adaptations, Illness Management

UNIT 12 Nursing Care of Clients with Endocrine Disorders

SECTIONS

› Diagnostic and Therapeutic Procedures
› Pituitary Disorders
› Thyroid Disorders
› Adrenal Disorders
› Diabetes Mellitus

NCLEX® CONNECTIONS

When reviewing the chapters in this unit, keep in mind the relevant sections of the NCLEX® outline, in particular:

Client Needs: Pharmacological and Parenteral Therapies	Client Needs: Reduction of Risk Potential	Client Needs: Physiological Adaptation
› Relevant topics/tasks include: » Adverse Effects/Contraindications/Side Effects/Interactions › Manage the client experiencing side effects and adverse reactions of medication. » Dosage Calculation › Use clinical decision making/critical thinking when calculating dosages. » Medication Administration › Titrate dosage of medication based on assessment and ordered parameters.	› Relevant topics/tasks include: » Diagnostic Tests › Apply knowledge of related nursing procedures and psychomotor skills when caring for clients undergoing diagnostic testing. » Laboratory Values › Notify the provider about laboratory test results. » Therapeutic Procedures › Educate the client about treatments and procedures.	› Relevant topics/tasks include: » Fluid and Electrolyte Imbalances › Apply knowledge of pathophysiology when caring for the client with fluid and electrolyte imbalances. » Illness Management › Educate the client about managing illness. » Pathophysiology › Identify pathophysiology related to an acute or chronic condition.

chapter 77

Overview

- The function of the endocrine system is evaluated primarily by using laboratory tests. These tests vary according to the organ or system under analysis.

- Many of these tests are blood tests used to determine an excess or lack of a particular hormone in the body. Some of these tests are used to stimulate a reaction in the body that will facilitate diagnosis of a particular disorder.

- Endocrine diagnostic procedures that nurses should be knowledgeable about include those used to diagnose disorders of the:

  ○ Posterior pituitary gland.

  ○ Adrenal cortex.

  ○ Adrenal medulla.

  ○ Metabolism of carbohydrates.

  ○ Thyroid and anterior pituitary glands.

Posterior Pituitary Gland

- The posterior pituitary gland secretes the hormone vasopressin (antidiuretic hormone [ADH]). ADH increases permeability of the renal distal tubules, causing the kidneys to reabsorb water.

  ○ A deficiency of ADH causes diabetes insipidus, which is characterized by the excretion of a large quantity of diluted urine.

  ○ Excessive secretion of ADH causes the syndrome of inappropriate antidiuretic hormone (SIADH). In SIADH, the kidneys retain water, urine becomes concentrated, urinary output decreases, and extracellular fluid volume is increased.

  ○ Diagnostic tests for the posterior pituitary gland include the water deprivation test, serum ADH, serum and urine electrolytes and osmolality, and urine-specific gravity.

- Water deprivation test
  - The water deprivation test measures the kidneys' ability to concentrate urine in light of an increased plasma osmolality and a low plasma vasopressin level. It is a specialized test that must be performed in a controlled setting, and the client should be observed throughout the test.
  - Indications
    - This test is performed for clients who have a diagnosis of diabetes insipidus.
    - It should only be conducted if the client's baseline serum sodium level is within the expected reference range and the osmolality of the urine is below 300 mOsm/kg H_2O.
    - This test should not be performed on clients who have renal insufficiency, uncontrolled diabetes mellitus, hypovolemia of any etiology, or untreated adrenal or thyroid hormone deficiency.
  - Interpretation of Findings – The test is positive for diabetes insipidus if the kidneys are unable to concentrate urine despite increased plasma osmolality.
  - Preprocedure
    - Nursing Actions
      - Instruct client to avoid smoking or the use of caffeine or alcohol prior to the test.
      - Begin test by withholding fluids for 8 to 12 hr, or until 3% to 5% of body weight is lost. Ensure someone remains with client during test.
      - Obtain IV access.
  - Intraprocedure
    - Nursing Actions
      - Place the client in a recumbent position for 30 min, during which the following steps can be performed. (The client may sit or stand during voiding and weight determination.)
        - ▸ Obtain 7 to 10 mL of heparinized blood in an iced tube and send to the laboratory for immediate processing to determine sodium level.
        - ▸ Ask the client to empty his bladder, record the amount, and send the specimen to the laboratory for immediate processing to determine osmolality.
        - ▸ Weigh the client to nearest tenth of a kilogram (0.1 kg). Record weight and obtain and record blood pressure and pulse.
      - Initiate a complete fluid restriction and have the client maintain a semi-recumbent position except to void if necessary.
      - Repeat the three steps – weigh, measure urine, obtain serum – hourly and record any findings.
      - Continue the steps until the serum sodium concentration or osmolality rises above the upper limit of the expected reference range.
  - Complications
    - Dehydration can occur due to a decrease in vascular volume.
      - Nursing Actions – Monitor the client closely for early indications of dehydration, including postural hypotension, tachycardia, and dizziness.

- Serum ADH, serum and urine electrolytes and osmolality, and urine-specific gravity tests are performed to diagnose SIADH.

TESTS TO DIAGNOSE SIADH	
SERUM ADH	
Normal Reference Range	1 to 5 pg/mL
Interpretation of Findings	› Increased serum ADH is indicative of SIADH.
Nursing Actions	› The client should fast and avoid stress for 12 hr prior to the test. › Some medications may interfere with the test. Review medications with the provider. › Blood is obtained and transported to the laboratory within 10 min.
SERUM ELECTROLYTES	
Normal Reference Range	› Sodium – 136 to 145 mEq/L › Potassium – 3.5 to 5.0 mEq/L › Chloride – 98 to 106 mEq/L › Magnesium – 1.3 to 2.1 mEq/L
Interpretation of Findings	› Low serum sodium and high urine sodium content are expected with SIADH. › Decreased serum osmolality and increased urine osmolality are indicative of SIADH.
Nursing Actions	› No pre/postprocedure care required. Serum samples of blood and urine are analyzed for electrolyte components.
URINE ELECTROLYTES AND OSMOLALITY	
Normal Reference Range	› Urine sodium – 75 to 200 mEq/day › Urine potassium – 26 to 123 mEq/day (intake dependent) › Urine chloride – 110 to 250 mEq/24 hr › Urine osmolality – 200 to 800 mOsm/kg
Interpretation of Findings	› Low serum sodium and high urine sodium content are expected with SIADH. › Decreased serum osmolality and increased urine osmolality are indicative of SIADH.
Nursing Actions	› No pre/postprocedure care required. Serum samples of blood and urine are analyzed for electrolyte components.
URINE-SPECIFIC GRAVITY	
Normal Reference Range	1.010 to 1.025
Interpretation of Findings	› A decrease in urine output and an increase in urine-specific gravity occur as a result of excess production of ADH.
Nursing Actions	› This test is usually performed in a laboratory but can be done in the clinical unit using a calibrated hydrometer or a temperature-compensated refractometer.

Adrenal Cortex

- Cushing's disease and Cushing's syndrome (hypercortisolism) are characterized by a hyperfunctioning adrenal cortex and an excess production of cortisol. Addison's disease is characterized by hypofunctioning of the adrenal cortex and a consequent lack of adequate amounts of serum cortisol.

    ○ Diagnostic tests for the adrenal cortex include the dexamethasone (Decadron) suppression test, plasma and salivary cortisol, 24-hr urine for cortisol, serum adrenocorticotropic hormone (ACTH), and ACTH stimulation tests.

    ○ A CT scan and/or an MRI may be performed to determine if there is atrophy of the adrenal glands causing hypofunction.

- Dexamethasone suppression test

    ○ This test is performed to determine if dexamethasone, which is a steroid similar to cortisol, has an effect on cortisol levels. Typically, the client takes a dose of dexamethasone by mouth, and a blood sample is obtained the next morning to determine if cortisol is present.

        ■ A low dose of dexamethasone is given to screen a client for Cushing's disease; high doses are given to determine the cause of the disease.

        ■ Some medications are withheld and stress is reduced prior to and during testing, as these can affect the outcome of the test results.

    ○ Indications – Cushing's disease

    ○ Interpretation of Findings

        ■ When decreased amounts of ACTH are produced by the pituitary gland, decreased amounts of cortisol are released by the adrenal glands.

        ■ When dexamethasone is given to clients who have Cushing's disease, there is no decrease in the production of ACTH and cortisol.

DIAGNOSTIC TESTS FOR THE ADRENAL CORTEX

PLASMA CORTISOL

Normal Reference Range	› Cortisol varies according to the time of day. Because it has a diurnal (daily) pattern, higher levels are present in the early morning, and the lowest levels occur around midnight, or 3 to 5 hr after the onset of sleep.
Interpretation of Findings	› Diurnal variations are not seen in a client who has Cushing's syndrome.
Nursing Actions	› Plasma cortisol is usually collected at midnight.

SALIVARY CORTISOL

Normal Reference Range	› A typical salivary cortisol value at midnight is less than 2.0 ng/mL.
Interpretation of Findings	› Higher levels indicate hypercortisolism.
Nursing Actions	› Salivary cortisol is usually collected at midnight. › A sample of saliva is obtained by placing a salivary cushion pad inside the client's cheek, directly over the salivary gland.

URINARY CORTISOL

Normal Reference Range	10 to 100 mcg/day
Interpretation of Findings	› Higher levels indicate hypercortisolism.
Nursing Actions	› Urinary cortisol is measured during 24-hr urine collection. » The client empties his bladder and then collects all urine excreted during the next 24-hr period. » The urine must be kept in a jug with boric acid added and kept on ice. » If the client is receiving spironolactone, this should be withheld for 7 days prior to the test.

SERUM ACTH

Normal Reference Range	› Typical early morning values are 25 to 200 pg/mL, and early evening values are usually 0 to 50 pg/mL.
Interpretation of Findings	› ACTH may be elevated with Addison's disease or decreased with Cushing's disease.
Nursing Actions	› Serum ACTH is most accurate if performed in the morning.

ACTH STIMULATION TEST

Normal Reference Range	› If no increase in cortisol occurs after administration of ACTH, the test is positive for Addison's disease or hypocortisolism.
Interpretation of Findings	› ACTH stimulation test determines the functioning of the pituitary gland in relation to stimulating the secretion of adrenal hormones of cortisol.
Nursing Actions	› Two consecutive collections of 24-hr urine are used, one prior to and one after the administration of ACTH.

Adrenal Medulla

- Disorders of the adrenal medulla may cause hypersecretion of catecholamines, resulting in stimulation of a sympathetic response, such as tachycardia, hypertension, and diaphoresis.
    - ○ Diagnostic tests for the adrenal medulla include vanillylmandelic acid (VMA) testing, clonidine suppression test, and phentolamine blocking test.
- VMA testing is a 24-hr urine collection for vanillylmandelic acid (VMA), a breakdown product of catecholamines. Analysis of other urinary catecholamines, such as dopamine and normetanephrine, also may be measured.
    - ○ Indications – diagnosis of pheochromocytoma
    - ○ Interpretation of Findings
        - Expected reference range for VMA is 2 to 7 mg/24 hr.
        - Elevated VMA levels at rest indicate pheochromocytoma.

    - ○ Preprocedure
        - Nursing Actions – Monitor/instruct the client regarding 24-hr urine collection. Urine is collected for 24 hr (in a container with a preservative) beginning with an empty bladder.
        - Client Education
            - □ Caffeine, vanilla, bananas, and chocolate may be restricted for 2 to 3 days before the test. The client may also be asked to withhold aspirin and antihypertensive medications.
            - □ Instruct the client to maintain a moderate level of activity.
- Clonidine suppression test – The client's plasma catecholamines levels are taken prior to and 3 hr after administration of clonidine (Catapres).
    - ○ Indications – Pheochromocytoma
    - ○ Interpretation of Findings
        - If a client does not have a pheochromocytoma, clonidine suppresses catecholamine release and decreases the serum level of catecholamines (decreases blood pressure).
        - If the client does have a pheochromocytoma, the clonidine has no effect (no decreased blood pressure).
    - ○ Pre/intraprocedure
        - Nursing Actions
            - □ Inform the client about the test.
            - □ Monitor the client for hypotension.
    - ○ Postprocedure
        - Client Education – Inform the client that fatigue may occur after the test.
- Phentolamine blocking test – Phentolamine (Regitine), an alpha blocker, is administered.
    - ○ Indications – pheochromocytoma
    - ○ Interpretation of Findings – A rapid decrease in systolic blood pressure of greater than or equal to 35 mm Hg and diastolic blood pressure of greater than or equal to 25 mm Hg with the administration of phentolamine is diagnostic for pheochromocytoma.
    - ○ Intraprocedure
        - Nursing Actions – Monitor blood pressure.

Carbohydrate Metabolism

- Dysfunction of carbohydrate metabolism may be caused by insulin deficiency, as in type 1 diabetes mellitus, or insulin resistance, as in type 2 diabetes mellitus, resulting in hyperglycemia.

  ○ Diagnostic tests to evaluate carbohydrate metabolism include fasting blood glucose, oral glucose tolerance testing, and glycosylated hemoglobin (HbA1c).

FASTING BLOOD GLUCOSE	
Normal Reference Range	› Less than 110 mg/dL
Interpretation of Findings	› Determines blood glucose when no foods or fluids (other than water) have been consumed for the past 8 hr.
Nursing Actions	› Ensure that the client has fasted (no food or drink other than water) for the 8 hr prior to the blood sample being obtained. › Antidiabetic medications should be postponed until after the level is drawn.
ORAL GLUCOSE TOLERANCE TEST	
Normal Reference Range	› Less than 140 mg/dL
Interpretation of Findings	› Determines ability to metabolize a standard amount of glucose.
Nursing Actions	› Instruct the client to consume a balanced diet for the 3 days prior to the test and fast for the 10 to 12 hr prior to the test. › A fasting blood glucose level is obtained at start of the test. › The client is then instructed to consume a specified amount of glucose. › Blood samples are obtained every 30 min for 2 hr. Clients must be assessed for hypoglycemia throughout the procedure.
GLYCOSYLATED HEMOGLOBIN (HbA1c)	
Normal Reference Range	› HbA1c of 5% or less indicates absence of diabetes mellitus; HbA1c of 5.7% to 6.4% indicates prediabetes mellitus, and HbA1c of 6.5% or higher indicates diabetes mellitus.
Interpretation of Findings	› HbA1c is the best indicator of an average blood glucose level for the past 120 days. › Assists in evaluating treatment effectiveness and compliance with the diet plan, medication regimen, and exercise schedule.
Nursing Actions	› No pre/postprocedure care is required. The test requires obtaining a random blood sample.

Thyroid and Anterior Pituitary Gland

- Hyperthyroidism and hypothyroidism are conditions in which there are inappropriate amounts of the thyroid hormones triiodothyronine (T_3) and thyroxine (T_4) circulating. These inappropriate amounts of T_3 and T_4 cause an increase or decrease in metabolic rate that affects all body systems.

- The anterior pituitary gland secretes thyroid stimulating hormone (TSH). Hyposecretion of TSH may lead to secondary hypothyroidism, and hypersecretion of TSH may cause secondary hyperthyroidism.
  - ○ Diagnostic tests to evaluate the function of the thyroid and anterior pituitary glands include serum T_3, serum T_4, serum TSH, serum thyrotropin-releasing hormone (TRH) stimulation test, and radioactive iodine uptake (RAIU).
  - ○ Ultrasounds or CT scans may be performed to determine the size, shape, and presence of nodules and masses on these glands.

TESTS TO EVALUATE THE FUNCTION OF THE THYROID AND ANTERIOR PITUITARY GLANDS	
T_3 and T_4	
Normal Reference Range	› T_3: 70 to 205 ng/dL › T_4: 4.0 to 12.0 mcg/dL
Interpretation of Findings	› Low and high levels of each indicate hypothyroidism and hyperthyroidism respectively; a high level of T_3 is more diagnostic of hyperthyroidism than is T_4.
Nursing Actions	› No pre/postprocedure care is required for either test. The laboratory requires a random blood sample.
TSH	
Normal Reference Range	0.3 to 5.0 microunits/mL
Interpretation of Findings	› It stimulates the release of thyroid hormone by the anterior pituitary gland. › TSH may be elevated or decreased, depending on the cause. An increased value indicates primary hypothyroidism or secondary hyperthyroidism. A decreased value indicates primary hyperthyroidism (Graves' disease) or secondary hypothyroidism.
Nursing Actions	› No pre/postprocedure care is required. The laboratory requires a random blood sample.
TRH	
Normal Reference Range	› Relative to baseline
Interpretation of Findings	› It is normal for the TSH to double the baseline value shortly after administration. › If the TSH increases twofold or more above baseline, this finding is indicative of hypothyroidism.
Nursing Actions	› The TRH is assessed by giving a bolus of thyrotropin-releasing hormone, and serum concentrations of TSH are assessed at intervals.
RAIU	
Normal Reference Range	› Less than 35% of injected amount of radioactive iodine (^{123}I)
Interpretation of Findings	› It measures the amount of ^{123}I that is absorbed by the thyroid gland. › Clients who have hyperthyroidism absorb high amounts (greater than 35%) of ^{123}I.
Nursing Actions	› The client is given an oral radioactive dose of ^{123}I, and the amount absorbed is measured by a scintillation counter. › This test cannot be done if the client is pregnant or has had another test done that used an iodine-containing dye.

APPLICATION EXERCISES

1. A client asks a nurse why the provider bases his medication regimen on his HbA1c instead of his log of morning fasting blood glucose results. Which of the following is an appropriate response by the nurse?

   A. "HbA1c measures how well insulin is regulating your blood glucose between meals."

   B. "HbA1c indicates how well your blood glucose has been regulated over the past 3 months."

   C. "A test of HbA1c is the first test to determine if an individual has diabetes."

   D. "A test of HbA1c determines if the dosage of insulin needs to be adjusted."

2. A nurse is reviewing the laboratory findings of a client who has suspected hyperthyroidism. An elevation of which of the following supports this diagnosis?

   A. Triiodothyronine (T_3)

   B. Vanillylmandelic acid (VMA)

   C. Adrenocorticotropic hormone (ACTH)

   D. Glycosylated hemoglobin (HbA1c)

3. A nurse is reviewing the health record of a client who has syndrome of inappropriate antidiuretic hormone (SIADH). Which of the following laboratory findings should the nurse anticipate? (Select all that apply.)

   ___X___ A. Low serum sodium

   _____ B. High serum potassium

   _____ C. Decreased urine osmolality

   ___X___ D. High urine sodium

   ___X___ E. Increased urine-specific gravity

4. A nurse is caring for a client who has primary adrenal insufficiency. Which of the following findings should the nurse anticipate after an IV injection of ACTH 1.0 mg?

   A. Decrease in serum plasma cortisol

   B. Elevated fasting serum blood glucose

   C. Decrease in serum sodium

   D. Increase in urinary output

5. A nurse is providing teaching to a client who is scheduled for a phentolamine blocking test. This test supports a diagnosis for which of the following disorders?

    A. Addison's disease

    B. Diabetes mellitus

    C. Cushing's disease

    D. Pheochromocytoma

6. A nurse is planning care for a client who is scheduled for a clonidine suppression test. What should be included in the plan of care? Use the ATI Active Learning Template: Diagnostic Procedure to complete this item to include the following:

    A. Indications

    B. Interpretation of Findings

    C. Pre/intraprocedure Nursing Actions: Describe two.

APPLICATION EXERCISES KEY

1. A. INCORRECT: Capillary glucose monitoring evaluates how well insulin is regulating blood glucose between meals.

    B. **CORRECT:** HbA1c measures the client's blood glucose control over the past 2 to 3 months.

    C. INCORRECT: A fasting blood glucose is the first test performed to diagnose diabetes mellitus.

    D. INCORRECT: Capillary glucose monitoring evaluates how well insulin regulates blood glucose.

    Ⓝ NCLEX® Connection: Reduction of Risk Potential, Laboratory Values

2. A. **CORRECT:** T_3 increases in a hyperthyroid state.

    B. INCORRECT: VMA is used to detect pheochromocytoma and reflects the amount of catecholamine byproducts.

    C. INCORRECT: ACTH is used to detect Cushing's disease.

    D. INCORRECT: HbA1c is used to identify blood glucose control over the past 2 to 3 months.

    Ⓝ NCLEX® Connection: Reduction of Risk Potential, Laboratory Values

3. A. **CORRECT:** SIADH results in water retention, causing a low serum sodium level.

    B. INCORRECT: SIADH does not affect serum potassium levels.

    C. INCORRECT: SIADH results in an increase in urine osmolality.

    D. **CORRECT:** SIADH results in water retention, causing a high urine sodium level.

    E. **CORRECT:** SIADH results in water retention, causing an increase in urine-specific gravity.

    Ⓝ NCLEX® Connection: Reduction of Risk Potential, Laboratory Values

4. A. **CORRECT:** A decrease in serum plasma cortisol is indicative of primary adrenal insufficiency due to inadequate production of aldosterone and cortisol.

    B. INCORRECT: An elevated fasting serum blood glucose is used to diagnose diabetes.

    C. INCORRECT: An increase in serum sodium is indicative of primary adrenal insufficiency.

    D. INCORRECT: A decrease in urinary output is indicative of primary adrenal insufficiency.

    (N) NCLEX® Connection: Pharmacological and Parenteral Therapies, Expected Actions/Outcomes

5. A. INCORRECT: Evaluation of plasma cortisol is used to identify Addison's disease.

    B. INCORRECT: A fasting blood glucose is used to identify diabetes.

    C. INCORRECT: An dexamethasone suppression test is used to identify Cushing's syndrome.

    D. **CORRECT:** Phentolamine, an alpha blocker, is administered and decreases the client's blood pressure when pheochromocytoma is present.

    (N) NCLEX® Connection: Reduction of Risk Potential, Diagnostic Tests

6. *Using the ATI Active Learning Template: Diagnostic Procedure*

    A. Indications
    - Confirms a diagnosis of a pheochromocytoma

    B. Interpretation of Findings
    - If client does not have a pheochromocytoma, clonidine suppresses catecholamine release and decreases the serum level of catecholamines (decreases blood pressure).
    - If client has a pheochromocytoma, clonidine has no effect (no decrease in blood pressure).

    C. Pre/intraprocedure Nursing Actions
    - Inform the client about the test.
    - Monitor the client for hypotension.

    (N) NCLEX® Connection: Reduction of Risk Potential, Diagnostic Tests

chapter **78**

Overview

- The posterior pituitary gland secretes the hormone vasopressin, or antidiuretic hormone (ADH).

  - Vasopressin increases permeability of the renal distal tubules, causing the kidneys to reabsorb water.

  - A deficiency of ADH causes diabetes insipidus (DI).

    - DI is characterized by the excretion of a large quantity of diluted urine.

  - Excessive secretion of ADH causes the syndrome of inappropriate antidiuretic hormone (SIADH).

    - In SIADH, the kidneys retain water, urine output decreases, and extracellular fluid volume is increased.

- Posterior pituitary disorders result in fluid and electrolyte imbalances.

DIABETES INSIPIDUS

Overview

- Diabetes insipidus results from a deficiency of ADH, which is secreted by the posterior lobe of the pituitary gland (neurohypophysis).

- Decreased ADH reduces the ability of collecting and distal renal tubules in the kidneys to concentrate urine, resulting in excessive diluted urination, excessive thirst, and excessive fluid intake.

- Types of diabetes insipidus

  - Neurogenic (also known as central or primary) – Caused by damage to the hypothalamus or pituitary gland from trauma, irradiation, or cranial surgery.

  - Nephrogenic – Inherited; renal tubules do not react to ADH.

  - Drug-induced – Lithium carbonate (Lithobid) or demeclocycline (Declomycin) may alter the way the kidneys respond to ADH.

Assessment

- Risk Factors

  - Clients who have a head injury, tumor or lesion, surgery near or around the pituitary gland, or infection (meningitis, encephalitis).

  - Clients who are taking lithium carbonate (Lithobid) or demeclocycline (Declomycin).

  - Older adult clients are at higher risk for dehydration due to lower water content of the body, decreased thirst response, decreased ability of the kidneys to concentrate urine, increased use of diuretics, swallowing difficulties, or poor food intake.

- Subjective Data
  - Polyuria (abrupt onset of excessive urination, urinary output of 4 to 20 L/day of dilute urine)
  - Polydipsia (excessive thirst, consumption of 2 to 20 L/day)
  - Nocturia
  - Fatigue
  - Dehydration, as evidenced by extreme thirst, weight loss, muscle weakness, headache, constipation, and dizziness
- Objective Data
  - Physical Assessment Findings
    - Sunken eyes
    - Tachycardia
    - Hypotension
    - Loss or absence of skin turgor
    - Dry mucous membranes
  - Laboratory Tests
    - Urine chemistry – Think DILUTE.
      - Decreased urine specific gravity (less than 1.005).
      - Decreased urine osmolality (less than 300 mOsm/L).
      - Decreased urine pH.
      - Decreased urine sodium.
      - Decreased urine potassium.
      - As urine volume increases, urine osmolality decreases.
    - Serum chemistry – Think CONCENTRATED.
      - Increased serum osmolality (greater than 300 mOsm/L).
      - Increased serum sodium.
      - Increased serum potassium.
      - As serum volume decreases, the serum osmolality increases.
    - Radioimmunoassay – decreased ADH
  - Diagnostic Procedures
    - Water deprivation test
      - This is an easy and reliable diagnostic test. Dehydration is induced by withholding fluids. Urine output is measured and tested hourly.
      - The test is positive for diabetes insipidus if the kidneys are unable to concentrate urine despite increased plasma osmolarity.
      - Nursing Actions
        - Obtain baseline weight, vital signs, serum electrolytes and osmolarity, and urine specific gravity and osmolarity.
        - Monitor hourly vital signs, urine specific gravity, and osmolarity.
        - Monitor for severe dehydration.
          - Early indications may be postural hypotension, tachycardia, and dizziness. Be prepared to discontinue the test if these indicators develop.

▫ Client Education

▸ Explain the test procedure to the client.

▸ Advise the client to report any dizziness, headache, or nausea.

▪ Vasopressin test

▫ A subcutaneous injection of vasopressin produces urine output with an increased specific gravity if the client has central diabetes insipidus. This differentiates central from nephrogenic diabetes insipidus.

▫ Nursing Actions – Monitor vital signs, urine specific gravity, and osmolarity hourly.

▫ Client Education – Explain the test procedure to the client. Advise the client to notify the nurse of any dizziness, headache, or nausea.

Patient-Centered Care

• Nursing Care

  ○ Monitor vital signs, urinary output, central venous pressure, I&O, specific gravity, and laboratory studies (potassium, sodium, BUN, creatinine, specific gravity, osmolarity).

  ○ Weigh daily.

  ○ Promote the prescribed diet (regular diet with restriction of foods that exert a diuretic effect, such as caffeine).

  ○ IV therapy – Hydration (intake and output must be matched to prevent dehydration), and electrolyte replacement.

  ○ Promote safety – Keep bedside rails up while client is in bed, and provide assistance with ambulation due to dizziness or muscle weakness. Ensure easy access to a bathroom or bedpan.

  ○ Add bulk foods and fruit juices to the diet if constipation develops. A laxative may be needed.

  ○ Assess skin turgor and mucous membranes.

  ○ Provide skin and mouth care, and apply a lubricant to cracked or sore lips. Use a soft toothbrush and mild mouthwash to avoid trauma to the oral mucosa. Use alcohol-free skin care products, and apply emollient lotion after baths.

  ○ Encourage the client to drink fluids in response to thirst.

  ○ Administer medications as prescribed.

• Medications

  ○ ADH replacement agents – desmopressin acetate (DDAVP) or aqueous vasopressin (Pitressin) administered intranasally, orally, or parenterally

    ▪ Used as a synthetic posterior pituitary hormone, which results in increased water absorption from kidneys and decreased urine output

    ▪ Nursing Considerations

      ▫ Monitor vital signs, urinary output, central venous pressure, I&O, specific gravity, and laboratory studies (potassium, sodium, BUN, creatinine, specific gravity, osmolarity).

      ▫ Dose may need to be adjusted to urine output.

- Client Education
  - For an intranasal dose, teach the client to clear nasal passage and sit upright prior to inhalation.
  - Instruct the client to monitor weight and notify the provider of a gain greater than 0.9 kg (2 lb) in 24 hr.
  - Instruct the client to restrict fluids if directed and notify the provider of headache or confusion.
- ADH stimulants – carbamazepine (Tegretol)
  - Anticonvulsants stimulate release of ADH. They may be effective in partial central diabetes insipidus.
  - Nursing Considerations
    - Monitor vital signs, urinary output, central venous pressure, I&O, specific gravity, and laboratory studies (potassium, sodium, BUN, creatinine, specific gravity, osmolarity).
    - Monitor for dizziness or drowsiness related to the medication.
    - Monitor for indications of thrombocytopenia (sore throat, bruising, fever).
  - Client Education
    - Take the medication with food to reduce gastric distress.
    - Use caution driving or operating heavy machinery until effects of the medication are established.
    - Notify the provider of sore throat, fever, or bleeding.
- Vasopressin (Pitressin)
  - Posterior pituitary hormone that causes an increase in water absorption from kidneys and a decrease in urine output
  - Nursing Considerations
    - Give vasopressin cautiously to clients who have coronary artery disease because the medication may cause vasoconstriction.
    - Monitor vital signs, urinary output, central venous pressure, I&O, specific gravity, and laboratory studies (potassium, sodium, BUN, creatinine, specific gravity, osmolarity).
    - Monitor for headache, confusion, or other indications of water intoxication.
  - Client Education
    - Educate the client regarding lifelong self-injection vasopressin therapy, daily weights, and the importance of reporting weight gain, polyuria, and polydipsia to the provider.
    - Instruct the client to restrict fluids if directed, and notify the provider of headache or confusion.
- Teamwork and Collaboration – Home assistance for fluid, medication, and dietary management may be required.
- Care After Discharge
  - Client Education
    - Instruct client on medications for home use.
    - Instruct the client to weigh daily, eat a diet that is high in fiber, wear a medical alert wristband, and monitor fluid intake.
    - Teach the client to monitor for indications of dehydration (weight loss; dry, cracked lips; confusion; weakness).
    - Advise the client to restrict fluids as prescribed to prevent water intoxication, and avoid consumption of alcohol.

Complications

- Untreated DI can cause hypovolemia, hyperosmolarity, hypernatremia, circulatory collapse, unconsciousness, central nervous system damage, and seizures.

  ○ Excessive urine output causing severe dehydration can lead to these complications.

  ○ Nursing Actions – Monitor fluid balance and prevent dehydration with providing proper fluid intake.

  ○ Client Education – Advise the client to seek early medical attention for any sign of diabetes insipidus and follow care instructions.

SYNDROME OF INAPPROPRIATE ANTIDIURETIC HORMONE (SIADH)

Overview

- Syndrome of inappropriate antidiuretic hormone (SIADH) is an excessive release of antidiuretic hormone (ADH), also known as vasopressin, secreted by the posterior lobe of the pituitary gland (neurohypophysis).

- Excess ADH leads to renal reabsorption of water and suppression of renin-angiotensin mechanism, causing renal excretion of sodium leading to water intoxication, cellular edema, and dilutional hyponatremia. Fluid shifts within compartments cause decreased serum osmolarity.

Assessment

- Risk Factors

  ○ Conditions that stimulate the hypothalamus to hypersecrete ADH include malignant tumors (the most common cause is oat-cell lung cancer), increased intrathoracic pressure (such as with positive pressure ventilation), head injury, meningitis, cardiovascular accident, medications (alcohol, lithium carbonate, phenytoin), trauma, pain, and stress.

  ○ Diuretics are sometimes used to treat conditions such as heart failure. Sodium losses due to diuretic use can further contribute to the problems caused by SIADH. A careful client history and medication review may help alert nurses to the possibility of SIADH.

- Subjective Data

  ○ Early manifestations of SIADH include headache, weakness, anorexia, muscle cramps, and weight gain (without edema because water, not sodium, is retained).

  ○ As the serum sodium level decreases, the client experiences personality changes, hostility, sluggish deep tendon reflexes, nausea, vomiting, diarrhea, and oliguria.

- Objective Data

  ○ Physical Assessment Findings

    ▪ Confusion, lethargy, and Cheyne-Stokes respirations herald impending crisis. When the serum sodium level drops further, seizures, coma, and death may occur.

    ▪ Manifestations of fluid volume excess include tachycardia, possible hypertension, crackles in lungs, distended neck veins, and taut skin. Intake is greater than output.

○ Laboratory Tests

- Urine chemistry – Think CONCENTRATED.

  □ Increased urine sodium.

  □ Increased urine osmolarity.

  □ As urine volume decreases, urine osmolarity increases.

- Blood chemistry – Think DILUTE.

  □ Decreased serum sodium.

  □ Decreased serum osmolarity (less than 270 mEq/L).

  □ As serum volume increases, serum osmolarity decreases.

  □ Radioimmunoassay – Increased ADH.

Patient-Centered Care

- Nursing Care

  ○ Restrict oral fluids to 500 to 1,000 mL/day to prevent further hemodilution (first priority). During fluid restriction, provide comfort measures for thirst, including mouth care, ice chips, lozenges, and staggered water intake.

  ○ Flush all enteral and gastric tubes with 0.9% sodium chloride, instead of water, to replace sodium and prevent further hemodilution.

  ○ Monitor I&O. Report decreased urine output.

  ○ Monitor vital signs for increased blood pressure, tachycardia, and hypothermia.

  ○ Monitor for decreased serum sodium/osmolarity and elevated urine sodium/osmolarity.

  ○ Weigh daily. A weight gain of 0.9 kg (2 lb) indicates a gain of 1 L of fluid.

  ○ Report altered mental status (headache, confusion, lethargy, seizures, coma).

  ○ Reduce environmental stimuli and position the client as needed.

  ○ Provide a safe environment for clients who have altered levels of consciousness. Maintain seizure precautions.

  ○ Monitor the client for indications of heart failure, which can occur from fluid overload. Use of a loop diuretic may be indicated.

- Medications

  ○ Demeclocycline (Declomycin)

  - Tetracycline derivative.

  - May cause drug-induced diabetes insipidus.

  - Nursing Considerations – Monitor for effective treatment, such as increased serum sodium/osmolarity and decreased urine sodium osmolarity.

  - Client Education

    □ Advise the client that it may take a week to see results.

    □ Advise the client to monitor for indications of a yeast infection, such as a white, cheese-like film inside the mouth.

    □ Have the client rinse toothbrush with a diluted bleach solution (10%), and increase consumption of yogurt.

- ○ Lithium (Lithium Carbonate)
  - Used to block the renal response to ADH
  - May induce diabetes insipidus
  - Nursing Considerations
    - □ Monitor for adverse effects (lithium toxicity, nausea, diarrhea, tremors ataxia).
    - □ Monitor blood glucose levels.
    - □ Monitor ECG for dysrhythmias.
    - □ Monitor for effective treatment (increased serum sodium/osmolarity, decreased urine sodium/osmolarity).
  - Client Education
    - □ Advise the client to monitor for symptoms of lithium toxicity.
    - □ Advise the client to take the medication with food.
    - □ Advise the client to allow 1 to 3 weeks to see effects.
- ○ Furosemide (Lasix)
  - A loop diuretic used to increase water excretion from kidneys
  - Nursing Considerations – Use with caution because loop diuretics cause sodium excretion and may worsen hyponatremia.
  - Client Education
    - □ Advise the client to change positions slowly in case of postural hypotension.
    - □ Advise the client to notify the provider of findings of hyponatremia, such as nausea, decreased appetite, and vomiting.
- • Teamwork and Collaboration
  - ○ Home care for may be required for fluid, medication, and dietary management.
- • Therapeutic Procedures
  - ○ Hypertonic sodium chloride IV fluid – The goal is to elevate the sodium level enough to alleviate neurologic compromise, not to raise the level to normal.
    - Nursing Actions
      - □ In severe hyponatremia/water intoxication, administration of 200 to 300 mL of hypertonic IV fluid (3% to 5% sodium chloride).
      - □ Monitor for fluid overload and heart failure (distended neck veins, crackles in lungs).
    - Client Education
      - □ Explain the procedure to the client.
      - □ Advise the client to report difficulty breathing or shortness of breath, which may indicate heart failure.
      - □ Include information about medications with discharge instructions.
      - □ Instruct the client to obtain daily weights, wear a medical alert wristband, and restrict fluid intake.

□ Advise the client to monitor for indications of hypervolemia (weight gain, difficulty breathing) and any neurological changes (tremors, disorientation), which may lead to seizures.

□ Advise the client to notify the provider of indications of hyponatremia, such as nausea, decreased appetite, and vomiting.

□ Advise the client to avoid consumption of alcohol.

Complications

- Water intoxication, cerebral edema, and severe hyponatremia

  ○ Without prompt treatment, SIADH may lead to these complications, with resultant coma and death.

  ○ Nursing Actions

    ▪ Monitor for early manifestations of water intoxication, such as lung crackles, distended neck veins, changes in neurological state (confusion, headaches, twitching, disorientation), edema, and decreased urinary output.

    ▪ Monitor neurologic status.

    ▪ Maintain seizure precautions.

    ▪ Administer medications as prescribed.

    ▪ Monitor serum sodium level.

  ○ Client Education

    ▪ Instruct the client and family about fluid restrictions, and offer information about the condition and treatment.

    ▪ Provide support to ease the client's fears.

- Central pontine myelinolysis (CPM)

  ○ Treatment for SIADH may result in CPM, a condition characterized by nerve damage that is caused by the destruction of the myelin sheath in the brainstem (pons). The most common cause is a rapid change in sodium levels in the body. This most commonly occurs when a client is being treated for hyponatremia and the sodium levels rise too fast.

  ○ Nursing Actions – During treatment with hypertonic saline or loop diuretics, plasma osmolarity and serum sodium should be monitored every 2 to 4 hr. Any deterioration in neurologic status should be reported immediately.

  ○ Client Education

    ▪ Inform the client and family about the condition.

    ▪ Explain all procedures and information about medication and treatment.

APPLICATION EXERCISES

1. A nurse is caring for a client who has primary diabetes insipidus. Which of the following manifestations should the nurse expect to find? (Select all that apply.)

___X___ A. Serum sodium of 155 mEq/L

___X___ B. Fatigue

_____ C. Serum osmolality of 250 mOsm/L

___X___ D. Polyuria

___X___ E. Nocturia

2. A nurse is caring for a client who has diabetes insipidus. Which of the following urinalysis laboratory findings should the nurse anticipate?

A. Absence of glucose

(B.) Decreased specific gravity

C. Presence of ketones

D. Presence of red blood cells

3. A nurse is caring for a client who has syndrome of inappropriate antidiuretic hormone (SIADH). Which of the following findings should the nurse expect? (Select all that apply.)

___X___ A. Decreased serum sodium

_____ B. Urine specific gravity 1.001

___X___ C. Serum osmolarity 230 mOsm/L

_____ D. Polyuria

_____ E. Increased thirst

4. A nurse is assessing a client who has SIADH. Which of the following findings indicate the client is experiencing a complication?

A. Decreased central venous pressure (CVP)

B. Increased urine output

(C.) Distended neck veins

D. Extreme thirst

5. A nurse is providing teaching to a client who has a new diagnosis of diabetes insipidus. Which of the following statements by the client requires further teaching?

A. "I can drink up to 2 quarts of fluid a day."

B. "I should expect to urinate frequently at night."

C. "I may experience headaches."

D. "I may experience a dry mouth."

6. A nurse is planning care for a client who has SIADH and has a new prescription for demeclocycline (Declomycin). What should be included in the plan of care? Use the ATI Active Learning Template: Medication to complete this item to include the following:

A. Therapeutic Use

B. Nursing Considerations: Describe one.

C. Client Education: Describe two.

APPLICATION EXERCISES KEY

1. A. **CORRECT:** Primary diabetes insipidus is caused by a reduction in the secretion of antidiuretic hormone (ADH), which can result in increased serum sodium.

    B. **CORRECT:** Primary diabetes insipidus is caused by a reduction in the secretion of ADH, which can result in fatigue due to electrolyte imbalance.

    C. INCORRECT: The serum osmolality is increased with primary diabetes insipidus. Serum osmolality will be greater than 300 mOsm/L.

    D. **CORRECT:** Primary diabetes insipidus is caused by a reduction in the secretion of ADH, which can result in polyuria.

    E. **CORRECT:** Primary diabetes insipidus is caused by a reduction in the secretion of ADH, which can result in nocturia.

    Ⓝ NCLEX® Connection: Physiological Adaptations, Pathophysiology

2. A. INCORRECT: Glucose in the urine is indicative of diabetes mellitus.

    B. **CORRECT:** The urine of a client who has diabetes insipidus will be dilute with a urine specific gravity of less than 1.005.

    C. INCORRECT: Ketones in the urine is indicative of diabetes mellitus.

    D. INCORRECT: Red blood cells in the urine is indicative of diabetes mellitus.

    Ⓝ NCLEX® Connection: Reduction of Risk Potential, Laboratory Values

3. A. **CORRECT:** A decrease in serum sodium is caused by an increase in the secretion of ADH.

    B. INCORRECT: A urine specific gravity greater than 1.030 is caused by an increase in the secretion of ADH.

    C. **CORRECT:** A decrease in serum osmolarity is caused by an increase in the secretion of ADH.

    D. INCORRECT: Reduced urine output is caused by the increase in the secretion of ADH.

    E. INCORRECT: Increased thirst is a finding in a client who has diabetes insipidus.

    Ⓝ NCLEX® Connection: Pharmacological and Parenteral Therapies, Expected Actions/Outcomes

4. A. INCORRECT: Decreased CVP is indicative of shock.

   B. INCORRECT: Increased urine output is indicative of diabetes insipidus.

   C. **CORRECT:** Distended neck veins are a manifestation of fluid overload, which can lead to pulmonary edema and heart failure.

   D. INCORRECT: Extreme thirst is indicative of diabetes insipidus.

   (N) NCLEX® Connection: Physiological Adaptations, Unexpected Response to Therapies

5. A. **CORRECT:** Excessive thirst is a manifestation of diabetes insipidus. Consumption of 4 to 30 L/day can be expected, and fluid intake should not be limited.

   B. INCORRECT: Nocturia is a manifestation of diabetes insipidus.

   C. INCORRECT: Headaches are a manifestation of diabetes insipidus.

   D. INCORRECT: Dry mouth is a manifestation of diabetes insipidus.

   (N) NCLEX® Connection: Physiological Adaptations, Illness Management

6. *Using the ATI Active Learning Template: Medication*

   A. Therapeutic Use
   - Demeclocycline (Declomycin) is a derivative of tetracycline and is used to treat SIADH.

   B. Nursing Considerations
   - Monitor effectiveness of treatment, such as increased serum sodium/osmolarity and decreased urine sodium osmolarity.

   C. Client Education
   - Advise the client that it may take several weeks to see results.
   - Advise the client to monitor for indications of a yeast infection, such as a white, cheese-like film inside the mouth.
   - Have the client rinse toothbrush with a diluted bleach solution (10%), and increase consumption of yogurt.

   (N) NCLEX® Connection: Pharmacological and Parenteral Therapies, Medication Administration

chapter 79

Overview

- The thyroid gland produces three hormones: thyroxine (T_4), triiodothyronine (T_3), and thyrocalcitonin (calcitonin). Secretion of T_3 and T_4 is regulated by the anterior pituitary gland through a negative feedback mechanism.

- When serum T_3 and T_4 levels decrease, thyroid-stimulating hormone (TSH) is released by the anterior pituitary. This stimulates the thyroid gland to secrete more hormones until normal levels are reached.

- T_3 and T_4 affect all body systems by regulating overall body metabolism, energy production, and fluid and electrolyte balance, and controlling tissue use of fats, proteins, and carbohydrates.

- Calcitonin inhibits mobilization of calcium from bone and reduces blood calcium levels.

- Hyperthyroidism is a clinical syndrome caused by excessive circulating thyroid hormones. Because thyroid activity affects all body systems, excessive thyroid hormone exaggerates normal body functions and produces a hypermetabolic state.

Health Promotion and Disease Prevention

- Client Education
  - Advise the client to
    - Take all medications as directed.
    - Check with the provider prior to taking over-the-counter medications.
    - Keep all follow-up appointments.
    - Adjust diet to increased metabolism when needed.
    - Seek measures to reduce stress, and get rest as needed.
    - Notify the provider of fever, increased restlessness, palpitations, or chest pain.

Assessment

- Risk Factors
  - Causes of hyperthyroidism
    - Graves' disease is the most common cause. Autoimmune antibodies result in hypersecretion of thyroid hormones.
    - Toxic nodular goiter, a less common form of hyperthyroidism, is caused by overproduction of thyroid hormone due to the presence of thyroid nodules.
    - Exogenous hyperthyroidism is caused by excessive dosages of thyroid hormone.

- Clinical Manifestations
  - Nervousness, irritability, hyperactivity, emotional lability, decreased attention span
  - Weakness, easy fatigability, exercise intolerance
  - Heat intolerance
  - Weight change (usually loss) and increased appetite
  - Insomnia and interrupted sleep
  - Frequent stools and diarrhea
  - Menstrual irregularities (amenorrhea/decreased menstrual flow)
  - Libido initially increased in both men and women, followed by a decrease in libido as the condition progresses
  - Warm, sweaty, flushed skin with velvety-smooth texture
  - Tremor, hyperkinesia, hyperreflexia
  - Exophthalmos (Graves' disease only)

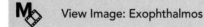
View Image: Exophthalmos

  - Vision changes, retracted eyelids, global lag
  - Hair loss
  - Goiter
  - Bruit over the thyroid gland
  - Elevated systolic blood pressure and widened pulse pressure
  - Tachycardia and dysrhythmias
  - Findings in older adult clients are often more subtle than those in younger clients.
  - Occasionally an older adult client who has hyperthyroidism will demonstrate apathy or withdrawal instead of the more typical hypermetabolic state.
  - Older adult clients who have hyperthyroidism often present with heart failure and atrial fibrillation.
  - Laboratory Tests
    - Serum TSH test – Decreased in the presence of Graves' disease (may be elevated in secondary or tertiary hyperthyroidism)
    - Free thyroxine index (FTI) and T_3 – Elevated in the presence of disease
    - Thyrotropin-releasing hormone (TRH) stimulation test – Failure of expected rise in TSH
  - Diagnostic Procedures
    - Ultrasound is used to produce images of the thyroid gland and surrounding tissue.
    - An electrocardiogram is used to evaluate the effects of excessive thyroid hormone on the heart (tachycardia, dysrhythmias).
    - Radioiodine (^{123}I) uptake and thyroid scan
      - Clarifies size and function of the gland.
      - The uptake of ^{123}I, administered orally 24 hr prior to the test, is measured. An elevated uptake is indicative of hyperthyroidism.

- Nursing Actions
  - □ Confirm that the client is not pregnant prior to the scan.
  - □ Take a medication history to determine the use of iodides.
  - □ Recent use of contrast media and client's use of oral contraceptives may cause falsely elevated serum thyroid hormone levels.
  - □ Severe illness; malnutrition; and the use of aspirin, corticosteroids, and phenytoin sodium may cause a false decrease in serum thyroid hormone levels.
  - □ Inform the provider if the client received any iodine contrast within 4 weeks of the test.
- Client Education
  - □ Advise the client to avoid foods high in iodine for 1 week prior to the test.
  - □ Suggest that the client use noniodized salt; avoid fish, shellfish, and medications that contain iodine; reduce milk intake; and avoid canned fruits and vegetables.

Patient-Centered Care

- Nursing Care
  - ○ Minimize the client's energy expenditure by assisting with activities as necessary and by encouraging the client to alternate periods of activity with rest.
  - ○ Promote a calm environment.
  - ○ Assess the client's mental status and decision-making ability. Intervene as needed to ensure safety.
  - ○ Monitor the client's nutritional status. Provide increased calories, protein, and other nutritional support as necessary.
  - ○ Monitor intake and output, and the client's weight.
  - ○ Provide eye protection (patches, eye lubricant, tape to close eyelids) for a client who has exophthalmos.
  - ○ Monitor vital signs and hemodynamic parameters (for a client who is actually ill) for findings of heart failure.
  - ○ Report a temperature increase of 1 degree or more to the provider immediately.
  - ○ Monitor ECG for dysrhythmias.
  - ○ Assure the family that any abrupt changes in the client's behavior are likely disease related and should subside with antithyroid therapy.
  - ○ Avoid excessive palpation of the thyroid gland.
  - ○ Administer antithyroid medications.
  - ○ Prepare the client for a total/subtotal thyroidectomy if the client is unresponsive to antithyroid medications or has an airway-obstructing goiter.

- Medications
  - ○ Thionamides – methimazole (Tapazole) and propylthiouracil (PTU) inhibit the production of thyroid hormone.
    - ▪ Thionamides are used to treat Graves' disease, as an adjunct to radioactive iodine therapy, to decease hormone levels in preparation for surgery, and to treat thyrotoxicosis.
    - ▪ Nursing Considerations
      - □ Monitor for manifestations of hypothyroidism, such as intolerance to cold, edema, bradycardia, increase in weight, or depression.
      - □ Monitor CBC for leukopenia or thrombocytopenia.
      - □ Monitor for indications of hepatotoxicity.
    - ▪ Client Education
      - □ Instruct the client to take the medication with meals.
      - □ Advise the client to take the medication in divided doses at regular intervals to maintain an even therapeutic drug level.
      - □ Remind the client that thionamides typically are taken for 1 to 2 years.
      - □ Advise the client to report fever, sore throat, or bruising to the provider.
      - □ Advise the client to report any evidence of jaundice (yellowing of skin or eyes, darkening of urine).
      - □ Advise the client to follow the provider's instructions about dietary intake of iodine.
  - ○ Propranolol (Inderal)
    - ▪ Beta-adrenergic blocker – Treats sympathetic nervous system effects (tachycardia, palpitations)
    - ▪ Nursing Considerations
      - □ Monitor blood pressure, heart rate, and ECG.
      - □ Monitor for hypoglycemia.
    - ▪ Client Education
      - □ Advise the client that the medication can cause dizziness and to sit on the side of the bed for a few minutes before standing.
      - □ Teach the client to check pulse prior to each dose. Advise the client to notify the provider of significant changes.
      - □ Advise the client to discontinue the medication only on the advice of the provider.
  - ○ Iodine solutions – Lugol's solution and saturated solution of potassium iodine (SSKI) inhibit release of thyroid hormone
    - ▪ Nursing Considerations
      - □ These medications are for short-term use only.
      - □ Administer 1 hr after an antithyroid medication.
      - □ Use of these medications is contraindicated in pregnancy.
    - ▪ Client Education
      - □ Instruct the client to notify the provider of fever, sore throat, and mouth ulcers.
      - □ Medication is available as a solution. Mix with juice or other liquid to mask the taste. Use a straw to avoid staining teeth. Take with food.

- Teamwork and Collaboration

  - An endocrinologist, radiologist, pharmacist, and dietitian may collaborate in providing care for the client.

- Therapeutic Procedures

  - Radioactive iodine therapy – Radioactive iodine is taken up by the thyroid and destroys some of the hormone-producing cells (^{131}I).

    - Nursing Actions

      - Radioactive iodine (^{131}I) therapy is contraindicated in women who are pregnant.

      - Monitor for manifestations of hypothyroidism, such as edema, intolerance to cold, bradycardia, increase in weight, and depression.

    - Client Education

      - Advise the client that the effects of therapy may not be evident for 6 to 8 weeks.

      - Advise the client to continue to take the medication as directed.

      - Advise the client to stay away from infants or small children for 2 to 4 days and to avoid becoming pregnant for 6 months following therapy.

      - Although a low dose of radiation is used, provide the client with precautions to prevent radiation exposure to others. Remind the client to follow directions from provider, which may include the following:

        ▸ Do not use same toilet as others for 2 weeks, sit down to urinate, and flush toilet three times.

        ▸ Take a laxative 2 to 3 days after treatment to help rid the body of stool contaminated with radiation.

        ▸ Wear clothing that is washable, wash clothing separate from clothing of others, and run the washing machine for a full cycle after washing contaminated clothing.

        ▸ Avoid contamination from saliva, do not share a toothbrush, and use disposable food service items (paper plates).

- Surgical Interventions

  - Total or subtotal thyroidectomy

    - A thyroidectomy is the surgical removal of part or all of the thyroid gland.

      - A subtotal thyroidectomy may be performed for the treatment of hyperthyroidism when medication therapy fails or radiation therapy is contraindicated. It may also be used to correct diffuse goiter and thyroid cancer. After a subtotal thyroidectomy, the remaining thyroid tissue usually supplies enough thyroid hormone for normal function.

      - If a total thyroidectomy is performed, the client will need thyroid hormone replacement therapy.

- Nursing Actions
  - Preprocedure
    - ▸ Explain the purpose of the thyroidectomy to the client. Tell the client that there will be an incision in the neck, a dressing, and possibly a drain in place. Tell the client that some hoarseness and a sore throat from intubation and anesthesia may be experienced.
    - ▸ The client is usually prescribed propylthiouracil or methimazole 4 to 6 weeks before surgery.
    - ▸ The client should receive iodine for 10 to 14 days before surgery. This reduces the gland's size and prevents excess bleeding.
    - ▸ Propranolol (Inderal) may be given to block adrenergic effects.
    - ▸ Notify the provider immediately if the client fails to follow the medication regimen.
  - Postprocedure
    - ▸ Keep the client in a high-Fowler's position. Support head and neck with pillows. Avoid neck extension.
    - ▸ Check surgical dressing and back of neck for excessive bleeding. Be aware that respiratory distress can occur from compression of trachea due to hemorrhage.
    - ▸ Respiratory distress also can occur due to edema. Ensure that tracheostomy supplies are immediately available. Humidify air, assist to cough and deep breathe, and provide oral and tracheal suction if needed.
    - ▸ Check for laryngeal nerve damage by asking the client to speak as soon as awake from anesthesia and every 2 hr thereafter.
    - ▸ Administer medication to manage pain. Reassure the client that discomfort will resolve within a few days.
    - ▸ Hypocalcemia and tetany can occur if parathyroid glands are damaged or removed. Indications are tingling of toes or around mouth, and muscle twitching. Check for positive Chvostek's and Trousseu's signs. Ensure that IV calcium gluconate or calcium chloride are immediately available.
    - ▸ If no drain is in place, prepare the client for discharge the day following surgery as indicated. However, if a drain is in place, the surgeon will usually remove it, along with half of the surgical clips, on the second day after surgery. The remaining clips are removed the following day before discharge.
- Client Education
  - Instruct the client to cough and breathe deeply while stabilizing her neck.
  - Show the client how to change positions while supporting the back of the neck.
  - Remind the client to be careful of the incisional drain if applicable.
  - Advise the client that the voice will become hoarse, and to expect pain.
  - Advise the client to notify the nurse of any tingling sensation of the mouth, tingling of the distal extremities, or muscle twitching.

      □ Remind the client that talking at intervals will be expected to check for nerve damage.

      □ Instruct the client to notify the surgeon of incisional drainage, swelling, or redness that may indicate infection.

      □ Advise the client and family to monitor for manifestations of hypothyroidism, such as hypothermia, lethargy, and weight gain.

      □ Instruct the client to take all medications as directed.

      □ Instruct clients who have had a total thyroidectomy that lifelong thyroid replacement medications will be required.

      □ Advise the client to check with the surgeon/provider prior to taking over-the-counter medications.

      □ Instruct the client to keep all follow-up appointments.

          ▸ Advise the client to notify the surgeon of fever, increased restlessness, palpitations, or chest pain.

- Medications

    ○ Calcium gluconate and calcium chloride

        ▪ Calcium supplement is used for for emergency treatment of hypocalcemia due to damage of the parathyroid glands.

        ▪ Nursing Considerations

            □ Keep emergency equipment near the bedside.

            □ Monitor the client for evidence of hypocalcemia, such as tingling, muscle twitching, and numbness of mouth or distal extremities.

        ▪ Client Education

            □ Advise the client to notify the nurse of any muscle twitching or tingling sensation of the mouth or distal extremities.

    ○ Prednisone (Deltasone)

        ▪ Corticosteroids reduce postoperative edema

        ▪ Nursing Considerations

            □ Monitor for swelling.

            □ Monitor the airway.

            □ Provide humidity to reduce swelling.

            □ Monitor blood pressure and serum glucose.

            □ When discontinuing medication, dose should be tapered gradually.

        ▪ Client Education

            □ Advise the client to take the medication with food.

            □ Instruct the client not to discontinue dosage abruptly.

- ○ Furosemide (Lasix)
  - ▪ A loop diuretic reduces swelling caused by fluid retention
  - ▪ Nursing Considerations
    - □ Monitor for swelling.
    - □ Monitor the airway.
    - □ Provide humidity to reduce swelling.
    - □ Monitor blood pressure and serum electrolytes.
    - □ Monitor urine output.
  - ▪ Client Education
    - □ Instruct the client to take dose in the morning.
    - □ Advise the client to stand upright slowly to prevent postural hypotension.

Complications

- Hemorrhage at the incision site due to a loosened surgical tie, excessive coughing, or movement
  - ○ Nursing Actions
    - ▪ Inspect the surgical incision and dressing for drainage and bleeding, especially at the back of the neck, and change the dressing as directed.
    - ▪ Expect about 50 mL of drainage in the first 24 hr.
    - ▪ If no drainage is found, check for drain kinking or the need to reestablish suction.
    - ▪ Expect only scant drainage after 24 hr.
    - ▪ Support the client's head and neck with pillows or sandbags. If the client is to be transferred from a stretcher to the bed, support the client's head and neck in good body alignment.
  - ○ Client Education
    - ▪ To avoid pressure on the suture line, encourage the client to avoid neck flexion or extension.
    - ▪ Instruct the client to cough and deep breath while supporting the neck.
    - ▪ Show the client how to change positions while supporting the back of the neck.
- Thyroid Storm/Crisis
  - ○ Thyroid storm/crisis results from a sudden surge of large amounts of thyroid hormones into the bloodstream, causing an even greater increase in body metabolism. This is a medical emergency with a high mortality rate.
  - ○ Precipitating factors include infection, trauma, emotional stress, diabetic ketoacidosis, and digitalis toxicity, all of which increase demands on body metabolism. It also can occur following a surgical procedure or a thyroidectomy as a result of manipulation of the gland during surgery.
  - ○ Findings are hyperthermia, hypertension, delirium, vomiting, abdominal pain, hyperglycemia, and tachydysrhythmias. Additional findings include chest pain, dyspnea, and palpitations.

- ○ Nursing Actions
  - Maintain a patent airway.
  - Provide continuous cardiac monitoring for dysrhythmias.
  - Administer acetaminophen to decrease the client's temperature.
    - □ Caution – Salicylate antipyretics are contraindicated because they release thyroxine from protein-binding sites and increase free thyroxine levels.
  - Provide cool sponge baths, or apply ice packs to decrease fever. If fever continues, obtain a prescription for a cooling blanket for hyperthermia.
  - Administer thionamides – methimazole or propylthiouracil (PTU) – to prevent further synthesis and release of thyroid hormones.
  - Administer propranolol to block sympathetic nervous system effects.
  - Administer glucocorticoids to treat shock.
  - Administer IV fluids to provide adequate hydration and prevent vascular collapse. Fluid volume deficit may occur because of increased fluid excretion by the kidneys or excessive diaphoresis. Monitor intake and output hourly to prevent fluid overload or inadequate replacement.
  - Administer sodium iodide as prescribed, 1 hr after administering PTU.
    - □ Caution – If given before PTU, sodium iodide can exacerbate manifestations in susceptible clients.
  - Administer small doses of insulin as prescribed to control hyperglycemia, which can occur because of the hypermetabolic state.
  - Administer supplemental O_2 to meet increased oxygen demands.
- ○ Client Education
  - Provide the client and family support and information about the client's condition and all procedures. Advise the client to notify the provider of fever, increased restlessness, palpitations, and chest pain.
- • Airway Obstruction
  - ○ Hemorrhage, tracheal collapse, tracheal mucus accumulation, laryngeal edema, and vocal cord paralysis can cause respiratory obstruction, with sudden stridor and restlessness.
  - ○ Nursing Actions
    - A tracheostomy tray should be kept near the client at all times during the immediate recovery period.
    - Maintain the bed in a high-Fowler's position to decrease edema and swelling of the neck.
    - If the client reports that the dressing feels tight, the provider should be alerted immediately.
    - Listen for respiratory stridor.
    - Provide humidified air.
    - Have suction equipment at the bedside.
    - Medicate as prescribed to reduce swelling.
  - ○ Client Education
    - Instruct the client to notify the nurse of tightness or difficulty breathing.

- Hypocalcemia and Tetany
  - ○ Damage to parathyroid gland causes hypocalcemia and tetany.
  - ○ Nursing Actions
    - Monitor for indications of hypocalcemia (tingling of the fingers and toes, carpopedal spasms, convulsions).
    - Assess for Chvostek's and Trousseau's signs, which are indicators of neuromuscular irritability from hypocalcemia.
    - Have IV calcium gluconate available for emergency administration.
    - Maintain seizure precautions.
  - ○ Client Education
    - Advise the client to notify the nurse of any tingling sensation of the mouth, tingling of distal extremities, or muscle twitching.
- Nerve Damage
  - ○ Nerve damage can lead to vocal cord paralysis and vocal disturbances.
  - ○ Incisional damage or swelling can cause nerve damage.
  - ○ Nursing Actions
    - Teach the client that he will be hoarse, he will be able to speak only rarely, and he will need to rest his voice for several days.
    - After the procedure, monitor the client's ability to speak with each measurement of vital signs.
    - Assess the client's voice tone and quality and compare it with the preoperative voice.
  - ○ Client Education
    - Remind the client that he will be asked to try to talk at intervals to check for nerve damage. Advise the client that a hoarse voice is not typically permanent.

APPLICATION EXERCISES

1. A nurse in a provider's office is reviewing the health record of a client who is being evaluated for Graves' disease. Which of the following is an expected laboratory finding for this client?

    A. Decreased thyrotropin receptor antibodies

    B. Decreased thyroid stimulating hormone (TSH)

    C. Decreased free thyroxine index

    D. Decreased triiodothyronine

2. A nurse is reviewing the clinical manifestations of hyperthyroidism with a client. Which of the following findings should the nurse include? (Select all that apply.)

    _____ A. Dry skin

    __X__ B. Heat intolerance

    _____ C. Constipation

    __X__ D. Palpitations

    __X__ E. Weight loss

    _____ F. Bradycardia

3. A nurse is providing instructions to a client who has Graves' disease and has a new prescription for propranolol (Inderal). Which of the following information should the nurse include?

    A. An adverse effect of this medication is jaundice.

    B. Take your pulse before each dose.

    C. The purpose of this medication is to decrease production of thyroid hormone.

    D. You should stop taking this medication if you have a sore throat.

4. A nurse is preparing to receive a client from the PACU who is postoperative following a thyroidectomy. The nurse should ensure that which of the following equipment is available? (Select all that apply.)

    __X__ A. Suction equipment

    __X__ B. Humidified air

    _____ C. Flashlight

    __X__ D. Tracheostomy tray

    __X__ E. Oxygen delivery equipment

5. A nurse in a provider's office is planning care for a client who has a new diagnosis of Graves' disease and a new prescription for methimazole (Tapazole). Which of the following should the nurse include in the plan of care? (Select all that apply.)

_____ A. Monitor CBC.

_____ B. Monitor triiodothyronine (T$_3$).

_____ C. Inform the client that the medication should not be taken for more than 3 months.

_____ D. Advise the client to take the medication at the same time every day.

_____ E. Inform the client that an adverse effect of this medication is iodine toxicity.

6. A nurse is assessing a client who is 12 hr postoperative following a thyroidectomy. Which of the following findings are indicative of thyroid crisis? (Select all that apply.)

_____ A. Bradycardia

_____ B. Hypothermia

_____ C. Tremors

_____ D. Abdominal pain

_____ E. Mental confusion

7. A nurse is reinforcing teaching with a client who is to have radioactive iodine therapy. What should be included in the teaching? Use the ATI Active Learning Template: Therapeutic Procedure to complete this item to include the following sections:

A. Description of Procedure: Provide a brief description of the procedure.

B. Client Education: Identify five client instructions the nurse should include.

APPLICATION EXERCISES KEY

1. A. INCORRECT: In the presence of Graves' disease, elevated thyrotropin receptor antibodies is an expected finding.

   B. **CORRECT:** In the presence of Graves' disease, low thyroid stimulating hormone (TSH) is an expected finding. The pituitary gland decreases the production of TSH when thyroid hormone levels are elevated.

   C. INCORRECT: In the presence of Graves' disease, elevated free thyroxine index is an expected finding.

   D. INCORRECT: In the presence of Graves' disease, elevated triiodothyronine is an expected finding.

   N NCLEX® Connection: Reduction of Risk Potential, Laboratory Values

2. A. INCORRECT: Moist skin is an expected finding for the client who has hyperthyroidism.

   B. **CORRECT:** Hyperthyroidism increases the client's metabolism. Therefore, heat intolerance is an expected finding.

   C. INCORRECT: Diarrhea is an expected finding for the client who has hyperthyroidism.

   D. **CORRECT:** Hyperthyroidism increases the client's metabolism. Therefore, palpitations are an expected finding for the client who has hyperthyroidism.

   E. **CORRECT:** Hyperthyroidism increases the client's metabolism. Therefore, weight loss is an expected finding for the client who has hyperthyroidism.

   F. INCORRECT: Hyperthyroidism increases the client's metabolism. Therefore, tachycardia is an expected finding for the client who has hyperthyroidism.

   N NCLEX® Connection: Physiological Adaptations, Pathophysiology

3. A. INCORRECT: Yellowing of the skin is an adverse effect of methimazole.

   B. **CORRECT:** Propranolol can cause bradycardia. The client should take his pulse before each dose. If there is a significant change, he should withhold the dose and consult his provider.

   C. INCORRECT: The purpose of this medication is to suppress tachycardia, diaphoresis, and other effects of Graves' disease.

   D. INCORRECT: Sore throat is not an adverse effect of this medication. The client should not discontinue taking this medication because this action can result in tachycardia and dysrhythmias.

   N NCLEX® Connection: Pharmacological and Parenteral Therapies, Medication Administration

4. A. **CORRECT:** The client may require oral or tracheal suctioning. Therefore, the nurse should ensure that this equipment is available.

    B. **CORRECT:** Humidified air thins secretions and promotes respiratory exchange. Therefore, this equipment should be available.

    C. INCORRECT: A flashlight is used to measure the reaction of the pupils to light for a client who has an intracranial disorder. This test is not indicated for this client.

    D. **CORRECT:** The client may experience respiratory obstruction. Therefore, this equipment should be available.

    E. **CORRECT:** The client may require supplemental oxygen due to respiratory complications. Therefore, this equipment should be available.

    Ⓝ NCLEX® Connection: Physiological Adaptations, Illness Management

5. A. **CORRECT:** Methimazole can cause a number of hematologic effects, including leukopenia and thrombocytopenia. Therefore, the nurse should monitor the client's CBC.

    B. **CORRECT:** Methimazole reduces thyroid hormone production. Therefore, the nurse should monitor the client's T3.

    C. INCORRECT: Methimazole can be prescribed for the client who has Graves' disease for 1 to 2 years.

    D. **CORRECT:** Methimazole should be taken at the same time every day to maintain blood levels.

    E. INCORRECT: Iodine toxicity is an adverse effect of Lugol's solution.

    Ⓝ NCLEX® Connection: Pharmacological and Parenteral Therapies, Medication Administration

6. A. INCORRECT: When thyroid crisis occurs, the client experiences an extreme rise in metabolic rate, which results in tachycardia.

    B. INCORRECT: When thyroid crisis occurs, the client experiences an extreme rise in metabolic rate, which results in a high fever.

    C. **CORRECT:** Excessive levels of thyroid hormone can cause the client to experience tremors.

    D. **CORRECT:** When thyroid crisis occurs, the client can experience gastrointestinal conditions, such as vomiting, diarrhea, and abdominal pain.

    E. **CORRECT:** Excessive thyroid hormone levels can cause the client to experience mental confusion.

    N NCLEX® Connection: Reduction of Risk Potential, Potential for Complications from Surgical Procedures and Health Alterations

7. *Using the ATI Active Learning Template: Therapeutic Procedure*

    A. Description of Procedure
    - Radioactive iodine (^{131}I) is administered orally 24 hr prior to a thyroid scan. The thyroid absorbs the radiation, which results in destruction of cells that produce thyroid hormone.

    B. Client Education
    - Advise the client that the effects of the therapy may not be evident for 6 to 8 weeks.
    - Advise the client to take medication as directed.
    - Advise female clients to avoid becoming pregnant for 6 months.
    - Provide the client with precautions to prevent radiation exposure to others. Remind the client to follow directions from provider, which may include the following:
      ○ Do not use same toilet as others for 2 weeks, sit down to urinate, and flush toilet three times.
      ○ Take a laxative 2 to 3 days after treatment to rid the body of stool contaminated with radiation.
      ○ Wear clothing that is washable, wash clothing separate from clothing of others, and run the washing machine for a full cycle after washing contaminated clothing.
      ○ Advise the client to avoid infants or small children for 2 to 4 days after the procedure.
      ○ Avoid contamination from saliva, do not share a toothbrush, and use disposable food service items (paper plates).

    N NCLEX® Connection: Reduction of Risk Potential, Therapeutic Procedures

chapter 80

Overview

- Hypothyroidism is a condition in which there is an inadequate amount of circulating thyroid hormones triiodothyronine (T_3) and thyroxine (T_4), causing a decrease in metabolic rate that affects all body systems.

- Classifications of hypothyroidism by etiology

  ○ Primary – Primary hypothyroidism stems from dysfunction of the thyroid gland. This is the most common type of hypothyroidism and is caused by disease (autoimmune thyroiditis – Hashimoto's disease) or loss of the thyroid gland (iodine deficiency, radioactive iodine treatment, surgical removal of the gland).

  ○ Secondary – Secondary hypothyroidism is caused by failure of the anterior pituitary gland to stimulate the thyroid gland or failure of the target tissues to respond to the thyroid hormones (pituitary tumors).

  ○ Tertiary – Tertiary hypothyroidism is caused by failure of the hypothalamus to produce thyroid-releasing factor.

- Hypothyroidism is also classified by age of onset.

  ○ Cretinism – Cretinism is a state of severe hypothyroidism found in infants. When infants do not produce normal amounts of thyroid hormones, central nervous system development and skeletal maturation are altered, resulting in retardation of cognitive development, physical growth, or both.

  ○ Juvenile hypothyroidism – Juvenile hypothyroidism is most often caused by chronic autoimmune thyroiditis and affects the growth and sexual maturation of the child. Clinical manifestations are similar to adult hypothyroidism, and the treatment reverses most of the clinical manifestations of the disease.

  ○ Adult hypothyroidism

Ⓖ - Because older adult clients who have hypothyroidism may have manifestations that mimic the aging process, hypothyroidism is often undiagnosed in older adult clients, which can lead to potentially serious adverse effects from medications (sedatives, opiates, anesthetics).

Assessment

- Risk Factors

  ○ The disorder is most prevalent in women, with the incidence rising significantly in people who are 30 to 60 years of age.

  ○ Many individuals who have mild hypothyroidism are frequently undiagnosed, but the hormone disturbance may contribute to an acceleration of atherosclerosis or complications of medical treatment (intraoperative hypotension, cardiac complications following surgery).

  ○ Use of medications (lithium [Lithobid], amiodarone [Cordarone])

  ○ Inadequate intake of iodine

- Subjective and Objective Data
  - Hypothyroidism is often characterized by vague and varied findings that develop slowly over time. Clinical manifestations can vary and are related to the severity of the condition.
  - Early findings
    - Fatigue, lethargy, irritabilily
    - Intolerance to cold
    - Constipation
    - Weight gain without an increase in caloric intake
    - Pale skin
    - Thin, brittle fingernails
    - Depression
    - Thinning hair
    - Joint and/or muscle pain
  - Late findings
    - Bradycardia, hypotension, dysrhythmias
    - Slow thought process and speech
    - Hypoventilation, pleural effusion
    - Thickening of the skin
    - Thinning of hair on the eyebrows
    - Dry, flaky skin
    - Swelling in face, hands, and feet (myxedema [non-pitting, mucinous edema])
    - Decreased acuity of taste and smell
    - Hoarse, raspy speech
    - Abnormal menstrual periods (menorrhagia/amenorrhea) and decreased libido
  - Laboratory Tests (The expected reference range for T_3 is 70 to 205 ng/dL, and the expected reference range for T_4 is 4 to 12 mcg/dL.)

LABORATORY TEST EXPECTED RESULTS WITH HYPOTHYROIDISM	
T_3	› Decreased
Serum thyroid-stimulating hormone (TSH)	› Increased with primary hypothyroidism › Decreased in secondary hypothyroidism
Free thyroxine index (FTI) and thyroxine (T_4) levels	› Decreased
T_3 resin uptake	› Decreased
Thyroid antibodies	› Increased titers
Serum cholesterol	› Increased
CBC	› Anemia

○ Diagnostic Procedures

▪ Skull x-ray, computed tomography scan, and magnetic resonance imaging

□ These procedures can locate pituitary or hypothalamic lesions that may be the underlying cause of hypothyroidism.

▪ Radioisotope (^{123}I) scan and uptake

□ Clients who have hypothyroidism have a low uptake of the iodine preparation.

▪ ECG

□ Sinus bradycardia, flat or inverted T waves, and ST deviations

Patient-Centered Care

• Nursing Care

○ Monitor for cardiovascular changes (low blood pressure, bradycardia, dysrhythmias).

○ If the client's mental status is compromised, orient periodically, and provide safety measures.

○ Increase the client's activity level gradually, and provide frequent rest periods to avoid fatigue and decrease myocardial oxygen demands.

○ Apply antiembolism stockings, and elevate the client's legs to assist venous return.

○ Encourage the client to cough and breathe deeply to prevent pulmonary complications.

○ Consult with dietitian. Provide a low-calorie, high-bulk diet, and encourage activity to prevent constipation and promote weight loss. Administer cathartics and stool softeners as needed. Avoid fiber laxatives, which interfere with absorption of levothyroxine.

○ Provide meticulous skin care. Turn and reposition the client every 2 hr if the client is on extended bed rest. Use alcohol-free skin care products and an emollient lotion after bathing.

○ Provide extra clothing and blankets for clients who have decreased cold tolerance. Dress the client in layers, adjust room temperature, and encourage intake of warm liquids if possible. Caution the client against using electric blankets or other electric heating devices because the combination of vasodilatation, decreased sensation, and decreased alertness may result in unrecognized burns.

○ Encourage the client to verbalize feelings and fears about changes in body image. Return to the euthyroid (normal thyroid gland function) state takes time. The client may need frequent reassurance that most of the physical manifestations are reversible.

○ Use caution due to alteration in metabolism.

▪ CNS depressants (barbiturates or sedatives) are contraindicated because of the risk of respiratory depression.

▪ If CNS depressants are prescribed, the dose should be significantly below the dose prescribed for a client who does not have hypothyroidism.

▪ Hypothyroidism alters the client's metabolism and excretion of medications. Therefore, the provider uses caution in prescribing medications to the client who has this condition.

- Medications
  - Thyroid hormone replacement therapy – levothyroxine (Synthroid)
    - Thyroid hormone replacement therapy is a treatment of choice.
    - It increases the effects of warfarin (Coumadin) and can increase the need for insulin and digoxin (Lanoxin).
    - Medications that decrease the absorption of levothyroxine include cimetidine (Tagamet), lansoprazole (Prevacid), and colestipol (Colestid).
    - Use caution when starting thyroid hormone replacement with older adult clients and those who have coronary artery disease to avoid coronary ischemia because of increased oxygen demands of the heart. It is preferable to start with much lower doses and increase gradually, taking 1 to 2 months to reach full replacement doses.
    - Nursing Considerations
      - Administer thyroid hormone replacement therapy.
      - Monitor for cardiovascular compromise (e.g., chest pain, palpitations, rapid heart rate, shortness of breath).
    - Client Education
      - Instruct the client that treatment begins slowly and that the dosage is increased every 2 to 3 weeks until the desired response is obtained. Serum TSH is monitored at scheduled times to ensure appropriate dosage.
      - Remind the client to take the dose prescribed by the provider. Do not stop taking the medication or increase/decrease the dose.
      - Tell the client to take the medication 1 to 2 hr before breakfast.
      - Inform the client that fiber supplements, calcium, iron, and antacids interfere with absorption.
      - Instruct the client to monitor for and report manifestations of hyperthyroidism, (irritability, tremors, tachycardia, palpitations, heat intolerance, rapid weight loss).
      - Inform the client that the treatment is considered to be lifelong, requiring ongoing medical assessment of thyroid function.
- Teamwork and Collaboration
  - A home health nurse may need to visit the client and assess for adverse effects during the first few weeks of therapy.

Complications

- Myxedema
  - Myxedema coma is a life-threatening condition that occurs when hypothyroidism is untreated or when a stressor (such as infection, heart failure, stroke, or surgery) affects an individual who has hypothyroidism. Clients who have been taking levothyroxine and suddenly stop the medication are also at risk.
  - Clinical Manifestations
    - Significantly depressed respirations (hypoxia, hypercapnia)
    - Decreased cardiac output
    - Worsening cerebral hypoxia
    - Lethargy, stupor, coma
    - Hypothermia
    - Bradycardia, hypotension
    - Hyponatremia
  - Nursing Actions
    - Maintain airway patency with ventilatory support if necessary.
    - Provide continuous ECG monitoring.
    - Monitor ABGs to detect hypoxia, hypercapnia, respiratory acidosis.
    - Warm the client with blankets.
    - Monitor the client's body temperature until stable.
    - Replace thyroid hormone by administering large doses of levothyroxine (Synthroid) IV bolus. Monitor vital signs because rapid correction of hypothyroidism can cause adverse cardiac effects.
    - Monitor intake and output, and daily weights. With treatment, urine output should increase, and body weight should decrease; failure to do so should be reported to the provider.
    - Treat hypoglycemia with glucose.
    - Administer corticosteroids.
    - Check for possible sources of infection (blood, sputum, urine) that may have precipitated the coma. Treat any underlying illness.

APPLICATION EXERCISES

1. A nurse in a provider's office is reviewing the laboratory findings of a client who is being evaluated for primary hypothyroidism. Which of the following laboratory findings is expected for a client who has this condition?

    A. Serum T_4 10 mcg/dL

    B. Serum T_3 200 ng/dL

    C. Hematocrit 34%

    D. Serum cholesterol 180 mg/dL

2. A nurse is collecting an admission history from a female client who has hypothyroidism. Which of the following findings are expected with this condition? (Select all that apply.)

    _____ A. Diarrhea

    ___X___ B. Menorrhagia

    ___X___ C. Dry skin

    _____ D. Increased libido

    ___X___ E. Hoarseness

3. A nurse is reinforcing teaching with a client who has been prescribed levothyroxine (Synthroid) to treat hypothyroidism. Which of the following should the nurse include in the teaching? (Select all that apply.)

    _____ A. Weight gain is expected while taking this medication.

    ___X___ B. Medication should not be discontinued without the advice of the provider.

    ___X___ C. Follow-up serum TSH levels should be obtained.

    ___X___ D. Take the medication on an empty stomach.

    _____ E. Use fiber laxatives for constipation.

4. A nurse in an intensive care unit is admitting a client who has myxedema coma. Which of the following should the nurse anticipate in caring for this client? (Select all that apply.)

_____X_____ A. Observe cardiac monitor for inverted T wave.

_____X_____ B. Observe for evidence of urinary tract infection.

_____X_____ C. Initiate IV fluids using 0.9% sodium chloride.

_____X_____ D. Expect a prescription for levothyroxine (Synthroid) IV bolus.

_____ E. Provide warmth using a heating pad.

5. A staff nurse is reviewing information about hypothyroidism with a newly licensed nurse. What should be included in the discussion? Use the ATI Active Learning Template: Systems Disorder to complete this item to include the following sections:

A. Description of the Disease/Disorder: Provide a brief description of the disorder.

B. Risk Factors: Identify two risk factors.

C. Diagnostic Procedures: Identify two laboratory tests that are used to diagnose hypothyroidism.

APPLICATION EXERCISES KEY

1. A. INCORRECT: A serum T_4 of 10 mcg/dL is within the expected reference range. A decreased serum T4 is an expected finding for a client who has hypothyroidism.

    B. INCORRECT: Serum T_3 of 200 ng/mL is within the expected reference range. A decreased serum T_3 is an expected finding for a client who has hypothyroidism.

    C. **CORRECT:** Hematocrit of 34% indicates anemia, which is an expected result for a client who has hypothyroidism.

    D. INCORRECT: Serum cholesterol of 180 mg/dL is within the expected reference range. An elevated serum cholesterol is an expected finding for a client who has hypothyroidism.

    Ⓝ NCLEX® Connection: Reduction of Risk Potential, Laboratory Values

2. A. INCORRECT: Constipation is a clinical manifestation of hypothyroidism.

    B. **CORRECT:** Abnormal menstrual periods, including menorrhagia and amenorrhea, are clinical manifestations of hypothyroidism.

    C. **CORRECT:** Dry skin is a clinical manifestation of hypothyroidism.

    D. INCORRECT: Decreased libido is a clinical manifestation of hypothyroidism.

    E. **CORRECT:** Hoarseness is a clinical manifestation of hypothyroidism.

    Ⓝ NCLEX® Connection: Physiological Adaptations, Pathophysiology

3. A. INCORRECT: Levothyroxine speeds up metabolism. Therefore, weight loss is an expected effect.

    B. **CORRECT:** The provider carefully titrates the dosage of this medication. It should be increased slowly until the client reaches an euthyroid state. Therefore, the client should not discontinue the medication unless directed to do so by the provider.

    C. **CORRECT:** Serum TSH levels are used to measure the effectiveness of the medication.

    D. **CORRECT:** The medication should be taken on an empty stomach to promote absorption.

    E. INCORRECT: Fiber laxatives reduce absorption of the medication and should be avoided.

    Ⓝ NCLEX® Connection: Pharmacological and Parenteral Therapies, Medication Administration

4. A. **CORRECT:** A client who has myxedema may have a flat or inverted T wave as well as ST deviations.

    B. **CORRECT:** An infection, such as in the urinary tract, may precipitate myxedema coma. Therefore, the nurse should observe the client for clinical manifestations of infection so that the underlying illness can be treated.

    C. **CORRECT:** Hyponatremia is a typical finding in the presence of myxedema coma. Therefore, intravenous therapy is administered using either isotonic or hypertonic fluids.

    D. **CORRECT:** Myxedema coma is a severe complication of hypothyroidism that if left untreated can lead to coma or death. Levothyroxine is administered IV bolus to treat the condition.

    E. **INCORRECT:** The nurse should provide warmth with extra clothing and blankets. Electric heating devices should be avoided because the combination of vasodilation, decreased sensation, and decreased alertness places the client at risk for burns.

     NCLEX® Connection: Physiological Adaptations, Medical Emergencies

5. *Using the ATI Active Learning Template: Systems Disorder*

    A. Description of the Disease
       - Hypothyroidism is a condition in which there is an inadequate amount of circulating thyroid hormones triiodothyronine (T_3) and thyroxine (T_4), causing a decrease in metabolic rate that affects all body systems.

    B. Risk Factors
       - Female age 30 to 60
       - Use of lithium (Lithobid) or amiodarone (Cordarone)

    C. Laboratory tests
       - Serum T_3
       - Serum T_4
       - Free T_4 index
       - T_3 resin uptake
       - Thyroid antibodies
       - THR stimulation test
       - TSH
       - Serum cholesterol
       - CBC

     NCLEX® Connection: Physiological Adaptations, Illness Management

chapter 81

Overview

- Cushing's disease and Cushing's syndrome are caused by an oversecretion of the adrenal cortex. Pituitary disease is caused by oversecretion of adrenocorticotropic hormone (ACTH) by the anterior pituitary gland. Adrenal Cushing's disease is caused by oversecretion of the adrenal cortex. Cushing's syndrome is caused by long-term use of glucocorticoids to treat other conditions, such as asthma or rheumatoid arthritis.

- The adrenal cortex produces:

  ○ Mineralocorticoids – Aldosterone (increases sodium absorption, causes potassium excretion in the kidney)

  ○ Glucocorticoids – Cortisol (affects glucose, protein, and fat metabolism; the body's response to stress; and the body's immune function)

  ○ Sex hormones – Androgens and estrogens

Health Promotion and Disease Prevention

- Advise the client to take prescribed medications as instructed and monitor for adverse reactions. Advise the client that medication therapy may be lifelong.

- Advise the client to eat foods high in calcium and vitamin D. The client should not use alcohol or caffeine. Advise the client to monitor for indications of gastric bleeding, such as coffee-ground emesis or black, tarry stools.

- Advise the client to avoid infection by using good hygiene and avoiding crowds or individuals who are infected.

- Advise the client that residual muscle weakness may be present, and home assistance may be needed.

- Instruct the client to monitor weight every day and report weight gain.

Assessment

- Risk Factors

  ○ Endogenous causes of increased cortisol (Cushing's disease)

    ▪ Adrenal hyperplasia

    ▪ Adrenocortical carcinoma

    ▪ Carcinomas of the lung, gastrointestinal (GI) tract, or pancreas (these tumors can secrete ACTH)

    ▪ Pituitary carcinoma that secretes adrenocorticotropic hormone (ACTH)

- Exogenous causes of increased cortisol (Cushing's syndrome) include the therapeutic use of glucocorticoids for:
  - Organ transplant
  - Chemotherapy
  - Autoimmune diseases
  - Asthma
  - Allergies
  - Chronic inflammatory diseases
- Clinical Manifestations
  - Weakness, fatigue, sleep disturbances
  - Back and joint pain
  - Altered emotional state (may include irritability or depression)
- Objective Data
  - Physical Assessment Findings
    - Evidence of decreased immune function and decreased inflammatory response (increased incidence of infections without the accompanying fever, swelling, drainage, and redness)
    - Thin, fragile skin
    - Bruising and petechiae (fragile blood vessels)
    - Hypertension (sodium and water retention)
    - Tachycardia
    - Gastric ulcers due to oversecretion of hydrochloric acid
    - Weight gain
    - Irregular menses
    - Dependent edema – Changes in fat distribution, including the characteristic fat distribution of moon face, truncal obesity, and fat collection on the back of the neck (buffalo hump)
    - Fractures (osteoporosis)
    - Bone pain/fractures with increased risk for falls
    - Muscle wasting (particularly in the extremities)
    - Impaired glucose tolerance
    - Frequent infections, poor wound healing
    - Hirsutism
    - Acne
    - Red cheeks
    - Striae (reddened lines on abdomen and thighs)
    - Emotional lability

- ○ Laboratory Tests

  - ▪ Elevated plasma cortisol levels in the absence of acute illness or stress are diagnostic for Cushing's disease/syndrome. Urine cortisol levels (24-hr urine collection) contain elevated levels of free cortisol.

  - ▪ Plasma adrenocorticotropic hormone (ACTH) levels:

    - □ Hypersecretion of ACTH by the anterior pituitary results in elevated ACTH levels.

    - □ Disorder of the adrenal cortex or medication therapy results in decreased ACTH levels.

  - ▪ Salivary cortisol levels are used to confirm the diagnosis of Cushing's disease. Cortisol levels are elevated in the presence of Cushing's disease.

  - ▪ Serum potassium and calcium levels – Decreased

  - ▪ Serum glucose level – Increased

  - ▪ Serum sodium level – Increased

  - ▪ Lymphocytes – Decreased

  - ▪ Dexamethasone suppression tests – Tests vary in length and amount of dexamethasone administered. 24-hr urine collections reveal suppression of cortisol excretion in clients without Cushing's disease. Nonsuppression of cortisol excretion is indicative of Cushing's disease. Medications are withheld and stress is reduced prior to and during testing. False positive results may occur in clients with acute illness and alcoholism.

- ○ Diagnostic Procedures

  - ▪ X-ray, magnetic resonance imaging, and CT scans may be performed to identify lesions of the pituitary gland, adrenal gland, lung, gastrointestinal tract, or pancreas.

  - ▪ Radiological imaging may be performed to determine the source of adrenal insufficiency (tumor, adrenal atrophy).

  - ▪ Nursing Actions

    - □ Establish an IV line if needed.

    - □ Determine allergies.

    - □ Explain the procedure to the client.

    - □ Provide padding, pillows, and/or blankets to provide comfort.

  - ▪ Client Education

    - □ Explain to the client that the tests are noninvasive and not painful.

Patient-Centered Care

- • Teamwork and Collaboration

  - ○ Request dietary consult. Dietary alterations include decreased sodium intake and increased intake of potassium, protein, and calcium.

  - ○ Monitor intake and output, and daily weight.

  - ○ Assess for indications of hypervolemia (edema, distended neck veins, shortness of breath, presence of adventitious breath sounds, hypertension, tachycardia).

  - ○ Maintain a safe environment to minimize the risk of pathological fractures and skin trauma.

- ○ Prevent infection by performing frequent hand hygiene.
- ○ Encourage physical activity within the client's limitations.
- ○ Provide meticulous skin care.
- ○ Monitor for and protect against skin breakdown and infection.
- Medications
  - ○ Treatment is dependent upon the cause. For Cushing's syndrome, tapering off glucocorticoids or managing the symptoms may be necessary.
  - ○ Aminoglutethimide (Cytadren)
    - Adrenal corticosteroid inhibitor
    - Aminoglutethimide decreases adrenal hormone synthesis to provide short-term symptom relief for clients with Cushing's syndrome.
    - Nursing Considerations
      - □ Use temporarily until surgery or other treatment is finished, usually no more than 3 months.
      - □ Monitor blood pressure for hypotension.
      - □ Monitor fluids and electrolytes for clients with gastric effects.
    - Client Education
      - □ Advise the client not to drive or operate heavy machinery until medication effects are known.
      - □ Advise the client that the medication may cause nausea, drowsiness, dizziness, or rash.
      - □ Advise the client relief is temporary. Symptoms will return if medication is discontinued.
      - □ Inform the client that the medication may be taken with food to relieve gastric effects.
  - ○ Ketoconazole (Nizoral)
    - Adrenal corticosteroid inhibitor
    - Ketoconazole is an antifungal agent that when taken in high dosages inhibits adrenal corticosteroid synthesis.
    - Nursing Considerations
      - □ Can be used in addition to radiation or surgery.
      - □ Monitor liver enzymes and for indications of liver toxicity (yellow sclera, dark-colored urine).
      - □ Monitor fluids and electrolytes for clients who have gastric effects.
    - Client Education
      - □ Advise the client that the medication can cause nausea, vomiting, or dizziness.
      - □ Advise the client relief is temporary. Symptoms will return if the medication is discontinued.
      - □ Inform the client that the medication may be taken with food to relieve gastric effects.
  - ○ Mitotane (Lysodren)
    - Suppresses action of adrenal cortex
    - Nursing Considerations
      - □ Used to treat inoperable adrenal carcinoma.
      - □ Monitor for indications of shock and hepatotoxicity.

- Client Education
  - Advise the client that the purpose of medication is to reduce the size of the tumor.
  - Inform the client to notify the provider if he experiences weakness, dizziness, nausea, vomiting, or weight loss.
  - Advise the client to use caution when driving or operating heavy machinery.
- Spironolactone (Aldactone)
  - Aldosterone antagonist.
  - Spironolactone is a potassium-sparing diuretic.
  - Used when bilateral adrenal hyperplasia is the underlying cause of the condition.
  - Nursing Considerations
    - Monitor electrolytes, especially sodium and potassium.
    - Monitor vital signs and weight.
  - Client Education
    - Advise the client to take with food to promote absorption.
    - Inform the client to restrict intake of high-potassium foods.
    - Advise the client not to use salt substitutes containing potassium.
    - Advise the client to report indications of hyperkalemia to provider (nausea, diarrhea, muscle weakness, numbness in arms and legs, tingling of hands and feet and around mouth).
    - Inform the client to report menstrual changes or impotence to the provider.
- Teamwork and Collaboration
  - A dietitian may be consulted to advise the client about restricting fluids and consuming a low-sodium, high-protein diet.
- Therapeutic Procedures
  - Chemotherapy with cytotoxic agents for Cushing's disease caused by a tumor.
    - Nursing Actions
      - Registered nurses who have advanced education in the administration of chemotherapy administer IV chemotherapy. However, other nurses who provide care to the client must monitor and manage the multitude of adverse effects of medications. For standards of care from the Oncology Nursing Society, see www.ons.org. The Occupational Safety & Health Administration regulations are available at www.osha.gov.
      - Monitor for adverse effects, such as thrombocytopenia or nausea and vomiting, depending on the chemotherapeutic agent.
      - Monitor WBC, absolute neutrophil count, platelet count, hemoglobin, and hematocrit.
      - Assess the client for bruising and bleeding gums.
      - Administer an antiemetic.
    - Client Education
      - Instruct the client to avoid crowds and contact with individuals who are infected.
      - Advise the client to monitor for bleeding, such as tarry stools or coffee-ground emesis.
      - Advise the client that alopecia may occur.

- ○ Radiation therapy
  - ▪ Nursing Actions
    - ▫ Provide skin care and assess for skin damage.
  - ▪ Client Education
    - ▫ Advise the client to
      - ▸ Avoid removing radiation markings.
      - ▸ Avoid applying lotions, other than those prescribed by the radiologist to affected areas.
      - ▸ Avoid exposing irradiated areas to sun.
      - ▸ Expect fatigue and altered taste due to radiation.
- • Surgical Interventions
  - ○ Hypophysectomy
    - ▪ Surgical removal of the pituitary gland (depending on the cause of Cushing's disease)
    - ▪ Nursing Actions
      - ▫ Monitor and correct electrolytes, especially sodium, potassium, and chloride. Monitor and adjust serum glucose levels. Monitor ECG.
      - ▫ Protect the client from developing an infection by using good hand hygiene and avoiding contact with individuals who have infections. Use caution to prevent a fracture by providing assistance getting out of bed and raising side rails.
      - ▫ Monitor for bleeding. Monitor nasal drainage for a possible cerebral spinal fluid (CSF) leak. Assess drainage for the presence of glucose or a halo sign (yellow on the edge and clear in the middle), which may indicate CSF.
      - ▫ Assess neurologic condition every hour for the first 24 hr and then every 4 hr.
      - ▫ Administer glucocorticoids to prevent an abrupt drop in cortisol level.
      - ▫ Administer stool softeners to prevent straining.
    - ▪ Client Education
      - ▫ Advise the client to use caution preoperatively to prevent infection or fractures.
      - ▫ Advise the client that a transsphenoidal hypophysectomy is accessed through the sphenoid sinus via the nasal cavity or under the upper lip. The client may have nasal packing postoperatively. A drip pad will be placed under the nose for bloody drainage. The client will need to breathe through his mouth. Advise the client to avoid coughing, blowing his nose, or sneezing.
      - ▫ Numbness at the surgical site and a diminished sense of smell may be experienced for 3 to 4 months after surgery.
      - ▫ Instruct the client to avoid bending over at the waist and straining to prevent increased intracranial pressure. If bending is required to pick up an object or to tie shoes, bend at the knees.
      - ▫ Instruct the client to avoid brushing teeth for 2 weeks. Advise the client to floss and rinse his mouth.

□ Advise the client to notify the health care provider of sweet-tasting drainage, drainage that makes a halo (yellow on the edge and clear in the middle), or clear drainage from the nose, which may indicate CSF leak. Another indication may include a headache.

□ Advise the client to notify the provider of excessive bleeding, confusion, or headache.

□ To avoid constipation, which contributes to increased intracranial pressure, the client should eat high-fiber food. Docusate sodium (Colace) also can be used to prevent constipation.

○ Adrenalectomy

▪ Surgical removal of the adrenal gland (may be unilateral [one gland] or bilateral [both glands])

▪ Nursing Actions

□ Provide glucocorticoid and hormone replacement as needed.

□ Monitor for adrenal crisis due to an abrupt drop in cortisol level. Findings may include hypotension, tachycardia, tachypnea, nausea, and headache.

□ Monitor vital signs and hemodynamic levels frequently initially (every 15 min).

□ Monitor fluids and electrolytes.

□ Monitor the incision site for bleeding.

□ Monitor bowel sounds.

□ Provide pain medication as needed. Administer stool softeners as needed.

□ Slowly introduce foods.

□ Assess the abdomen for distention and tenderness. Monitor the incision site for redness, discharge, and swelling.

▪ Client Education

□ Teach the client about postoperative pain management, deep breathing, and antiembolism care.

□ Advise the client of the need to take glucocorticoids, mineralocorticoids, and hormone replacements.

Complications

• Perforated viscera/ulceration

○ Decreases production of protective mucus in the lining of the stomach due to an increase in cortisol

○ Nursing Actions

▪ Monitor for evidence of GI bleeding (tarry, black stool, coffee-ground emesis).

▪ Administer antiulcer medications as prescribed.

○ Client Education

▪ Advise the client to monitor for GI bleeding and to avoid alcohol, caffeine, and smoking.

- Risk for bone fractures due to hypocalcemia

  ○ Nursing Actions
    ▪ Use caution when moving the client.
    ▪ Provide assistance when ambulating.
    ▪ Clear floors to prevent falls.
  ○ Client Education
    ▪ Encourage a diet high in calcium and vitamin D.
    ▪ Advise the client to avoid dangerous activities.
- Risk for infection due to immunosuppression
  ○ Immunosuppression and reduced inflammatory response occur due to elevated glucocorticoid levels
  ○ Nursing Actions
    ▪ Monitor for subtle indications of infection, (fatigue, fever, localized swelling or redness).
  ○ Client Education
    ▪ Instruct the client about measures to minimize exposure to infectious organisms (avoid ill people and crowds, use good hand hygiene).
    ▪ Report indications of infection to the provider.
- Risk for adrenal crisis (also known as acute adrenal insufficiency)
  ○ Sudden drop in corticosteroids due to sudden withdrawal of medication or tumor removal
  ○ May develop with abrupt withdrawal of steroid medication
  ○ Nursing Actions
    ▪ Indications include hypotension, hypoglycemia, hyperkalemia, abdominal pain, weakness, and weight loss.
    ▪ Administration of glucocorticoids treats acute adrenal insufficiency.
  ○ Client Education
    ▪ Instruct the client to gradually taper the medication.
    ▪ During times of stress, additional glucocorticoids may be needed to prevent adrenal crisis.

APPLICATION EXERCISES

1. A nurse is planning care for a client who has Cushing's disease. In planning care, the nurse should recognize that clients who have Cushing's disease are at increased risk for which of the following? (Select all that apply.)

___X___ A. Infection ~ immunosuppressant

___X___ B. Gastric ulcer · ↓ hydrochic acid

_____ C. Renal calculi

___X___ D. Bone fractures - hypocalcemia

_____ E. Dysphagia

2. A nurse is reviewing the laboratory findings of a client who has Cushing's disease. Which of the following findings are expected for this client? (Select all that apply.)

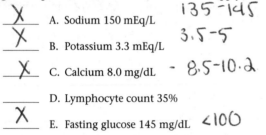

___X___ A. Sodium 150 mEq/L   135-145

___X___ B. Potassium 3.3 mEq/L   3.5-5

___X___ C. Calcium 8.0 mg/dL   - 8.5-10.2

_____ D. Lymphocyte count 35%

___X___ E. Fasting glucose 145 mg/dL   <100

3. A nurse at the beginning of a shift is assessing a client who has Cushing's disease. Which of the following is the priority assessment?

(A.) Daily weights

B. Fatigue

C. Fragile skin

D. Joint pain

4. A nurse is caring for a client who is 6 hr postoperative following a transsphenoidal hypophysectomy. The nurse should test the client's nasal drainage for the presence of which of the following?

A. RBCs

B. Ketones

(C.) Glucose ~ spinal fluid contains glucose

D. Streptococcus

5. A nurse is providing discharge instructions to a client who had a transsphenoidal hypophysectomy. Which of the following instructions should the nurse include? (Select all that apply.)

_____ A. Brush teeth after every meal or snack.

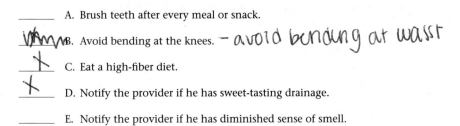 B. Avoid bending at the knees. — avoid bending at waist

_____ C. Eat a high-fiber diet.

_____ D. Notify the provider if he has sweet-tasting drainage.

_____ E. Notify the provider if he has diminished sense of smell.

6. A nurse is reinforcing teaching to a client who bilateral adrenal hyperplasia and has a new prescription for spironolactone (Aldactone). Use the ATI Active Learning Template: Medication to complete this item to include the following sections:

A. Therapeutic Uses: Explain why this medication has been prescribed for this client.

B. Client Education: Identify three facts to be included about this medication.

APPLICATION EXERCISES KEY

1. A. **CORRECT:** Suppression of the immune system places the client at risk for infection.

    B. **CORRECT:** Overproduction of gastric acid places the client at risk for gastric ulcers.

    C. INCORRECT: Clients who have Cushing's disease are not at risk for renal calculi.

    D. **CORRECT:** Client's who have Cushing's disease are at risk for bone fracture because decreased calcium absorption leads to osteoporosis.

    E. INCORRECT: Clients who have Cushing's disease are not at risk for dysphagia.

     NCLEX® Connection: Reduction of Risk Potential, Potential for Complications from Surgical Procedures and Health Alterations

2. A. **CORRECT:** This finding is above the expected reference range. Hypernatremia is an expected finding for clients who have Cushing's disease.

    B. **CORRECT:** This finding is below the expected reference range. Hypokalemia is an expected finding for clients who have Cushing's disease.

    C. **CORRECT:** This finding is below the expected reference range. Hypocalcemia is an expected finding for clients who have Cushing's disease.

    D. INCORRECT: This finding is within the expected reference range. A decreased lymphocyte count is an expected finding for clients who have Cushing's disease.

    E. **CORRECT:** This finding is above the expected reference range. Clients who have Cushing's disease have an elevated fasting blood glucose because glucose metabolism is affected.

     NCLEX® Connection: Reduction of Risk Potential, Laboratory Values

3. A. **CORRECT:** The greatest risk to a client who has Cushing's disease is fluid retention, which can lead to hypertension and heart failure. Therefore, this is the priority assessment.

    B. INCORRECT: Although the client who has Cushing's disease should be assessed for fatigue, this is not the priority assessment.

    C. INCORRECT: Although the client who has Cushing's disease should be assessed for fragile skin, this is not the priority assessment.

    D. INCORRECT: Although the client who has Cushing's disease should be assessed for joint pain, this is not the priority assessment.

     NCLEX® Connection: Reduction of Risk Potential, Potential for Alterations in Body Systems

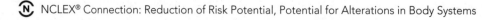

4. A. INCORRECT: The nurse should not test for the presence of RBC as an indication of cerebral spinal fluid leak.

    B. INCORRECT: The nurse should not test for the presence of ketones as an indication of cerebral spinal fluid leak.

    C. **CORRECT:** Cerebral spinal fluid contains glucose. Therefore, the nurse should test nasal drainage for glucose to determine whether the nasal drainage contains glucose.

    D. INCORRECT: The nurse should not test for the presence of streptococcus as an indication of cerebral spinal fluid leak.

     NCLEX® Connection: Reduction of Risk Potential, Laboratory Values

5. A. INCORRECT: The client should avoid brushing his teeth for 2 weeks to allow time for the incision to heal.

    B. INCORRECT: The client should avoid bending at the waist. If bending is necessary, he should bend at the knees.

    C. **CORRECT:** To avoid constipation, which contributes to increased intracranial pressure, the client should eat a high-fiber diet. Docusate sodium (Colace) can be used to prevent constipation.

    D. **CORRECT:** Sweet-tasting fluid is an indication of a cerebral spinal fluid leak. The client should notify the provider.

    E. INCORRECT: Diminished sense of smell is an expected finding after surgery.

     NCLEX® Connection: Reduction of Risk Potential, Therapeutic Procedures

6. *Using the ATI Active Learning Template: Medication*

    A. Therapeutic Uses
    - Spironolactone is an aldosterone antagonist that blocks the effectiveness of aldosterone. Hyperaldosteronism is a clinical manifestation of Cushing's disease.

    B. Client Eduction
    - Take with food to promote absorption.
    - Restrict intake of high-potassium foods.
    - Do not use salt substitutes containing potassium.
    - Report indications of hyperkalemia (nausea, diarrhea, muscle weakness, numbness in arms and legs, tingling of hands and feet and around mouth) to provider.

     NCLEX® Connection: Pharmacological and Parenteral Therapies, Medication Administration

chapter 82

Overview

- Addison's disease is an adrenocortical insufficiency. It is caused by damage or dysfunction of the adrenal cortex. The adrenal cortex produces:

  - Mineralocorticoids – aldosterone (increases sodium absorption, causes potassium excretion in the kidney)

  - Glucocorticoids – cortisol (affects glucose, protein, and fat metabolism; the body's response to stress; and the body's immune function)

  - Sex hormones – androgens and estrogens

- With Addison's disease, the production of mineralocorticoids and glucocorticoids is diminished, resulting in decreased aldosterone and cortisol.

- Acute adrenal insufficiency, also known as Addisonian crisis, has a rapid onset. It is a medical emergency. If it is not quickly diagnosed and properly treated, the prognosis is poor.

- Ⓖ Older adult clients are less able to tolerate the complications of Addison's disease and acute adrenal insufficiency and need more frequent monitoring.

Assessment

- Risk Factors

  - Causes of primary Addison's disease

    - Idiopathic autoimmune dysfunction (majority of cases)

    - Tuberculosis

    - Histoplasmosis

    - Adrenalectomy

    - Cancer

  - Causes of secondary Addison's disease

    - Steroid withdrawal

    - Hypophysectomy

    - Pituitary neoplasm

○ Acute adrenal insufficiency is a life-treating event that left untreated can lead to death. Factors that precipitate acute adrenal insufficiency are as follows.

- Sepsis
- Trauma
- Stress (myocardial infarction, surgery, anesthesia, hypothermia, volume loss, hypoglycemia)
- Adrenal hemorrhage
- Steroid withdrawal

• Subjective and Objective Data

○ Physical Assessment Findings

- Clinical manifestations of chronic Addison's disease develop slowly.
- Clinical manifestations of acute adrenal insufficiency develop rapidly.
- Clinical manifestations:
  □ Weight loss
  □ Craving for salt
  □ Hyperpigmentation
  □ Weakness and fatigue
  □ Nausea and vomiting
  □ Dizziness with orthostatic hypotension
  □ Severe hypotension (acute adrenal insufficiency)
  □ Dehydration
  □ Hyponatremia
  □ Hyperkalemia
  □ Hypoglycemia
  □ Hypercalcemia

○ Laboratory Tests

- Serum electrolytes – increased K^+, decreased Na^+, and increased calcium
- BUN and creatinine – increased
- Serum glucose – decreased
- Serum cortisol – decreased
- Adrenocorticotropic hormone (ACTH) stimulation test – ACTH is infused, and the cortisol response is measured 30 min and 1 hr after the injection. With primary adrenal insufficiency, plasma cortisol levels do not rise.

○ Diagnostic Procedures

- ECG is used to assess for ECG changes or dysrhythmias associated with electrolyte imbalance.
  □ Client Education – Explain procedures to the client.
- X-ray, CT scan, and magnetic resonance imaging (MRI) scan
  □ Radiological imaging to determine source of adrenal insufficiency, such as a tumor or adrenal atrophy
  □ Client Education – Explain to the client that tests are noninvasive and not painful.

Patient-Centered Care

- Nursing Care

  - Monitor the client for fluid deficits and electrolyte imbalances. Administer saline infusions to restore fluid volume. Observe for dehydration. Obtain orthostatic vital signs.

  - Administer hydrocortisone IV bolus and a continuous infusion or intermittent IV bolus.

  - Monitor for and treat hyperkalemia:

    - Obtain a serum potassium and ECG.

    - Administer sodium polystyrene sulfonate (Kayexalate), insulin, calcium, glucose, and sodium bicarbonate.

  - Monitor for and treat hypoglycemia:

    - Perform frequent checks of the client's neurologic status, monitor for hypoglycemia, and check serum glucose.

    - Administer food and/or supplemental glucose.

  - Maintain a safe environment:

    - Provide assistance ambulating.

    - Raise side rails.

    - Prevent falls by keeping floors clear.

- Medications

  - Hydrocortisone (Cortef), prednisone (Deltasone), and cortisone

    - Glucocorticoid is used as an adrenocorticoid replacement for adrenal insufficiency and as an anti-inflammatory.

    - Nursing Considerations

      - Monitor weight, blood pressure, and electrolytes.

      - Increase dosage during periods of stress or illness if necessary.

      - Taper dose if discontinuing to avoid acute adrenal insufficiency.

      - Give with food to reduce gastric effects.

    - Client Education

      - Advise the client to:

        - Take medication as directed.

        - Avoid discontinuing the medication abruptly.

        - Report symptoms of Cushing's syndrome (round face, edema, weight gain).

        - Advise the client to take the medication with food.

        - Report symptoms of adrenal insufficiency (fever, fatigue, muscle weakness, anorexia).

○ Fludrocortisone (Florinef) is a mineralocorticoid used as a replacement in adrenal insufficiency.

■ Nursing Considerations

□ Monitor weight, blood pressure, and electrolytes.

□ Hypertension is a potential adverse effect.

□ Dosage may need to be increased during periods of stress or illness.

■ Client Education

□ Advise the client to take the medication as directed.

□ Warn the client to expect mild peripheral edema.

• Teamwork and Collaboration – Home assistance for fluid, medication, and dietary management may be required.

• Care After Discharge

○ Client Education

■ Advise the client to:

□ Take prescribed medications as instructed and monitor for adverse reactions.

□ Avoid using alcohol and caffeine.

□ Monitor for signs of gastric bleeding (coffee-ground emesis; tarry, black stool).

□ Monitor for hypoglycemia (diaphoresis, shaking, tachycardia, headache).

□ Report symptoms of adrenal insufficiency (fever, fatigue, muscle weakness, dizziness, anorexia).

□ To prevent acute adrenal insufficiency, instruct clients who have Addison's disease to increase corticosteroid doses as directed by a provider during times of stress.

■ Inform the client that medication therapy may be lifelong.

Complications

• Acute adrenal insufficiency (Addisonian crisis)

○ Acute adrenal insufficiency (Addisonian crisis) occurs when there is an acute drop in adrenocorticoids due to sudden discontinuation of glucocorticoid medications or when induced by severe trauma, infection, or stress.

○ Nursing Actions

■ Administer insulin to move potassium into cell. Glucose often is given with insulin.

■ Administer calcium to counteract the effects of hyperkalemia and protect the heart, as well as sodium polystyrene sulfonate (Kayexalate), a resin that absorbs potassium.

■ If acidosis occurs, administer sodium bicarbonate to promote alkalinity and increase uptake of and move potassium into cells.

■ Loop or thiazide diuretics are used to manage hyperkalemia.

■ Establish an IV line and initiate a rapid infusion of 0.9% sodium chloride.

- Monitor vital signs and monitor for clinical manifestations of hyperkalemia such as bradycardia, heart block, high T wave, and prolonged PR interval.

- Monitor electrolytes.

- Administer hydrocortisone sodium succinate (Solu-Cortef) as replacement therapy.

○ Client Education

- Advise the client to notify the provider of any infection, trauma, or stress that may increase the need for adrenocorticoids.

- Advise the client to take the medication as directed.

- Advise the client not to discontinue the medication abruptly.

- Hypoglycemia

○ Insufficient glucocorticoid causes increased insulin sensitivity and decreased glycogen, which leads to hypoglycemia.

○ Nursing Actions – Monitor glucose levels.

○ Client Education

- Advise the client and family to monitor for hypoglycemia.

□ Symptoms may include diaphoresis, shaking, tachycardia, and headache.

- Instruct the client to have a 15 g carbohydrate snack readily available.

- Hyperkalemia/Hyponatremia

○ Decrease in aldosterone levels can cause an increased excretion of sodium and a decreased excretion of potassium.

○ Nursing Actions – Monitor electrolytes and ECG.

○ Client Education

- Advise the client to take the medications as directed.

- Instruct the client to report signs of hyperkalemia (muscle weakness, tingling sensation, irregular heart beat).

APPLICATION EXERCISES

1. A nurse is caring for a client who has Addison's disease and is taking hydrocortisone (Cortef). Which of the following medication instructions is appropriate for the nurse to include? (Select all that apply.)

_____ A. Take the medication on an empty stomach.

___X___ B. Notify the provider of any illness or stress.

___X___ C. Report any symptoms of weakness or dizziness.

___X___ D. Do not discontinue the medication suddenly.

_____ E. Eat a low-sodium diet.

2. A nurse is reviewing serum laboratory results for a client who has Addison's disease. Which of the following findings are typical for a client who has this condition? (Select all that apply.)

___X___ A. Sodium 130 mEq/L

___X___ B. Potassium 6.1 mEq/L

___X___ C. Calcium 11.6 mg/dL

_____ D. Magnesium 2.5 mg/dL

___X___ E. Glucose 65 mg/dL

3. A nurse is admitting a client who has acute adrenal insufficiency to the intensive care unit. Which of the following prescriptions should the nurse anticipate? (Select all that apply.)

_____ A. IV therapy with 0.45% sodium chloride

___X___ B. Regular insulin

___X___ C. Hydrocortisone sodium succinate (Solu-Cortef)

___X___ D. Sodium polystyrene sulfonate (Kayexalate)

___X___ E. Furosemide (Lasix)

4. A nurse is planning to teach a client who is being evaluated for Addison's disease about the adrenocorticotropic hormone (ACTH) stimulation test. The nurse should base her instructions to the client on which of the following?

A. The ACTH stimulation test measures the response by the kidneys to ACTH.

B. In the presence of primary adrenal insufficiency, plasma cortisol levels rise in response to administration of ACTH.

C. ACTH is a hormone produced by the pituitary gland.

D. The client is instructed to take a dose of ACTH by mouth the evening before the test.

5. A nurse in provider's office is reviewing the health care history of a client who has Addison's disease. Use the ATI Active Learning Template: Systems Disorder to complete this item to include the following sections:

A. Risk Factors: Identify the most common cause and two additional causes of primary Addison's disease.

B. Objective and Subjective Data: Identify three manifestations of Addison's disease.

APPLICATION EXERCISES KEY

1. A. INCORRECT: The client should take hydrocortisone with food to decrease GI distress.

    B. **CORRECT:** Physical and emotional stress increase the need for cortisone. Therefore, the provider may increase the dosage when stress occurs.

    C. **CORRECT:** Weakness and dizziness are indications of adrenal insufficiency, and the client should report these indications to the provider.

    D. **CORRECT:** Rapid discontinuation can result in adverse effects, including acute adrenal insufficiency. If hydrocortisone is to be discontinued, the dose should be tapered.

    E. INCORRECT: Clients who have Addison's disease are typically hyponatremic. Therefore, a low-sodium diet is not advised.

    Ⓝ NCLEX® Connection: Pharmacological and Parenteral Therapies, Medication Administration

2. A. **CORRECT:** This finding is below the expected reference range. In the presence of Addison's disease insufficient glucose can cause sodium and water excretion. Therefore, this is an expected finding.

    B. **CORRECT:** This finding is above the expected reference range. Hyperkalemia is an expected finding for a client who has Addison's disease.

    C. **CORRECT:** This finding is above the expected reference range. Hypercalcemia is an expected finding for a client who has Addison's disease.

    D. INCORRECT: Although this finding is above the expected reference range, it is not an expected finding for a client who has Addison's disease.

    E. **CORRECT:** This finding is below the expected reference range. Hypoglycemia is an expected finding for a client who has Addison's disease.

    Ⓝ NCLEX® Connection: Reduction of Risk Potential, Laboratory Values

3.   A. INCORRECT: 0.45% sodium chloride is hypotonic. Clients who have acute adrenal insufficiency are hyponatremic. Therefore, a solution that contains 0.9% sodium chloride is administered.

   B. **CORRECT:** Clients who have acute adrenal insufficiency are hyperkalemic. Insulin is administered to shift potassium into the cells.

   C. **CORRECT:** Hydrocortisone sodium succinate is administered as replacement therapy of both glucocorticoid and mineralocorticoid.

   D. **CORRECT:** Clients who have acute adrenal insufficiency are hyperkalemic. Sodium polystyrene sulfonate is administered because it absorbs potassium.

   E. **CORRECT:** Loop and thiazide diuretics promote potassium excretion and are administer to treat hyperkalemia.

   Ⓝ NCLEX® Connection: Physiological Adaptations, Alterations in Body Systems

4.   A. INCORRECT: The ACTH stimulation test measures the response by the adrenal glands to ACTH.

   B. INCORRECT: In the presence of primary adrenal insufficiency, plasma cortisol levels do not rise in response to administration of ACTH.

   C. **CORRECT:** Secretion of corticotropin-releasing hormone from the hypothalamus prompts the pituitary gland to secrete ACTH

   D. INCORRECT: ACTH is administered IV during the testing process, and plasma cortisol levels are measured 30 min and 1 hr after the injection.

   Ⓝ NCLEX® Connection: Reduction of Risk Potential, Diagnostic Tests

5.   *Using the ATI Active Learning Template: Systems Disorder*

   A. Risk Factors
   • Most common – autoimmune dysfunction
   • Additional causes – tuberculosis, histoplasmosis, adrenalectomy, cancer

   B. Objective and Subjective Data

• Hyperpigmentation	• Weakness	• Vomiting
• Weight loss	• Fatigue	• Dizziness upon standing or moving from lying to sitting position
• Craving for salt	• Nausea	

   Ⓝ NCLEX® Connection: Physiological Adaptations, Pathophysiology

chapter 83

NURSING CARE OF CLIENTS WITH ENDOCRINE DISORDERS
SECTION: DIABETES MELLITUS

CHAPTER 83 Diabetes Mellitus Management

Overview

- Diabetes mellitus is characterized by chronic hyperglycemia due to inadequate insulin secretion and/or the effectiveness of endogenous insulin (insulin resistance).

- Diabetes mellitus is a contributing factor to development of cardiovascular disease, hypertension, kidney disease, neuropathy, retinopathy, peripheral vascular disease, and stroke as individuals age.

- Diabetes mellitus is significantly more prevalent in African Americans, American Indians, and Hispanic populations, possibly due to obesity and inactivity.

- Type 1 diabetes mellitus is an autoimmune dysfunction involving the destruction of beta cells, which produce insulin in the islets of Langerhans of the pancreas. Immune system cells and antibodies are present in circulation and may also be triggered by certain genetic tissue types or viral infections.

- Type 1 diabetes mellitus usually occurs at a young age, and there are no successful interventions to prevent the disease.

- Type 2 diabetes mellitus is a progressive condition due to increasing inability of cells to respond to insulin (insulin resistance) and decreased production of insulin by the beta cells. It often occurs later in a client's life due to obesity, inactivity, and heredity.

Health Promotion and Disease Prevention

- Diabetic Screening

  ○ Determine risk factors – obesity, hypertension, inactivity, hyperlipidemia, cigarette smoking, genetic history, elevated C-reactive protein (CRP), ethnic group, and women who have delivered infants weighing more than 9 lb

  ○ American Diabetes Association (ADA) recommends screening a client who has a BMI greater than 24 and age greater than 45 years, or if a child is overweight and has additional risk factors.

  ○ Test urine for glucose and ketones during routine examinations to evaluate the need for further testing.

- Client Education

  ○ Teach the client that exercise and good nutrition are necessary for preventing or controlling diabetes.

  ○ Instruct the client to limit calories and decrease total fat intake to 30% of total daily calories.

  ○ Encourage a diet low in saturated fats to decrease low-density lipoprotein (LDL), assist with weight loss for secondary prevention of diabetes, and reduce risk of heart disease.

  ○ Modify diet to include omega-3 fatty acids and fiber to lower cholesterol levels, improve blood glucose for clients who have diabetes, for secondary prevention of diabetes, and to reduce the risk of heart disease.

RN ADULT MEDICAL SURGICAL NURSING

Assessment

- Risk Factors

  - Obesity, physical inactivity, high triglycerides (greater than 250 mg/dL), and hypertension may lead to the development of insulin resistance and type 2 diabetes.

  - Pancreatitis and Cushing's syndrome are secondary causes of diabetes.

  - Vision and hearing deficits may interfere with the understanding of teaching, reading of materials, and preparation of medications.

  - Tissue deterioration secondary to aging may impact the client's ability to prepare food, care for self, perform ADLs, perform foot/wound care, and perform glucose monitoring.

  - A fixed income may mean that there are limited funds for buying diabetic supplies, wound care supplies, insulin, and medications. This may result in complications.

  - Older adult clients may not be able to drive to the provider's office, grocery store, or pharmacy. Assess support systems available for older adult clients.

  - The older adult is at risk for altered metabolism of medication due to decreased kidney and liver function because of the aging process.

  - The older adult may have visional alterations (yellowing of lens, decreased depth perception, cataracts), which can affect ability to read information and attend to medication administration.

- Clinical Manifestations

  - Hyperglycemia – blood glucose level usually greater than 250 mg/dL

  - Polyuria (excess urine production and frequency) from osmotic diuresis

  - Polydipsia (excessive thirst) due to dehydration

    - Loss of skin turgor, skin warm and dry

    - Dry mucous membranes

    - Weakness and malaise

    - Rapid weak pulse and hypotension

  - Polyphagia (excessive hunger and eating) caused from inability of cells to receive glucose (cells are starving)

    - Client may display weight loss.

    - Ketones accumulate in the blood due to breakdown of fatty acids when insulin is not available, resulting in metabolic acidosis.

    - Kussmaul respirations – increased respiratory rate and depth in attempt to excrete carbon dioxide and acid due to metabolic acidosis.

  - Other manifestations can include acetone/fruity breath odor due to accumulation of ketones, headache, nausea, vomiting, abdominal pain, inability to concentrate, decreased level of consciousness, and seizures leading to coma.

  - Laboratory Tests

    - Diagnostic criteria for diabetes include two findings (on separate days) of one of the following:

      - Manifestations of diabetes plus casual blood glucose concentration greater than 200 mg/dL (without regard to time since last meal)

      - Fasting blood glucose greater than 126 mg/dL

      - 2-hr glucose greater than 200 mg/dL with an oral glucose tolerance test

- Fasting blood glucose

  - □ Nursing Actions – Postpone administration of antidiabetic medication until after the level is drawn.

  - □ Client Education – Instruct the client to fast (no food or drink other than water) for the 8 hr prior to the blood test.

- Oral glucose tolerance test

  - □ A fasting blood glucose level is drawn at the start of the test. The client is then instructed to consume a specified amount of glucose. Blood glucose levels are obtained every 30 min for 2 hr. The clients must be assessed for hypoglycemia throughout the procedure.

  - □ Client Education – Instruct the client to consume a balanced diet for 3 days prior to the test. Then instruct the client to fast for 10 to 12 hr prior to the test.

- Glycosylated hemoglobin (HbA1c)

  - □ The expected reference range is 4% to 6%, but an acceptable target for clients who have diabetes may be 6.5% to 8%, with a target goal of less than 7%.

  - □ HbA1c is the best indicator of the average blood glucose level for the past 120 days. It assists in evaluating treatment effectiveness and compliance.

○ Client Education

- Instruct the client that the test evaluates treatment effectiveness and compliance.

- Recommended quarterly or twice yearly depending on the glycemic levels.

○ Urine Ketones

- High ketones in the urine associated with hyperglycemia (exceed 300 mg/dL) is a medical emergency.

○ Diagnostic Procedures

- Self-monitored blood glucose (SMBG)

  - □ Nursing Action – Ensure that the client follows the proper procedure for blood sample collection and use of a glucose meter. Supplemental short-acting insulin may be prescribed for elevated pre-meal glucose levels.

  - □ Client Education

    - ▸ Instruct the client to check the accuracy of the strips with the control solution provided.

    - ▸ Instruct the client to use the correct code number in the meter to match the strip bottle number.

    - ▸ Instruct the client to store strips in the closed container in a dry location.

    - ▸ Instruct the client to obtain an adequate amount of blood sample when preforming the test.

    - ▸ Encourage appropriate hand hygiene.

    - ▸ Encourage use of fresh lancets, and avoid sharing glucose monitoring equipment to prevent infection.

    - ▸ Advise the client to keep a record of the SMBG that includes time, date, serum glucose level, insulin dose, food intake, and other events that may alter glucose metabolism, such as activity level or illness.

- Medications
  - Insulin regimens are established for clients who have type 1 diabetes mellitus and are as follows:
    - More than 1 type of insulin (rapid, short, intermediate, and long-acting).
    - Given one or more times a day based on blood glucose results.
    - Insulin may be required by some clients who have type 2 diabetes or women who have gestational diabetes if glycemic control is not obtained with diet, exercise, and oral hypoglycemic agents.
      - Continuous infusion of insulin may be accomplished using a small pump that is worn externally. The pump is programmed to deliver insulin through a needle in subcutaneous tissue. The needle should be changed at least every 2 to 3 days to prevent infection.
      - Complications of the insulin pump are accidental cessation of insulin administration, obstruction of the tubing/needle, pump failure, and infection.
  - Insulin pens are prefilled cartridges of 150 to 300 units of insulin in a programmable device with disposable needles.
    - Used if only one insulin is given at a time
    - Convenient for travel
  - Oral hypoglycemics are used by clients who have type 2 diabetes, along with diet and exercise, to regulate their blood glucose.
  - Types of Insulin (also see the *Diabetes Mellitus* chapter in the *Pharmacology Review Module*)
    - Rapid-acting insulin
      - Lispro insulin (Humalog), aspart insulin (Novolog), glulisine insulin (Apidra).
      - Administer before meals to control postprandial rise in blood glucose.
      - Onset is rapid, 10 to 30 min depending on which insulin is administered.
      - Administer in conjunction with intermediate- or long-acting insulin to provide glycemic control between meals and at night.
    - Short-acting insulin
      - Regular insulin (Humulin R, Novolin R).
      - Administer 30 to 60 min before meals to control postprandial hyperglycemia.
      - Available in two concentrations.
        - U-500 is reserved for the client who has insulin resistance and is never administered IV.
        - U-100 is prescribed for most clients and may be administered IV.
    - Intermediate-acting insulin
      - NPH insulin (Humulin N), detemir insulin (Levemir).
      - Administered for glycemic control between meals and at night.
      - Not administered before meals to control postprandial rise in blood glucose.
      - Contains protamine (a protein), which causes a delay in the insulin absorption or onset and extends the duration of action of the insulin.
      - Administer NPH insulin subcutaneous only and as the only insulin to mix with short-acting insulin.
      - Administer detemir insulin subcutaneous only and is never mixed with other insulin.

□ Detemir insulin is a dose-dependent, intermediate-acting insulin. The greater units/kg the client receives, the longer the duration of the insulin. In some cases, the client can receive up to 0.4 units/kg, resulting in a duration of 20 to 24 hr, making it a long-acting insulin.

- Long-acting insulin

  □ Glargine insulin (Lantus)

  □ Administered once daily, anytime during the day but always at the same time each day.

  □ Glargine insulin forms microprecipitates that dissolves slowly over 24 hr and maintains a steady blood sugar level with no peaks or troughs.

  □ Administer glargine insulin subcutaneous only and never administer IV.

- Nursing Considerations – Observe the client perform self-administration of insulin and offer additional instruction as indicated.

- Client Education

  □ Provide information regarding self-administration of insulin.

    ‣ Rotate injection sites (prevent lipohypertrophy) within one anatomic site (prevent day-to-day changes in absorption rates).

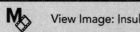

View Image: Insulin Subcutaneous Injection Sites

    ‣ Inject at a 90° angle (45° angle if thin). Aspiration for blood is not necessary.

    ‣ When mixing a rapid- or short-acting insulin with a longer-acting insulin, draw up the shorter-acting insulin into the syringe first and then the longer-acting insulin (this reduces the risk of introducing the longer-acting insulin into the shorter-acting insulin vial).

○ Advise the client to eat at regular intervals, avoid alcohol intake, and adjust insulin to exercise and diet to avoid hypoglycemia.

○ Hypoglycemia Manifestations and Management

- Teach the client measures to take in response to hypoglycemia (mild shakiness, mental confusion, sweating, palpitations, headache, lack of coordination, blurred vision, seizures, and coma).

- Hypoglycemia preventive measures are to avoid excess insulin, exercise, and alcohol consumption on an empty stomach.

- A decrease in food intake or delay in food absorption can also cause hypoglycemia.

- Check blood glucose level.

- Follow guidelines outlined by the provider/diabetes educator. Guidelines may include:

  □ Instruct the client who has hypoglycemia (glucose of 70 mg/dL or less) to take 15 to 20 g of a readily absorbable carbohydrate (4 to 6 oz of fruit juice or regular soft drink, 3 to 4 glucose tablets, 8 to 10 hard candies, or 1 tbsp of honey) and recheck blood glucose in 15 min.

  □ Repeat the administration of carbohydrates if not within normal limits, and recheck blood glucose in 15 min.

  □ If blood glucose is within normal limits, have a snack containing a carbohydrate and protein (if the next meal is more than 1 hr away).

    ‣ Blood glucose increases approximately 40 mg/dL over 30 min following ingestion of 10 g of absorbable carbohydrate.

- If the client is unconscious or unable to swallow, administer glucagon subcutaneous or IM (repeat in 10 min if still unconscious) and notify the provider.

- In acute care, the nurse should administer 50% dextrose if IV access is available. Consciousness should occur within 20 min.

- Once consciousness occurs and the client is able to swallow, have the client ingest oral carbohydrates.

○ Hyperglycemia Manifestations and Management

- Teach the client manifestations of hyperglycemia (hot, dry skin and fruity breath) and measures to take in response to hyperglycemia.

- Encourage oral fluid intake of sugar-free fluids to prevent dehydration.

- Administer insulin as prescribed.

- Restrict exercise when blood glucose levels are greater than 250 mg/dL.

- Test urine for ketones and report if outside of expected reference range.

- Consult the provider if manifestations progress.

○ Encourage the client to wear a medical identification wristband.

○ Oral hypoglycemics

BIGUANIDES METFORMIN HCI (GLUCOPHAGE)	
Action	› Reduces the production of glucose by the liver (gluconeogenesis). › Increases tissue sensitivity to insulin.
Nursing Considerations	› Monitor significance of gastrointestinal (GI) effects (flatulence, anorexia, nausea, vomiting). › Monitor for lactic acidosis, especially in clients who have renal insufficiency or liver dysfunction. › Stop medication for 48 hr before any type of radiographic test with iodinated contrast dye – may cause lactic acidosis.
Client Education	› Take with food to decrease adverse GI effects. › Instruct the client to take vitamin B_{12} and folic acid supplements. › Contact the provider if manifestations of lactic acidosis develop (myalgia, sluggishness, somnolence, and hyperventilation). › May take during pregnancy for gestational diabetes. › Never crush or chew the medication.
SECOND-GENERATION SULFONYLUREAS GLIPIZIDE (GLUCOTROL), GLIMEPIRIDE (AMARYL), GLYBURIDE (DIABETA, GLYNASE PRESTAB)	
Action	› Stimulates insulin release from the pancreas causing a decrease in blood sugar levels. › Increases tissue sensitivity to insulin.
Nursing Considerations	› Monitor for hypoglycemia. › Beta-blockers can mask tachycardia typically seen during hypoglycemia.
Client Education	› Administer 30 min before meals. › Monitor for hypoglycemia and report frequent episodes to the provider. › Instruct the client to avoid alcohol due to disulfiram effect.

MEGLITINIDES REPAGLINIDE (PRANDIN), NATEGLINIDE (STARLIX)	
Action	› Stimulates insulin release from pancreas. › Administered for postmeal hyperglycemia.
Nursing Considerations	› Monitor for hypoglycemia. › Monitor HbA1c every 3 months to determine effectiveness.
Client Education	› Administer 15 to 30 min before a meal. › Omit the dose if skipped a meal to prevent hypoglycemic crisis.
THIAZOLIDINEDIONES PIOGLITAZONE (ACTOS)	
Action	› Reduces the production of glucose by the liver (gluconeogenesis). › Increases tissue sensitivity to insulin.
Nursing Considerations	› Monitor for fluid retention, especially in clients who have a history of heart failure. › Monitor for elevation of the client's LDL and triglycerides levels.
Client Education	› Report rapid weight gain, shortness of breath, decreased exercise tolerance. › Use additional contraception methods because the medication reduces the blood levels of oral contraceptives and stimulate ovulation. › Have liver function tests every 2 months the first year.
ALPHA-GLUCOSIDASE INHIBITORS ACARBOSE (PRECOSE), MIGLITOL (GLYSET)	
Action	› Slow carbohydrate absorption from the intestinal tract. › Reduces postmeal hyperglycemia.
Nursing Considerations	› Alert the client that GI discomfort (abdominal distention, cramps, excessive gas, diarrhea) is common with these medications. › Monitor liver function every 3 months. › Treat hypoglycemia with dextrose, not table sugar (prevents table sugar from breaking down).
Client Education	› Instruct the client to have liver function tests performed every 3 months or as prescribed. › Take the medication with the first bite of each meal in order for the medication to be effective. › Have available dextrose paste to treat hypoglycemia.
DIPEPTIDYL PEPTIDASE-4 (DPP-4) INHIBITORS SITAGLIPTIN (JANUVIA), SAXAGLIPTIN (ONGLYZA)	
Action	› Augments naturally occurring intestinal incretin hormones, which promote release of insulin and decrease secretion of glucagon › Lowers fasting and postprandial glucose levels
Nursing Considerations	› Few side effects, but upper respiratory symptoms (nasal and throat inflammation) may be present. › Alert the client of GI discomforts (nausea, vomiting, and diarrhea).
Client Education	› Instruct the client to report persistent upper respiratory symptoms. › Medication only works when blood sugar is rising.

INCRETIN MIMETIC EXENATIDE (BYETTA)	
Action	› Mimics the function of intestinal incretin hormone by decreasing glucagon secretion and gastric emptying. › Decrease insulin demand by reducing fasting and postprandial hyperglycemia.
Nursing Considerations	› Administer subcutaneously 60 min before morning and evening meal. › Monitor for gastrointestinal distress.
Client Education	› Do not administer after a meal. › Oral antibiotic, oral contraceptive, or acetaminophen (Tylenol) should never be given within 1 hr of oral exenatide or 2 hr after an injection of exenatide. › May have decreased appetite and weight loss. › Wait for next scheduled dose if the scheduled medication is missed.
AMYLIN MIMETIC PRAMLINTIDE (SYMLIN)	
Action	› A synthetic amylin hormone found in the beta cells of the pancreas, it suppresses glucagon secretion and controls postprandial blood glucose levels.
Nursing Considerations	› Administer subcutaneously immediately before each major meal. › Do not administer if HbA1c is greater than 9%. › May administered with insulin therapy or oral hypoglycemic agent.
Client Education	› Monitor and report frequent periods of hypoglycemia. › Monitor for injection site reactions.

Patient-Centered Care

- Nursing Care
  - Monitor
    - Blood glucose levels and factors affecting levels (other medications)
    - I&O and weight
    - Skin integrity and healing status of any wounds for presence of recurrent infections
      □ Feet and folds of the skin should be monitored.
    - Sensory alterations (tingling, numbness)
    - Visual alterations
    - Dietary practices
    - Exercise patterns
    - The client's SMBG skill proficiency
    - The client's self-medication administration proficiency
  - Client Education
    - Teach the client appropriate techniques for SMBG, including obtaining blood samples, recording and responding to results, and correctly handling supplies and equipment.
    - Provide information regarding self-administration of insulin.
    - Rotate injection sites to prevent lipohypertrophy (increased swelling of fat) or lipoatrophy (loss of fat tissue) within one anatomic site (prevents day-to-day changes in absorption rates).

○ Foot Care

- Inspect feet daily. Wash feet daily with mild soap and warm water. Test water temperature with hands before washing feet.

- Pat feet dry gently, especially between the toes, and avoid lotions between toes to decrease excess moisture and prevent infection.

- Use mild foot powder (powder with cornstarch) on sweaty feet.

- Do not use commercial remedies for the removal of calluses or corns, which may increase the risk for tissue injury and infection.

- Consult a podiatrist.

- The best time to perform nail care is after a bath/shower, when toenails are soft and easier to trim.

- Separate overlapping toes with cotton or lamb's wool.

- Avoid open-toe, open-heel shoes. Leather shoes are preferred to plastic. Wear shoes that fit correctly. Wear slippers with soles. Do not go barefoot.

- Wear clean, absorbent socks or stockings that are made of cotton or wool and have not been mended.

- Do not use hot water bottles or heating pads to warm feet. Wear socks for warmth.

- Avoid prolonged sitting, standing, and crossing of legs.

- Teach the client to follow facility policies or recommendations of a podiatrist for nail care. Some protocols allow for trimming toenails straight across with clippers and filing edges with an emery board or nail file to prevent soft tissue injury. If clippers or scissors are contraindicated, the client should file the nails straight across.

- Teach the client to cleanse cuts with warm water and mild soap, gently dry, and apply a dry dressing. Instruct the clients to monitor healing and to seek intervention promptly.

○ Nutritional Guidelines

- Consult dietician for collaborative education with the client and family on meal planning to include food intake, weight management, and lipid and glucose management.

- Plan meals to achieve appropriate timing of food intake, activity, onset, and peak of insulin. Calories and food composition should be similar each day.

- Eat at regular intervals, and do not skip meals.

- Count grams of carbohydrates consumed for glycemic control.

- Recognize that 15 g of carbohydrates are equal to 1 carbohydrate exchange.

- Restrict calories and increase physical activity as appropriate to facilitate weight loss (for clients who are obese) or to prevent obesity.

- Include fiber in the diet to increase carbohydrate metabolism and to help control cholesterol levels.

- Use artificial sweeteners.

- Read and interpret fat content information on food labels to keep saturated fats within 7% of the recommendations of the daily total caloric intake.

○ Teach the client guidelines to follow when sick.

- Monitor blood glucose every 3 to 4 hr.

- Continue to take insulin or oral hypoglycemic agents.

- Consume 4 oz of sugar-free, noncaffeinated liquid every 30 min to prevent dehydration.

- Meet carbohydrate needs through soft food (custard, cream soup, gelatin, graham crackers) six to eight times per day, if possible. If not, consume liquids equal to usual carbohydrate content.

- Test urine for ketones and report to provider if they are outside the expected reference range. (The level should be negative to small.)

- Rest.

- Call the provider if:

  □ Blood glucose is greater than 240 mg/dL. Test urine for ketones, if prescribed.

  □ Fever is greater than 38.6° C (101.5° F), does not respond to acetaminophen, or lasts more than 24 hr.

  □ Feeling disoriented or confused.

  □ Experiencing rapid breathing.

  □ Vomiting occurs more than once.

  □ Diarrhea occurs more than five times or for longer than 24 hr.

  □ Unable to tolerate liquids.

  □ Illness lasts longer than 2 days.

- Teamwork and Collaboration

  ○ Refer the client to a diabetes educator for comprehensive education in diabetes management.

Complications

- Consistent maintenance of blood glucose within the expected reference range is the best protection against the complications of diabetes mellitus. Expected reference ranges may vary.

- Cardiovascular and cerebrovascular disease

  ○ Hypertension, myocardial infarction, and stroke

  ○ Nursing Actions – Monitor blood pressure.

  ○ Client Education

    - Encourage checks of cholesterol (HDL, LDL, and triglycerides) yearly and monitoring of blood pressure (below 130/80 mm Hg), and HbA1c every 3 months.

    - Encourage participation in regular activity for weight loss and control.

    - Encourage a diet of low-fat meals that are high in fruits, vegetables, and whole-grain foods.

    - Teach the client to report shortness of breath, headaches (persistent and transient), numbness in distal extremities, swelling of feet, infrequent urination, and changes in vision.

    - Encourage a dietary consult.

- Diabetic retinopathy

  ○ Impaired vision and blindness

  ○ Client Education

    - Encourage yearly eye exams to ensure the health of the eyes and to protect vision.

    - Encourage management of blood glucose levels.

- Diabetic neuropathy
  - ○ Caused from damage to sensory nerve fibers resulting in numbness and pain.
  - ○ Is progressive, may affect every aspect of the body, and can lead to ischemia and infection.
  - ○ Nursing Actions
    - Monitor blood glucose levels to keep within an acceptable range to slow progression.
    - Provide foot care.
  - ○ Client Education
    - Encourage annual exams by a podiatrist.
    - Encourage regular follow-up with provider to assess and treat neuropathy.
- Diabetic nephropathy
  - ○ Damage to the kidneys from prolonged elevated blood glucose levels and dehydration
  - ○ Nursing Actions
    - Monitor hydration and kidney function (I&O, serum creatinine).
    - Report an hourly output of less than 30 mL/hr.
    - Monitor blood pressure.
  - ○ Client Education
    - Encourage yearly urine analysis, BUN, and serum creatinine.
    - Encourage the client to avoid soda, alcohol, and toxic levels of acetaminophen or NSAIDS.
    - Teach the client to consume 2 to 3 L of fluid per day from food and beverage sources, and to drink an adequate amount of water.
    - Tell the client to report decrease in output to the provider.

View Images
  › Diabetic Retinopathy   › Diabetic Foot Ulcers

APPLICATION EXERCISES

1. A nurse is caring for a client who has blood glucose of 52 mg/dL. The client is lethargic but arousable. Which of the following actions should the nurse perform first?

    A. Recheck blood glucose in 15 min.

    B. Provide a carbohydrate and protein food.

    C. Provide 4 oz grape juice.

    D. Report findings to the provider.

2. A nurse is preparing to administer a morning dose of aspart insulin (NovoLog) to a client who has type 1 diabetes mellitus. Which of the following is an appropriate action by the nurse?

    A. Check the client's blood glucose immediately after breakfast.

    B. Administer the insulin when breakfast arrives.

    C. Hold breakfast for 1 hr after insulin administration.

    D. Clarify the prescription because insulin should not be administered at this time.

3. A nurse is preparing to administer the morning doses of glargine (Lantus) insulin and regular (Humulin R) insulin to a client who has a blood glucose of 278 mg/dL. Which of the following is an appropriate nursing action?

    A. Draw up the regular insulin and then the glargine insulin in the same syringe.

    B. Draw up the glargine insulin then the regular insulin in the same syringe.

    C. Draw up and administer regular and glargine insulin in separate syringes.

    D. Administer the regular insulin, wait 1 hr, and then administer the glargine insulin.

4. A nurse is presenting information to a group of clients about nutrition habits that prevent type 2 diabetes mellitus. Which of the following should the nurse include in the information? (Select all that apply.)

    _____ A. Eat less meat and processed foods.

    _____ B. Decrease intake of saturated fats.

    _____ C. Increase daily fiber intake.

    _____ D. Limit saturated fat intake to 15% of daily caloric intake.

    _____ E. Include omega-3 fatty acids in the diet.

5. A nurse is teaching foot care to a client who has diabetes mellitus. Which of the following information should the nurse include in the teaching? (Select all that apply.)

_____ A. Remove calluses using over-the-counter remedies.

_____ B. Apply lotion between toes.

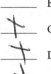 C. Perform nail care after bathing.

_____ D. Trim toenails straight across.

_____ E. Wear closed-toe shoes.

6. A nurse is providing guidelines to a client who has type 1 diabetes mellitus. What information should the nurse include in the guidelines? Use the ATI Active Learning Template: Systems Disorder to complete this item to include the following:

A. Description of Disorder/Disease Process

B. Client Education: Describe six teaching points.

APPLICATION EXERCISES KEY

1. A. INCORRECT: Blood glucose is rechecked in 15 min after a rapidly absorbed carbohydrate is ingested, but is not the priority nursing action.

   B. INCORRECT: A carbohydrate and protein food is given to the client if the next meal is more than 1 hr away after the blood glucose returns to a normal range. This is not the priority nursing action.

   C. **CORRECT:** The client's acute need for a rapidly absorbed carbohydrate, such as grape juice, takes priority when treating the blood glucose of 52 mg/dL.

   D. INCORRECT: Reporting the findings to the provider is not the priority action.

    NCLEX® Connection: Physiological Adaptations, Unexpected Response to Therapies

2. A. INCORRECT: Blood glucose should be checked prior to insulin administration to prevent an episode of hypoglycemia.

   B. **CORRECT:** Administer aspart insulin when breakfast arrives to avoid a hypoglycemic episode. Aspart insulin is rapid-acting, and should be administered 5 to 10 min before breakfast.

   C. INCORRECT: Aspart insulin is rapid-acting and is administered 5 to 10 min before breakfast. Breakfast should be available at the time of the injection.

   D. INCORRECT: Aspart insulin is administered at breakfast time and may be prescribed for administration 2 to 3 times a day.

    NCLEX® Connection: Pharmacological and Parenteral Therapies, Medication Administration

3. A. INCORRECT: These insulins are not compatible. They should not be drawn up in the same syringe.

   B. INCORRECT: These insulins are not compatible. They should not be drawn up in the same syringe.

   C. **CORRECT:** Administer each insulin as a separate injection. These insulins are not compatible and should not be drawn up in the same syringe.

   D. INCORRECT: These insulins should be administered at the same time. Regular insulin is short-acting and should lower the blood glucose level in a short period of time. Glargine insulin is long-acting and administered once a day.

    NCLEX® Connection: Pharmacological and Parenteral Therapies, Dosage Calculation

4. A. **CORRECT:** Healthy nutrition should include decreasing the consumption of meats and processed foods, which can prevent diabetes and hyperlipidemia.

    B. **CORRECT:** Healthy nutrition should include lowering LDL by decreasing intake of saturated fats, which can prevent diabetes and hyperlipidemia.

    C. **CORRECT:** Healthy nutrition should include increasing dietary fiber to control weight gain and decrease the risk of diabetes and hyperlipidemia.

    D. **INCORRECT:** The recommendation for saturated fat intake is no more than 7% of total daily caloric intake.

    E. **CORRECT:** Healthy nutrition should include omega-3 fatty acids for secondary prevention of diabetes and heart disease.

     NCLEX® Connection: Basic Care and Comfort, Nutrition and Oral Hydration

5. A. **INCORRECT:** A podiatrist should remove calluses or corns. Commercial over-the-counter remedies may increase the risk for tissue injury and an infection.

    B. **INCORRECT:** Applying lotion between the toes increases moisture for growth of micro-organisms, which can lead to infection.

    C. **CORRECT:** Perform nail care after bathing, when toenails are soft and easier to trim.

    D. **CORRECT:** Trim toenails straight across to prevent injury to soft tissue of the toes.

    E. **CORRECT:** Wear closed-toe shoes to prevent injury to soft tissue of the toes and feet.

    NCLEX® Connection: Reduction of Risk Potential, Potential for Complications of Diagnostic Tests/ Treatments/Procedures

6. *Using the ATI Active Learning Template: Systems Disorder*

    A. Description of Disorder/Disease Process

    • Type 1 diabetes mellitus is an autoimmune dysfunction involving the destruction of beta cells in the pancreas triggered by a certain genetic tissue type or viral infection.

    B. Client Education

    • Monitor blood glucose every 3 to 4 hr.

    • Continue to take insulin as prescribed.

    • Prevent dehydration by drinking sugar-free fluids.

    • Call provider if unable to tolerate liquids.

    • If unable to eat soft foods, consume liquids equal to usual carbohydrate content.

    • Call provider if ill for longer than 2 days, having more than five episodes of diarrhea, or for longer than 24 hr.

    • Call provider if fever is greater than 38.6° C (101.5° F), does not respond to acetaminophen or lasts more than 24 hr.

    NCLEX® Connection: Physiological Adaptations, Illness Management

chapter 84

Overview

- Diabetic ketoacidosis (DKA) is an acute, life-threatening condition characterized by hyperglycemia (greater than 300 mg/dL) resulting in the breakdown of body fat for energy and an accumulation of ketones in the blood and urine. The onset is rapid, and the mortality rate of DKA is less than 5%.

- Hyperglycemic-hyperosmolar state (HHS) is an acute, life-threatening condition characterized by profound hyperglycemia (greater than 600 mg/dL), hyperosmolarity that leads to dehydration, and an absence of ketosis. The onset generally occurs gradually over several days, and if left untreated can lead to coma and death.

- This condition leads to an alteration in the sense of awareness (sensorium), caused by insulin resistance, which results in loss of fluids and electrolytes.

Assessment

- Risk Factors

  - DKA

    - Lack of sufficient insulin related to undiagnosed or untreated type 1 diabetes mellitus or nonadherence to a diabetic regimen

    - Reduced or missed dose of insulin (insufficient dosing of insulin or error in dosage)

    - Any condition that increases carbohydrate metabolism, such as physical or emotional stress, illness, infection (No. 1 cause of DKA), surgery, or trauma that requires an increased need for insulin

      - Increased hormone production (e.g., cortisol, glucagon, epinephrine) stimulates the liver to produce glucose and decreases the effect of insulin.

  - HHS

    - Older adult who has residual insulin secretion, which is enough to prevent the production of ketone bodies in the blood, but not enough to prevent excess blood glucose. The client manifests type 2 diabetes mellitus and is unaware of any finding.

    - Older adults who have inadequate fluid intake and become dehydrated experience osmotic diuresis due to high blood glucose.

    - Older adults who have decreased kidney function are unable to excrete the excess glucose into urine, with resulting high blood glucose.

    - Medical conditions such as myocardial infarction, cerebral vascular injury, or sepsis.

    - Certain medications – glucocorticoids, diuretics, phenytoin (Dilantin), propranolol (Inderal), and calcium channel blockers.

    - Infection or stress.

- Clinical Manifestations

CLINICAL MANIFESTATIONS	CAUSE OF MANIFESTATIONS	DKA	HHS
Polyuria	› Osmotic diuresis resulting in excess urine production	✓	✓
Polydipsia (excess thirst)	› Osmotic diuresis causing excess loss of fluids resulting in increased thirst	✓	✓
Polyphagia	› Cell starvation due to inability to receive glucose resulting in increased appetite	✓	
Weight loss	› Cells are unable to use glucose because of insulin deficiency. The body is placed in a catabolic state.	✓	
GI effects (nausea, vomiting, abdominal pain)	› Increased ketones and acidosis lead to nausea, vomiting, and abdominal pain	✓	
Blurred vision, headache, weakness	› Fluid volume depletion caused from osmotic diuresis resulting in dehydration	✓	✓
Orthostatic hypotension	› Fluid volume depletion caused by osmotic diuresis resulting in dehydration	✓	✓
Fruity odor of breath	› Elevated ketone bodies (small fatty acids) used for energy that collect in the blood, which leads to metabolic acidosis	✓	
Kussmaul respirations	› Deep rapid respirations occur in an attempt to excrete carbon dioxide and acid when in metabolic acidosis	✓	
Metabolic acidosis	› Caused from the breakdown of stored glucose, protein, and fat to produce ketone bodies	✓	
Mental status changes	› Alert, sleepy, or comatose	✓	✓
Seizures, myoclonic jerking	› Related to serum osmolarity greater than 350 mOsm/L		✓
Reversible paralysis	› Related to how elevated the serum osmolarity becomes (greater than 350 mOsm/L)		✓

- Laboratory Tests
  - ○ Therapeutic management is guided by serial laboratory analysis.

DIAGNOSTIC PROCEDURE	DKA	HHS
› Serum glucose	› Greater than 300 mg/dL	› Greater than 600 mg/dL
› Serum electrolytes » Sodium (Na⁺) » Potassium (K⁺)	› Na⁺ – increased due to water loss › K⁺ – initially decreased due to diuresis, which may increase due to acidosis	› Na⁺ – increased due to water loss › K⁺ – initially decreased due to diuresis
› Serum renal studies » BUN » Creatinine	› Increased secondary to dehydration › BUN greater than 30 mg/dL › Creatinine greater than 1.5 mg/dL	› Increased secondary to dehydration › BUN greater than 30 mg/dL › Creatinine greater than 1.5 mg/dL
› Ketones » Serum » Urine	› Present in serum and urine	› Absent in serum and urine
› Serum osmolarity	› High	› Greater than 320 mOsm/L
› Serum pH (ABG)	› Metabolic acidosis with respiratory compensation (Kussmaul respirations) › pH less than 7.3	› Absence of acidosis › pH greater than 7.4

Patient-Centered Care

- Nursing Care
  - ○ Always treat the underlying cause (infectious process).
    - ■ Provide rapid isotonic fluid (0.9% sodium chloride) replacement to maintain perfusion to vital organs. Monitor the client for evidence of fluid volume excess (urine output, kidney function, pulmonary status, jugular venous distention, and body weight) due to the need for large quantities of fluid.
    - ■ Physiological changes in cardiac and pulmonary function may place older adult clients at greater risk for fluid overload (precipitate heart failure exacerbation) from fluid replacement therapy.
  - ○ Follow with a hypotonic fluid (0.45% sodium chloride) to continue replacing losses to total body fluid.
  - ○ When serum glucose levels approach 250 mg/dL, add glucose to IV fluids to minimize the risk of cerebral edema associated with drastic changes in serum osmolarity and prevent hypoglycemia.
  - ○ Administer regular insulin (Humulin R) 0.1 unit/kg as an IV bolus dose and then follow with a continuous IV infusion of regular insulin at 0.1 unit/kg/hr.
    - ■ IV regular insulin is administered because of the 4-min half-life of the insulin infusion, avoiding delay in onset.

○ Monitor blood glucose hourly. Blood glucose of less than 200 mg/dL is the goal for resolution.

○ Monitor serum potassium levels. Potassium levels will initially be increased with insulin therapy, but potassium will shift into cells and the client will need to be monitored for hypokalemia.

 ▪ Provide potassium replacement therapy in all replacement IV fluids, as indicated by laboratory values.

 ▪ Make sure urinary output is adequate before administering potassium.

○ Administer sodium bicarbonate by slow IV infusion for severe acidosis (pH of less than 7.0). Monitor potassium levels because a correcting acidosis too quickly may lead to hypokalemia.

○ Considerations for older adult clients

 ▪ Teach older adult clients to monitor blood glucose every 1 to 4 hr when ill.

 ▪ Emphasize the importance of not skipping an insulin dose when ill.

 ▪ Maintain hydration because older adult clients may have a diminished thirst sensation.

 ▪ Changes in mental status may keep older adult clients from seeking treatment.

• Client Education

 ○ Provide the client with education to prevent reoccurrence.

 ▪ Encourage all clients to wear a medical alert bracelet.

 ▪ Take measures to decrease the risk of dehydration. Drink at least 3 L of water/day unless contraindicated by other health problems.

 ▪ Monitor glucose every 4 hr when ill and continue to take insulin.

 ▪ Consume liquids with carbohydrates and electrolytes (sports drinks) when unable to eat solid food.

 ▪ Notify the provider if:

  □ Illness lasts more than 1 day.

  □ Blood glucose is greater than 240 mg/dL.

  □ Client is unable to tolerate food or fluids.

  □ Ketones are found in urine for more than 24 hr.

  □ Temperature for 24 hr of 38.6° C (101.5° F).

APPLICATION EXERCISES

1. A nurse is reviewing the health record of a client who has hyperglycemic-hyperosmolar state (HHS). Which of the following data confirms this diagnosis? (Select all that apply.)

_____ A. Evidence of recent myocardial infraction

_____ B. BUN 35 mg/dL

_____ C. Takes a calcium channel blocker

_____ D. Age 77 years

_____ E. No insulin production

2. A nurse is assessing a client who has diabetic ketoacidosis and ketones in the urine. Which of the following are expected findings? (Select all that apply.)

_____ A. Weight gain

_____ B. Fruity odor of breath

_____ C. Abdominal pain

_____ D. Kussmaul respirations

_____ E. Metabolic acidosis

3. A nurse is reviewing laboratory reports of a client who has hyperglycemic-hyperosmolar state (HHS). Which of the following is an expected finding?

A. Serum pH 7.2

B. Serum osmolarity 350 mOsm/L

C. Serum potassium 3.8 mg/dL

D. Serum creatinine 0.8 mg/dL

4. A nurse is preparing to administer IV fluids to a client who has diabetic ketoacidosis. Which of the following is an appropriate nursing action?

A. Administer an IV infusion of regular insulin at 0.3 unit/kg/hr.

B. Administer an IV infusion of 0.45% sodium chloride.

C. Rapidly administer an IV infusion of 0.9% sodium chloride.

D. Add glucose to the IV infusion when serum glucose is 350 mg/dL.

5. A nurse is providing discharge teaching to a client who experienced diabetic ketoacidosis. Which of the following should the nurse include in the teaching? (Select all that apply.)

    ✗   A. Drink 3 L of fluids daily.

    ✗   B. Monitor blood glucose every 4 hr when ill.

    ✗   C. Administer insulin as prescribed when ill.

    ✗   D. Notify the provider when blood glucose is 200 mg/dL. → > 240

    ✗   E. Report ketones in the urine after 24 hr of illness.

6. A nurse is planning care for a client who has diabetic ketoacidosis. What should the nurse include in the plan of care? Use the ATI Active Learning Template: Basic Concept to complete this item to include the following:

    A. Related Content: List three treatments.

    B. Underlying Principles: Describe the nursing actions for each treatment.

APPLICATION EXERCISES KEY

1. A. **CORRECT:** The client who has type 2 diabetes mellitus and had a myocardial infraction is at risk for developing HHS. This is due to the increased hormone production during illness or stress, which can stimulate the liver to produce glucose and decrease the effects of insulin.

    B. **CORRECT:** The client who has type 2 diabetes mellitus may be at risk for developing HHS when the BUN is 35 mg/dL because it is an indication of decreased kidney function and inability of the kidney to filter high levels of blood glucose into the urine.

    C. **CORRECT:** A calcium channel blocker is one of several medications that increase the risk for HHS in a client who has type 2 diabetes mellitus.

    D. **CORRECT:** The older adult client is at risk for developing type 2 diabetes mellitus and may be unaware of associated symptoms, increasing the risk for HHS.

    E. INCORRECT: The client who has type 2 diabetes mellitus can produce enough insulin to prevent ketoacidosis but not enough to control blood glucose, resulting in HHS.

     NCLEX® Connection: Physiological Adaptations, Pathophysiology

2. A. INCORRECT: Weight loss occurs when the cells are unable to use glucose because of insulin deficiency and places the body in a catabolic state.

    B. **CORRECT:** Fruity odor of breath is a manifestation of elevated ketone levels that lead to metabolic acidosis.

    C. **CORRECT:** Abdominal pain is a GI manifestation of increased ketones and acidosis.

    D. **CORRECT:** Kussmaul respirations are an attempt to excrete carbon dioxide and acid when in metabolic acidosis.

    E. **CORRECT:** Metabolic acidosis is caused from glucose, protein, and fat breakdown, which produces ketones.

     NCLEX® Connection: Physiological Adaptations, Pathophysiology

3. A. INCORRECT: A client who has a serum pH of 7.2 is an indication of diabetic ketoacidosis and is not an expected finding for HHS.

    B. **CORRECT:** A client who has HHS would have a serum osmolarity greater than 320 mOsm/L.

    C. INCORRECT: This finding is within the expected reference range. A client who has HHS would initially have a decreased serum potassium due to diuresis.

    D. INCORRECT: This finding is within the expected reference range. A client who has HHS would have a serum creatinine of greater than 1.5 mg/dL, secondary to dehydration.

     NCLEX® Connection: Reduction of Risk Potential, Laboratory Values

4. A. **INCORRECT:** The nurse should administer an IV infusion of regular insulin at 0.1 unit/kg/hr to gradually lower blood glucose to prevent cerebral edema.

    B. **INCORRECT:** The administration of an IV infusion of 0.45% sodium chloride should follow the isotonic fluid and is used as maintenance fluids.

    C. **CORRECT:** The nurse should rapidly administer an IV infusion of 0.9% sodium chloride, an isotonic fluid, as prescribed to maintain blood perfusion to vital organs.

    D. **INCORRECT:** The nurse should add glucose to the IV infusion when the serum glucose is 250 mg/dL, not 350 mg/dL, to prevent hypoglycemia and minimize cerebral edema.

     NCLEX® Connection: Pharmacological and Parenteral Therapies, Parenteral/Intravenous Therapies

5. A. **CORRECT:** Drinking 3 L of fluids daily may prevent dehydration if the client develops diabetic ketoacidosis.

    B. **CORRECT:** Blood glucose tend to increase during illness. Blood glucose should be monitored every 4 hr.

    C. **CORRECT:** Illness often causes blood glucose to increase. Regular doses of insulin should be administered.

    D. **INCORRECT:** Notify the provider when blood glucose is greater than 240 mg/dL.

    E. **CORRECT:** The provider should be notified if there are ketones in the urine after 24 hr of illness.

     NCLEX® Connection: Physiological Adaptations, Illness Management

6. *Using the ATI Active Learning Template: Basic Concept*

    A. Related Content/B. Underlying Principles
    - Fluid replacement
      - Rapidly infuse the prescribed amount of IV 0.9% sodium chloride.
      - Follow with IV infusion of 0.45% sodium chloride as maintenance fluids.
    - Monitor laboratory tests
      - Monitor and replace potassium as prescribed.
      - Review BUN and creatinine levels for expected improvement.
      - Monitor serum osmolarity.
      - Evaluate blood glucose hourly.
    - Insulin administration
      - Administer regular insulin IV bolus dose as prescribed.
      - Follow with regular insulin IV infusion as prescribed.

     NCLEX® Connection: Physiological Adaptations, Illness Management

Nursing Care of Clients with Immune System Disorders

SECTIONS

› Diagnostic and Therapeutic Procedures
› Immune Disorders
› Autoimmune Disorders
› Cancer-Related Disorders

NCLEX® CONNECTIONS

When reviewing the chapters in this unit, keep in mind the relevant sections of the NCLEX® outline, in particular:

Client Needs: Health Promotion and Maintenance	Client Needs: Pharmacological and Parenteral Therapies	Client Needs: Reduction of Risk Potential

› Relevant topics/tasks include:
 	
» Health Promotion/Disease Prevention
 	
  › Educate the client on actions to promote/ maintain health and prevent disease.
 	
» Health Screening
 	
  › Apply knowledge of pathophysiology to health screening.
 	
» High-Risk Behaviors
 	
  › Provide information for the prevention of high-risk health behaviors.
	› Relevant topics/tasks include:
	
	» Medication Administration
	
	  › Administer and document medications given by parenteral routes.
	
	» Parenteral/Intravenous Therapy
	
	  › Monitor the use of an infusion pump.
	
	» Pharmacological Pain Management
	
	  › Administer and document pharmacological pain management appropriate for client age and diagnoses.
		› Relevant topics/tasks include:
		
		» Alterations in Body Systems
		
		  › Identify signs, symptoms, and incubation periods of infectious diseases.
		
		  › Provide care for the client with an infectious disease.
		
		  › Evaluate the client's response to treatment for an infectious disease.

chapter 85

Overview

- Diagnostic procedures for immune and infectious disorders involve identification of pathogenic micro-organisms. The most accurate and definitive way to identify micro-organisms and cell characteristics is by examining blood, body fluids, and tissue samples under a microscope.

- Immune and infectious disorders diagnostic procedures that nurses should be knowledgeable about

  - Serum WBC count with differential

  - Radioallergosorbent test

  - Skin testing for allergens

- Effective treatment of infectious disease begins with identification of the pathogenic micro-organism.

White Blood Cells

- WBCs, or leukocytes, stimulate the inflammatory response and offer protection against various types of infection and foreign antigens.

- There are five types of WBCs. Laboratory analysis of circulating WBCs is called the differential. The differential is listed so the percentages of the types of WBCs totals 100%. This number is arrived at by counting the number of each type of cell in a representative sample of 100 WBCs and multiplying it by 100. If the percentage of one type of cell increases, the percentages of other types decrease accordingly.

- Interpretation of Findings

  - The normal reference range for WBCs is 5,000 to 10,000/mm³. A healthy older adult can have a range of 3,000 to 9,000/mm³.

  - Leukopenia is a total WBC count of less than 4,500/mm³. It may indicate a compromised inflammatory response or viral infection.

  - Leukocytosis is a total WBC count of greater than 10,000/mm³. It may indicate an inflammatory response to a pathogen or a disease process.

  - Neutropenia is a neutrophil count of less than 2,000/mm³. Neutropenia occurs in clients who are immunocompromised, are undergoing chemotherapy, or have a process that reduces the production of neutrophils. A client who has neutropenia is at an increased risk for infection.

    - The absolute neutrophil count (ANC) of a client who has neutropenia is calculated by multiplying the total WBC count by the summed number of neutrophils and bands and then dividing by 100. Neutropenic precautions (a private room; designated equipment; restricted exposure to live plants, ingestion of fresh fruits, and vegetables) should be instituted if the client's ANC is 1.0 or less.

  - The term "left shift" indicates an increase in "banded" or immature neutrophils, which occurs in a client who has an infectious process. Neutrophil production is increased when infection is present, allowing the release of immature neutrophils which have not reached their full potential.

TYPE OF WBC

NEUTROPHILS

Percent of circulating WBCs	55% to 75%
Increased in relation to:	› Acute bacterial infection › Fungal infection
Decreased in relation to:	› Sepsis › Radiation therapy, aplastic anemia, chemotherapy, and influenza
Additional information	› The majority of neutrophils are segmented (mature) with a lesser amount being banded (not fully mature). › Immature neutrophils (bands) should not be found.

LYMPHOCYTES (T CELLS AND B CELLS)

Percent of circulating WBCs	20% to 40%
Increased in relation to:	› Chronic bacterial or viral infection › Bacteria such as hepatitis › Viruses such as mononucleosis, › Lymphocytic leukemia, mumps, and measles multiple myeloma
Decreased in relation to:	› Leukemia › Sepsis
Additional information	› T-lymphocytes initiate cell-mediated immunity. › B-lymphocytes initiate humoral immunity.

MONOCYTES

Percent of circulating WBCs	2% to 8%
Increased in relation to:	› Chronic inflammation › Viral infections such as › Protozoal infections mononucleosis, mumps, › Tuberculosis and measles
Decreased in relation to:	› Corticosteroids

EOSINOPHILS

Percent of circulating WBCs	1% to 4%
Increased in relation to:	› Allergic reaction › Chronic inflammation › Parasitic infection › Hodgkin's disease
Decreased in relation to:	› Stress › Corticosteroids

BASOPHILS

Percent of circulating WBCs	0.5% to 1%
Increased in relation to:	› Leukemia
Decreased in relation to:	› Acute allergic/hypersensitivity reaction › Hyperthyroidism

Radioallergosorbent Test

- A radioallergosorbent test (RAST) is a blood test to determine sensitivity to various allergens. It may be done in conjunction with skin testing or as an alternative when the risk of a hypersensitivity reaction to an allergen exists.

- The advantage to RAST testing is that it will not precipitate a dangerous allergic reaction in the client and is quicker to administer.

- The disadvantage to RAST testing is that it is available for fewer antigens, may be less sensitive than skin testing, and is more expensive.

- Indications
  - Potential Diagnoses – suspected environmental and food allergies
  - Client Presentation
    - Report of hypersensitivity reactions
    - Presence of hives, asthma, and/or gastrointestinal dysfunction

- Interpretation of Findings
  - During the test, various radiolabeled allergens are exposed to the client's blood, and the amount of the client's immunoglobulin E (IgE) that is attracted to each specific allergen is measured according to standardized values. If an allergen is not attracted, this is considered a negative result. If a client's IgE is attracted to an allergen, the amount is measured on a scale of 0 to 5, with the higher number indicating a higher level from sensitivity.

- Intraprocedure
  - Nursing Actions – Obtain a blood sample.

- Postprocedure
  - Nursing Actions – Inform the client when to expect results (usually at least a week).

Skin Testing for Allergens

- Skin testing for allergens involves the use of intradermal injections or scratching the superficial layer (scratch or prick test) of the skin with small amounts of suspected allergens.

- Intradermal testing runs a higher risk of hypersensitivity reactions and is usually done if the scratch test is inconclusive.

- Indications
  - Potential Diagnoses – suspected environmental and food allergies
  - Client Presentation – presence of hives, asthma, and/or gastrointestinal dysfunction

- Interpretation of Findings
  - Allergens that provoke a localized reaction (wheal and flare) are considered a positive reaction to that allergen.
  - The larger the reaction the worse the allergy.

- Preprocedure
  - Nursing Actions
    - Prepare the skin for application of various allergens using soap and water (client's back or forearm are usually used for testing).

    - Alcohol may be used to remove oil.
    - Have equipment available for a possible anaphylaxis reaction.
  - Client Education – Instruct the client to avoid taking corticosteroids and antihistamines 5 days prior to the testing.
- Intraprocedure
  - Nursing Actions
    - The skin is scratched or pricked with a needle after application of a drop of an allergen.
    - Standard pattern of application should be used so identification of the allergen can be done according to the location of the reaction.
    - Application of saline (negative control for reaction) and histamine (positive control for reaction) should be done as a baseline for expected reactions.
    - An assessment of reactions is done after 15 to 20 min.
- Postprocedure
  - Nursing Actions
    - Assess the skin for areas of reaction, and document the allergen that is responsible.
    - Remove all solutions from the skin.
    - Inform the client when results will be available.
    - Recommend an antihistamine or topical corticosteroid if the client experiences itching secondary to the testing.
  - Client Education
    - Teach desensitizing options and avoidance therapies to the client related to identifying allergens.
    - Advise the client to follow a special diet that eliminates allergens (gluten-free).

APPLICATION EXERCISES

1. A nurse is reviewing the laboratory findings of a client who has a WBC count of 20,000/mm³. Based on these findings, the nurse should conclude that the client has which of the following?

    A. Neutropenia

    B. Leukocytosis

    C. Hemolysis

    D. Leukopenia

2. A nurse is reviewing the laboratory findings of a client who has the measles. The nurse should expect to find an increase in which of the following types of WBCs?

    A. Neutrophils

    B. Basophils

    C. Monocytes

    D. Eosinophils

3. A nurse is preparing to administer a scratch test to a client who has suspected food and environmental allergies. Which of the following actions should the nurse perform prior to the procedure? (Select all that apply.)

    _____ A. Cleanse the client's skin with povidone-iodine (Betadine).

    _____ B. Ask the client about previous reactions to allergens.

    _____ C. Ask the client about medications taken over the past several days.

    _____ D. Inform the client to expect itching at one site.

    _____ E. Obtain emergency resuscitation equipment.

4. A nurse is caring for a client who is scheduled to have a radioallergosorbent test (RAST) completed. Use the ATI Active Learning Template: Diagnostic Procedure to complete this item to include the following:

    A. Indications: Describe two.

    B. Interpretation of Findings: Describe one.

    C. Postprocedure Nursing Actions: Describe one.

APPLICATION EXERCISES KEY

1. A. INCORRECT: Neutropenia is a neutrophil count of less than 2,000/mm³.

    B. **CORRECT:** Leukocytosis is a WBC count of greater than 10,000/mm³, which can indicate an inflammatory response to a pathogen or a disease process.

    C. INCORRECT: Hemolysis is the breakdown of red blood cells.

    D. INCORRECT: Leukopenia is a total WBC count of less than 4,300/mm³, which can indicate a compromised inflammatory response or a viral infection.

     NCLEX® Connection: Reduction of Risk Potential, Laboratory Values

2. A. INCORRECT: Neutrophils are increased when an acute bacterial or fungal infection is present.

    B. INCORRECT: Basophils are increased when leukemia is present.

    C. **CORRECT:** Monocytes are increased when a viral infection such as measles occurs and chronic inflammation is present.

    D. INCORRECT: Eosinophils are increased when an allergic reaction occurs or chronic inflammation is present.

     NCLEX® Connection: Reduction of Risk Potential, Laboratory Values

3. A. INCORRECT: The nurse should use soap and water to cleanse the skin. Povidone-iodine could interfere with an allergen and elicit a response.

    B. **CORRECT:** The nurse should ask the client about any previous reactions to allergens, which could indicate an increased risk of an anaphylactic reaction.

    C. **CORRECT:** The nurse should ask the client about medications taken over the past several days. Antihistamines and corticosteroids should not be taken within the past 5 days due to their ability to suppress reactions.

    D. **CORRECT:** Histamine will be applied as a control site so the client will experience itching at this site.

    E. **CORRECT:** Emergency equipment should be available, even if the client denies experiencing an anaphylactic reaction.

     NCLEX® Connection: Reduction of Risk Potential, Diagnostic Tests

4. *Using the ATI Active Learning Template: Diagnostic Procedure*

A. Indications
   - Suspected environmental and food allergies
   - Report of hypersensitivity reactions
   - Presence of hives, asthma, and/or gastrointestinal dysfunction

B. Interpretation of Findings
   - During the test, various radiolabeled allergens are exposed to the client's blood, and the amount of the client's immunoglobulin E (IgE) that is attracted to each specific allergen is measured according to standardized values. If an allergen is not attracted, this is considered a negative result. If a client's IgE is attracted to an allergen, the amount is measure on a scale of 0 to 5, with the higher number indicating a higher level from sensitivity.

C. Postprocedure Nursing Actions
   - Inform the client when to expect results (usually takes at least a week).

   (N) NCLEX® Connection: Reduction of Risk Potential, Diagnostic Tests

chapter 86

Overview

- Administration of a vaccine causes production of antibodies that prevent illness from a specific microbe.

- Vaccines may be made from killed viruses or live, attenuated (or weakened) viruses.

- Adaptive immunity allows the body to make antibodies in response to a foreign organism. Adaptive immunity can be active or passive, or natural or artificial.

- Active-natural immunity develops when the body produces antibodies in response to exposure to a live pathogen.

- Active-artificial immunity develops when a vaccine is given and the body produces antibodies in response to exposure to a killed or attenuated virus.

- Passive-natural occurs when antibodies are passed from the mother to the fetus/newborn through the placenta and breast milk.

- Passive-artificial immunity occurs after antibodies in the form of immune globulins are administered to an individual who requires immediate protection against a disease where exposure has already occurred. After several weeks or months, the individual is no longer protected.

Medication Classification: Immunization

- The 2013 Centers for Disease Control and Prevention (CDC) immunization recommendations for adults (18 years and older) (Go to www.cdc.gov/vaccines for updates.)

  ○ Tetanus, diphtheria (Td) booster – Give booster every 10 years. For adults 19 to 64 years of age who did not receive a dose of tetanus, diphtheria, pertussis (Tdap) previously, substitute one dose with Tdap.

    ■ Adults age 65 years or older who have not received Tdap and have contact with children younger than age 12 months should be immunized.

    ■ Pregnant women after 20 weeks gestation may receive the vaccine.

  ○ Measles, mumps, and rubella vaccine (MMR) – Give one to two doses at ages 19 to 49 and one dose after age 50.

  ○ Varicella vaccine – Give two doses to adults who do not have evidence of a previous infection. A second dose should be given to adults who have had only one previous dose.

Ⓖ
- ○ Pneumococcal polysaccharide vaccine (PPSV) – Immunize adults who are immunocompromised, who have a chronic disease, who smoke cigarettes, or who live in a long-term care facility. CDC guidelines should be followed for reimmunization. Give one dose to adults older than 65 years of age who have not previously been immunized nor have history of disease. Administer a second dose if 5 years have elapsed since the first dose.

- ○ Hepatitis A – Two doses for high-risk individuals.

- ○ Hepatitis B – Three doses for high-risk individuals.

  - ▪ Recommended for adults age 60 years or younger who have diabetes mellitus, adults who have a new diagnosis of diabetes mellitus, and clients older than 60 years who are at risk for needing assistance with blood glucose monitoring.

- ○ Influenza vaccine – Give one dose annually. Recommended for all adults annually and to all people who lack documentation of immunization or have no evidence of previous infection. Note that the live attenuated vaccine (LAIV), given as a nasal spray, is indicated only for adults under age 50 or for those who are not pregnant or immunocompromised.

- ○ Meningococcal conjugate vaccine (MCV4) – One or two doses are recommended for students entering college and living in dormitories if not previously immunized. Also recommended for adults if another risk factor is present (medical, occupational, lifestyle). Reimmunization may be recommended after 5 years for those at high risk for infection (military, splenectomy, travel to a hyperendemic or epidemic country).

- ○ Human papilloma virus (HPV2 or HPV4) vaccine – Given in three doses and recommended for females up to age 26 who were not immunized as children. The second dose should be administered 2 months after the first dose, and the third dose should be administered 6 months after the first dose.

  - ▪ HPV4 – This vaccine is given to males up to age 21. Recommended to age 26 in the presence of other risk factors (medical, occupational, lifestyle).

Ⓖ
- ○ Herpes zoster vaccine – Recommended for all adults older than 60 years.

Purpose

- • Expected Pharmacological Action

  - ○ Immunizations produce antibodies that provide active immunity. Immunizations may take months to have an effect, but they provide long-lasting protection against infectious diseases.

- • Therapeutic Uses

  - ○ Eradication of infectious diseases (polio, smallpox)

  - ○ Prevention of childhood and adult infectious diseases and their complications (measles, diphtheria, mumps, rubella, tetanus, H. influenza)

Contraindications/Precautions

- An anaphylactic reaction to a vaccine is a contraindication for further doses of that vaccine.
- An anaphylactic reaction to a vaccine is a contraindication to use of other vaccines containing the same substance.
- Moderate or severe illnesses with or without fever are contraindications for use of a vaccine. With acute febrile illness, immunization is deferred until symptoms resolve. The common cold and other minor illnesses are not contraindications.
  - Contraindications to immunizations require the provider to analyze data and weigh the risks that come with and without immunizations.
  - Individuals who are immunocompromised are defined by the CDC as those who have hematologic or solid tumors, who have congenital immunodeficiency, are HIV-positive, or are receiving long-term immunosuppressive therapy, including corticosteroids.

ADVERSE EFFECTS	CONTRAINDICATIONS
Td or DTaP	
› Local reaction at injection site	› Severe febrile illness › A history of prior anaphylactic reaction to the DTaP vaccine › An occurrence of encephalopathy 7 days after the administration of the DTaP immunization › An occurrence of seizures within 3 days of the immunization › Guillain-Barré syndrome less than 6 weeks after previous dose of tetanus toxoid-containing vaccine
MMR	
› Local reactions such as rash; fever; and swollen glands in cheeks, neck, and under the jaw › Possibility of joint pain lasting for days to weeks › Risk for anaphylaxis and thrombocytopenia	› Pregnancy › Allergy to gelatin and neomycin › Clients who are immunocompromised › Recent transfusion with antibody-containing blood products
Varicella (two doses)	
› Varicella-like rash that may be local or generalized, such as vesicles on the body › Fever, malaise, and anorexia	› Pregnancy – Women who are pregnant should avoid close proximity to children who are recently immunized. › Allergy to gelatin and neomycin › Severe allergy (anaphylaxis) after previous dose or any vaccine component › Severe immunodeficiency › Recent transfusion with antibody-containing blood products
Pneumococcal (PCV) (one or two doses)	
› Mild local reactions, fever, and no serious adverse effects	› Pregnancy › Severe allergy (anaphylaxis) after previous dose, any vaccine component, or any diptheria toxoid-containing vaccine

ADVERSE EFFECTS	CONTRAINDICATIONS
Hepatitis A (two doses); Hepatitis B (three doses)	

› Local reaction at injection site
› Headache
› Loss of appetite
› Mild fatigue
	› Hepatitis A
	  » Severe allergy (anaphylaxis) after previous dose or any vaccine component
	  » Hypersensitivity to neomycin
	  » Pregnancy may be a contraindication.
	› Hepatitis B
	  » Severe allergy (anaphylaxis) after previous dose, or any vaccine component

Influenza (one dose annually)	
› Inactivated – mild local reaction, and fever › Live attenuated – headache, cough, and fever › Rare – risk for Guillain-Barré syndrome	› Live attenuated influenza vaccine administered as a nasal spray is contraindicated for adults who are older than 50, are immunocompromised or have a chronic disease, or women who are pregnant › History of Guillain-Barré syndrome › Allergy to egg protein › Severe allergy (anaphylaxis) after previous dose or any vaccine component
Meningococcal Conjugate (MCV4) (one or more doses)	
› Mild local reaction and rare risk of allergic response › Possible mild fever	› History of Guillain-Barré syndrome › History of latex hypersensitivity › Severe allergy (anaphylaxis) after previous dose or any vaccine component
Herpes zoster	
› Local reaction at injection site › Rare – headache	› Clients who are immunocompromised › Severe allergy (anaphylaxis) after previous dose or any vaccine component › Pregnancy › Allergies to neomycin and gelatin
Human papilloma virus (HPV2 or HPV4) (Three doses – second dose should be administered 2 months after the first dose; third dose should be administered 6 months after the first dose.)	
› Mild local reaction and fever › Headache › Fainting has occurred shortly after receiving vaccine › Rare – risk for Guillain-Barré syndrome	› Pregnancy › Severe allergy (anaphylaxis) after previous dose or any vaccine component › Yeast hypersensitivity

Medication/Food Interactions

- None significant

Nursing Administration

- For adults
  - ○ Give subcutaneous immunizations in outer aspect of the upper arm or anterolateral thigh.
  - ○ Give intramuscular immunizations into the deltoid muscle.
- For clients of all ages
  - ○ Have emergency medications and equipment on standby in case the client experiences an allergic response such as anaphylaxis (rare) or serious reaction at injection site.
  - ○ Follow storage and reconstitution directions. If reconstituted, use within 30 min.
  - ○ Provide written, up-to-date immunization information, and review the content with clients.
    - ▪ Antipyretic for fever, cool compress for localized tenderness, and mobilize the affected extremity.
  - ○ Instruct clients to observe for complications and to notify the provider if adverse effects occur.
  - ○ Document administration of vaccines to include date, route, site, type, manufacturer, lot number, and expiration date of vaccine. Also document the client's name, address, and signature.
  - ○ Include the name, title of the person administering the vaccine, and the address of the facility where the permanent record is located.

Nursing Evaluation of Medication Effectiveness

- Depending on the therapeutic intent of the immunization, effectiveness may be evidenced by:
  - ○ Improvement of local reaction with absence of pain, fever, and swelling at the site of injection.

APPLICATION EXERCISES

1. A nurse is reviewing strategies to promote comfort with a client who received an immunization. Which of the following information should the nurse include? (Select all that apply.)

_____ A. Massage the injection site.

_____ B. Apply a cool compress to the injection site.

_____ C. Take acetaminophen or ibuprofen.

_____ D. Use the affected extremity.

_____ E. Apply an antimicrobial ointment to the injection site.

2. A nurse is preparing to administer an IM injection of immune globulin to a client who has been exposed to hepatitis A. Which of the following statements by the nurse is appropriate?

A. "This medication offers permanent immunity to hepatitis A."

B. "This medication involves receiving three injections over several months."

C. "This medication provides you with an immune response more quickly than your body can produce it."

D. "This medication contains an attenuated virus to help your body create antibodies."

3. A nurse is preparing to administer a varicella immunization to a client. Which of the following questions by the nurse is appropriate?

A. "Are you allergic to eggs?"

B. "Are you allergic to baker's yeast?"

C. "Are you pregnant?"

D. "Do you have a history of Guillain-Barré syndrome?"

4. A nurse is preparing to document the administration of a meningococcal vaccine to a client. Which of the following should the nurse include in the documentation? (Select all that apply.)

_____ A. Time of administration

_____ B. Name of vaccine manufacturer

_____ C. Vaccine expiration date

_____ D. Date of administration

_____ E. Serial number of the vaccine

5. A nurse in a clinic is caring for a client who is to receive an immunization. The client asks about contraindications to immunizations. Which of the following is an appropriate response by the nurse? (Select all that apply.)

_____ A. "The use of corticosteroid medications is a contraindication."

_____ B. "An anaphylactic reaction is a contraindication for administration of any type of immunization."

_____ C. "The common cold is a contraindication for receiving an immunization."

_____ D. "Your provider will weigh the risks if you have experienced any contraindications."

_____ E. "HIV is a contraindication for receiving any immunization."

6. A nurse is developing a plan of care related to immunizations for an older adult client. Which immunizations should the nurse include in the plan? Use the ATI Active Learning Template: Basic Concept to complete this item. Include the following:

A. Related Content: Summary statement

B. Underlying Principles: Identify four immunizations recommended for the older adult client.

C. Nursing Interventions: Describe one adverse effect and one intervention for each immunization that should be reviewed with the client.

APPLICATION EXERCISES KEY

1. A. INCORRECT: Massaging the injection site for any extended period of time can increase localized discomfort.

    B. **CORRECT:** Applying a cool compress to the injection site can relieve discomfort from the localized reaction.

    C. **CORRECT:** Taking an antipyretic can relieve a low-grade fever and localized discomfort at the injection site.

    D. **CORRECT:** Mobilizing the affected extremity will help relieve discomfort due to a localized reaction.

    E. INCORRECT: Applying an antimicrobial ointment at the injection site is not indicated.

    Ⓝ NCLEX® Connection: Pharmacological and Parenteral Therapies, Parenteral/Intravenous Therapies

2. A. INCORRECT: The statement by the nurse is not appropriate because this medication produces passive-artificial immunity that lasts only several weeks or months.

    B. INCORRECT: This statement by the nurse is not appropriate because this medication produces passive-artificial immunity and is given one time after exposure to hepatitis A.

    C. **CORRECT:** This statement by the nurse is appropriate because this medication produces passive-artificial immunity and contains antibodies to help protect against hepatitis A for several weeks or months.

    D. INCORRECT: This statement by the nurse is not appropriate because this medication contains antibodies, not an attenuated virus.

    Ⓝ NCLEX® Connection: Pharmacological and Parenteral Therapies, Parenteral/Intravenous Therapies

3. A. INCORRECT: This question by the nurse is not appropriate because an allergy to eggs should be reviewed if the client is to receive an influenza immunization. The nurse should ask about allergy to gelatin and neomycin, which may be used in the ingredients of the varicella vaccine.

    B. INCORRECT: This question by the nurse is not appropriate because an allergy to yeast should be reviewed if the client is to receive HPV. The nurse should ask about allergy to gelatin and neomycin, which may be used in the ingredients of the varicella vaccine.

    C. **CORRECT:** The nurse should ask whether the client is pregnant because the varicella immunization is contraindicated during pregnancy.

    D. INCORRECT: This question by the nurse is not appropriate because Guillain-Barré syndrome is not a contraindication for varicella immunization, but it is a contraindication for other immunizations.

    Ⓝ NCLEX® Connection: Pharmacological and Parenteral Therapies, Adverse Effects/Contraindications/ Side Effects/Interactions

4. A. INCORRECT: Documentation of the time the vaccine was administered is not included.

    B. **CORRECT:** The nurse should document the name of the vaccine manufacturer.

    C. **CORRECT:** The nurse should document the expiration date of the vaccine.

    D. **CORRECT:** The nurse should document the date the vaccine was administered.

    E. INCORRECT: The nurse should document the lot number, not the serial number, of the vaccine.

    Ⓝ NCLEX® Connection: Pharmacological and Parenteral Therapies, Adverse Effects/Contraindications/ Side Effects/Interactions

5. A. **CORRECT:** The client should not receive immunizations if taking corticosteroids, which are immunosuppressant medications.

    B. INCORRECT: The client who has experienced an anaphylactic reaction can receive other immunizations that contain different substances.

    C. INCORRECT: The client who has a common cold may receive an immunization because the client is not immunosuppressed.

    D. **CORRECT:** The client who has experienced contraindications should inform the provider so the provider can weigh the risks of an immunization.

    E. **CORRECT:** HIV is considered a contraindication for receiving an immunization because of immunosuppression.

    Ⓝ NCLEX® Connection: Pharmacological and Parenteral Therapies, Adverse Effects/Contraindications/ Side Effects/Interactions

6. *Using the ATI Active Learning Template: Basic Concept*

A. Related Content
- Immunizations recommended for an older adult client.

B. Underlying Principles
- Tetanus diphtheria booster
- Pneumococcal polysaccharide
- Hepatitis B
- Influenza, live attenuated virus

C. Nursing Interventions
- Tetanus Diphtheria booster: localized reaction at the injection site; encourage mobilization of the affected extremity.
- Pneumococcal polysaccharide: fever; take an antipyretic medication.
- Hepatitis B: localized reaction at the injection site and fatigue; apply a cold compress and rest.
- Influenza, live attenuated virus: headache; take a mild analgesic.

Ⓝ NCLEX® Connection: Health Promotion and Maintenance, Aging Process

chapter 87

Overview

- Human immunodeficiency virus (HIV) is a retrovirus that is transmitted through blood and body fluids (semen, vaginal secretions).
- HIV targets CD4+ lymphocytes, also known as T-cells or T-lymphocytes.
  - T-cells work in concert with B-lymphocytes. Both are part of specific acquired (adaptive) immunity.
  - HIV integrates its RNA into host cell DNA through reverse transcriptase, reshaping the host's immune system.
- HIV is found in feces, urine, tears, saliva, cerebrospinal fluid, cervical cells, lymph nodes, corneal tissue, and brain tissue, but epidemiologic studies indicate that these are unlikely sources of infection.
- All women who are pregnant should be screened for HIV.
- HIV infection is one continuous disease process with three stages.
  - Progression of HIV infection
    - Manifestations occur within 2 to 4 weeks of infection.
    - Symptoms are similar to those of influenza and can include a rash and a sore throat.
    - This stage is marked by a rapid rise in the HIV viral load, decreased CD4+ cells, and increased CD8 cells.
    - The resolution of clinical manifestations coincides with the decline in viral HIV copies.
    - Lymphadenopathy persists throughout the disease process.
  - Chronic asymptomatic infection
    - This stage may be prolonged and clinically silent (asymptomatic).
    - The client may remain asymptomatic for 10 years or more.
    - Anti-HIV antibodies are produced (HIV positive).
    - Over time, the virus begins active replication using the host's genetic machinery.
      - CD4+ cells are destroyed.
      - The viral load increases.
      - Dramatic loss of immunity begins.
  - AIDS
    - This stage is characterized by life-threatening opportunistic infections.
    - This is the end stage of HIV infection. Without treatment, death occurs within 5 years.
    - All people with AIDS have HIV, but not all people with HIV have AIDS.

Health Promotion and Disease Prevention

- Teach the client how the virus is transmitted and ways to prevent infection, such as the use of condoms, abstinence, and avoiding sharing needles.

- Encourage the client to maintain up-to-date immunizations, including yearly seasonal influenza and pneumococcal polysaccharide vaccine (PPSV).

- Health care providers should use standard precautions when caring for the client.

Assessment

- Risk Factors

  - Unprotected sex (vaginal, anal, oral)

  - Multiple sex partners

  - Occupational exposure (health care workers)

  - Perinatal exposure

  - Blood transfusions (not a significant source of infection in the U.S.)

  - Intravenous drug use with a contaminated needle

  - HIV infection may go undiagnosed in older adult clients due to the similarity of its manifestations to other illnesses that are common in this age group.

  - Older adults are more susceptible to fluid and electrolyte imbalances, malnutrition, skin alterations, and wasting syndrome than younger adults.

  - Older women experience vaginal dryness and thinning of the vaginal wall, increasing their susceptibility to HIV infection.

- Subjective Data

  - Chills

  - Rash

  - Anorexia, nausea, weight loss

  - Weakness and fatigue

  - Headache and sore throat

  - Night sweats

- Objective Data
  - Physical Assessment Findings and Laboratory Data
    - A confirmed case classification meets the laboratory criteria for a diagnosis of HIV infection and one of the four HIV infection stages.
      - Stage 4 has no data available concerning CD4+ T-cell counts and percentages, and no information on the AIDS-defining illness of the client.

STAGE	DEFINING CONDITIONS	CD4+ T-LYMPHOCYTE COUNT	CD4+ T-LYMPHOCYTE PERCENTAGE OF TOTAL LYMPHOCYTES
Stage 1	› None	500 cells/mm³ or more	29 or more
Stage 2	› None	200 to 499 cells/mm³	14 to 28
Stage 3 (AIDS)*	› One or more of the following: » Candidiasis of the esophagus, bronchi, trachea, or lungs » Herpes simplex – Chronic ulcers (of more than 1 month duration) » HIV-related encephalopathy » Disseminated or extrapulmonary histoplasmosis » Kaposi's sarcoma » Burkitt's lymphoma » Mycobacterium tuberculosis of any site » Pneumocystis jirovecii pneumonia » Recurrent pneumonia » Progressive multifocal leukoencephalopathy » Recurrent Salmonella septicemia » Wasting syndrome attributed to HIV	Less than 200 cells/mm³	Less than 14
Stage 4	› No information available	› No information available	› No information available

*Documentation of an AIDS-defining condition supersedes a CD4+ T-lymphocyte count of 200 cells/mm³ or more and a CD4+ T-lymphocyte percentage of total lymphocytes of more than 14.

To read more about HIV, go to www.cdc.gov.

- CBC and differential – Abnormal (anemia, thrombocytopenia, leukopenia)
- Platelet count – Decreased less than 150,000/mm³

○ Diagnostic Procedures

- HIV determination

  □ Positive result from an HIV antibody screening test (enzyme-linked immunosorbent assay [ELISA]) confirmed by a positive result from a supplemental HIV antibody test (Western blot or indirect immunofluorescence assay test)

  □ Positive result or report of a detectable quantity from any of the following HIV virologic (viral load) testing:

    ▸ HIV nucleic acid (DNA or RNA) detection test (reverse transcriptase [RT-PCR])

    ▸ Branched DNA (bDNA) method

    ▸ Nucleic acid sequenced-based assay (NASBA)

- Liver profile, biopsies, and testing of stool for parasites

  □ Nursing Actions

    ▸ Prepare the client for the test.

  □ Client Education

    ▸ Inform the client about the details of the test, such as length and what to expect.

- Brain or lung MRI or CT scan

  □ Detailed image of the brain or lung to detect abnormalities

  □ Nursing Actions

    ▸ Prepare the client for the procedure.

  □ Client Education

    ▸ Inform the client about the length of time the test takes (sometimes up to 1 hr).

Patient-Centered Care

- Nursing Care

  ○ Assess risk factors (sexual practices, IV drug use).

  ○ Monitor fluid intake/urinary output.

  ○ Obtain daily weights to monitor weight loss.

  ○ Monitor nutritional intake.

  ○ Monitor electrolytes.

  ○ Assess skin integrity (rashes, open areas, bruising).

  ○ Assess the client's pain status.

  ○ Monitor vital signs (especially temperature).

  ○ Assess lung sounds/respiratory status (diminished lung sounds).

  ○ Assess neurological status (confusion, dementia, visual changes).

  ○ Encourage activity alternated with rest periods.

  ○ Administer supplemental oxygen as needed.

  ○ Provide analgesia as needed.

  ○ Provide skin care as needed.

- Medications
  - Highly active antiretroviral therapy (HAART) involves using three to four HIV medications in combination with other antiretroviral medications to reduce medication resistance, adverse effects, and dosages.
    - Infusion inhibitors – enfuvirtide (Fuzeon)
      - □ Blocks the fusion of HIV with the host cell
    - Entry inhibitors – maraviroc (Selzentry)
    - Nucleoside reverse transcriptase inhibitors (NRTIs) – zidovudine (Retrovir)
      - □ Interfere with the virus's ability to convert RNA into DNA
    - Non-nucleoside reverse transcriptase inhibitors (NNRTIs) – delavirdine (Rescriptor) and efavirenz (Sustiva)
      - □ Inhibit viral replication in cells
    - Protease inhibitors – atazanavir (Reyataz), nelfinavir (Viracept), saquinavir (Invirase), and indinavir (Crixivan)
      - □ Inhibit an enzyme needed for the virus to replicate
    - Integrase inhibitors – raltegravir (Isentress)
    - Antineoplastic medication – interleukin (Interferon)
      - □ Immunostimulant that enhances the immune response and reduces the production of cancer cells (used commonly with Kaposi's sarcoma)
  - Nursing Considerations
    - Monitor laboratory results (CBC, WBC, liver function tests). Antiretroviral medications may increase alanine aminotransferase (ALT), aspartate aminotransferase (AST), bilirubin, mean corpuscular volume (MCV), high-density lipoproteins (HDLs), total cholesterol, and triglycerides.

  - Client Education
    - Educate the client about the side effects of the medications and ways to decrease the severity of the side effects.
    - Educate the client about the need to take medications on a regular schedule and to not miss doses. Missed medication doses can cause drug resistance.
- Teamwork and Collaboration
  - Infectious disease services may be consulted to manage HIV.
  - Respiratory services may be consulted to improve respiratory status.
  - Nutritional services may be consulted for dietary supplementation.
  - Rehabilitation services may be consulted for strengthening and improving the client's level of energy.

- Alternative Therapy
  - ○ Vitamins, herbal products, and shark cartilage may help alleviate the symptoms of HIV.
    - Ask the client if she is taking herbal products. These can alter the effects of the prescribed medications.

- Care After Discharge
  - ○ Refer the client to local AIDS support groups as appropriate.
  - ○ Home health service may be indicated for clients who need help with strengthening and assistance regarding ADLs.
  - ○ Home health services may also provide assistance with IVs, dressing changes, and total parenteral nutrition (TPN).
  - ○ Respiratory services may be consulted for providing portable oxygen.
  - ○ Long-term care facilities may be indicated for clients with chronic HIV.
  - ○ Hospice services may be indicated for clients who have a late stage of HIV.
  - ○ Food services may be indicated for clients who are homebound and need meals prepared.
  - ○ Client Education
    - Instruct the client to practice good hygiene and frequent hand hygiene to reduce the risk of infection.
    - Instruct the client to avoid crowded areas or traveling to countries with poor sanitation.
    - Encourage the client to avoid raw foods, such as vegetables and meats.
    - Instruct the client to avoid cleaning pet litter boxes to reduce the risk of toxoplasmosis.
    - Encourage the client to keep the home environment clean and to avoid being exposed to family and friends who have colds or flu viruses.
    - Provide client teaching.
      - □ Transmission, infection control measures, and safe sex practices
      - □ The importance of maintaining a well-balanced diet
      - □ Self-administration of prescribed medications and potential side effects
      - □ Signs/symptoms that need to be reported immediately (infection)
    - Instruct the client to adhere to the antiretroviral dosing schedules.
    - Instruct the client about the need for frequent follow-up monitoring of CD4+ and viral load counts.
    - Encourage the use of constructive coping mechanisms.
    - Assist the client with identifying primary support systems.
    - Teach the client to report signs of infection immediately to the health care provider.

Complications

- Opportunistic Infections
  - Bacterial diseases, such as tuberculosis, bacterial pneumonia, and septicemia (blood poisoning)
  - HIV-associated malignancies, such as Kaposi's sarcoma, lymphoma, and squamous cell carcinoma
  - Viral diseases, such as those caused by cytomegalovirus, herpes simplex, and herpes zoster virus
  - Fungal diseases, such as PCP, candidiasis, cryptococcosis, and penicilliosis
  - Protozoal diseases, such as pneumocystis jiroveci pneumonia (PCP), toxoplasmosis, microsporidiosis, cryptosporidiosis, isosporiasis, and leishmaniasis
  - Nursing Actions
    - Implement and maintain antiretroviral medication therapy as prescribed.
    - Administer antineoplastics, antibiotics, analgesics, antifungals, and antidiarrheals as prescribed.
    - Administer appetite stimulants (to enhance nutrition).
    - Monitor for skin breakdown.
    - Maintain fluid intake.
    - Maintain nutrition.
  - Client Education
    - Teach the client to report signs of infection immediately to the health care provider.
- Wasting Syndrome
  - Nursing Actions
    - Maintain nutrition orally or by TPN if indicated.
    - Provide between-meal supplements/snacks.
    - Serve at least six small feedings with high protein value.
- Fluid/Electrolyte Imbalance
  - Nursing Actions
    - Monitor fluid/electrolyte status.
    - Report abnormal laboratory data promptly.
    - Maintain IV fluid replacement.
    - Make dietary adjustments to reduce diarrhea.
- Seizures (HIV encephalopathy)
  - Nursing Actions
    - Maintain client safety.
    - Implement seizure precautions.

APPLICATION EXERCISES

1. A nurse working in an outpatient clinic is assessing a client who reports night sweats and fatigue. He states he has had a cough along with nausea and diarrhea. His temperature is 38.1° C (100.6° F) orally. The client is afraid he has HIV. Which of the following actions should the nurse take? (Select all that apply.)

_____ A. Perform a physical assessment.

_____ B. Determine when current symptoms began.

_____ C. Teach the client about HIV transmission.

_____ D. Draw blood for HIV testing.

_____ E. Obtain a sexual history.

2. A nurse is caring for a client who is suspected of having HIV. Which of the following diagnostic tests and laboratory values are used to confirm HIV infection? (Select all that apply.)

_____ A. Western blot

_____ B. Indirect immunofluorescence assay

_____ C. CD4+ T-lymphocyte count

_____ D. CD4+ T-lymphocyte percentage of total lymphocytes

_____ E. Cerebrospinal fluid (CSF) analysis

3. A nurse is assessing a client for HIV. Which of the following are risk factors associated with this virus? (Select all that apply.)

_____ A. Perinatal exposure

_____ B. Pregnancy

_____ C. Monogamous sex partner

_____ D. Older adult woman

_____ E. Occupational exposure

4. A nurse is completing discharge instructions with a client who has AIDS. Which of the following statements by the client indicates an understanding of the teaching?

    A. "I will wear gloves while changing the pet litter box."

    B. "I will rinse raw fruits with water before eating them."

    C. "I will wear a mask when around family members who are ill."

    D. "I will cook vegetables before eating them."

5. A nurse is caring for a client who has HIV and has been newly diagnosed with Burkitt's lymphoma. Which of the following HIV infection stages is the client in?

    A. Stage 1

    B. Stage 2

    C. Stage 3

    D. Stage 4

6. A nurse is planning care for a client who has AIDS. Use the ATI Active Learning Template: Systems Disorder to complete this item to include the following: Patient-Centered Care: Describe at least three nursing interventions.

APPLICATION EXERCISES KEY

1.   A. **CORRECT:** The nurse should perform a physical assessment to gather data about the client's condition. This is an appropriate action by the nurse.

    B. **CORRECT:** The nurse should gather more data to determine whether the clinical manifestations are acute or chronic. This is an appropriate action by the nurse.

    C. INCORRECT: Teaching the client about HIV transmission is not an appropriate action by the nurse at this time. This is not a priority action for the nurse to include at this time.

    D. INCORRECT: Drawing blood for HIV testing is not an appropriate action by nurse at this time. This is not a priority action for the nurse to include at this time.

    E. **CORRECT:** The nurse should obtain a sexual history to determine how the virus was transmitted. This is an appropriate action by the nurse.

    Ⓝ NCLEX® Connection: Physiological Adaptations, Illness Management

2.   A. **CORRECT:** Positive results of a Western blot test confirm the presence of HIV infection.

    B. **CORRECT:** Positive results of an indirect immunofluorescence assay confirm the presence of HIV infection.

    C. INCORRECT: CD4+ T-lymphocyte count assists with classifying the stage of HIV infection.

    D. INCORRECT: CD4+ T-lymphocyte percentage of total lymphocytes assists with classifying the stage of HIV infection.

    E. INCORRECT: CSF analysis can be used to confirm meningitis.

    Ⓝ NCLEX® Connection: Reduction of Risk Potential, Diagnostic Tests

3.   A. **CORRECT:** Perinatal exposure is a risk factor associated with HIV. Women who are pregnant should take cautionary measures to prevent HIV exposure.

    B. INCORRECT: Women who are pregnant should be tested for HIV, but pregnancy is not a risk factor associated with this virus.

    C. INCORRECT: Having a monogamous sex partner is not a risk factor associated with the HIV virus.

    D. **CORRECT:** Being an older adult woman is a risk factor associated with the HIV virus due vaginal dryness and the thinning of the vaginal wall.

    E. **CORRECT:** Occupational exposure, such as being a health care worker, is a risk factor associated with the HIV virus.

    Ⓝ NCLEX® Connection: Health Promotion and Maintenance, Health Promotion/Disease Prevention

4. A. INCORRECT: A client who has AIDS should avoid changing the pet litter box to prevent acquiring toxoplasmosis.

    B. INCORRECT: A client who has AIDS should avoid consuming raw fruits due to the presence of bacteria that can cause opportunistic infections.

    C. INCORRECT: Due to compromised immune response, a client who has AIDS should avoid contact with family members who are ill.

    D. **CORRECT:** A client who has AIDS should cook vegetables before eating to kill bacteria that cause opportunistic infections.

    Ⓝ NCLEX® Connection: Physiological Adaptations, Illness Management

5. A. INCORRECT: In stage 1, there are no defining conditions.

    B. INCORRECT: In stage 2, there are no defining conditions.

    C. **CORRECT:** In stage 3, there are one or more defining conditions present. These can include candidiasis of the esophagus, bronchi, trachea, or lungs; chronic ulcers of herpes simplex; HIV-related encephalopathy; disseminated or extrapulmonary histoplasmosis; Kaposi's sarcoma; and Burkitt's lymphoma.

    D. INCORRECT: In stage 4, there is no information available.

    Ⓝ NCLEX® Connection: Physiological Adaptations, Illness Management

6. *Using ATI Active Learning Template: Systems Disorder*
    - Patient-Centered Care
        - Assess risk factors (sexual practices, IV drug use).
        - Monitor fluid intake/urinary output.
        - Obtain daily weights to monitor weight loss.
        - Monitor nutritional intake.
        - Monitor electrolytes.
        - Assess skin integrity (rashes, open areas, bruising).
        - Assess the client's pain status.
        - Monitor vital signs (especially temperature).
        - Assess lung sounds/respiratory status (diminished lung sounds).
        - Assess neurological status (confusion, dementia, visual changes).

    Ⓝ NCLEX® Connection: Physiological Adaptations, Alterations in Body Systems

chapter 88

Overview

- Systemic lupus erythematosus (SLE) is an autoimmune disorder in which an atypical immune response results in chronic inflammation and destruction of healthy tissue.

  - In autoimmune disorders, small antigens may bond with healthy tissue. The body then produces antibodies that attack the healthy tissue. This may be triggered by toxins, medications, bacteria, and/or viruses.

  - Control of manifestations and a decrease in the number and frequency of exacerbations is the goal of treatment, because there is no cure for autoimmune disorders.

  - Other autoimmune disorders include rheumatoid arthritis, vasculitis, multiple sclerosis, scleroderma (including Raynaud's phenomenon), and psoriasis.

  - Ⓖ Occurrence of autoimmune disorders increases with age.

- SLE varies in severity and progression. It is generally characterized by periods of exacerbations (flares) and remissions.

- SLE is classified as discoid or systemic. A temporary form of SLE may be medication-induced.

  - Discoid SLE primarily affects the skin. It is characterized by an erythematosus butterfly rash over the nose and cheeks and is generally self-limiting.

  - Systemic SLE affects the connective tissues of multiple organ systems and can lead to major organ failure.

  - Medication-induced SLE can be caused by medications (procainamide, hydralazine, isoniazid). Findings resolve when the medication is discontinued, and it does not cause renal or neurologic disease.

- SLE may be difficult to diagnose because of the vague nature of early manifestations.

Assessment

- Risk Factors

  - Females between the ages of 20 and 40

  - African American, Asian, or Native American descent

  - The incidence of lupus declines in women following menopause but remains steady in men.

  - Ⓖ Diagnosis of SLE may be delayed in older adult clients because many of the clinical manifestations mimic other disorders or may be associated with reports common to the normal aging process.

    - Joint pain and swelling may significantly limit ADLs in older adult clients who have comorbidities.

    - Older adult clients are at an increased risk for fractures if corticosteroid therapy is used.

- Subjective Data
  - Fatigue/malaise
  - Alopecia
  - Blurred vision
  - Malaise
  - Pleuritic pain
  - Anorexia/weight loss
  - Depression
  - Joint pain, swelling, tenderness
- Objective Data
  - Physical Assessment Findings
    - Fever (also a major symptom of exacerbation)
    - Anemia
    - Lymphadenopathy
    - Pericarditis (presence of a cardiac friction rub or pleural friction rub)
    - Raynaud's phenomenon (arteriolar vasospasm in response to cold/stress)
    - Findings consistent with organ involvement (kidney, heart, lungs, and vasculature)
    - Butterfly rash on face

	View Images	
	› Butterfly Rash	› Raynaud's Syndrome

  - Laboratory Tests
    - Autoantibodies
      - Antinuclear antibody (ANA) titer (antibody produced against one's own DNA) – positive ANA titer in 90% of clients who have lupus (expected finding is negative ANA titer at 1:20 dilution)
    - Anti-DNA – positive (not specific for SLE but positive in the vast majority of clients who have SLE)
    - Extractable nuclear antibodies (ENAs) specific for selected parts of a cell's nucleus
      - Anti-Smith (anti-Sm) – positive (highly specific for SLE)
      - Anti-RO (SSA) – positive
      - Anti-LA (SSB) – positive
      - Anti-RNP – positive
      - Anti-phospholipids (AP) – positive
    - Serum complement (C3, C4) – decreased
      - The complement system is made up of proteins (there are nine major complement proteins). These proteins work with the immune system and play a role in the development of inflammation. C3 and C4 are diagnostic for SLE because they decrease due to depletion secondary to an exaggerated inflammatory response.
    - BUN and serum creatinine – increased (with kidney involvement)
    - Urinalysis – positive for protein and RBCs (kidney involvement)
    - CBC – pancytopenia

Patient-Centered Care

- Nursing Care
  - Assess/Monitor
    - Pain, mobility, and fatigue
    - Vital signs (especially blood pressure)
    - Systemic manifestations
      - Hypertension and edema (renal compromise)
      - Urine output (renal compromise)
      - Diminished breath sounds (pleural effusion)
      - Tachycardia and sharp inspiratory chest pain (pericarditis)
      - Rubor, pallor, and cyanosis of hands/feet (vasculitis/vasospasm, Raynaud's phenomenon)
      - Arthralgias, myalgias, and polyarthritis (joint and connective tissue involvement)
      - Changes in mental status that indicate neurologic involvement (psychoses, paresis, seizures)
      - BUN, serum creatinine, and urinary output for renal involvement
      - Nutritional status
  - Provide small, frequent meals if anorexia is a concern. Offer between-meal supplements.
  - Encourage the client to limit salt intake for fluid retention secondary to steroid therapy.
  - Provide emotional support to the client and family.
- Medications
  - NSAIDs
    - Used to reduce inflammation and arthritic pain.
    - Nursing Considerations
      - NSAIDs are contraindicated for clients who have renal compromise.
      - Monitor for NSAID-induced hepatitis.
  - Corticosteroids (prednisone [Deltasone])
    - Used for immunosuppression and to reduce inflammation.
    - Nursing Considerations – Monitor for fluid retention, hypertension, and renal dysfunction.
    - Client Education – Do not stop taking steroids or decrease the dose abruptly.

  - Immunosuppressant agents – methotrexate and azathioprine (Imuran)
    - Used to suppress the immune response.
    - Nursing Considerations – Monitor for toxic effects (bone marrow suppression, increased liver enzymes).
  - Antimalarial – hydroxychloroquine (Plaquenil)
    - Used for suppression of synovitis, fever, and fatigue.
    - Nursing Considerations – Encourage frequent eye examinations.

- Teamwork and Collaboration
  - Physical and occupational therapy services may be used for strengthening exercises and adaptive devices as needed.
  - Refer clients to support groups as appropriate.
- Care After Discharge
  - Client Education
    - Avoid UV and sun exposure. Use sunscreen when outside and exposed to sunlight.
    - Use mild protein shampoo and avoid harsh hair treatments.
    - Use steroid creams for skin rash.
    - Report peripheral and periorbital edema promptly.
    - Report evidence of infection related to immunosuppression.
    - Avoid crowds and individuals who are sick, because illness can precipitate an exacerbation.
    - Educate client of childbearing age regarding risks of pregnancy with lupus and treatment medications.

Complications

- Lupus nephritis (renal failure/glomerulonephritis)
  - Clients whose SLE is unable to be managed with immunosuppressants and corticosteroids may experience renal failure secondary to glomerulonephritis. This is a major cause of death, and a renal transplant may be necessary.
  - Nursing Actions – Monitor for periorbital and lower extremity swelling and hypertension. Monitor the client's renal status (creatinine, BUN).
  - Client Education
    - Teach the client the importance of taking immunosuppressants and corticosteroids as prescribed.
    - Teach the client the importance of avoiding stress and illness.
- Pericarditis and myocarditis (instruct the client to report chest pain)
  - Inflammation of the heart, its vessels, and the surrounding sac can occur secondary to SLE.
  - Nursing Actions – Monitor for chest pain, fatigue, arrhythmias, and fever.
  - Client Education
    - Take immunosuppressants and corticosteroids as prescribed.
    - Avoid stress and illness.
    - Report chest pain to the provider.

APPLICATION EXERCISES

1. A nurse is reviewing the plan of care for a client who has systemic lupus erythematosus (SLE). The client reports fatigue, joint tenderness, swelling, and difficulty urinating. Which of the following laboratory findings should the nurse anticipate ? (Select all that apply.)

_____ A. Positive ANA

_____ B. Increased hemoglobin

_____ C. 2+ urine protein

_____ D. Increased serum C3 and C4 complement

_____ E. Elevated BUN

2. A nurse is providing teaching about self-care to a client who has SLE. Which of the following statements by the client indicates a need for further teaching?

A. "I should avoid sun exposure."

B. "I will apply powder to any skin rash."

C. "I should use a mild hair shampoo."

D. "I will call my doctor if I have a cough."

3. A nurse is providing teaching to a client who has a new prescription for prednisone (Deltasone). Which of the following should be included in the teaching? (Select all that apply.)

_____ A. Hypotension can occur.

_____ B. Weight gain is expected.

_____ C. Abdominal striae may appear.

_____ D. Loss of appetite may be present.

_____ E. Moon facies may be evident.

4. A nurse is admitting a client who has suspected SLE. Which of the following clinical findings supports this diagnosis?

A. Weight loss

B. Petechiae on thighs

C. Increased hair growth

D. Alopecia

5. A nurse is caring for a client who has SLE and is experiencing an episode of Raynaud's phenomenon. Which of the following clinical findings should the nurse anticipate?

    A. Swelling of joints of the fingers

    B. Pallor of toes with cold exposure

    C. Feet become reddened with ambulation

    D. Client report of intense feeling of heat in the fingers

6. A nurse is discussing care for a client who has systemic lupus erythematosus (SLE) with a newly hired nurse. What should be included in the teaching? Use the ATI Active Learning Template: Systems Disorder to complete this item to include the following:

    A. Description of Disorder/Disease

    B. Assessment: Describe two risk factors and three objective data.

    C. Laboratory Tests: Describe two that are specific to SLE.

APPLICATION EXERCISES KEY

1. A. **CORRECT:** A positive antinuclear antibody (ANA) titer is an expected finding in a client who has SLE. The ANA test identifies the presence of antibody produced against the client's own DNA.

   B. INCORRECT: Increased hemoglobin is not an expected finding in a client who has SLE.

   C. **CORRECT:** Increased urine protein is an expected finding due to renal involvement as a result of SLE.

   D. INCORRECT: Increased serum C3 and C4 are not expected findings in a client who has SLE. Findings would be decreased.

   E. **CORRECT:** Elevated BUN is an expected finding due to renal involvement in a client who has SLE.

   Ⓝ NCLEX® Connection: Reduction of Risk Potential, Laboratory Values

2. A. INCORRECT: A client who has SLE should avoid sun exposure.

   B. **CORRECT:** This statement requires further teaching because the client should apply steroid-based creams to skin rashes.

   C. INCORRECT: A client who has SLE should use a mild hair shampoo that does not irritate the scalp.

   D. INCORRECT: A client who has SLE should notify the provider about a cough due to the increased risk of infection while being immunocompromised.

   Ⓝ NCLEX® Connection: Physiological Adaptations, Illness Management

3. A. INCORRECT: Increased blood pressure is an adverse effect while taking this medication.

   B. **CORRECT:** Prednisone causes fluid retention which results in weight gain.

   C. **CORRECT:** Prednisone causes weight gain, especially in the abdomen, and can result in the appearance of abdominal striae.

   D. INCORRECT: An increase in appetite is an adverse effect while taking this medication.

   E. **CORRECT:** Moon facies (rounding of the face due to an accumulation of fatty tissue) is an adverse effect while taking this medication.

   Ⓝ NCLEX® Connection: Pharmacological and Parenteral Therapies, Medication Administration

4. A. INCORRECT: Weight gain may occur in the client who has SLE and is being treated with corticosteroids.

   B. INCORRECT: A butterfly rash on the face is a clinical finding in a client who has SLE.

   C. INCORRECT: Alopecia is an expected clinical finding in a client who has SLE

   D. **CORRECT:** Areas of hair loss are an expected finding in a client who has SLE.

   Ⓝ NCLEX® Connection: Physiological Adaptations, Pathophysiology

5. A. **INCORRECT:** Swelling, pain, and joint tenderness are clinical findings in a client who has SLE and is not specific to an episode of Raynaud's phenomenon.

    B. **CORRECT:** Pallor of the extremities occurs in Raynaud's phenomenon in a client who has SLE and has been exposed to cold or stress.

    C. **INCORRECT:** The extremities becoming red, white, and blue when exposed to cold or stress is characteristic of an episode of Raynaud's phenomenon in a client who has SLE.

    D. **INCORRECT:** A client report of intense pain in the hands and feet is characteristic of an episode of Raynaud's phenomenon in a client who has SLE.

    Ⓝ NCLEX® Connection: Physiological Adaptations, Pathophysiology

6. *Using the ATI Active Learning Template: Systems Disorder*
    A. Description of Disorder/Disease
    - SLE is an autoimmune disorder in which an atypical immune response results in chronic inflammation and destruction of healthy tissue.
      - In autoimmune disorders, small antigens may bond with healthy tissue. The body then produces antibodies that attack the healthy tissue. This may be triggered by toxins, medications, bacteria, and/or viruses.
      - Control of symptoms and decrease in number of exacerbations is the goal of treatment, because there is no cure for autoimmune disorders.
      - Occurrence of autoimmune disorders increases with age.

    B. Assessment
    - Risk Factors
      - Females between the ages of 20 and 40.
      - African American, Asian, or Native American descent.
      - The incidence of lupus drops in women following menopause but remains steady until then.
      - Diagnosis of SLE may be delayed in older adult clients because many of the clinical manifestations mimic other disorders or may be associated with reports common to the normal aging process.
        - Joint pain and swelling may significantly limit ADLs in older adult clients who have comorbidities.
        - Older adult clients are at an increased risk for fractures if corticosteroid therapy is used.
    - Objective Data
      - Physical Assessment Findings
        - Fever (also a major manifestation of exacerbation)
        - Pericarditis (cardiac or pleural friction rub may be present)
        - Anemia
        - Lymphadenopathy
        - Raynaud's phenomenon (arteriolar vasospasm in response to cold/stress)
        - Findings consistent with organ involvement (kidney, heart, lungs and vasculature)
        - Butterfly rash on face

    C. Laboratory Tests
    - Antinuclear antibody (ANA) titer
    - Anti-Smith extractible nuclear antibody
    - Serum complement (C3, C4)

    Ⓝ NCLEX® Connection: Physiological Adaptations, Illness Management

chapter 89

Overview

- Rheumatoid arthritis (RA) is a chronic, progressive inflammatory disease that can affect tissues and organs but principally attacks the joints producing an inflammatory synovitis. It involves joints bilaterally and symmetrically, and it typically affects several joints at one time. RA typically affects upper joints first.

- RA is an autoimmune disease that is precipitated by WBCs attacking synovial tissue. The WBCs cause the synovial tissue to become inflamed and thickened. The inflammation can extend to the cartilage, bone, tendons, and ligaments that surround the joint. Joint deformity and bone erosion may result from these changes, decreasing the joint's range of motion and function.

- RA is also a systemic disease that can affect any connective tissue in the body. Common structures that are affected are the blood vessels, pleura surrounding the lungs, and pericardium. Iritis and scleritis can also develop in the eyes.

- The natural course of the disease is one of exacerbations and remissions.

Health Promotion and Disease Prevention

- Use adaptive devices that prevent development of deformity of inflamed joints during ADLs.
- Continue using affected joints and ambulating to maintain function and range of motion.

Assessment

- Risk Factors
  - Female gender (3:1)
  - Age 20 to 50 years
  - Genetic predisposition
  - Epstein-Barr virus
  - Stress
  - Environmental factors
  - Early signs of RA (fatigue, joint discomfort) are vague and may be attributed to other disorders in older adult clients.
  - Joint deformities are late signs of RA.
  - Joint pain and dysfunction may have a greater effect on older adult clients than on younger adult clients due to the presence of other chronic conditions.
  - Older adult clients may be less able to overcome and/or cope with joint pain/deformity.

- Subjective Data
  - Pain at rest and with movement
  - Morning stiffness
  - Pleuritic pain (pain upon inspiration)
  - Xerostomia (dry mouth)
  - Anorexia/weight loss
  - Fatigue
  - Paresthesias
  - Recent illness/stressor
  - Joint pain
  - Lack of function
- Objective Data
  - Clinical findings depend on the area affected by the disease process.
  - Joint swelling and deformity
    - Joint swelling, warmth, and erythema.
    - Finger, hands, wrists, knees, and foot joints are generally affected.
    - Finger joints affected are the proximal interphalangeal and metacarpophalangeal joints.
    - Joints may become deformed merely by completing ADLs.
    - Ulnar deviation, swan neck, and boutonnière deformities are common in the fingers.

  M View Image: Rheumatoid Arthritis Changes

  - Subcutaneous nodules
  - Fever (generally low grade)
  - Muscle weakness/atrophy
  - Reddened sclera and/or abnormal shape of pupils
  - Lymph node enlargement
  - Laboratory Tests
    - Anti-CCP antibodies – Positive
      - This test detects antibodies to cyclic citrullinated peptide (anti-CCP). The result is positive in most people who have rheumatoid arthritis, even years before symptoms develop. The test is more sensitive for RA than rheumatoid factor (RF) antibodies.
    - RF antibody
      - Diagnostic level for rheumatoid arthritis is 1:40 to 1:60 (expected reference range 1:20 or less).
      - High titers correlate with severe disease.
      - Other autoimmune diseases also can increase RF antibody.

- Erythrocyte sedimentation rate (ESR) – Elevated

  □ The increase is associated with the inflammation or infection in the body.

  □ 20 to 40 mm/hr is mild inflammation.

  □ 40 to 70 mm/hr is moderate inflammation.

  □ 70 to 150 mm/hr is severe inflammation.

  □ Other autoimmune diseases also can increase ESR antibody.

- C-reactive protein (may be done in place of ESR) – Positive

  □ This test is useful for diagnosing disease or monitoring disease activity, and for monitoring the response to anti-inflammatory therapy.

- Antinuclear antibody (ANA) titer (antibody produced against one's own DNA)

  □ A positive ANA titer is associated with RA (it is normally negative at 1:20 dilution).

  □ Other autoimmune diseases also can increase ANA.

- Elevated WBCs

  □ WBC count may be elevated during an exacerbation secondary to the inflammatory response.

  □ Decreased RBCs due to anemia.

○ Diagnostic Procedures

- Arthrocentesis

  □ Synovial fluid aspiration by needle

  □ With RA, increased WBCs and RF are present in fluid.

  □ Nursing Actions

    ▸ Monitor for bleeding or a synovial fluid leak from the needle biopsy site.

  □ Client Education

    ▸ Take acetaminophen (Tylenol) for pain.

- X-ray

  □ X-rays are used to determine the degree of joint destruction and monitor its progression. They may provide adequate visualization and reveal bony erosions and narrowed joint spaces. This negates the need for more expensive radiologic tests, such a CT scan or magnetic resonance imaging (MRI).

  □ Nursing Actions

    ▸ Assist the client into position.

  □ Client Education

    ▸ Instruct the client about the need to minimize movement during the procedure.

Patient-Centered Care

- Nursing Care
  - Apply heat or cold to the affected areas as indicated based on client response.
    - Morning stiffness (hot shower)
    - Pain in hands/fingers (heated paraffin)
    - Edema (cold therapy)
  - Assist with and encourage physical activity to maintain joint mobility (within the capabilities of the client).
  - Monitor the client for indications of fatigue.
  - Teach the client measures to
    - Maximize functional activity
    - Minimize pain
    - Monitor skin closely
    - Conserve energy (space out activities, take rest periods, ask for additional assistance when needed)
    - Promote coping strategies
    - Encourage routine health screenings
  - Provide a safe environment.
    - Provide referrals for physical therapy and occupational therapy.
    - Provide information for support organizations.
    - Facilitate the use of assistive devices.
    - Remove unnecessary equipment and supplies.
  - Use progressive muscle relaxation.
  - Administer medications and proper positioning as prescribed.
  - Monitor for medication effectiveness (reduced pain, increased mobility).
  - Teach the client regarding signs/symptoms that need to be reported immediately (fever, infection, pain upon inspiration, pain in the substernal area of the chest).
- Nutritional Teaching
  - Encourage foods high in vitamins, protein, and iron.
  - Eat small, frequent meals.

- Medications
  - NSAIDs (Treatment begins with NSAIDs.)
    - NSAIDs provide analgesic, antipyretic, and anti-inflammatory effects. NSAIDs can cause considerable gastrointestinal (GI) distress.
    - Nursing Considerations
      - Request a concurrent prescription for a GI-acid lowering agent (histamine$_2$-receptor antagonist, proton pump inhibitor) if GI distress is reported.
      - Monitor for fluid retention, hypertension, and renal dysfunction.
    - Client Education
      - Instruct the client to
        - Take the medication with food or with a full glass of water or milk. If taking routinely, H$_2$-receptor antagonist may also be prescribed.
        - Observe for GI bleeding (coffee ground emesis; dark, tarry stools).
        - Avoid alcohol, which can increase the risk of GI complications.
  - COX-2 Enzyme Blockers
    - Cause less GI distress but carry a risk of cardiac disease.
  - Corticosteroids
    - Corticosteroids (prednisone) are strong anti-inflammatory medications that may be given for acute exacerbations or advanced forms of the disease. They are not given for long-term therapy due to significant adverse effects (osteoporosis, hyperglycemia, immunosuppression, cataracts).
    - Nursing Considerations
      - Observe for Cushingoid changes.
      - Monitor weight and blood pressure.
    - Client Education
      - Instruct the client to observe for changes in vision, blood glucose, and impaired healing.
      - Instruct the client to avoid crowds.
      - Instruct the client to follow the provider's prescription, such as alternate day dosing, tapering, and discontinuing medication.
  - Disease modifying anti-rheumatic drugs (DMARDs)
    - DMARDs work in a variety of ways to slow the progression of RA and suppress the immune system's reaction to RA that causes pain and inflammation. Relief of symptoms may not occur for several weeks.
    - Antimalarial agent – hydroxychloroquine (Plaquenil)
    - Antibiotic – minocycline (Minocin)
    - Sulfonamide – sulfasalazine (Azulfidine)
    - Biologic response modifiers – etanercept (Enbrel), infliximab (Remicade), adalimumab (Humira), and chelator penicillamine (Cuprimine)
    - Cytotoxic medications – methotrexate (Rheumatrex), leflunomide (Arava), cyclophosphamide (Cytoxan), and azathioprine (Imuran). These medications can cause severe adverse effects.

- Teamwork and Collaboration
  - Refer the client to support groups as appropriate.
  - Refer the client to occupational therapy for adaptive devices that can facilitate carrying out ADLs and prevent deformities.
  - A home health aide may be necessary for assistance with ADLs.
- Therapeutic Procedures
  - Plasmapheresis
    - Removes circulating antibodies from plasma, decreasing attacks on the client's tissues
  - May be done for a severe, life-threatening exacerbation
- Surgical Interventions
  - Total joint arthroplasty
    - Surgical repair and replacement of a joint may be done for a severely deformed joint that has not responded to medication therapy.

Complications

- Sjögren's syndrome (triad of symptoms – dry eyes, dry mouth, and dry vagina)
  - Caused by obstruction of secretory ducts and glands
  - Nursing Actions
    - Provide the client with eye drops and artificial saliva, and recommend vaginal lubricants as needed.
    - Provide fluids with meals.
- Secondary osteoporosis
  - Immobilization caused by arthritis can contribute to the development of osteoporosis.
  - Nursing Actions
    - Encourage weight-bearing exercises as tolerated.
- Vasculitis (organ ischemia)
  - Inflammation of arteries can disrupt blood flow, causing ischemia. Smaller arteries in the skin, eyes, and brain are most commonly affected in RA.
  - Nursing Actions
    - Monitor for skin lesions, decrease in vision, and symptoms of cognitive dysfunction.

APPLICATION EXERCISES

1. A nurse working in an outpatient clinic is assessing a client who has rheumatoid arthritis (RA). The client reports increased joint tenderness and swelling. Which of the following findings should the nurse expect? (Select all that apply.)

_____ A. Recent influenza

_____ B. Decreased range of motion

_____ C. Hypersalivation

_____ D. Decreased blood pressure

_____ E. Pain at rest

2. A nurse is caring for a client who has rheumatoid arthritis. Which of the following laboratory tests are used to diagnose this disease? (Select all that apply.)

_____ A. Urinalysis

_____ B. Erythrocyte sedimentation rate (ESR)

_____ C. BUN

_____ D. Antinuclear antibody (ANA) titer

_____ E. WBC count

3. A nurse is providing information to a client newly diagnosed with rheumatoid arthritis (RA). Which of the following statements by the nurse is appropriate?

A. "You may experience morning stiffness when you get out bed."

B. "You may experience abdominal pain."

C. "You may experience weight gain."

D. "You may experience low blood sugar."

4. A nurse is providing information about the adverse effects of prednisone (Deltasone) to a client who has rheumatoid arthritis. Use the ATI Active Learning Template: Medication and the ATI Pharmacology Review Module to complete this item. Include Adverse Effects: Identify three adverse effects of this medication.

APPLICATION EXERCISES KEY

1. A. **CORRECT:** Exacerbating factors, such as a recent illness, are indicative of RA.

   B. **CORRECT:** Decreased ange of motion is indicative of RA.

   C. INCORRECT: Xerostomia is indicative of RA.

   D. INCORRECT: Blood pressure changes are not indicative of RA.

   E. **CORRECT:** Pain at rest is characteristic of RA.

    NCLEX® Connection: Physiological Adaptations, Pathophysiology

2. A. INCORRECT: A urinalysis is not a laboratory test used to diagnose rheumatoid arthritis. This test can used for detecting kidney failure.

   B. **CORRECT:** ESR is a laboratory test used to diagnose rheumatoid arthritis. This laboratory test will show an elevated result in clients who have rheumatoid arthritis.

   C. INCORRECT: A BUN is not a laboratory test used to diagnose rheumatoid arthritis. This test can be used for detecting kidney failure.

   D. **CORRECT:** ANA titer is a laboratory test used to diagnose rheumatoid arthritis. This laboratory test will show a positive result in clients who have rheumatoid arthritis.

   E. **CORRECT:** WBC count is a laboratory test used to diagnose rheumatoid arthritis. This laboratory test will show a decreased result in clients who have rheumatoid arthritis.

    NCLEX® Connection: Reduction of Risk Potential, Diagnostic Tests

3. A. **CORRECT:** The client can experience stiffness in her joints upon rising. This is an appropriate statement for the nurse to give.

   B. INCORRECT: This is not an appropriate statement for the nurse to give. The client who has RA may experience pleuritic pain (upon inspiration).

   C. INCORRECT: This is not an appropriate statement for the nurse to give. The client who has RA may experience weight loss.

   D. INCORRECT: This is not an appropriate statement for the nurse to give. The client who has RA does not experience a low blood sugar.

    NCLEX® Connection: Physiological Adaptations, Illness Management

4. *Using the ATI Active Learning Template: Medication*
    - Adverse Effects
      ○ Risk of infection (fever and/or sore throat): Advise clients to notify the provider immediately if symptoms occur.
      ○ Osteoporosis: Advise clients to take calcium supplements, vitamin D, and/or bisphosphonate (etidronate).
      ○ Adrenal suppression
      ○ Advise clients to observe for symptoms and to notify the provider if symptoms occur.
      ○ Administer fluids such as normal saline, salt, and hydrocortisone IV. Advise clients not to discontinue the medication suddenly.
      ○ Fluid retention: Monitor for signs of fluid excess, such as crackles, weight gain, edema.
      ○ GI discomfort
      ○ Advise clients to observe for symptoms and to notify the provider if symptoms occur.
      ○ H_2 antagonists can be used prophylactically.
      ○ Advise clients to report symptoms of GI bleeding (coffee-ground emesis; or black, tarry stools).
      ○ Hyperglycemia: Monitor blood glucose level. Clients who have diabetes mellitus may need to adjust hypoglycemic agent.
      ○ Hypokalemia
      ○ Monitor serum potassium levels.
      ○ Advise clients to eat potassium-rich foods.
      ○ Administer potassium supplements.

      ⓝ NCLEX® Connection: Pharmacological and Parenteral Therapies, Medication Administration

chapter 90

Overview

- Cancer is a neoplastic disease process that involves abnormal cell growth and differentiation.
- The exact cause of cancer is unknown, but viruses, physical and chemical agents, hormones, genetics, and diet are thought to be factors that trigger abnormal cell growth.
- Cancer cells can invade surrounding tissues and/or spread to other areas of the body through lymph and blood vessels (metastasis).
- Metastasis is usually diagnosed when there is onset of new clinical findings (bone pain indicative of bone metastasis; change in bowel or bladder tone indicative of nervous system involvement).
- Cancers may arise from almost any tissue in the body: epithelial tissue (carcinomas), glandular organs (adenocarcinomas), mesenchymal tissue (sarcomas), blood-forming cells (leukemias), lymph tissue (lymphomas), or plasma cells (myelomas).
- Screening and early diagnosis are the most important aspects of health education and care. The nurse should prevent, recognize, and treat complications associated with carcinoma.

Health Promotion and Disease Prevention

- Consume a healthy diet (low-fat diet with increased consumption of fruits, vegetables, and lean protein foods).
- Limit intake of sugar and salt.
- Maintain a healthy body weight/body mass index (BMI).
- Avoid smoking and alcohol consumption.
- Avoid risky lifestyle choices (recreational drug use, needle sharing, unprotected sexual intercourse).
- Avoid exposure to environmental hazards (radiation, chemicals). Use proper protection when unavoidable.
- Breast feed infant exclusively for the first 6 months of life.
- Engage in physical activity or exercise routinely.

Risk Factors

Ⓖ
- Age – The highest incidence of cancer occurs in older adults.
  - ○ Older adult women most commonly develop colorectal, breast, lung, pancreatic, and ovarian cancers.
  - ○ Older adult men most commonly develop lung, colorectal, prostate, pancreatic, and gastric cancers.
- Race
  - ○ Caucasian women over the age of 40 are more likely to develop breast cancer than are African-American, American-Indian, and Hispanic women. However, the death rate for each of these groups is higher than for Caucasian women.
  - ○ Caucasian men are at an increased risk for testicular cancer, whereas African-American men are at an increased risk for prostate cancer.
- Genetic predisposition
- Exposure to chemicals, tobacco, and alcohol
- Exposure to certain viruses and bacteria
  - ○ Liver cancer can develop after many years of infection with hepatitis B or hepatitis C.
  - ○ Infection with human T-cell leukemia virus increases the risk of lymphoma and leukemia (indigenous to certain areas of the world, such as Africa and Melanesia).
  - ○ Infection with Epstein-Barr virus has been linked to an increased risk of lymphoma.
  - ○ Human papillomavirus (HPV) infection is the main cause of cervical cancer.
  - ○ HIV increases the risk of lymphoma and Kaposi's sarcoma.
  - ○ *Helicobacter pylori* may increase the risk of stomach cancer and lymphoma of the stomach lining.
- A diet high in fat and red meat, and low in fiber
- Sun, ultraviolet light, or radiation exposure (radon)
- Sexual lifestyles (multiple sexual partners or STIs)
- Poverty, obesity, and chronic GERD
- Chronic disease

Staging of Cancer

- The tumor-node-metastasis (TNM) system is used to stage cancer.
  - ○ Tumor (T)
    - ▪ TX – unable to evaluate the primary tumor
    - ▪ T0 – no evidence of primary tumor
    - ▪ Tis – tumor in situ
    - ▪ T1, T2, T3, and T4 – size and extent of tumor
  - ○ Node (N)
    - ▪ NX – unable to evaluate regional lymph nodes
    - ▪ N0 – no evidence of regional node involvement
    - ▪ N1, N2, and N3 – number of nodes that are involved and/or extent of spread

- Metastasis (M)
  - MX – unable to evaluate distant metastasis
  - M0 – no evidence of distant metastasis
  - M1 – presence of distant metastasis

Prognosis

- Early diagnosis of cancer usually results in a better prognosis. Many cancers spread or metastasize before any manifestations are noted.
- Minority populations tend to have a worse prognosis for cancer related to several factors (low socioeconomic status, lack of access to health care, or reluctance to seek treatment).

Complications and Nursing Implications

- Malnutrition
  - Clients who have cancer are at increased risk for weight loss and anorexia.
    - The presence of carcinoma in the body increases the amount of energy required for metabolic function.
    - Cancer can impair the body's ability to ingest, digest, and absorb nutrients.
    - Adverse effects of cancer treatment can affect the desire for food or the ability to eat. Findings include nausea and vomiting, changes in taste, anorexia, pain, diarrhea, early satiety, dry mouth, thickened saliva, and irritation to the gastrointestinal tract.
    - Nursing Actions
      - Educate the client about managing the expected effects of treatment.
      - Administer antiemetics and antacids as prescribed.
      - Monitor relevant laboratory data (albumin, ferritin, transferrin).
      - Encourage frequent oral hygiene.
      - Incorporate client preferences into meal planning, when possible.
      - Teach the client to consume adequate protein and calories.
- Paraneoplastic syndromes
  - Paraneoplastic syndromes result when T cells in the body attack normal cells rather than cancerous ones. They result in changes in neurological function (movement, sensation, mental function).
    - Management includes minimizing the immune system response by administration of steroids, immune factors, plasmapheresis, or irradiation.
    - Nursing Actions
      - Recognize manifestations of paraneoplastic syndrome.
      - Administer medications as prescribed.
      - Provide a safe environment until client returns to baseline mental status.
      - Use aids for vision or hearing deficits, as indicated.

- Oncologic Emergencies
  - Syndrome of inappropriate antidiuretic hormone (SIADH)
    - SIADH occurs when excessive levels of antidiuretic hormones are produced. Because antidiuretic hormones help the kidneys and body to conserve the correct amount of water, SIADH causes the body to retain water. This results in a dilution of electrolytes (such as sodium) in the blood. It is most commonly associated with lung and brain cancers. Key findings include nausea and vomiting (early); lethargy, hostility, seizures, and coma.
    - Nursing Actions
      - Monitor the client for hyponatremia and low serum osmolality.
      - Administer furosemide (Lasix), 0.9% sodium chloride IV, and/or hypertonic sodium chloride solution as prescribed for severe hyponatremia.
      - Monitor vital signs and serum sodium as Lasix promotes sodium excretion and hypertonic sodium chloride can cause fluid overload.
  - Hypercalcemia
    - A common complication of breast, lung, head, and neck cancers; leukemias and lymphomas; multiple myelomas; and bony metastases of any cancer.
    - Manifestations include anorexia, nausea, vomiting, shortened QT interval, kidney stones, bone pain, and changes in mental status.
    - Nursing Actions – Administer 0.9% sodium chloride IV, furosemide (Lasix), pamidronate, and phosphates as prescribed.
  - Superior vena cava syndrome
    - Results from obstruction (metastases from breast or lung cancers) of venous return and engorgement of the vessels from the head and upper body. Manifestations include periorbital and facial edema, erythema of the upper body, dyspnea, and epistaxis.
    - Nursing Actions – Position the client in a high-Fowler's position initially to facilitate lung expansion. Use high-dose radiation therapy for emergency temporary relief.
  - Disseminated intravascular coagulation – a complication secondary to leukemia or adenocarcinomas
    - Nursing Actions
      - Observe the client for bleeding, and apply pressure as needed.
      - Be prepared to administer blood clotting factors that have been lost through bleeding and may need to be replaced with plasma transfusions. Heparin also can be used to slow the cascade of events that makes the body overuse its blood clotting factors.

APPLICATION EXERCISES

1. A nurse is teaching a client about the risk for cancer. Which of the following client statements indicates the need for further teaching?

    A. "I see a dermatologist regularly for the mole on my thigh."

    B. "I take Milk of Magnesia for occasional constipation."

    C. "I tan using an indoor tanning lotion instead of laying out in the sun."

    D. "I used to smoke but switched to chewing tobacco 3 years ago."

2. A nurse is teaching a client about maintaining a diet that may prevent certain cancers. The nurse should inform the client that the intake of which of the following may be beneficial? (Select all that apply.)

    _____ A. Low saturated fats

    _____ B. Fiber

    _____ C. Red meats

    _____ D. Simple carbohydrates

    _____ E. Fish

3. A nurse is caring for a client who has lung cancer and is exhibiting manifestations of syndrome of inappropriate antidiuretic hormone (SIADH). Which of the following findings should the nurse report to the provider? (Select all that apply.)

    _____ A. Behavioral changes

    _____ B. Client report of headache

    _____ C. Urine output 40 mL/hr

    _____ D. Client report of nausea

    _____ E. Increased urine specific gravity

4. A nurse in an oncology clinic is reviewing the health record of a client who had surgery to stage ovarian cancer. The nurse reviews the following diagnostic notation on the pathology report: T2-N3-MX. Which of the following is an expected finding that supports this diagnosis?

    A. The tumor is 4 cm in size involving the ovary and adjacent tissues.

    B. No lymph nodes contain cancer cells.

    C. The tumor is receptive to current medication therapy.

    D. The cancer has metastasized to other areas in the body.

5. A nurse is planning care for a client who has malnutrition due to cancer. Which of the following interventions should the nurse include in the plan of care? (Select all that apply.)

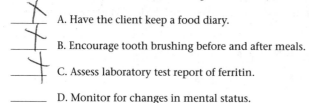

_____ A. Have the client keep a food diary.

_____ B. Encourage tooth brushing before and after meals.

_____ C. Assess laboratory test report of ferritin.

_____ D. Monitor for changes in mental status.

_____ E. Explain that fluid intake should occur between meals.

6. A nurse is preparing a poster about risk factors for cancer to be displayed at a community health fair. What information should be included in this poster? Use the ATI Active Learning Template: Systems Disorder to include the following:

A. Types of Cancer:
- Identify two with increased incidence in older adult women.
- Identify two with increased incidence in older adult men.
- Identify one with increased risk in Caucasian men and women.

B. Viruses/Bacteria: Describe at least three and the type of cancer they can cause.

C. Diet-Related Risk Factors: Describe three.

D. Lifestyle-Related Risk Factors: Describe at least three.

APPLICATION EXERCISES KEY

1. A. INCORRECT: This statement indicates understanding of the risk of skin exposure to environmental effects as a cause of cancer.

    B. INCORRECT: This statement indicates awareness of potential changes in bowel habits as a risk factor for cancer.

    C. INCORRECT: This statement indicates understanding of the risk of skin exposure to environmental effects as a cause of cancer.

    D. **CORRECT:** Chewing tobacco is a cause of oral cancer, and places the client at the same risk as smoking tobacco.

    Ⓝ NCLEX® Connection: Health Promotion and Maintenance, Health Promotion/Disease Prevention

2. A. **CORRECT:** Foods that are low in saturated fats provide protection against certain types of cancers.

    B. **CORRECT:** A diet high in fiber provides protection against certain types of cancers.

    C. INCORRECT: The consumption of red meat can increase the risk of cancer.

    D. INCORRECT: Eating simple carbohydrates can increase the risk of cancer.

    E. **CORRECT:** Eating fish can provide protection against certain types of cancers.

    Ⓝ NCLEX® Connection: Health Promotion and Maintenance, Health Promotion/Disease Prevention

3. A. **CORRECT:** Behavioral changes indicate cerebral edema due to SIADH. This finding should be reported to the provider.

    B. **CORRECT:** A client report of headache indicates cerebral edema due to SIADH. This finding should be reported to the provider.

    C. INCORRECT: Urine output of 40 mL/hr is a finding consistent with suspected SIADH and does not need to be reported to the provider.

    D. **CORRECT:** A client report of nausea can indicate cerebral edema due to SIADH and should be reported to the provider.

    E. INCORRECT: An increased urine specific gravity is a finding consistent with SIADH and does not need to be reported to the provider.

    Ⓝ NCLEX® Connection: Physiological Adaptations, Illness Management

4.   A. **CORRECT:** A T2 designation describes the size and extent of the ovarian tumor using the tumor-node-metastasis (TNM) staging system.

   B. INCORRECT: A N3 designation indicates that three adjacent lymph nodes show evidence of spread of cancer using the TNM staging system.

   C. INCORRECT: The TNM diagnostic notation of the staging system is not used to indicate the response of a tumor to a medication therapy regimen used for treatment.

   D. INCORRECT: The MX designation indicates there is no evidence of distant metastasis to other areas of the body using the TNM staging system.

    NCLEX® Connection: Physiological Adaptations, Pathophysiology

5.   A. **CORRECT:** The use of a food diary assists in monitoring the client's changes in eating habits that occur in malnutrition due to cancer.

   B. **CORRECT:** Oral hygiene before and after meals promotes increased salivation and improves the client's taste perception.

   C. **CORRECT:** Ferritin is an indicator of the protein intake of a client who has malnutrition due to cancer.

   D. INCORRECT: The nurse should monitor the client who has malnutrition due to cancer for changes related to the desire for food and the ability to eat.

   E. INCORRECT: Fluid intake should be encouraged with meals due to the dry mouth and thickened saliva that are present in the client who has malnutrition due to cancer.

    NCLEX® Connection: Basic Care and Comfort, Nutrition and Oral Hydration

6. *Using the ATI Active Learning Template: Systems Disorder*

A. Types of Cancer
- Highest incidence of cancer in older adult women: colorectal, breast, lung, pancreatic, and ovarian cancers
- Highest incidence of cancer in older adult men: lung, colorectal, prostate, pancreatic and gastric cancers
- Caucasian men: testicular; Caucasian women: breast cancer

B. Viruses/Bacteria
- Hepatitis B or C – liver cancer
- Human T-cell leukemia virus – lymphoma and leukemia
- Epstein-Barr virus – lymphoma
- Human papilloma virus (HPV) – cervical cancer
- HIV– lymphoma and Kaposi's sarcoma
- *Helicobacter pylori* – stomach cancer and lymphoma of the stomach lining

C. Diet-Related Risk Factors
- Diet high in fat and red meat, low in fiber

D. Lifestyle-Related Risk Factors
- Multiple sexual partners or STIs
- Sun, ultraviolet light, and radiation exposure
- Use of tobacco and alcohol

Ⓝ NCLEX® Connection: Health Promotion and Maintenance, Health Promotion/Disease Prevention

chapter 91

Overview

- Screening and diagnostic procedures provide objective and subjective client data.

- Screening and diagnosis for cancer can involve the use of hands-on assessment techniques, invasive procedures, radiography and imaging studies, and laboratory testing.

  - The type and location of the suspected cancer dictate which methods are used.

- Identification of tumor cells is required for definitive diagnosis and the development of a targeted treatment plan.

Procedures

- Assessment

  - Subjective data indicative of cancer includes altered body function (fatigue, weakness, anorexia), change in body structure (weight loss, masses), change in body symmetry or onset of recent clinical findings (pain, nausea, vomiting).

  - Subjective data indicative of metastasis includes:

    - Secondary sites of discomfort

    - Swelling and/or tenderness of lymph nodes or areas of the body

    - Presence of masses

    - Altered function of another body system

    - Bone pain

  - Nursing Actions

    - Complete a health history and physical assessment including client report of findings and family history of cancer or genetic disorder.

    - Provide for privacy. Consider the client's cultural preference for examination (a professional of the same or opposite gender).

    - Inspect for changes in color, symmetry, movement, or body function.

    - Auscultate for adventitious sounds that indicate altered body system function.

      - Heart, lung, and bowel sounds

      - Main arteries (carotid, femoral, renal, iliac)

      - Masses or areas of discomfort

- Palpate to detect masses or tissue abnormalities.
    - Use light, medium, and deep pressure as appropriate.
    - Some palpation assessments should be performed by the provider only (digital rectal exam for colorectal cancer).
- Percuss for changes in expected sound over organs.
    - Dullness in the lungs or bowel can indicate areas of consolidation or tumor.
    - Increased liver size (noted by measurement of borders [dullness]) can indicate inflammation or tumor.
  - Client Education
    - Explain all procedures prior to assessment.
    - Report unexpected findings to the provider.
    - Provide explanation when there is need for further testing or evaluation of unexpected findings.
    - Instruct the client on self-examination practices to continue at home (breast or testicular self-examination).
    - Instruct client on seven warning signs (CAUTION) clients should watch for:
        - C – Change in bowel or bladder habits
        - A – A sore that doesn't heal
        - U – Unusual bleeding or discharge
        - T – Thickening or lump in the breast or elsewhere
        - I – Indigestion or difficulty swallowing
        - O – Obvious change in warts or moles
        - N – Nagging cough or hoarseness
- Biopsy – provides definitive diagnosis indicating the site of origin (specific cell type) and cell characteristics (special receptors on cell surface).
  - May be obtained during other procedures (endoscopy, laparoscopy, thoracotomy).
  - Types include:
    - Shave biopsy (basal or squamous cell skin cancer) – sampling of outer skin layers (raised lesions) using a scalpel or razor blade.
    - Needle biopsy (fine or core) – aspiration of tumor close to the skin surface for fluid and tissue sampling.
        - Bone marrow aspiration is a form of needle biopsy used to diagnose leukemia and lymphoma.
    - Incisional or excisional (open) biopsy – cutting through skin to remove part of (incisional) or all of (excisional) a tumor.
        - Punch biopsy is a form of excisional biopsy used to diagnose skin cancer. A circular instrument "punches" a 2 to 6 mm sample of subcutaneous fat.
    - Sentinel lymph node biopsy – removal of lymph node in proximity to the cancer. Dye is used to create a "map" of affected nodes.
        - If lymph nodes are negative, the cancer has not likely spread.
        - If lymph nodes are positive, surgical excision of remaining lymph nodes in the area is performed (lymph node dissection).

- ○ Nursing Actions

  - ▪ Obtain signed informed consent form from the client.

  - ▪ Assemble supplies and facilitate aseptic technique.

  - ▪ Prevent bleeding (withhold anticoagulants, as prescribed). Monitor findings of coagulation studies.

  - ▪ Monitor for bleeding (visible staining of dressing, hypotension, tachycardia).

  - ▪ Provide a safe environment until effects of sedation are minimal (maintain bedrest, withhold oral intake).

  - ▪ Ensure adequate oxygenation during the recovery period.

  - ▪ Position the client in a recovery position appropriate to the procedure (lay on right side following liver biopsy).

- • Laboratory testing

  - ○ Performed to assess for possible cancer or effects on the body (electrolyte imbalance, altered function).

    - ▪ Elevated liver function tests (LFTs) can indicate primary liver cancer or metastasis of another cancer (colorectal cancer).

  - ○ Tumor marker assays – detect the presence of normal body proteins at higher than expected levels (carcinoembryonic antigen [CEA], prostate-specific antigen [PSA], alpha fetoprotein [AFP]).

    - ▪ Samples of urine, stool, tissue, blood, or other body fluids are tested for an excess of specific proteins or DNA patterns.

    - ▪ Used to detect cancer, measure the severity of cancer, or monitor for a positive response to the cancer treatment regimen (expected finding is a decrease in the tumor marker or return to expected reference range).

  - ○ Other testing may be done in addition to biopsy to identify tumor cell type (sputum analysis, cytology of fluid sampling).

    - ▪ Nursing Action – Explain the purpose of testing, as appropriate.

    - ▪ Client Education – Inform the client that laboratory testing can continue throughout treatment (to monitor progress) and following treatment (to screen for return of cancer).

- • Genetic testing – to identify the presence of certain genes in a sample of blood or saliva

  - ○ Genetic overexpression or the existence of extra genes can increase the risk of cancer or cause rapid tumor growth.

  - ○ Genetic mutations can be inherited. Positive results indicate the client is at high risk for development of certain types of cancer (presence of BRCA1 and BRCA2 genes associated with breast cancer).

  - ○ In most states, informed consent is required for genetic testing to protect the client from discrimination by providers or insurance company.

  - ○ Nursing Action – Consult a genetic counselor to clarify misconceptions regarding positive results and cancer risk.

  - ○ Client Education – Assure the client that genetic information is protected.

Imaging Studies

- Common imaging techniques are used as secondary tools to assist in treatment of cancer. Imaging is completed around the time of diagnosis to measure the severity of cancer. Computerized tomography (CT) scan, magnetic resonance imaging (MRI), positron emission tomography (PET) scan, ultrasound (US), and x-ray are used to:
  - ○ Provide more accurate visualization of tumors and their borders.
  - ○ Detect metastasis to organs and other body structures.
  - ○ Monitor the client during remission.
- Digital imaging is usually more accurate. Digital storage of images and results allows for information to be easily shared among members of the interprofessional treatment team.
- X-rays – provide visualization of body structures (chest x-ray, mammogram)
  - ○ Clients may be given dye (intravenous pyelogram) or contrast (barium enema) to enhance visualization.
  - ○ With angiography the client is injected with dye and then x-rays are taken to "map" vascular structures such as arterial, venous, or lymphatic mapping.
  - ○ Nursing Actions
    - ▪ Obtain signed informed consent form.
    - ▪ Monitor for allergic reaction to contrast dye (dyspnea, tachycardia, restlessness).
    - ▪ Monitor incision or puncture site for infection or bleeding.
    - ▪ Instruct the client about wound care.
- Nuclear imaging – evaluates the function of organs and structures by detecting the presence of radiation in the body after the client is given a radioactive tracer (intravenous or oral). Used for detection and staging of cancer.
  - ○ Cancerous tissues may absorb more or less tracer than expected. These tissues are distinguishable by nuclear imaging.
- Positron emission tomography (PET) measures positrons released with tissue uptake of radioactive sugar (more rapid in cancer). Mammography can be performed this way (PEM). CT may be used with PET scans.
- A multigated acquisition (MUGA) scan is used to evaluate heart function prior to cancer treatment or to identify damage following chemotherapy or radiation to the upper body.
- Other types of imaging include bone scan, gallium scan, and thyroid scan.
  - ○ Nursing Actions – Prepare the client as indicated according to the type of procedure.
- Endoscopy – permits visualization inside the body using flexible scopes and cameras
  - ○ Tumors may be visualized in the joints (arthroscopy), respiratory system (laryngoscopy, bronchoscopy), body cavity (mediastinoscopy, thoracoscopy), or gastrointestinal system (enteroscopy, sigmoidoscopy). Organs may be visualized as well (hysteroscopy, cystoscopy).
  - ○ Nursing Actions
    - ▪ Obtain signed informed consent form.
    - ▪ Prepare the client as indicated for the type of procedure to be performed.
    - ▪ Provide a safe environment until effects of sedation are minimal (maintain bedrest, withhold oral intake).
    - ▪ Ensure adequate oxygenation during the recovery period.

Summary

- Findings which indicate or increase suspicion of cancer must be further evaluated.
- A variety of imaging and laboratory tests can be used to detect:
  - Degree of tumor involvement
  - Type of tumor
  - Areas of metastasis
  - Complications of cancer
- Nursing Actions
  - Maintain knowledge of screening and diagnostic procedures.
  - Educate the client about routine cancer screenings as part of health promotion and disease prevention.
  - Prepare the client for testing, as indicated.
    - Withhold or restrict food or fluids.
    - Withhold medications which may alter test results or harm the client.
    - Administer preprocedure/testing medication (sedatives, IV or PO fluids, analgesics, barium).
    - Maintain appropriate monitoring, as indicated (ECG, arterial line).
    - Position the client and promote comfort.
  - Provide education to the client regarding the purpose and process of procedures.
  - Provide a safe environment pre-, intra-, and post-procedure.
  - Provide teaching and resources for client about self-care in the home environment.

APPLICATION EXERCISES

1. A nurse in a clinic is caring for a client who has suspected uterine cancer. Which of the following assessment techniques should the nurse anticipate the provider will perform on this client?

    A. Bimanual pelvic examination

    B. Papanicolaou (Pap) test with cultures

    C. Digital rectal examination

    D. Percussion of the upper abdominal quadrants for tympany

2. A nurse at a health fair is reviewing possible warning signs of cancer that a client should watch for. Which of the following information should be included in this review? (Select all that apply.)

    _____ A. Presence of a fever of 102° F (38.9° C) for more than 48 hr

    _____ B. A sore that does not heal

    _____ C. Difficulty swallowing

    _____ D. Presence of unusual discharge

    _____ E. Weight gain of 4 lb (1.8 kg) in 2 weeks

3. A nurse is reviewing preoperative teaching with a client who will undergo a shave biopsy for suspected cancer. Which of the following statements by the client indicates understanding of the procedure?

    A. "A test of my bone marrow will be performed."

    B. "A lymph node will be removed."

    C. "A needle will be inserted into the mass."

    D. "A small skin sample will be obtained."

4. A nurse is completing preprocedure teaching for a client who will undergo nuclear imaging for suspected cancer. Which of the following is an appropriate statement by the nurse?

    A. "The presence of a liver enzyme will be identified."

    B. "You will be given an injection of a radioactive substance."

    C. "An endoscope will be inserted through your mouth."

    D. "The tumor will be aspirated."

5. A nurse is planning care for a client who will undergo genetic testing for suspected cancer. Which of the following interventions should be included in the plan of care?

A. Obtain a signed informed consent form.

B. Withhold all medications prior to the procedure.

C. Verify the prescription for a tumor marker assay.

D. Ensure the client is placed in a recovery position after testing.

6. A nurse educator is discussing collection of objective and subjective data as part of screening for cancer with a group of oncology nurses. What should be included in the discussion? Use the ATI Active Learning Template: Diagnostic Procedures to include the following sections:

A. Subjective Data: Describe at least three indicating the presence of metastasis.

B. Objective Data: Describe four assessment techniques and possible findings.

C. Client Education: Describe two self-assessment techniques that can identify data.

APPLICATION EXERCISES KEY

1. A. **CORRECT:** Due to the location of uterine cancer, a bimanual pelvic examination will need to be performed to assess for uterine size, shape, and contour, which may be altered by a mass.

    B. INCORRECT: A Pap test with cultures is performed when screening for cervical cancer.

    C. INCORRECT: A digital rectal examination is performed when screening for prostate or rectal cancer.

    D. INCORRECT: Percussion of the upper abdominal quadrants for tympany is a screening tool for detecting an abdominal mass.

    (N) NCLEX® Connection: Health Promotion and Maintenance, Health Promotion/Disease Prevention

2. A. INCORRECT: Presence of a fever for an extended period is not a warning sign for cancer.

    B. **CORRECT:** A sore that does not heal is a warning sign for cancer.

    C. **CORRECT:** Difficulty swallowing is a warning sign for cancer.

    D. **CORRECT:** The presence of unusual discharge is a warning sign for cancer.

    E. INCORRECT: Weight gain is not a warning sign for cancer.

    (N) NCLEX® Connection: Health Promotion and Maintenance, Health Promotion/Disease Prevention

3. A. INCORRECT: A bone marrow aspiration is a type of needle biopsy.

    B. INCORRECT: A sentinel node biopsy involves excision of a lymph node.

    C. INCORRECT: A needle biopsy involves aspiration of a tumor for fluid and tissue sampling.

    D. **CORRECT:** A shave biopsy is a sampling of the outer skin layer using a scalpel or razor blade.

    (N) NCLEX® Connection: Physiological Adaptations, Illness Management

4. A. INCORRECT: Liver function tests involve the identification of altered liver enzymes, which may be present in a client who has cancer. They are not nuclear imaging tests.

    B. **CORRECT:** Nuclear imaging involves the administration of an oral or IV radioactive tracer to identify cancerous tissue.

    C. INCORRECT: Endoscopy permits visualization inside the body and is not a form of nuclear imaging.

    D. INCORRECT: A needle biopsy is performed to aspirate fluid and tissue samples for cancer cells and is not a form of nuclear imaging.

    (N) NCLEX® Connection: Physiological Adaptations, Pathophysiology

5. A. **CORRECT:** A signed informed consent form should be obtained prior to the procedure.

   B. INCORRECT: Medication does not affect the results of genetic testing.

   C. INCORRECT: A tumor marker assay is a laboratory test to identify the presence of specific body proteins in blood, body secretions and tissue and is not a component of genetic testing.

   D. INCORRECT: Genetic testing involves collection of blood or saliva and a recovery positioning is not required following testing.

   Ⓝ NCLEX® Connection: Basic Care and Comfort, Nutrition and Oral Hydration

6. *Using the ATI Active Learning Template: Diagnostic Procedures*

   A. Subjective Data
      - Discomfort at secondary sites
      - Swelling and/or tenderness of lymph nodes or areas of the body
      - Presence of masses
      - Altered function of another body system
      - Bone pain

   B. Objective Data
      - Inspection for changes in color, symmetry, movement or body function
      - Auscultation for adventitious sounds which may indicate altered body system function
      - Palpation to detect masses or tissue abnormalities
      - Percussion to detect changes in expected sound over organs, which may indicate inflammation or tumor

   C. Client Education
      - Testicular and breast self-examinations

   Ⓝ NCLEX® Connection: Health Promotion and Maintenance, Health Promotion/Disease Prevention

chapter 92

Overview

- Cancer treatment is based on the cell of origin of the cancer. When metastasis occurs, treatment is still based on the primary tumor origin even though the malignancy is located elsewhere in the body.

- Cancer treatment options focus on removing or destroying cancer cells and preventing the continued abnormal cell growth and differentiation. Treatments may be curative or palliative.

- The treatment plan is guided by many client factors (age, childbearing desire, pregnancy, current state of health expected lifespan) and may involve several treatment methods.

- Adjuvant treatment is what is given in addition to the primary treatment standard, and can include hormone, radiation, and targeted therapies; immunotherapy; and chemotherapy.

- Many cancers are curable when diagnosed early.

- Nursing care for clients who have cancer should include collaboration with supportive therapies and services, counseling, and transfer of care to another provider at discharge.

Procedures

- Cancer treatment includes manipulation or removal of the tumor.

  - Tumors may be reduced through topical procedures (cryosurgery, laser therapy, ablation) or by destruction of the main arteries that provide blood flow to the tumor (artery embolization).

  - Tumor excision may be open or endoscopic (curettage and electrodissection for skin cancer).

    - The tumor and tissue immediately surrounding it (tumor margin) are removed. The goal is that all of the outermost tissue that was removed does not contain cancer cells (a negative margin).

    - Surgery may be done for excision, biopsy (diagnosis and staging), or for relief (palliation) based on clinical findings.

    - Lymph node dissection or sentinel lymph node biopsy is done if the cancer spreads or there is added risk of spread.

    - More extensive surgeries (tumors involving multiple organs or structures, lymph node involvement, deep lesions) increase the risk of complications and typically require longer recovery periods. Intensive care may be required.

    - Nursing Actions:

      - Obtain signed informed consent form.

      - Prepare the client for procedures (NPO status, withhold or administer medications, as prescribed, monitor laboratory findings).

      - Provide postoperative care as indicated by tumor location and procedure type.

      - Prevent general postoperative complications (infection, fluid or electrolyte imbalance, hemorrhage, thromboembolism, inadequate oxygenation, shock).

  □ Prevent and treat pain as prescribed using pharmacological and nonpharmacological measures.

  □ Educate the client on care for drains, wounds, and implanted devices.

  □ Teach the client to monitor for complications after discharge.

Chemotherapy

- Chemotherapy involves the administration of systemic or local cytotoxic medications that damage a cell's DNA or destroy rapidly dividing cells.

  ○ Chemotherapeutic agents are often selected in relation to their effect on various stages of cell division. Subsequently, combinations of anticancer medications are used to enhance destruction of cancer cells.

  ○ Most chemotherapy agents are cytotoxic. The adverse effects of these agents are related to the unintentional harm done to normal rapidly proliferating cells, such as those found in the mucous membranes of the gastrointestinal tract, hair follicles, and bone marrow.

  ○ Targeted therapy is a type of chemotherapy that is not cytotoxic. It blocks or slows actions that cause cell replication.

  ○ Chemotherapy can be administered in a health care setting, provider's office, clinic, or home.

  ○ Depending on the agent, it can be given by the oral, parenteral, IV, intracavitary, or intrathecal route. Special training/certification is necessary for the administration of some agents.

    ▪ Implanted port – used when therapy is intended to be given on a long-term basis

      □ The port is comprised of a small reservoir that is covered by a thick septum.

    ▪ A central catheter is usually placed for chemotherapy administration or laboratory blood testing. Types include nontunneled percutaneous central catheter (triple lumen), peripherally inserted central catheter (PICC), tunneled percutaneous central catheter (Hickman, Groshong), and implanted port. (Refer to the chapter on *Cardiovascular Diagnostic and Therapeutic Procedures*.)

    ▪ Nursing Actions – Instruct the client/family in the proper use of vascular access devices.

  ○ Extravasation of agents that are vesicants requires special, immediate attention to minimize tissue damage. Selection of a neutralizing solution is dependent on vesicant. Closely monitor the infusion site for evidence of infiltration.

- Intracavitary chemotherapy involves the administration of chemotherapy directly into a body cavity (pleural space, bladder). A small catheter may be used.

  ○ Local irritation may be increased, but systemic adverse effects are usually prevented.

  ○ In some cases, the medication may be removed following a "dwell time."

  ○ Nursing Actions

    ▪ Inform client that some discomfort may be present during infusion.

    ▪ Instruct the client to monitor for evidence of infection at the site of administration.

- Indications

  ○ Chemotherapy can be used to cure a disease, help control its progression, or as palliative treatment for individuals who have a terminal disease.

  ○ Chemotherapy is most commonly used for treatment of cancer, but it may also be used for other disorders, such as autoimmune diseases.

- Preprocedure
  - Because administration of chemotherapeutic medications is limited to certified individuals, management of adverse effects is the primary focus of health care personnel.
  - Instruct client on findings which indicate potential complications. Client should report findings immediately.
- Complications
  - Immunosuppression due to bone marrow suppression by cytotoxic medications is the most significant adverse effect of chemotherapy.
    - Nursing Actions
      - Monitor temperature and white blood cell (WBC) count.
      - A fever greater than 37.8° C (100° F) should be reported to the provider immediately.
      - Monitor skin and mucous membranes for infection (breakdown, fissures, abscess).
      - Cultures should be obtained prior to initiating antimicrobial therapy.
      - If the client's WBC drops below 1,000/uL, place the client in a private room and initiate neutropenic precautions.
        - ▸ Have the client remain in his room unless he needs to leave for a diagnostic procedure or therapy. In this case, place a mask on him during transport.
        - ▸ Protect the client from possible sources of infection (plants, change water in equipment daily).
        - ▸ Have client, staff, and visitors perform frequent hand hygiene. Restrict visitors who are ill.
        - ▸ Avoid invasive procedures that could cause a break in tissue unless necessary (rectal temperatures, injections).
        - ▸ Keep dedicated equipment in the client's room (blood pressure machine, thermometer, stethoscope).
        - ▸ Administer colony-stimulating factors filgrastim (Neupogen, Neulasta) as prescribed to stimulate WBC production.
    - Client Education
      - Encourage the client to avoid crowds while undergoing chemotherapy.
      - Take temperature daily. Report elevated temperature to the provider.
      - Avoid food sources that could contain bacteria (fresh fruits and vegetables; undercooked meat, fish, and eggs; pepper and paprika).
      - Avoid yard work, gardening, or changing a pet's litter box.
      - Avoid fluids that have been sitting at room temperature for longer than 1 hr.
      - Wash all dishes in hot, soapy water or dishwasher. Always wash glasses and cups after one use.
      - Wash toothbrush daily in dishwasher or rinse in bleach solution.
      - Do not share toiletry or personal hygiene items with others.
      - Report fever greater than 37.8° C (100° F) or other manifestations of bacterial or viral infections immediately to the provider.

○ Nausea and vomiting/anorexia

- Many of the medications used for chemotherapy are emetogenic (induce vomiting) or cause anorexia as well as an altered taste in the mouth.

- Serotonin blockers, such as ondansetron (Zofran), have been found to be effective and are often administered with corticosteroids, phenothiazines, and antihistamines.

- Nursing Actions

  □ Administer antiemetic medications at times that are appropriate for a chemotherapeutic agent (prior to treatment, during treatment, after treatment).

  □ Administer antiemetic medications for several days after each treatment as needed.

  □ Remove vomiting cues, such as odor and supplies associated with nausea.

  □ Implement nonpharmacological methods to reduce nausea (visual imagery, relaxation, acupuncture, distraction).

  □ Perform calorie counts to determine intake. Provide liquid nutritional supplements as needed. Add protein powders to food or tube feedings.

  □ Administer megestrol (Megace) to increase the appetite if prescribed.

  □ Assess for findings of dehydration or fluid and electrolyte imbalance.

  □ Perform mouth care prior to serving meals to enhance the client's appetite.

- Client Education

  □ Instruct the client about the administration of antiemetics and schedule them prior to meals.

  □ Encourage the client to eat several small meals a day if better tolerated. Low-fat and dry foods (crackers, toast) and avoiding drinking liquids during meals can prevent nausea.

  □ Suggest that the client select foods that are served cold and do not require cooking, which can emit odors that stimulate nausea.

  □ Encourage consumption of high-protein, high-calorie, nutrient-dense foods and avoidance of low- or empty-calorie foods. Use meal supplements as needed.

  □ Encourage the use of plastic eating utensils, sucking on hard candy, and avoiding red meats to prevent or reduce the sensation of metallic taste.

  □ Teach the client to create a food diary to identify items that can trigger nausea.

○ Alopecia is an adverse effect of certain chemotherapeutic medications related to their interference with the life cycle of rapidly proliferating cells.

- Nursing Actions

  □ Discuss the impact of alopecia on self-image. Discuss options such as hats, turbans, and wigs to deal with hair loss.

  □ Recommend soliciting information from the American Cancer Society regarding products for clients experiencing alopecia.

  □ Inform client that hair loss occurs 7 to 10 days after treatment begins (select agents). Encourage client to select hairpiece before treatment starts.

  □ Reinforce that alopecia is temporary, and hair should return when chemotherapy is discontinued.

- Client Education
  - Instruct the client to avoid the use of damaging hair-care measures, such as electric rollers and curling irons, hair dye, and permanent waves. Use of a soft hair brush or wide-tooth comb for grooming is preferred.
  - Suggest that the client cut her hair short before treatment to decrease weight on the hair follicle.
  - After hair loss, the client should protect the scalp from sun exposure and use a diaper rash ointment/cream for itching.
- Mucositis (stomatitis) is inflammation of tissues in the mouth, such as the gums, tongue, roof and floor of the mouth, and inside the lips and cheeks.
  - Nursing Actions
    - Examine the client's mouth several times a day, and inquire about the presence of oral lesions.
    - Document the location and size of lesions that are present. Lesions should be cultured and reported to the provider.
    - Avoid using glycerin-based mouthwashes or mouth swabs. Nonalcoholic, anesthetic mouthwashes are recommended.
    - Administer a topical anesthetic prior to meals.
    - Discourage consumption of salty, acidic, or spicy foods.
    - Offer oral hygiene before and after each meal. Use lubricating or moisturizing agents to counteract dry mouth.
  - Client Education
    - Encourage the client to rinse mouth with a solution of half 0.9% sodium chloride and half peroxide at least twice a day, and to brush teeth using a soft-bristled toothbrush.
    - Instruct client to take medications to control infection as prescribed (nystatin [Mycostatin], acyclovir [Zovirax]).
    - Encourage the client to eat soft, bland foods and supplements that are high in calories (mashed potatoes, scrambled eggs, cooked cereal, milk shakes, ice cream, frozen yogurt, bananas, and breakfast mixes).
- Anemia and thrombocytopenia occur secondary to bone marrow suppression (myelosuppression).
  - Nursing Actions for Anemia
    - Monitor for fatigue, pallor, dizziness, and shortness of breath.
    - Help the client manage anemia-related fatigue by scheduling activities with rest periods in between and using energy saving measures (sitting during showers and ADLs).
    - Administer erythropoietic medications such as epoetin alfa (Epogen) and antianemic medications such as ferrous sulfate (Feosol) as prescribed.
    - Monitor Hgb values to determine response to medications. Be prepared to administer blood if prescribed.

- Nursing Actions for Thrombocytopenia

    □ Monitor for petechiae, ecchymosis, bleeding of the gums, nosebleeds, and occult or frank blood in stools, urine, or vomitus.

    □ Institute bleeding precautions (avoid IVs and injections, apply pressure for approximately 10 min after blood is obtained, handle client gently and avoid trauma).

    □ Administer thrombopoietic medications such as oprelvekin (Interleukin 11, Neumega) to stimulate platelet production. Monitor platelet count, and be prepared to administer platelets if the count falls below 30,000/mm³.

- Client Education

    □ Instruct the client and family how to manage active bleeding.

    □ Instruct the client about measures to prevent bleeding (use electric razor and soft-bristled toothbrush, avoid blowing nose vigorously, ensure that dentures fit appropriately).

    □ Instruct the client to avoid the use of NSAIDs.

    □ Teach the client to prevent injury when ambulating (wear closed-toes shoes, remove tripping hazards in the home) and apply cold if injury occurs.

Radiation Therapy

- Radiation therapy involves the use of ionizing radiation to target tissues and destroy cells.

    ○ Adverse effects include skin changes, hair loss, and debilitating fatigue.

    ○ Can be administered internally with an implant(s) (brachytherapy) or externally with a radiation beam.

    ○ The client's body fluids are contaminated with radiation and should be disposed of appropriately, as directed by the facility.

    ○ Radiation therapy can be given preoperatively to decrease the size of a tumor.

    ○ Radiation exposure to health care personnel and visitors is reduced by limiting indirect contact time, maintaining indicated distances from sources of radiation, and preventing direct contact with the source.

- Internal Radiation Therapy

    ○ Brachytherapy describes internal radiation that is placed close to the target tissue. This is done via placement in a body orifice (vagina) or body cavity (abdomen) or delivered via IV such as with radionuclide iodine, which is absorbed by the thyroid.

    ○ Nursing Actions

        - Place the client in a private room away from other clients when possible.

        - Place appropriate sign on the door warning of the radiation source.

        - Wear a dosimeter film badge that records personal amount of radiation exposure.

        - Limit visitors to 30-min visits, and have visitors maintain a distance of 6 ft from the source.

        - Visitors and health care personnel who are pregnant or under the age of 16 should not come into contact with the client or radiation source.

        - Keep a lead container in the client's room if the delivery method could allow spontaneous loss of radioactive material. Tongs are available for placing radioactive material into this container.

        - Precautions listed above should be carried out at home if the client is discharged during therapy.

- ○ Client Education

  - ▪ Inform client of the need to remain in an indicated position to prevent dislodgement of the radiation implant.

  - ▪ Instruct the client to call the nurse for assistance with elimination.

  - ▪ Instruct client and family about radiation precautions needed in the health care and home environments.

- • External Radiation Therapy

  - ○ External radiation or teletherapy is delivered over the course of several weeks and aimed at the body from an external source.

  - ○ Nursing Actions

    - ▪ The client's skin over the targeted area is marked with "tattoos" that guide the positioning of the external radiation source.

    - ▪ Provide a well-balanced diet that does not contain red meat. Radiation can cause dysgeusia, making foods such as red meat unpalatable.

    - ▪ Help the client manage fatigue by scheduling activities with rest periods in between and using energy-saving measures (sitting during showers and ADLs).

    - ▪ Monitor for radiation injury to skin and mucous membranes and implement a skin care regimen.

      - ▫ Skin – blanching, erythema, desquamation, sloughing, hemorrhage

      - ▫ Mouth – mucositis, xerostomia (dry mouth)

      - ▫ Neck – difficulty swallowing

      - ▫ Abdomen – gastroenteritis

    - ▪ Monitor CBC (possible decreased platelets and WBCs).

  - ○ Client Education

    - ▪ Review nutrition considerations related to mucositis (avoid spicy, salty, acidic foods; hot foods may not be tolerated).

    - ▪ Gently wash the skin over the irradiated area with mild soap and water. Dry the area thoroughly using patting motions.

    - ▪ Do not remove or wash off radiation "tattoos" (markings) that are used to guide therapy. Do not apply powders, ointments, lotions, deodorants, or perfumes to the irradiated skin.

    - ▪ Wear soft clothing and avoid tight or constricting clothes.

    - ▪ Do not expose the irradiated skin to sun or a heat source.

    - ▪ Inspect skin for evidence of damage and report to the provider.

Hormonal Therapy

- Hormone therapy is effective against tumors that are supported or suppressed by hormones.

- By giving a similar hormone, uptake of the support hormone is blocked, or production reduced. Hormone agonists, gonadotropin-releasing hormone agonists (GnRH) like leuprolide (Eligard, Lupron) are effective against tumors that require a particular hormone for support.

  - The use of androgenic hormones in a client who has estrogen-dependent cancer can suppress growth of this type of cancer.

  - Conversely, the use of estrogenic hormones for a testosterone-dependent cancer can suppress growth of this type of cancer.

- Hormone antagonists compete with the support hormone for binding sites on or in the tumor cell and are effective against tumors that require a particular hormone for support.

  - The use of an anti-estrogen hormone in a client who has estrogen-dependent cancer can suppress growth of this type of cancer.

  - The same is true for anti-testosterone hormones.

- Nursing Actions

  - GnRH – Monitor cardiac status, along with blood pressure and for the occurrence of pulmonary edema.

    - Client Education

      - Inform male clients about the impact on sexual functions (decreased libido, erectile dysfunction) and feminizing effects of hormone therapy (gynecomastia, hot flashes, bone loss).

      - Instruct the client to increase intake of calcium and vitamin D.

      - Inform female clients of masculinizing effects (chest and facial hair growth, amenorrhea, decreased breast tissue).

  - Androgen antagonists (flutamide [Eulexin]) – Monitor laboratory findings (CBC [anemia], calcium, increased liver enzymes).

    - Client Education

      - Alert the male client about the feminizing effects of hormone therapy (gynecomastia, erectile dysfunction).

      - Advise the client to notify the provider of sore throat or bruising.

  - Estrogen antagonists – tamoxifen (Nolvadex), anastrozole (Arimidex), trastuzumab (Herceptin)

    - Ongoing Care

      - Monitor CBC, clotting times, lipid profiles, calcium and cholesterol serum levels, and liver function for medication-related changes.

      - Neurologic and cardiovascular functioning is monitored for changes.

    - Client Education

      - Inform the client of adverse effects, which include nausea, vomiting, hot flashes, weight gain, vaginal bleeding, and increased risk of thrombosis.

      - Reinforce the need for yearly gynecologic exams and the need to take calcium and vitamin D supplements.

Immunotherapy

- Immunotherapy (biotherapy) uses biologic response modifiers (BRMs), which alter a client's biological response to cancerous tumor cells. Antibodies, cytokines, and other immune substances normally produced by the immune system are administered to increase the body's defense against cancer.

  - Interleukins and interferons are the two primary cytokines (immune response modulators) used in immunotherapy.

    - Interleukins help coordinate the inflammatory and immune responses of the body, in particular, the lymphocytes.

    - Interferons, when stimulated, can exert an antitumor effect by activating a variety of responses.

  - Cytokines are the primary BRMs currently used, and they work to enhance the immune system. They help the client's immune system recognize cancer cells and use the body's natural defenses to destroy them.

- Nursing Actions

  - Interleukins – Monitor for influenza-like symptoms and edema.

  - Interferons – Monitor for altered mental status and lethargy.

    - Monitor for peripheral neuropathy that may affect vision, hearing, balance, and gait.

    - Take precautions for orthostatic hypotension.

    - Client Education

      - Instruct the client to immediately report influenza-like manifestations or changes consistent with peripheral neuropathy.

      - Alert the client that skin rashes are common and use of a perfume-free moisturizer may be helpful.

      - Instruct the client to avoid sun exposure and swimming if skin manifestations develop.

Photodynamic Therapy

- Photodynamic therapy involves the injection of a photosensitizing agent that is absorbed by all the cells in the body. One to three days later when the agent remains in only the cancer cells, the tumor is exposed to a specific wavelength of light via an endoscope. Cells are subsequently destroyed and tumors are eliminated or reduced in size.

  - Used to treat non-small cell lung cancer and esophageal cancer.

  - Effective with small tumors close to body surface (within 1 cm).

  - Adverse effects are related to the area of the body being treated.

  - Nursing Actions – Instruct the client to avoid sun exposure for 6 weeks (limit time outdoors, wear sunglasses).

Supportive Treatment

- In addition to cancer treatment, the client may require assistance for altered body function or to meet emotional and spiritual needs.

- Clients who have cancer are at risk for inadequate nutrition related to diagnosis or treatment. (Refer to the chapter on *Cancer and Immunosuppression Disorders* in the *Nutrition Review Module*.)

  ○ Nursing Actions

    ▪ Administer nutritional supplements or substitutes as prescribed.

    ▪ Monitor feeding tube or central line as appropriate.

    ▪ Encourage the addition of protein- and calorie-dense foods.

    ▪ Monitor for effectiveness of nutrition modifications (laboratory values, urine and bowel elimination, absence of GI upset).

    ▪ Monitor weight.

    ▪ Consult nutrition services.

- Clients may experience altered elimination.

  ○ Nursing Actions

    ▪ Assist with alternate means of elimination (insert indwelling or intermittent urinary catheter, apply drainage devices) as indicated.

    ▪ Monitor urine and bowel output.

    ▪ Instruct the client on self-management of elimination.

- Body image changes are a factor in clients where surgery is disfiguring, especially cancers of the face or sexual organs (breasts or genitalia).

  ○ Nursing Actions

    ▪ Encourage the client to express feelings.

    ▪ Encourage the client to look at or touch affected body areas.

    ▪ Assist the client with prosthetic devices, as indicated.

    ▪ Encourage the client to use positive measures to promote proper body image (makeup, clothing).

- Altered sexuality results from functional impairment or body image changes related to cancer treatments. Pain with sexual intercourse can also be a factor.

  ○ Nursing Actions

    ▪ Encourage the client and partner to communicate feelings to each other.

    ▪ Administer hormone therapy, as prescribed.

    ▪ Instruct the client about medications to promote erection or manage pain sensation, as prescribed.

- The client's ability to cope with the diagnosis and prognosis may be ineffective.

  ○ Nursing Actions

    ▪ Administer medications for anxiety or depression, as prescribed.

    ▪ Encourage the client to express feelings verbally or through journaling and blogging.

    ▪ Encourage the client to participate in a support group (physical or online) for clients who have similar cancers. Make a referral to a community resource.

- Make a referral to counseling services for the client and family, as needed.

- Educate the client on anticipatory grief and the stages of grief.

- Consult palliative services, as indicated.

- Incorporate client's beliefs and preferences regarding spirituality and illness/death.

- Cancer or cancer treatment may place the client in an immunocompromised state.

  ○ Nursing Actions – Teach the client to avoid individuals with colds/infections/viruses.

- Other supportive nursing actions

  ○ Facilitate safe activity, providing assistive devices when necessary for clients who have altered mobility or require assistance with self-care activities.

  ○ Coordinate transfer of client care to home health, hospice, or tertiary care setting (rehabilitation center) as appropriate.

  ○ Provide alternate means of communication for clients who have cancer affecting the mouth, throat, larynx, or vocal cords.

  ○ Use assistive aids and devices for clients who have visual or hearing impairment.

  ○ Consult physical therapy, and genetic or other counseling services as indicated.

  ○ Consult pain management for persistent or uncontrolled pain. (See the chapter on *Pain Management for Clients with Cancer*.)

APPLICATION EXERCISES

1. A nurse is planning care for a client who is undergoing chemotherapy and is placed on neutropenic precautions. Which of the following interventions should be included in the plan of care? (Select all that apply.)

_____ A. Encourage a high-fiber diet.

_____ B. Remove plants from the room.

_____ C. Have the client wear a mask when leaving the room.

_____ D. Have client-specific equipment remain in the room.

_____ E. Eliminate raw foods from the client's diet.

2. A nurse is caring for a client who is undergoing chemotherapy and reports severe nausea. Which of the following statements is appropriate for the nurse to make?

A. "Your nausea will lessen with each course of chemotherapy."

B. "Hot food is better tolerated because of the aroma."

C. "Try eating several small meals throughout the day."

D. "Increase your intake of red meat as tolerated."

3. A nurse is planning care for a client who has a platelet count of 25,000/mm³. Which of the following interventions should be included in the plan of care?

A. Apply prolonged pressure to puncture site after blood sampling.

B. Administer epoetin alfa (Epogen) as prescribed.

C. Place the client in a private room.

D. Have the client use an oral topical anesthetic before meals.

4. A nurse is caring for a client who has cervical cancer and undergoing brachytherapy. Which of the following are appropriate nursing interventions? (Select all that apply.)

_____ A. Permit visitors to stay 30 min at a time.

_____ B. Place the client on bed rest.

_____ C. Insert an indwelling urinary catheter.

_____ D. Administer fiber laxatives.

_____ E. Allow the skin "tattoo" guides for therapy to remain in place.

5. A nurse is caring for a client who has mucositis due to chemotherapy to treat cancer. Which of the following actions should the nurse take?

    A. Use a glycerin-soaked swab to clean the client's teeth.

    B. Encourage increased intake of citrus fruit juices.

    C. Obtain a culture of the lesions.

    D. Provide an alcohol-based mouthwash for oral hygiene.

6. A nurse is leading a discussion with a group of female clients who have alopecia and are undergoing chemotherapy. What should be included in the discussion? Use the Active Learning Template: Systems Disorder to complete this item to include the following sections:

    A. Pathophysiology of the Problem

    B. Client Education: Describe at least four teaching points.

    C. Nursing Interventions: Describe at least two.

APPLICATION EXERCISES KEY

1. A. INCORRECT: There is no benefit in placing a client who has neutropenia on a high-fiber diet.

    B. **CORRECT:** Neutropenic precautions include the client not having contact with flowers and plants due to the presence of surface infectious agents in the water and soil.

    C. **CORRECT:** Neutropenic precautions include having the client wear a mask when leaving the room to reduce the incidence of infection.

    D. **CORRECT:** Neutropenic precautions include having equipment available that is only for use in caring for the client to reduce the incidence of infection.

    E. **CORRECT:** A client who is neutropenic should avoid consuming raw foods due to the presence of surface infectious agents on peeling and rind.

    (N) NCLEX® Connection: Pharmacological and Parenteral Therapies, Pharmacological Pain Management

2. A. INCORRECT: Nausea usually occurs to the same extent with each session of chemotherapy.

    B. INCORRECT: Cold foods are better tolerated than warm/hot foods because odors from heated foods can induce nausea.

    C. **CORRECT:** Several small meals a day are usually better tolerated by the client who has nausea.

    D. INCORRECT: Red meat is not tolerated well by the client undergoing chemotherapy because the taste of meat is frequently altered and unpalatable.

    (N) NCLEX® Connection: Pharmacological and Parenteral Therapies, Pharmacological Pain Management

3. A. **CORRECT:** Bleeding precautions should be implemented for the client who has thrombocytopenia.

    B. INCORRECT: Epoetin alfa (Epogen) is administered to the client who has anemia.

    C. INCORRECT: The client who is neutropenic is placed in a private room.

    D. INCORRECT: A topical oral anesthetic is used for the client who has mucositis.

    (N) NCLEX® Connection: Reduction of Risk Potential, Therapeutic Procedures

4.   A. **CORRECT:** The client who has cervical cancer will have a vaginal radiation implant, so visitors should remain for 30 min at a time and maintain a distance of 6 ft.

   B. **CORRECT:** The client who has cervical cancer will have a vaginal radiation implant, and bed rest is needed to prevent displacement of the implant.

   C. **CORRECT:** The client who has cervical cancer will have a vaginal radiation implant, and a catheter is needed to prevent displacement of the implant during ambulation.

   D. INCORRECT: Fiber laxatives, which stimulate bowel movements, are not used to prevent displacing the vaginal radiation implant.

   E. INCORRECT: Skin "tattoo" guides are used for the client undergoing external radiation therapy, not brachytherapy.

   Ⓝ NCLEX® Connection: Physiological Adaptations, Alterations in Body Systems

5.   A. INCORRECT: Glycerin-based swabs should be avoided when providing oral hygiene to the client who has mucositis.

   B. INCORRECT: Acidic foods should be discouraged for the client who has oral mucositis.

   C. **CORRECT:** A culture of oral lesions is obtained to identify pathogens and determine appropriate treatment.

   D. INCORRECT: Nonalcoholic mouthwashes are recommended for the client who has mucositis.

   Ⓝ NCLEX® Connection: Physiological Adaptations, Unexpected Response to Therapies

6.   *Using the Active Learning Template: Systems Disorder*

   A. Pathophysiology of the Problem
   • Alopecia occurs as an adverse effect of chemotherapy medications. They interfere with the life cycle of rapidly proliferating cells, such as those found in hair follicles, resulting in hair loss.

   B. Client Education
   • Wear hats, turbans, and wigs.
   • Avoid the use of damaging hair-care measures, such as electric rollers and curling irons, hair dye, and permanent waves.
   • Use a soft hair brush or wide-tooth comb for grooming.
   • Avoid sun exposure. Use a diaper rash ointment or cream for itching.
   • Alopecia is temporary, and hair will return when chemotherapy is discontinued.

   C. Nursing Interventions
   • Discuss the impact of alopecia on self-image. Encourage the client to express feelings.
   • Recommend use of information from the American Cancer Society on managing alopecia.
   • Provide referral to a cancer support group.

   Ⓝ NCLEX® Connection: Physiological Adaptations, Alterations in Body Systems

chapter 93

Overview

- The various types of cancer share general cancer principles: abnormal cell growth, tumor formation, and potential for invasion to other locations.
- Each type of cancer has distinguishing characteristics related to risk, clinical manifestations, screening, and diagnosis.
- The prognosis and treatment of cancer varies by type.

SKIN CANCER

Overview

- Sunlight exposure is the leading cause of skin cancer. The most effective strategy for prevention of skin cancer is avoidance or reduction of skin exposure to sunlight.
- Precancerous skin lesions, called actinic keratoses, are common in people with chronically sun-damaged skin, such as older adults.
- There are three types of skin cancer.

SKIN CANCER TYPE	ASSESSMENT	CHARACTERISTICS
Squamous cell (epidermis)	› Rough, scaly lesion with central ulceration and crusting › Bleeding (possible)	› Localized; may metastasize.
Basal cell (basal epidermis or nearby dermal cells)	› Small, waxy nodule with superficial blood vessels, well-defined borders › Erythema and ulcerations	› Invades local structures (nerves, bone, cartilage, lymphatic and vascular tissue); rarely metastatic but high rate of recurrence.
Malignant melanoma (cancer of melanocytes)	› New moles or change in an existing mole (can occur in intestines or any other body structure that contains pigment cells) › Cracks, ulcerations, or bleeding (possible)	› Teach clients the "ABCDE" system to evaluate moles.

View Images

› Basal Cell Cancer   › Squamous Cell Cancer

Health Promotion and Disease Prevention

- Limit exposure to sunlight, especially between 1000 and 1500 hr.
- Apply sunscreen when near reflective surfaces (sand, snow, water, concrete).
- Use sunblock that has an SPF of at least 15, with both UVA and UVB protection. Apply 30 min before exposure to sun. Sunblock should be reapplied at least every 2 hr.
- Wear protective clothing, hats, sunglasses, and lip balm that has an SPF of at least 15.
- Avoid indoor tanning (tanning beds, booths, sunlamps).

Assessment

- Risk Factors
  - Immunosuppression therapy
  - Exposure to ultraviolet light (natural light or indoor tanning) over long periods of time
  - Chronic skin inflammation, burns, or scars
  - Fair complexion (blonde or red hair, fair skin, freckles, blue eyes) with a tendency to burn easily
  - Presence of several large or many small moles
  - Family or personal history of melanoma
  - Residing in higher elevations or in close proximity to equator (thinner layer of ozone)
  - Age over 50 years
- Subjective Data – Report of change in appearance of mole or lesion
- Screening and Diagnostic Procedures

METHOD	EXPECTED FINDINGS	NURSING ACTIONS
Assessment (self or clinician)	› New or suspicious lesions	› Instruct client to develop a body map (diagram of scars or lesions) and monitor monthly for changes. Inspect skin between fingers and toes and on scalp.
Biopsy (punch, shave, or excisional)	› Cancerous cells	› Instruct client to monitor for infection. › Teach client wound care, including care of sutures (punch, excisional biopsy).

  - If melanoma is diagnosed, blood tests are prescribed (CBC, CMP, liver) to check for organ involvement.
  - ABCDEs of suspicious lesions
    - A – Asymmetry: One side does not match the other
    - B – Borders: Ragged, notched, irregular, or blurred edges
    - C – Color: Lack of uniformity in pigmentation (shades of tan, brown, or black)
    - D – Diameter: Width greater than 6 mm, or about the size of a pencil eraser or a pea
    - E – Evolving: Or change in appearance (shape, size, color, height, texture) or condition (bleeding, itching)

M◇ View Images: Melanomas

- G
- Q
  PCC

○ Because of the cumulative effects of sun damage over the lifespan, screening for suspicious lesions is an essential part of the routine physical assessment of older adult clients.

○ In clients who have dark skin, lesions may appear on the palms or soles of feet. The nurse should assess suspicious lesions or skin patches for change in texture, tautness, or elasticity (color change is not always evident).

Patient-Centered Care

- Therapeutic Procedures

  ○ Cryosurgery to freeze and destroy isolated lesions by applying liquid nitrogen (-200° C).

    ▪ Skin becomes edematous and tender.

    ▪ Client Education – Teach the client to cleanse with hydrogen peroxide and apply a topical antimicrobial until healed.

  ○ Topical chemotherapy with 5-fluorouracil cream for treatment of actinic keratoses or for widespread superficial basal cell carcinoma.

    ▪ Client Education

      □ Prepare the client for extended treatment that will cause the lesion to weep, crust, and erode.

      □ Reassure the client that the appearance of the lesion will improve after treatment.

  ○ Interferon for postoperative treatment of stage III or greater melanomas

    ▪ Nursing Actions

      □ Report and provide relief for adverse or toxic effects of chemotherapy.

      □ Encourage adequate nutrition and fluid intake.

- Surgical Interventions

  ○ Excision

    ▪ The incision will be closed with sutures if possible. A skin graft may be necessary for large areas.

    ▪ Client Education – Advise the client about postoperative wound care and care of the skin graft if used.

- Complications – skin abscess and cellulitis

LEUKEMIAS AND LYMPHOMAS

Overview

- Leukemias are cancers of white blood cells or of cells that develop into white blood cells.

    - In leukemia, the white blood cells are not functional. They invade and destroy bone marrow, and they can metastasize to the liver, spleen, lymph nodes, testes, and brain.

    - Leukemias are divided into acute (acute lymphocytic leukemia and acute myelogenous leukemia) and chronic (chronic lymphocytic leukemia and chronic myelogenous leukemia) and are further classified by the type of white blood cells primarily affected.

    - The goal of treatment is to eliminate all leukemic cells.

- The exact cause of leukemia is not known.

- Overgrowth of leukemic cells prevents growth of other blood components (platelets, erythrocytes, mature leukocytes).

    - Lack of mature leukocytes leads to immunosuppression. Infection is the leading cause of death among clients who have leukemia.

    - Lack of platelets increases the client's risk of bleeding.

- Leukemia Incidence and Cure Rates

    - Acute lymphocytic leukemia (ALL) – Various factors influence the prognosis for children, but the 5-year survival rate is approximately 85% (age at diagnosis, gender, cell type involved); less than 50% of adults can be cured.

    - Acute myelogenous leukemia (AML) – Most common leukemia among adults; prognosis is poor.

    - Chronic lymphocytic leukemia (CLL) – Most cases involve people older than 60. This disease does not occur in children; disease progresses slowly in three phases over time.

    - Chronic myelogenous leukemia (CML) – Most cases involve young adults. The disease is uncommon in children; prognosis is less than 2 years of survival from the time of diagnosis.

- Lymphomas are cancers of lymphocytes (a type of white blood cell) and lymph nodes (which produce antibodies and fight infection).

    - There are two types of lymphoma.

        - Hodgkin's lymphoma (HL)

            □ Most cases involve young adults.

            □ Possible causes include viral infections and exposure to chemical agents.

        - Non-Hodgkin's lymphoma (NHL)

            □ More common in clients older than 50.

            □ Possible causes include gene damage, viral infections, autoimmune disease, and exposure to radiation or toxic chemicals.

    - Lymphomas can metastasize to almost any organ.

Health Promotion and Disease Prevention

- Use protective equipment, such as a mask, and ensure proper ventilation while working in environments that contain carcinogens or particles in the air.

- Influenza and pneumonia vaccinations are important for all clients who are immunosuppressed.

Assessment

- Risk Factors

  - Immunosuppression

  - Exposure to chemotherapy agents or medications that suppress bone marrow

  - Genetic factors (hereditary)

  - Ionizing radiation (radiation therapy, environmental)

  - Older adult clients often have diminished immune function and decreased bone marrow function, which increase the risk of complications of leukemia and lymphoma.

  - Older adult clients have decreased energy reserves and can tire more easily during treatment. Safety is a concern with ambulation.

- Subjective and Objective Data

  - Acute leukemia

    - Bone pain

    - Joint swelling

    - Enlarged liver and spleen

    - Weight loss

    - Fever

    - Poor wound healing (infected lesions)

    - Manifestations of anemia (fatigue, pallor, tachycardia, dyspnea on exertion)

    - Evidence of bleeding (ecchymoses, hematuria, bleeding gums)

  - HL and NHL

    - Most clients only experience an enlarged lymph node (usually in the neck with HL), which is a typical finding in client's with indolent (slow-growing) lymphomas.

    - Other possible manifestations include fever, fatigue, and infections.

  - Screening and Diagnostic Procedures

METHOD	EXPECTED FINDINGS	NURSING ACTIONS
CBC	› WBC may be high, low, or normal (leukemia) › Hemoglobin, hematocrit, and platelets decreased	› Explain unexpected findings to client.
Coagulation time	› Increased	› Monitor for bleeding
Biopsy of bone marrow (core or fine-needle aspiration)	› Large quantities of immature leukemic blast cells (diagnosis) › Typing of protein markers (to differentiate myeloid or lymphoid leukemia)	› Administer pain medication, as prescribed. › Apply pressure for 5 to 10 min, then a pressure dressing. › Monitor for bleeding and infection for 24 hr.

METHOD	EXPECTED FINDINGS	NURSING ACTIONS
CT scan (always used for HL staging)	› Guide for lymphoma staging procedures – identify presence, size, and shape of nodes, tumors.	› Prepare the client for the procedure.
Biopsy of lymph nodes	› Hodgkin's lymphoma – presence of Reed-Sternberg cells (cancerous B-lymphocytes) › Non-Hodgkin's Lymphoma – any other lymph node malignancy	› Provide client information specific to the diagnosis.

- Staging of lymphoma involves extensive testing to ensure proper treatment is prescribed. HL has two main subtypes; "classic" HL is further distinguished into four categories. NHL has more than 60 subtypes. Treatment must be specific to the client's needs.

Patient-Centered Care

- Nursing Care
  - Monitor for evidence of infection.
    - Assess for other physiological indicators of infection (lung crackles, cough, urinary frequency or urgency, oliguria, lesions of skin or mucous membrane).
  - Manifestations that stem from the immune response (increased WBC, fever, pus, redness, inflammation) are not likely due to immunosuppression.
  - Prevent infection. (Implement neutropenic precautions.) These interventions are especially important during chemotherapy induction and for clients who have received a bone marrow transplant.
    - Frequent, thorough hand hygiene is a priority intervention.
    - Place the client in a private room.
    - Allow only well visitors; when unavoidable, visitors who are ill must wear a mask.
    - Screen visitors carefully.
    - Restrict foods that may be contaminated with bacteria (no fresh or raw fruits, vegetables).
    - Monitor WBC.
    - Prevent transmission of bacteria and viruses (no live plants, flowers; use high-efficiency particulate air [HEPA] filtration). Eliminate standing water (humidifiers, denture cups, vases) to prevent bacteria breeding.
    - Encourage good personal hygiene.
    - Avoid crowds.
  - Prevent injury.
    - Monitor platelets.
    - Assess frequently for obvious and occult bleeding.
    - Protect the client from trauma (avoid injections and venipunctures, apply firm pressure, increase vitamin K intake).
    - Teach the client how to avoid trauma (use electric shaver, soft bristled toothbrush, avoid contact sports).

○ Conserve the client's energy.

- Encourage rest, adequate nutrition, and fluid intake.

- Ensure the client gets adequate sleep.

- Assess the client's energy resources/capability.

- Plan activities as appropriate.

• Medications

○ Chemotherapy

- Chemotherapy may be used to treat lymphoma in combination with other therapies.

- There are three phases of chemotherapy used to treat leukemia.

PHASE	GOAL	PROCEDURE	LENGTH OF TIME
Induction therapy – intensive combination therapy	Induce remission – absence of all findings of leukemia, including less than 5% blasts in bone marrow	Aggressive treatment (possible continuous infusion); IV infusion; CNS and CSF infusion prophylaxis (ALL)	4 to 6 weeks (hospitalization required due to increased risk for infection and hemorrhage)
Consolidation or intensification therapy	Cure by eradicating any residual leukemic cells	Same medications as induction phase at lower dosage or different combination of medications	About 6 months
Maintenance therapy	Prevent relapse	Lower doses of oral or IV chemotherapy	2 to 3 years
Reinduction therapy – for the client who relapses	Place the client back in remission	Combinations of chemotherapy used to achieve remission	Probability of relapse occurring decreases over time

- Client Education – Report manifestations of infection or illness immediately to the provider.

○ Colony-stimulating medications such as filgrastim (Neupogen) stimulate the production of leukocytes.

- Nursing Considerations – Monitor for report of bone pain. Monitor CBC twice weekly to check leukocytes. Use cautiously with clients who have bone marrow cancer.

- Client Education – Encourage client to report bone discomfort.

• Radiation

○ External lymph node radiation is the primary form of treatment for HL. Radiation therapy or radiolabeled antibodies may be used as part of treatment for NHL.

○ Radiation is not typically a treatment used for clients who have leukemia.

- Teamwork and Collaboration
  - ○ Bone marrow transplantation – Bone marrow is destroyed or "ablated" using radiation or chemotherapy and later replaced with healthy stem cells. The body is able to resume normal production of blood cells.
    - Autologous cells are the client's own cells that are collected before chemotherapy.
    - Matching of donor to recipient stem cells compares certain human leukocyte antigens (HLA) to reduce risk of rejection.
      - □ Syngeneic cells are donated from the client's identical twin (HLA identical).
      - □ Allogeneic cells are obtained from an HLA-matched donor, such as a relative or from umbilical cord blood (closely matched HLA).
    - Without transplantation, the client will likely die from infection or bleeding.
    - Following transplantation, the client is at high risk for infection and bleeding until the transfused stem cells begin producing white blood cells again.

Complications

- Pancytopenia – decrease in white and red blood cells and platelets
  - ○ Neutropenia secondary to disease and/or treatment greatly increases the client's risk for infection.
    - An absolute neutrophil count (ANC) less than 2,000/mm³ suggests an increased risk of infection. An ANC of less than 500/mm³ indicates a severe risk of infection.
    - Nursing Actions
      - □ Maintain a hygienic environment and encourage the client to do the same.
      - □ Monitor for infection (cough, alterations in breath sounds, urine, or feces). Report temperature greater than 37.8° C (100° F).
      - □ Administer antimicrobial, antiviral, and antifungal medications as prescribed.
      - □ Administer blood products (granulocytes) as needed.
  - ○ Thrombocytopenia secondary to disease and/or treatment greatly increases the client's risk for bleeding.
    - The greatest risk is at platelet counts less than 50,000/mm³, and spontaneous bleeding can occur at less than 20,000/mm³.
    - Nursing Actions
      - □ Minimize the risk of trauma (safe environment).
      - □ Administer blood products (platelets) as needed.
  - ○ Anemia secondary to disease and/or treatment significantly increases the client's risk for hypoxemia.
    - Nursing Actions
      - □ Plan client care to balance rest and activity and use assistive devices, as indicated.
      - □ Monitor RBC.
      - □ Provide a diet high in protein and carbohydrates.
      - □ Administer colony-stimulating factors, such as epoetin alfa (Procrit), as prescribed.
      - □ Administer blood products (packed red blood cells) as needed.

- Bone Marrow Transplant Complications
  - Failure of stem cells to engraft (grow) – Bone marrow transplant must be repeated.
  - Graft-versus-host disease (graft rejection)
    - Nursing Actions – Administer immunosuppressants as prescribed.
  - Phlebitis (hepatic) may occur up to 1 month after bone marrow transplant.
    - Nursing Actions
      - Monitor for jaundice, abdominal pain, and liver enlargement.
      - Monitor daily weights and abdominal girth to assess for fluid retention.

THYROID CANCER

Overview

- There are four types of thyroid cancer:
  - Papillary carcinoma grows slowly and is the most common form.
  - Follicular carcinoma affects blood vessels, bone, and lung tissues. It often attaches to the trachea, muscles, vasculature, and skin.
  - Medullary carcinoma is often the result of an endocrine disorder, which causes multiple tumors.
  - Anaplastic carcinoma replicates quickly, invading the area surrounding the tumor. It usually metastasizes before diagnosis.
- As thyroid tumors increase in size or spread, they impact the function of surrounding structures (larynx, pharynx, esophagus).

Health Promotion and Disease Prevention

- Avoid or stop smoking.
- Wear a thyroid guard to protect the neck during upper body x-rays.

Assessment

- Risk Factors
  - Female gender
  - Diet low in iodine (follicular carcinoma)
  - Radiation exposure
  - Older adults have higher incidence of follicular and medullary carcinoma.
- Subjective and Objective Data
  - Dyspnea
  - Dysphasia
  - Stridor

- ○ Change in size, shape of thyroid
- ○ Palpable nodules or irregularities
- ○ Dehydration (hormone imbalance)
- ○ Thyroid bruits (possible with enlargement)
- ○ Screening and Diagnostic Procedures

METHOD	EXPECTED FINDINGS	NURSING ACTIONS
Thyroid stimulation or suppression testing	› Altered TSH, T3, or T4 levels	› Confirm that client has not had other tests involving iodine or radiation in the last 6 weeks (may alter results).
24-hr urine	› Altered TSH, T3, T4, or iodine levels	› Instruct client to discard the first void, then save all urine for the next 24 hr.
Laryngoscopy	› Presence of cancer on vocal cords	› Instruct client to not eat or drink after midnight prior to the procedure.
Other laboratory testing	› Increased calcitonin, adrenocorticotropic hormone, prostaglandins, serotonin (medullary carcinoma)	› Explain unexpected findings to client.
BRAF gene mutation	› Presence indicates carcinoma, possible thyroid papillary cancer	› Consult genetic counseling services, if indicated.
RET/PTC gene alterations	› Presence indicates high probability of papillary carcinoma	› Consult genetic counseling services, if indicated.
Carcinoembryonic agent (CEA)	› Positive indicates cancer, possible medullary carcinoma	› Inform client that CEA can represent many types of cancer.
Biopsy (fine-needle plus open or core, if indicated)	› To identify presence of cancer cells in thyroid nodules or lymph nodes	› Instruct client that lesions greater than 1 cm and suspicious lymph nodes are tested. › Administer pain medication, as prescribed. › Apply pressure for 5 to 10 min, then a pressure dressing. › Monitor for bleeding and infection for 24 hr.
Ultrasound (US)	› Used to guide biopsy; reveals whether nodules are fluid-filled (typically benign) or solid (typically cancerous).	› Instruct and prepare client for the procedure.
Radioiodine scan	› Presence of radioactive cells (cells that retained radioiodine); not useful with medullary carcinoma	› Inform client that dye will be administered (injection or oral) then the thyroid and other suspicious areas are scanned.

- ▪ MRI or PET scan may be used to visualize the thyroid. CT scan is avoided due to iodine in the contrast dye.

Patient-Centered Care

- Nursing Care
  - Monitor airway patency in client who has a tumor affecting or compressing the trachea.
  - Assess swallowing in client who has a tumor affecting or compressing the esophagus.
  - Administer medications to treat hypertension, dysrhythmia, or tachycardia as prescribed.
- Medications
  - Thyroid suppression therapy
    - Involves administration of synthetic thyroxine (T4; levothyroxine sodium [Synthroid]).
    - Suppression therapy replaces T4 needed for body function. It also prevents or slows growth of cancerous thyroid cells.
    - Therapy is typically prescribed for several months following thyroid surgery.
    - Client Education

      - Instruct the client to never stop taking levothyroxine sodium (Synthroid), unless instructed by the provider.
      - Instruct the client to take levothyroxine sodium (Synthroid) on an empty stomach.
- Teamwork and Collaboration
  - Care After Discharge
    - Clients who are treated for thyroid cancer are hypothyroid.
    - Nursing Actions
      - Monitor vital signs for impaired oxygenation, hypotension, or bradycardia.
      - Use ECG monitoring to detect dysrhythmias.
      - Assess mental status and provide a safe environment.
- Therapeutic Procedures
  - Radiation is used to treat anaplastic carcinoma.
  - Radioactive iodine (RAI) therapy is used to destroy papillary or follicular carcinoma and can be used to treat hyperthyroidism.
    - RAI therapy works similarly to radioactive scanning (used to diagnose thyroid cancer).
    - The client ingests RAI in liquid or tablet form, which is absorbed by thyroid cells which are then destroyed.
    - Client may benefit from RAI therapy following thyroid suppression therapy.
    - Nursing Actions
      - Teach the client about radioactive precautions to reduce risk of radiation exposure.
      - Instruct the client to chew gum or hard candy to relieve dry mouth or reduced salivation.
      - Provide information on nutrition supplements for client experiencing altered taste. Consult nutrition services.

- Surgical Interventions
  - Papillary, follicular, and medullary carcinoma are treated surgically. Thyroidectomy (total or partial) or thyroid lobectomy is the treatment of choice for papillary carcinoma that is limited to the thyroid gland.
  - Involved lymph nodes in the neck are removed during surgery.
  - During surgery, the parathyroid glands or laryngeal nerve may be damaged.
  - A wound drain may be placed intraoperatively.
  - Nursing Actions
    - Monitor and treat cardiac abnormalities as prescribed.
    - Support neck with pillows or sandbags.
    - Maintain a humidifier to promote airway clearance.
    - Monitor for hemorrhage (incision site, hypotension, tachycardia, increased swallowing or throat "tickling").
    - Monitor for respiratory distress (caused by tetany, swelling, or laryngeal nerve damage).
    - Monitor for parathyroid injury (decreased PTH, hypocalcemia, tetany).
    - Monitor for thyroid storm (excessive release of thyroid hormone).
  - Client Education
    - Teach the client to place both hands behind the neck when moving or coughing (reduces strain on the incision).
    - Teach the client that thyroid suppression therapy is typically prescribed for 3 months following surgery.

Complications

- Myxedema coma is a rare, potentially lethal form of hypothyroidism resulting in decreased respiratory function (respiratory depression and cerebral hypoxia), altered cardiovascular function (bradycardia, hypotension, decreased cardiac output), endocrine abnormalities (hypoglycemia and hyponatremia), hypothermia, and stupor.
  - Nursing Actions
    - Notify provider of suspected myxedema coma.
    - Provide continuous monitoring of telemetry and vital signs.
    - Administer fluids, electrolytes, and medications as prescribed.
- Thyroid storm is caused by excess thyroid hormone release following surgery. This is a life-threatening emergency.
  - Key findings are fever, tachycardia, and systolic hypertension. Other manifestations include GI disturbance (nausea, vomiting, diarrhea, abdominal pain), anxiety, restlessness, confusion (progresses to psychosis), and neurological alterations (tremors or seizure).
- Nursing Actions
  - Notify the provider immediately.
  - Administer antithyroid drugs, sodium iodide, beta-adrenergic blocking agents, and glucocorticoids as prescribed.
  - Monitor cardiac rhythm and central venous pressure.
  - Reduce fever (administer antipyretics, apply cooling blanket).

LUNG CANCER

Overview

- Lung cancer is one of the leading causes of cancer-related deaths for both men and women. It most commonly occurs between the ages of 45 and 70.

- Prognosis of lung cancer is poor because it is often diagnosed in an advanced stage, when metastasis has occurred. Palliative care is often the focus at the advanced stage (III-IV).

- Bronchogenic carcinomas (arising from the bronchial epithelium) account for 90% of primary lung cancers.

- Most lung cancers are non-small cell lung cancer (NSCLC), which includes squamous, adeno, and large cell carcinomas.

- Small cell lung cancer (SCLC) is fast-growing and is consistently linked to a history of cigarette smoking.

Health Promotion and Disease Prevention

- Promote smoking cessation.

- Use protective equipment (mask) and ensure proper ventilation while working in environments that can contain carcinogens or particles in the air.

Assessment

- Risk Factors

  ○ Cigarette smoking (both firsthand and secondhand smoke)

  ○ Radiation exposure

  ○ Chronic exposure to inhaled environmental irritants (air pollution, asbestos, other talc dusts)

  ○ Older adult clients have decreased pulmonary reserves due to normal lung changes (decreased lung elasticity and thickening alveoli), contributing to impaired gas exchange.

  ○ Structural changes in the skeletal system decrease diaphragmatic expansion thereby restricting ventilation.

- Subjective Data

  ○ Orthopnea

  ○ Chronic cough

  ○ Chronic dyspnea

  ○ Chest wall pain

  ○ Fatigue, weight loss, or anorexia

- Objective Data

  ○ Clients may experience few clinical findings early in the disease. Monitor for manifestations that often appear late in the disease.

    ▪ Persistent cough, with or without hemoptysis (rust-colored or blood-tinged sputum)

    ▪ Hoarseness

- Altered breathing pattern: dyspnea, prolonged exhalation alternated with shallow breaths (obstruction), rapid, shallow breaths (pleuritic chest pain, elevated diaphragm)
- Altered breath sounds (wheezing), diminished, or absent breath sounds (obstruction)
- Chest wall masses
- Muffled heart sounds
- Pleural friction rub
- Clubbing of fingers
- Increased work of breathing (retractions, use of accessory muscle, stridor, nasal flaring)

○ Screening and Diagnostic Procedures

METHOD	EXPECTED FINDINGS	NURSING ACTIONS
Biopsy (bronchoscopy)	› Presence of tumor	› Keep client NPO after midnight. › Provide throat lozenges or sprays for report of a sore throat once the gag reflex returns following the procedure.
X-ray, CT scan	› Presence of tumor	› Explain and prepare client for the procedure.

M View Image: Lung Cancer Chest X-ray

Patient-Centered Care

- Nursing Care
  - Determine the pack-year history (number of packs of cigarettes smoked per day times the number of years smoked) for clients who smoke.
  - Evaluate use of other tobacco products (cigars, pipes, and chewing tobacco).
  - Ask about exposure to secondhand smoke.
  - Monitor for a cough that changes in pattern.
  - Monitor nutritional status, weight loss, and anorexia.
    - Promote adequate nutrition to provide needed calories for increased work of breathing and prevention of infection.
    - Encourage fluids to promote adequate hydration.
  - Maintain a patent airway and suction as needed.
  - Position the client in Fowler's position to maximize ventilation.
- Medications
  - Chemotherapy is the primary choice of treatment for lung cancers. It is often used in combination with radiation and/or surgery. Platinum compounds such as cisplatin (Platinol AQ) are commonly used.
  - Bronchodilators and corticosteroids can be given to help decrease inflammation and to dry secretions.

- Therapeutic Procedures
  - Targeted Therapy
    - Photodynamic therapy is performed through bronchoscopy to treat small, accessible tumors.
  - Radiation therapy is effective for lung cancer that has not spread beyond the chest wall and is used as an adjuvant therapy.
- Teamwork and Collaboration
  - Respiratory services should be consulted for inhalers, breathing treatments, and suctioning for airway management.
  - Rehabilitation care may be consulted if the client has prolonged weakness and needs assistance with increasing the level of activity.
- Surgical Interventions
  - The goal of surgery is to remove all tumor cells, including involved lymph nodes.
    - Often involves removal of a lung (pneumonectomy), lobe (lobectomy), segment (segmentectomy), or peripheral lung tissue (wedge resection).
  - Nursing Actions
    - Monitor vital signs, oxygenation (SaO$_2$, ABG values), and for evidence of hemorrhage.
    - Manage the chest tube and drainage system.
    - Administer oxygen and manage the ventilator if appropriate.
  - Client Education – Teach the client about the surgical procedure and chest tube placement.
- Care After Discharge
  - Client Education
    - Encourage the client to take rest periods as needed.
    - Encourage the client to eat high-calorie foods to promote energy.
    - Promote smoking cessation if the client smokes.

Complications

- Superior vena cava syndrome results from pressure placed on the vena cava by a tumor. It is a medical emergency.
  - Radiation and stent placement provide temporary relief. Prepare the client for radiation and stent placement.
  - Nursing Actions
    - Monitor for manifestations of superior vena cava syndrome and report to the provider immediately.
      - Early findings include facial edema, edema in neck, nosebleeds, peripheral edema, and dyspnea.
      - Late findings include mental status changes, cyanosis, hemorrhage, and hypotension.
    - Monitor vital signs and oxygenation during and after the procedure.

OROPHARYNGEAL CANCER

Overview

- Oral and pharyngeal carcinoma are more lethal than many types of cancer (cervical, testicular, thyroid, Hodgkin's lymphoma).
- There are three main types of oropharyngeal cancer:
    - Squamous cell carcinoma is the most common oral cancer and can be present on the lips, tongue, buccal mucosa, and oropharynx.
    - Basal cell carcinoma affects the lips and skin around the mouth.
    - Kaposi's sarcoma can be found on the hard palate, gums, tongue, or tonsils. Lesions appear as raised, purple nodules or plaques.
- Mouth lesions that do not heal within 2 weeks may be cancerous and should be reported to a provider.
- Oropharyngeal cancer has a high rate of recurrence.

Health Promotion and Disease Prevention

- Schedule dental visits twice yearly for cleaning and inspection of mouth tissues.
- Limit exposure to ultraviolet rays (mid-day sun exposure, indoor tanning).

Assessment

- Risk Factors
    - Tobacco use
    - Alcohol consumption
    - Radiation exposure, including x-rays of head and neck
    - Inadequate oral hygiene
    - Lack of fruits and vegetables in the diet
    - Occupation in textile, coal, metal, and plumbing industries
    - Age over 40 years
    - Human papilloma virus (HPV16) infection
    - Periodontal disease with mandibular bone loss
    - TP53 gene mutation
- Subjective and Objective Data
    - Mucosal erythroplasia (red patches) – earliest finding
    - Oral bleeding
    - Difficulty chewing or swallowing
    - Speech changes
    - Thick or absent saliva

- ○ Palpable masses
- ○ Facial paresthesia
- ○ Screening and Diagnostic Procedures

METHOD	EXPECTED FINDINGS	NURSING ACTIONS
Biopsy – fine-needle, incisional, excisional	› Presence of cancer	› Provide diagnosis-specific information to client.
Cell brushing (Oral CDx)	› Presence of cancer	› Inform client that a brush will be used to collect cells from suspicious areas in the mouth.
Toluidine blue 1% staining	› Malignant oral lesions retain blue stain	› Inform client that false positives are possible with inflammatory lesions.
MRI	› Presence of cancer › Thickness of lesion › Presence of nerve involvement	› Instruct and prepare client for procedure.

Patient-Centered Care

- • Protecting the airway and providing adequate nutrition are priority interventions in managing oropharyngeal cancer.
- • Nursing Care
  - ○ Monitor for adequate clearance of secretions (have the client turn, cough, deep breathe; suction as needed).
  - ○ Auscultate for adventitious lung sounds: wheezes (due to aspiration) or stridor (due to obstruction).
  - ○ Consult respiratory therapy to provide chest physiotherapy, as indicated.
  - ○ Position the client in semi- or high-Fowler's position to promote chest expansion.
  - ○ Use a cool mist face tent to promote clearance of secretions and reduce inflammation.
  - ○ Assess for difficulty swallowing.
  - ○ Perform oral hygiene every 2 hr (use an ultra-soft brush for a client who has a platelet count below 40,000/mm³).
- • Medications
  - ○ Targeted therapy
    - ▪ Body cells use growth factor (GF) for replication. In some types of cancer, cells have a greater number of GF receptors.
    - ▪ Medications that block GF receptors prevent tumor growth (cetuximab [Erbitux], erlotinib [Tarceva]).
  - ○ Antibiotics – for infection, as indicated
- • Teamwork and Collaboration
  - ○ Provide alternate means of communication for clients who have impaired communication (pen and paper, picture boards). Consult speech therapy, as indicated.
  - ○ Consult nutrition services to assess swallowing and provide nutrition recommendations, as needed.
- • Therapeutic Procedures
  - ○ Radiation, chemotherapy, or a combination of the two is used to treat oral lesions.
  - ○ Ablation (laser therapy, cryotherapy, or photodynamic therapy) is used to remove lesions.

- ○ Radiation (external, implanted, or both) is commonly used prior to surgery to reduce tumor size.
    - ▪ External radiation is used cautiously to minimize radiation dose to the brain and spinal cord.
    - ▪ Implanted radiation is used to cure early lesion on the floor of the mouth or anterior tongue.
    - ▪ Hospitalization is typically required until radiation dosing is complete.
- • Surgical Interventions
    - ○ Tumor excision is used to remove lesions through the inside of the mouth or through external entry into the head and neck.
        - ▪ The larger the tumor, the greater the risk to the client for disfigurement and loss of function.
        - ▪ Composite resections are the most extensive form of oral carcinoma surgery. They can include partial or total glossectomy and partial mandibulectomy.
        - ▪ Combined neck dissection, mandibulectomy, and oropharyngeal resection can be utilized ("commando" procedure).
        - ▪ Radical neck dissection can include removal of the sternocleidomastoid muscle, internal jugular vein, cranial nerve XI (accessory nerve), and all cervical lymph nodes on the affected side.
        - ▪ Surgery to remove large lesions may also include placement of a tracheostomy or wound drain.
    - ○ Nursing Actions
        - ▪ Provide clear liquid diet for 24 hr (clients having small lesions removed locally).
        - ▪ Maintain NPO status until intraoral suture lines heal (clients who have large tumors).
        - ▪ Provide routine tracheostomy care and suctioning, as appropriate.
        - ▪ Monitor wounds, incision sites, and donor grafting sites for evidence of infection.
        - ▪ Consult a speech language pathologist for clients who have slurred speech or difficulty speaking, as indicated.
        - ▪ Provide comfort to clients who have permanent loss of voice or disfigurement. Make a referral to counseling services, as indicated.
        - ▪ Teach clients to avoid mouthwashes containing alcohol or lemon-glycerin swabs (acidic) to prevent pain and worsening of condition.
        - ▪ Encourage the client to rinse mouth frequently with warm sodium bicarbonate or 0.9% sodium chloride solution.
    - ○ Client Education
        - ▪ Teach the client about the need and options for alternate communication following surgery.
        - ▪ Teach the client to keep the head of the bed elevated to reduce edema.
        - ▪ Instruct the client to report leakage of fluid from the suture line, swallowing difficulty, or coughing once oral intake is resumed.
        - ▪ Encourage the client to perform swallowing exercises regularly, as prescribed.
        - ▪ Teach the client and family how to thicken liquids prior to consumption, as indicted.
        - ▪ Instruct the client and family to continue thorough, frequent oral hygiene at home, cleansing the toothbrush after each use.
        - ▪ Instruct the client about possible temporary or permanent loss or changes in taste (dislike of meats, metallic taste).

Complications

- • Osteonecrosis (bone death) and issues related to motor impairment of jaw structure

---

ESOPHAGEAL CANCER

Overview

- Esophageal cancer is a fast-growing and metastasizing type of cancer.

- Cancers of the upper esophagus are typically squamous cell, and cancers of the lower esophagus are typically adenomas.

- Early findings are often vague, and the client's prognosis is significantly affected by a delay in seeking medical attention.

- Treatment often involves several weeks of chemotherapy and radiation therapy followed by surgery.

Health Promotion and Disease Prevention

- Avoid alcohol consumption.

- Promote smoking cessation.

- Avoid foods containing nitrites.

- Treat gastroesophageal reflux disease (GERD) with diet, positioning, and medications.

Assessment

- Risk Factors
  - Smoking
  - Alcohol use
  - Nitrites
  - GERD
  - Barrett's esophagus
- Subjective Data
  - Dysphagia
  - Odynophagia (painful swallowing)
  - Feeling of a lump in the throat
- Objective Data
  - Physical Assessment Findings
    - Weight loss
    - Chronic cough
    - Hoarseness
    - Halitosis
    - Regurgitation
    - Hiccups

○ Screening and Diagnostic Procedures

METHOD	EXPECTED FINDINGS	NURSING ACTIONS
Barium swallow (to evaluate dysphagia)	› Presence of tumor	› Administer stimulant laxative following procedure as prescribed (facilitates evacuation of barium, which may harden in the intestine).
Biopsy	› Cancerous cells	› Provide client with diagnosis-specific information.
Endoscopy (biopsy performed); esophagogastroduodenoscopy (EGD)	› Presence of tumor	› Instruct client not to eat or drink after midnight prior to procedure.

Patient-Centered Care

- Nursing Care
  - Obtain daily weight.
  - Support nutrition with a high-calorie diet, semi-soft foods and thickened liquids, and supplements. Maintain calorie count.
  - Monitor for aspiration during meals. Enteral feedings through a gastrostomy tube may be needed.
  - Keep the client's head elevated at least 30° at all times and higher after meals.
- Medications
  - Chemotherapy may be given prior to surgery to aid in shrinking the tumor, in place of surgery if the tumor is too extensive, or for palliation. Chemotherapy can make the tumor cells more susceptible to radiation.
    - Traditional chemotherapy (5-fluorouracil, cisplatin) may be used.
  - Targeted medication therapy – Monoclonal antibodies (MABs) may be used in conjunction with chemotherapy.
    - Angiogenesis inhibitors (inhibit growth of new blood vessels to tumors): bevacizumab (Avastin)
    - Tyrosine kinase inhibitors (decrease cell proliferation and increase cell death of certain cancers): cetuximab (Erbitux) and panitumumab (Vectibix)
- Therapeutic Procedures
  - Radiation can be effective in reducing the size of the tumor, making swallowing easier. Esophageal dilation may be needed after treatment in relation to esophageal strictures caused by scarring.
  - Antibiotics may be prescribed (prevention of endocarditis).
  - Photodynamic therapy (PDT)
    - Nursing Actions
      - Treat chest pain with opioids.
      - Treat nausea with antiemetic.
      - Monitor for difficulty breathing or swallowing.
    - Client Education
      - Instruct the client to avoid sun exposure for at least 6 weeks.
      - Instruct the client to consume a liquid diet for several days until pain subsides.

- Surgical Interventions
  - Esophagectomy/esophagogastrostomy
    - Some of the intestine may be used as an anatomic graft for the missing length of the esophagus. A more minimally invasive procedure may be done using a laparoscope, but esophageal cancer is usually too extensive for this type of surgery.
    - Pulmonary complications are common due to the location of the surgical incision.
    - Nursing Actions (pre, post)
      - Encourage the client to cough, deep breathe, and use the incentive spirometer every 1 to 2 hr (premedicate).
      - Instruct the client about tubes postoperatively.
      - Maintain the client in a semi-Fowler's position or higher.
      - Monitor chest tube and drainage.
      - Maintain NG tube patency and monitor drainage; do not replace NG tube if it comes out.
      - Do not manipulate or irrigate NG tube unless prescribed by the provider.
      - Provide enteral feedings if jejunostomy tube is placed.
      - Keep the client NPO until anastomosis has been determined to be patent (barium swallow).
      - Monitor for anastomotic leak (fever, saliva seeping through incision).
      - Provide the client with suction for oral secretions.

Complications

- Tracheoesophageal fistula formation and complete esophageal obstruction

---

COLORECTAL CANCER

Overview

- Colorectal cancer (CRC) is cancer of the rectum or colon. Most CRCs are adenocarcinoma, a tumor that arises from a gland in the epithelial layer of the colon.
- CRC occurs in stages from 0 to IV according to the tissue depth of the lesion and whether it has spread to local or distant sites.
- Adenocarcinoma begins as a polyp and is benign in the early stages. If left untreated, the polyp will grow and the risk of malignancy increases.
- CRC can metastasize (through blood or lymph) to the liver (most common site), lungs, brain, or bones. Spreading can occur as a result of peritoneal seeding (during surgical resection of tumor).
- The most common location of CRC is the rectosigmoidal region.

Health Promotion/Disease Prevention

- Consume a diet rich in calcium (calcium binds to free fatty acids and bile salts in the lower gastrointestinal tract).

Assessment

- Risk Factors
  - CRC is more common in women; rectal cancer is more common in men.
  - Adenomatous colon polyps
  - African American
  - Inflammatory Bowel Disease (ulcerative colitis, Crohn's disease)
  - High-fat, low-fiber diet
  - Older than 50 years of age
- Subjective and Objective Data
  - Blood in stool (many times the only clinical finding)
    - Left-sided tumors are more likely to produce frank bleeding and change in bowel pattern, consistency.
    - Right-sided tumors cause stools to be darker due to ulceration of the colon and intermittent bleeding.
  - Cramps and/or gas
  - Palpable mass (elicited by provider only through abdominal palpation or digital rectal exam)
  - Weight loss and fatigue
  - Vomiting
  - Abdominal distention
  - Abnormal bowel sounds indicative of obstruction (high-pitched tinkling bowel sounds)
  - Screening and Diagnostic Procedures

METHOD	EXPECTED FINDINGS	NURSING ACTIONS
Biopsy (endoscopic)	› Definitive diagnosis	› Provide client with diagnosis-specific information.
CT scan – traditional or CT guided colonoscopy	› Visualization of lesions (CT guided scan more accurate)	› Prepare client for procedure. › Instruct client on diet regimen (clear liquids then NPO after midnight) and bowel preparation for colonoscopy.
Endoscopy – colonoscopy, sigmoidoscopy	› Visualization of polyps or lesions	› Recommend screening between ages 50 and 75 (colonoscopy every 10 years, sigmoidoscopy every 5 years)
Barium enema	› Visualization and location of tumor	› Administer stimulant laxative following procedure as prescribed (facilitates evacuation of barium, which may harden in the intestine).
CBC	› Decreased hemoglobin, hematocrit	› Explain unexpected findings to the client.

METHOD	EXPECTED FINDINGS	NURSING ACTIONS
Carcinoembryonic antigen (CEA)	› Positive (denotes malignancy; not specific to CRC)	› Inform client that positive CEA can be indicative of many types of cancer.
Fecal occult blood testing (FOBT)	› Two positive stools within 3 days	› Do not use stool from digital rectal examination to avoid false-positive results. › Instruct client to avoid red meat, anti-inflammatory medications, and vitamin C for 48 hr prior to testing (to prevent false positives). › Recommend annual FOBT for clients ages 50 to 75.

- Virtual colonoscopy may be performed using CT scan or MRI. Imaging is performed after air is injected into the colon. The procedure is otherwise noninvasive. No sedation is required.
- Screening guidelines for individuals with polyps or a family history of CRC should be initiated at an earlier age and possibly performed more frequently.

Patient-Centered Care

- Surgical Interventions
  - ○ Colon resection (colectomy) involves the removal of a portion of the colon to excise the tumor. The remaining colon may be reconnected by (end-to-end) anastomosis or a colostomy can be created (temporary or permanent).
- Nursing Actions
  - ○ Assess the client's stoma (should be reddish pink, moist, small amount of blood postoperatively) and report ischemia, necrosis, or frank bleeding.

 View Image: Healthy Stoma

  - ○ Maintain nasogastric suction (decompression).
  - ○ Progress the diet slowly after suctioning is discontinued and monitor the client's response (bowel sounds present, no nausea or vomiting).
  - ○ Instruct the client to avoid heavy lifting.
  - ○ Instruct the client on the use of stool softeners as prescribed to avoid straining.
  - ○ Provide ostomy teaching (findings of ischemia to be reported to the provider, expected output, appliance management) if applicable.
  - ○ Management of a colostomy may be more difficult for the older adult client because of impaired vision and the decline in fine motor skills.
- Client Education
  - ○ Preoperatively
    - Educate the client regarding preoperative diet (clear liquids several days prior to surgery).
    - Instruct the client to complete bowel prep with cathartics as prescribed.
    - Inform the client of the administration of antibiotics (neomycin, metronidazole [Flagyl]) to eradicate intestinal flora.

- ○ Postoperatively
  - ▪ Educate the client regarding the care of the incision, activity limits, and ostomy care, if applicable.
- Teamwork and Collaboration
  - ○ Ostomy nurse referral for instruction on care of colostomy
  - ○ Referral to ostomy support group
- Therapeutic Procedures
  - ○ Chemotherapy is given for stage IV cancer.
  - ○ Adjuvant therapy may be given to decrease the chance of metastases for stage II and distant metastases for type III cancers.
  - ○ Targeted medication therapy – Monoclonal antibodies (MABs)
    - ▪ Angiogenesis inhibitors (inhibit growth of new blood vessels to tumors): bevacizumab (Avastin)
    - ▪ Tyrosine kinase inhibitors (decrease cell proliferation and increase cell death of certain cancers): cetuximab (Erbitux) and panitumumab (Vectibix)
  - ○ Radiation therapy is given in conjunction with chemotherapy to improve prognosis (usually used for rectal cancer to prevent lymph node involvement and recurrence).

Complications

- Second primary colorectal tumor or complete intestinal obstruction.

PANCREATIC CANCER

Overview

- Pancreatic carcinoma has vague manifestations and is usually diagnosed in late stages after liver or gall bladder involvement.
- Tumors are usually adeocarcinoma, originate in the pancreatic head, and grow rapidly in glandular patterns.
- It has a high mortality rate. Less than 20% live longer than 1 year after diagnosis.

Assessment

- Risk Factors
  - ○ Possible inherited risk
  - ○ 60 and 80 years of age
  - ○ Tobacco use
  - ○ Chronic pancreatitis
  - ○ Cirrhosis
  - ○ High intake of red meat (especially processed)
  - ○ Long-term exposure to gasoline and pesticides
  - ○ Diabetes mellitus

- Subjective Data
  - Pain that radiates to the back and is unrelieved by change in position, and is more severe at night
  - Fatigue
  - Anorexia
  - Pruritus
- Objective Data
  - Physical Assessment Findings
    - Weight loss
    - Palpable abdominal mass, enlarged gallbladder and liver
    - Hepatomegaly
    - Jaundice (late finding)
    - Clay colored stools
    - Dark, frothy urine
    - Ascites
    - Pruritus (buildup of bile salt)
    - Early satiety or anorexia
  - Screening and Diagnostic Procedures

METHOD	EXPECTED FINDINGS	NURSING ACTIONS
Biopsy (percutaneous or laparoscopic)	› Presence of cancer cells; holds some risk of seeding (not always performed if imaging shows tumor can be surgically removed)	› Provide diagnosis-specific information to the client.
Endoscopic retrograde cholangiopancreatography (ERCP)	› Definitive diagnosis of tumor	› Inform client that a biliary drain or stent may be placed during the procedure.
Abdominal paracentesis	› Presence of malignant cells in abdominal fluid	› Instruct client on care of dressing at puncture site and activity restrictions, as prescribed.
Carcinoembryonic antigen (CEA)	› Positive (denotes non-specific malignancy)	› Inform client that CEA can indicate many types of cancer.
Other laboratory testing	› Amylase, lipase, alkaline phosphatase, and bilirubin-elevated	› Elevated liver enzymes, albumin, and bilirubin can indicate primary or metastatic cancer.
Imaging	› Ultrasound or computerized tomography-visualization of the tumor during biopsy	› Prepare client and explain unexpected findings.

Patient-Centered Care

- Nursing Care
  - Care of a client who has pancreatic cancer usually focuses on palliation and not curative measures. Pain management is the priority intervention.
    - Advise client to ask for analgesics before the pain becomes severe.
  - Monitor blood glucose and administer insulin as prescribed.
  - A jejunostomy is often placed to provide enteral feedings (prevents reflux, promotes absorption). Provide nutritional support (enteral supplements, TPN).
- Nursing Actions – Increase feeding as tolerated, monitoring frequency of diarrhea.
- Therapeutic Procedures
  - Chemotherapy may be used to shrink tumor size. Several medications are given to improve the results.
  - Targeted therapy may be included.
  - Radiation may be used to shrink tumor size.
- Surgical Interventions – May be open or laparoscopic.
  - Partial pancreatectomy – small tumors
  - Whipple procedure – Removal of the head of the pancreas, duodenum, parts of the jejunum and stomach, gallbladder, and possibly the spleen. The pancreatic duct is connected to the common bile duct, and the stomach is connected to the jejunum.
  - Nursing Actions
    - Monitor NG tube and surgical drains for color and amount.
    - Monitor for bloody or bile-tinged drainage, which could indicate anastomotic disruption.
    - Place the client in semi-Fowler's position to facilitate lung expansion and to prevent stress on the suture line.
    - Monitor blood glucose and administer insulin as needed.
  - Client Education – Instruct the client about support measures for pain, anorexia, weight loss, and community resources.

Complications

- Fistulas – breakdown of a site of anastomosis
  - Nursing Actions – Report drainage that is not serosanguineous from the drain, or drainage from the wound to the provider immediately.
- Peritonitis – internal leakage of corrosive pancreatic fluid
  - Nursing Actions – Monitor for manifestations of peritonitis (elevated fever, WBC, abdominal pain, abdominal tenderness/rebound tenderness, alteration in bowel sounds, shoulder pain).
  - Administer antibiotics as prescribed.
- Thromboembolism – due to hypercoagulable state caused by release of necrotic products from the tumor, immobility postoperatively
  - Nursing Actions
    - Report findings of thromboembolism to the provider.
    - Administer anticoagulants as prescribed.
    - Maintain bedrest as indicated.

LIVER CANCER

Overview

- Hepatocellular carcinoma (HCC) is the most frequently occurring type of primary liver cancer. Primary liver cancer may also originate in the bile duct or liver vasculature.

Health Promotion and Disease Prevention

- Avoid excessive alcohol intake.
- Eat a low-fat diet and maintain a BMI less than 30.
- Receive a hepatitis B vaccination.
- Take precautions against hepatitis B and C (recognize that multiple sexual partners, IV drug use, and the sharing of needles all increase risk).

Assessment

- Risk Factors
  - Older age
  - Cirrhosis
    - Chronic hepatitis B or C infection
    - Alcoholic liver disease
    - Hemochromatosis (inability to breakdown iron)
  - Male gender
  - Tobacco use
  - Mediterranean or Asian heritage (particularly Vietnamese)
- Subjective Data
  - Abdominal pain
  - Loss of appetite
  - Weakness and fatigue
- Objective Data
  - Physical Assessment Findings
    - Weight loss
    - Enlarged liver upon palpation
    - Jaundice
    - Ascites
    - Pruritus
    - Encephalopathy
    - Bleeding or bruising

○ Screening and Diagnostic Procedures

METHOD	EXPECTED FINDINGS	NURSING ACTIONS
Biopsy – percutaneous or through the jugular to the hepatic veins (via fluoroscopy)	› Presence of cancerous cells	› Inform client that biopsy through venous route reduces the risk of hemorrhage. › Position the client to the right side for 1 to 2 hr to ensure hemostasis. › Monitor for hemorrhage (coagulation studies, frank bleeding).
Alpha fetoprotein (AFP)	› Elevated AFP – high probability of cancer (false positive – cirrhosis, hepatitis); elevated CEA along with elevated AFP can discriminate metastatic from primary cancer.	› Educate client about potential for false positives.
Other laboratory testing	› Alkaline phosphatase (ALP), serum aspartate aminotransferase (AST), albumin, and bilirubin – elevated	› Educate client about other reasons liver function tests might be elevated.
Imaging – contrast-enhanced ultrasound or CT scan	› Visualization of tumor	› Educate and prepare the client for procedure.

Patient-Centered Care

- Nursing Care

  ○ Observe for potential bleeding complications (frank bleeding, decreased hemoglobin and hematocrit, altered coagulation findings).

  ○ Administer blood products (packed red blood cells and fresh frozen plasma) to replace blood volume and clotting factors as prescribed by the provider.

  ○ Encourage the client to consume small, frequent meals that are high-calorie, moderate fat.

  ○ Replace vitamins due to the inability of the liver to store them (vitamin pills or vitamin-enriched supplements [Ensure, Boost]).

  ○ Restrict fluids for clients who have ascites.

  ○ Instruct the client on the benefits of avoiding alcohol (prevents further damage, allows for healing and regeneration of the liver, decreases risk of bleeding and other life-threatening complications).

  ○ Measure abdominal girth daily (indicates increased ascites).

  ○ Assess for adequate nutrition (fluid and electrolytes, weight loss, anorexia).

  ○ Monitor for worsening hepatic function (liver function tests, jaundice).

  ○ Assess and treat pain and abdominal discomfort.

  ○ Provide medications as prescribed.

    ▪ Medications are administered sparingly (especially opioids, sedatives, and barbiturates) due to impaired liver function (reduced ability to metabolize medications).

- Medications
  - Systemically delivered chemotherapy has been found to be largely ineffective in treating tumors of the liver or prolonging life. Therefore, more direct delivery methods are used.
  - Hepatic arterial infusion (HAI) is the direct infusion of chemotherapy via a catheter into the tumor. The client may go home with a catheter in place if continuous infusion is desired. Systemic adverse effects of chemotherapy are avoided through this delivery method.
    - Client Education – Instruct the client to watch for evidence of infection at the catheter site, hepatic toxicity (jaundice, liver function tests), and immunosuppression (fatigue, decreased WBC).
- Therapeutic Procedures
  - Hepatic artery embolization: Using a catheter threaded through the femoral artery and up to the liver, particles are injected into the arteries that supply blood to the tumor to block blood flow. If a chemotherapeutic drug is included, this procedure is called chemoembolization.
    - Nursing Actions – Monitor the client for bleeding.
  - Ablation procedures may be used to destroy cancerous cells.
    - Radiofrequency ablation delivers an electric current directly to the tumor via thin needles. This current is converted into heat waves that kill the cancer cells.
  - Percutaneous alcohol injections directly into the tumor mass cause cell death.
  - Cryotherapy uses liquid nitrogen injected directly into the tumor to destroy the tumor.
    - Nursing Actions
      - Monitor for hypothermia, bile leak, and hemorrhage.
      - Monitor urine for myoglobinuria.
  - External radiation is not generally used because healthy liver tissue does not tolerate high doses of radiation. Selective internal radiation therapy can be helpful for some clients.
- Surgical Interventions
  - Surgical resection or liver transplantation is required for long-term survival.
  - If liver cancer involves only one lobe of the liver, surgical removal may be indicated. A liver-lobe resection can result in a survival rate of up to 5 years. Most liver tumors are not resectable.
    - Nursing Actions
      - Inform the client about diagnostic tests that are done to determine if the liver cancer has metastasized (chest x-ray, PET scan, MRI, laparoscopy).
      - Monitor for altered blood glucose due to stress on the liver caused by surgery.
      - Monitor for bleeding and replace fluids and blood as necessary.
  - Liver transplantation may be an option for clients who have small primary tumors.
    - Immunosuppressants that are given after the transplant may increase the risk for recurrence of cancer and for development of secondary infection.

Complications

- Acute graft rejection post liver transplantation
- Liver failure or kidney failure (due to impaired blood flow to the kidneys)

RENAL CANCER

Overview

- Adenocarcinoma of the kidney, or renal cell cancer (RCC), is the most common form of kidney cancer.
- Paraneoplastic syndromes (syndromes resulting from cancer in the body) can occur with RCC. The tumor can produce hormones or prevent hormone production, causing imbalance in the body. Effects include:
  - Anemia (reduced erythropoietin)
  - Erythrocytosis (excess erythropoietin)
  - Hypercalcemia (tumor production of parathyroid hormone)
  - Liver dysfunction
  - Decreased libido and changes in secondary sex characteristics (increased human chronic gonadotropin [hCG])
  - Increased sedimentation rate
  - Hypertension (increased renin)
- RCC may be discovered when imaging studies or exploratory surgery are performed for other reasons.
- RCC that spreads to the inferior vena cava has a poor prognosis.

Health Promotion and Disease Prevention

- Minimize exposure to chemicals (environmental).

Assessment

- Risk Factors
  - Von Hippel-Lindau syndrome
  - Exposure to lead, cadmium, or phosphate
  - Age (55 to 60 years – highest incidence)
  - Family history of pelvic cancer
- Subjective and Objective Data
  - Smoky or cola-colored urine
  - Hematuria (late finding)
  - Inability to urinate or weak urine stream (urinary tract obstruction)
  - Flank pain (often dull, aching)
  - Nipple darkening
  - Gynecomastia (males)
  - Palpable mass
  - Renal bruit (possible)
  - Weight loss

○ Fever

○ Hypertension

○ Hypercalcemia

○ Screening and Diagnostic Procedures

METHOD	EXPECTED FINDINGS	NURSING ACTIONS
Biopsy (percutaneous through the flank)	› Positive for cancer	› Provide client with diagnosis-specific information. › Maintain client activity restrictions as prescribed (bedrest laying prone for at least 6 hr).
Urinalysis	› Hematuria (possible)	› Inform client of other reasons for hematuria.
CBC	› Hemoglobin and hematocrit – decreased	› Teach client about the role of the kidneys in red blood cell production.
ESR	› Increased (possible)	› Inform client of other reasons for elevated ESR.
Nuclear imaging – IV urogram with nephrograms	› Presence of tumor	› Prepare client for the procedure (keep NPO, assess for contrast dye allergy).
LFT	› Increased (possible)	› Inform client of other reasons for increased LFTs.
Imaging – CT, MRI, PET scans	› Identify tumor borders and presence in surrounding tissue	› Prepare client for imaging.

Patient-Centered Care

- Nursing Care

  ○ Monitor urine output and laboratory findings (BUN, serum creatinine, urinalysis) to assess renal function of the unaffected kidney.

- Therapeutic Procedures

  ○ Radiofrequency ablation is used to slow tumor growth in clients who have a single kidney or are poor candidates for surgery.

  ○ Biotherapy (interleukin-2, interferon, tumor necrosis factor) is not curative but is used to increase the client's lifespan.

  ○ Radiation is used to embolize arteries supplying blood to the tumor prior to surgery or as a palliative measure for clients who are not surgical candidates.

  ○ Chemotherapy, hormone therapy, and immunotherapy can also be prescribed.

- Surgical Interventions

  ○ Clients undergoing surgery for RCC are at increased risk for bleeding due to the highly vascular nature of RCC.

  ○ Nephrectomy is the standard of treatment for RCC.

    ▪ Ribs may be removed during surgery to allow better access to the kidney or tumor.

    ▪ Surgical entry may be transthoracic, lumbar, or abdominal. A wound drain may be placed.

- Adrenal glands are left intact, when possible.
- The unaffected kidney must be able to sustain adequate renal function.
- Nursing Actions
  □ Monitor for evidence of bleeding (hypotension, decreased urine output, altered level of consciousness). Blood may pool under client's back.
  □ Monitor hemoglobin and hematocrit every 6 to 12 hr for first 24 to 48 hr.
  □ Monitor urine output to evaluate remaining kidney function (25 to 30 mL/hr).
  □ Administer opioid analgesics for pain, as prescribed.
- Client Education
  □ Avoid lifting more than 5 lb or engaging in strenuous activity.
  □ Teach the client about measures to protect the function of the remaining kidney (control blood pressure, drink adequate fluids, limit NSAID use, stop smoking).

Complications

- Adrenal insufficiency
  - Manifestations of adrenal insufficiency are similar to those of hemorrhage (hypotension, decreased urine output, altered level of consciousness). This is a life-threatening emergency.
    - Hypotension and decreased volume of urine output are preceded by an increased volume in urine output.
    - Other manifestations include hyperkalemia, abdominal pain, and weakness.
  - Nursing Actions
    - Notify the provider of suspected adrenal insufficiency.
    - Administer corticosteroids, as prescribed.
    - Monitor ECG for dysrhythmia.
    - Administer medications to remove excess potassium and avoid potassium-sparing medications, as prescribed.
    - Monitor capillary blood glucose hourly.
    - Prevent and treat hypoglycemia (administer glucose, glucagon, or IV fluids containing dextrose) as prescribed.
    - Administer IV fluids as prescribed to offset volume depletion.
- Spinal cord decompression
  - RCC may expand and compress the spinal cord.
  - Key manifestations include sharp, severe pain that is "band like."
  - Nursing Actions
    - Report pain findings to the provider.
    - Prepare the client for imaging studies to assess for spinal cord decompression.

UROTHELIAL CANCER

Overview

- Cancer that can affect the urinary tract system or kidneys includes urothelial cancer, squamous cell cancer, and adenocarcinoma.

- Urothelial cancer affects the urinary tract, including portions of the kidney, renal pelvis, ureters, urinary bladder, and urethra. It is caused by changes to the urothelium (transitional cells which line these structures).

    ○ The bladder is the most common site of urothelial cancer.

    ○ Urothelial cancer typically has a multifocal origin and is highly invasive. Recurrence may occur up to 10 years after remission.

- Urothelial cancer is typically discovered when a cystoscopy is performed to evaluate painless hematuria.

Health Promotion and Disease Prevention

- Use personal protective equipment (PPE) when handling chemicals, paints, fertilizers, gasses, or items that contain certain environmental chemicals.

- When working with chemicals is unavoidable, shower and don clean clothing after task completion.

Assessment

- Risk Factors

    ○ Occupation: hairdresser or textile industry worker

    ○ Frequent contact with rubber, paint, or electric cable

    ○ Inhalation of gas, fumes, or chemical compounds

    ○ Tobacco use

    ○ Schistosoma haematobium (parasite) infection

    ○ Long-term cyclophosphamide (Cytoxan) use

    ○ Male gender

    ○ Chronic urinary tract inflammation

- Subjective and Objective Data

    ○ Hematuria

    ○ Dysuria, frequency, urgency (infection or obstruction present)

    ○ Weight loss

    ○ Anorexia

○ Screening and Diagnostic Procedures

METHOD	EXPECTED FINDINGS	NURSING ACTIONS
Biopsy (cystoscopic)	› Presence of cancer	› Prepare client for cystoscopy.
Bladder wash	› Presence of cancerous cells in saline "wash" solution (definitive diagnosis)	› Inform client that saline will be instilled into the bladder, then retrieved for microscopic examination.
Imaging – CT and MRI scan	› CT scan – extent of tumor invasion › MRI – depth and spread of tumor	› Prepare client for imaging.
Nuclear imaging – IV (excretory) urography and pyelography	› Possible changes in structure or function of the urinary tract	› Prepare client for procedure (keep NPO, assess for contrast allergy).
Urinalysis	› Microscopic or gross hematuria	› Inform the client of other possible reasons for hematuria.

Patient-Centered Care

- Medications

  ○ Bacillus Calmette-Guérin (BCG) (TheraCys BCG)

    ▪ BCG is a live virus compound commonly used to vaccinate high-risk individuals against tuberculosis.

    ▪ For urothelial cancer, BCG is infused into the bladder and retained for 2 hr.

    ▪ Nursing Actions

      ▫ Have the client void, then insert an indwelling urinary catheter for therapy infusion.

      ▫ After infusion, position the client on the back, abdomen, and each side for 15 min in each position.

      ▫ Assist the client to a standing position; ensure the client can safely stand for the second hour.

      ▫ After the 2 hr dwell time, the urinary catheter is removed and the client is instructed to sit to void. This position prevents urine splashing, reducing the risk of contamination.

      ▫ Provide or assist in perineal cleansing.

    ▪ Client Education

      ▫ Restrict fluids for 4 hr prior to infusion therapy.

      ▫ Teach the client precautions to prevent exposure of others to BCG over the following 24 hr. After each voiding (sitting position), the client should:

        ▸ Cleanse the genitals.

        ▸ Disinfect the urine by pouring 10% bleach solution (in an amount equal to the void) into the toilet prior to flushing.

        ▸ Cleanse the seat and toilet surfaces.

      ▫ Teach the client to wash clothing and linen that comes in contact with urine for 24 hr following infusion.

      ▫ Instruct the client to avoid sexual intercourse for 24 hr following the infusion.

- Therapeutic Procedures
  - Intravesical (inside the bladder) chemotherapy is used to treat carcinoma that has not metastasized.
  - Systemic chemotherapy or radiation is used to prolong the lifespan for clients who have metastatic carcinoma.
  - Radiation is the treatment of choice when surgery is not an option (client condition or advanced disease).
- Surgical Interventions
  - Surface excision, transurethral resection of bladder tumors, and partial cystectomy (removal of part of the bladder) are used to treat small, confined tumors.
  - Cystectomy with removal of surrounding tissue or muscle is used for large, invasive, or recurrent tumors. Intensive care may be required following extensive bladder repair. Ureters are diverted to another location.

SURGICAL INTERVENTION	URETER DIVERSION	PORTAL OF EXIT	URINARY ELIMINATION
Ileal conduit	› Ileum	› Abdominal stoma	› Continuous drainage into external pouch
Continent pouch	› Pouch created from large intestine	› Abdominal stoma › Penrose drain to collect lymph and secretions	› Client performs intermittent urinary catheterization. › Medena catheter remains until sutures heal.
Bladder reconstruction (neobladder)	› Pouch created from small intestine	› Urethra	› Client performs intermittent urinary catheterization.
Ureterosigmoidostomy	› Small intestine	› Anus	› During bowel movement

  - Internal or external drains or catheters can be placed intraoperatively.
  - Clients who have neobladder surgery are at risk for extreme weight loss.
  - Radical cystectomy with lymph node dissection includes the removal of other pelvic structures:
    - In males, the removal of the seminal vesicles and prostate with possible urethrectomy.
    - In females, the removal of the ovaries, fallopian tubes, uterus, cervix, anterior vaginal wall, and urethra.
  - Nursing Actions
    - Consult enterostomal therapy to assist with management and client/family education related to urinary diversion.
    - Provide adequate nutrition, snacks, and supplements to clients who have bladder reconstruction. Consult nutrition services as needed.
    - Monitor output from drains or catheters for expected color and amount.
    - Notify the provider if urine is decreased or absent in a client who has an external pouch.
    - Secure the client's external drainage catheter; notify the provider if it becomes dislodged or removed.

- ○ Client Education
    - ▪ Instruct the client to self-catheterize and plan procedure at timed intervals since there is no sensation of bladder fullness (neobladder, continent pouch).
    - ▪ Teach the client to monitor peristomal skin for redness, excoriation, or infection (ileal conduit, continent pouch).

Complications

- Hydronephrosis
    - ○ Inability to eliminate urine causes dilation of the renal pelvis.
    - ○ A tumor which blocks the urinary tract can prevent urinary elimination.
    - ○ Nursing Actions – Notify the provider if urine output is decreased or absent.

BREAST CANCER

Overview

- Breast cancer is the second-leading cause of cancer deaths in women in the United States.

Health Promotion and Disease Prevention

- Consume at least five servings of fruits and vegetables daily.

Assessment

- Risk Factors
    - ○ High genetic risk
        - ▪ First-degree relative with breast cancer (parent, sibling, child)
        - ▪ Early age at diagnosis
    - ○ Female gender (less than 1% of males develop breast cancer)
    - ○ Age over 40
    - ○ Early menarche
    - ○ Late menopause
    - ○ First pregnancy after age 30
    - ○ Early or prolonged use of oral contraceptives
    - ○ High-fat diet (possible risk)
    - ○ Low-fiber diet (possible risk)
    - ○ Excessive alcohol intake (possibly related to folic acid depletion)

- ○ Cigarette smoking
- ○ Exposure to low-level radiation
- ○ Hormone replacement therapy
- ○ Obesity
- ○ History of endometrial or ovarian cancer
- ○ Breast cancer rates are expected to increase over the next 50 years due to the increase of the older adult population.
- ○ Older adult clients are at greater risk of complications following surgery for cancer.
- • Subjective Data
  - ○ Breast change (appearance, texture, presence of lumps)
  - ○ Breast pain or soreness
- • Objective Data
  - ○ Physical Assessment Findings
    - ▪ Skin changes (peau d'orange)

 View Image: Breast Changes – Peau d'orange

    - ▪ Dimpling
    - ▪ Breast tumors (usually small, irregularly shaped, firm, nontender, and nonmobile)
    - ▪ Increased vascularity
    - ▪ Nipple discharge
    - ▪ Nipple retraction or ulceration
    - ▪ Enlarged lymph nodes
  - ○ Screening and Diagnostic Procedures
    - ▪ Breast cancer in men is often diagnosed later, with a poorer prognosis. Males at increased risk should discuss a screening plan with the provider.

METHOD	EXPECTED FINDINGS	NURSING ACTIONS
Biopsy (open or fine-needle)	› Definitive diagnosis of cancer cell type	› Provide diagnosis-specific information to the client.
Genetic testing	› BRCA1 and BRCA2 – presence of gene mutation increases breast cancer risk › HER2 – presence of excess HER2 (normal gene that causes cell replication) indicates the need for targeted therapy.	› Recommend genetic testing for BRCA1 and BRCA2 to clients at risk (two first-degree relatives diagnosed with breast cancer prior to age 50 or family history of breast and ovarian cancer).
MRI	› Better visualization of lesions in clients who have dense breasts.	› Prepare client for imaging.

 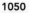

METHOD	EXPECTED FINDINGS	NURSING ACTIONS
Nuclear imaging – breast-specific gamma imaging (BSGI)	› Visualization of the lesion	› Inform client that scanning will display the "uptake" of the radioactive substance injected prior to the procedure.
Positron emission mammography (PEM) – type of PET scan	› Visualization of the lesion	› Inform client that PEM provides consistent images despite hormone fluctuations.
Ultrasound (US)	› Visualization of the lesion	› Inform client that US provides better visualization of lesions in clients who have dense breasts.
X-ray	› Visualization of the lesion (digital mammography is more accurate)	› Instruct clients over 40 years to schedule an annual mammogram.
Self-breast exam (SBE), clinical breast exam (CBE)	› Palpable tumors or lesions	› Instruct client to perform SBE monthly. › Instruct client to have regular CBE (every 3 years age 20 to 39; yearly over 40 years of age).

- Women with breast changes or at high risk should be screened earlier and more frequently. These clients should also have an MRI performed.

Patient-Centered Care

- Therapeutic Procedures
  - Adjuvant therapy follows surgery to decrease the risk of reoccurrence.
    - Hormone therapy – most effective in cancer cells with estrogen or progesterone receptors. This type of cancer has a better prognosis.
      - Gonadotropin-releasing hormone (GnRH)-leuprolide (Lupron)
        - Inhibits estrogen synthesis.
        - May be used in premenopausal women to stop or prevent the growth of breast tumors.
      - Selective estrogen receptor modulators (SERMs) – tamoxifen (Nolvadex) and raloxifene (Evista)
        - Used in women who are at high risk for breast cancer or who have advanced breast cancer.
        - Suppress the growth of remaining cancer cells postmastectomy or lumpectomy.
        - Tamoxifen has been found to increase the risk of endometrial cancer, deep-vein thrombosis, and pulmonary embolism. Raloxifene does not share these adverse effects.
    - Chemotherapy/radiation therapy
      - Chemotherapy and/or radiation may augment or replace a mastectomy, depending on several factors (client's age, hormone status related to menopause, genetic predisposition, and staging of disease).
      - Clients who undergo chemotherapy are usually given a combination of several medications (Cytoxan, Adriamycin, and fluorouracil).

    □ Radiation therapy is usually reserved for clients who had a lumpectomy or breast-conserving procedure.

      ▸ Whole or partial breast radiation may be prescribed. Skin care is a priority concern due to radiation damage as well as generalized fatigue.

      ▸ Brachytherapy with radioactive seeds may also be an option.

      ▸ Intraoperative radiation therapy allows an intense dose of radiation to be delivered directly to the surgical site.

- Other Medications

    □ Clients who have the HER2/neu gene may receive trastuzumab (Herceptin).

    □ Clients who have metastatic cancer may receive a vascular endothelial growth factor inhibitor, such as bevacizumab (Avastin).

- Other Procedures

    □ Stem-cell transplants are being researched in regard to treating clients who are at high risk of recurrence.

- Surgical Interventions

  ○ Surgical procedures include lumpectomy (breast-conserving), wide excision or partial mastectomy, total mastectomy, modified radical mastectomy (lymph nodes removed), radical mastectomy (lymph nodes and muscle removed), and reconstructive surgery.

M View Image: Total Mastectomy with Lymph Node Dissection

  ○ Nursing Actions

- Have the client sit with the head of the bed elevated 30° when awake and support her arm on a pillow. Laying on the unaffected side can relieve pain.

- Have the client wear a sling while ambulating (to support arm).

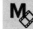

- Avoid administering injections, taking blood pressure, or obtaining blood from the client's affected arm. Place a sign above the client's bed regarding these precautions.

- Emphasize the importance of a well-fitting breast prosthesis for a client who had a mastectomy.

- Provide emotional support to the client and her family.

- Encourage the client to express feelings related to perception of sexuality and body image.

  ○ Client Education

- Teach the client how to care for her incision and drainage tubes. (Drains are usually left in for 1 to 3 weeks.)

- Advise the client to avoid placing her arm in a dependent arm position. This position will interfere with wound healing.

- Encourage early arm and hand exercises (squeezing a rubber ball, elbow flexion and extension, and hand-wall climbing) to prevent lymphedema and to regain full range of motion.

- Teach the client not to wear constrictive clothing and to avoid cuts and injuries to the affected arm.

- Teach/reinforce teaching regarding breast self-examination (BSE).

- Instruct the client to report numbness, pain, heaviness, or impaired motor function of the affected arm to the surgeon.

- Encourage the client to discuss breast reconstruction alternatives with the surgeon.

  □ Reconstruction may begin during the original breast removal procedure or after some healing has occurred.

  □ A tissue expander (a saline-filled implant that has a port through which additional saline can be injected, gradually expanding the tissue prior to permanent implant) is often placed during the original procedure.

  □ Saline or silicone implants are used for permanent placement.

  □ Autologous flaps may also be used for reconstruction.

  □ Nipple reconstruction may be done using tissue from the labia, abdomen, or inner thigh.

- Genetic counseling for clients who test positive for the BRCA1/BRCA2 genetic mutation includes recommendation of bilateral mastectomy and oophorectomy to prevent cancer occurrence. Clients who do not choose this option should have early, frequent, thorough screening for breast and ovarian cancer.

Complications

- Destruction of part of the chest wall and mastitis.

OVARIAN CANCER

Overview

- The exact etiology of ovarian cancer is unknown. However, the more times a woman ovulates in her lifetime seems to be a risk factor because ovarian cancer is more prevalent in women with early menarche, late-onset menopause, nulliparity, and those who use infertility agents.

- Metastases frequently occur before the primary ovarian malignancy is diagnosed.

Health Promotion and Disease Prevention

- Birth control pills and pregnancy may offer protection against ovarian cancer (reduced estrogen exposure).

Assessment

- Risk Factors

  ○ Over 40 years of age

  ○ Nulliparity or first pregnancy after 30 years of age

  ○ Family history of ovarian, breast, or colon cancer

  ○ History of dysmenorrhea or heavy bleeding

  ○ Endometriosis

  ○ High-fat diet (possible risk)

- ○ Hormone replacement therapy
- ○ Use of infertility medications
- ○ Older adult clients following surgery for cancer
- Subjective Data
  - ○ Abdominal pain or swelling
  - ○ Abdominal discomfort (dyspepsia, indigestion, gas, distention)
  - ○ Abdominal mass
  - ○ Urinary frequency
- Objective Data
  - ○ Screening and Diagnostic Procedures

METHOD	EXPECTED FINDINGS	NURSING ACTIONS
Physical assessment	› Enlarged ovary (possible if tumor is at least 4 inches)	› Inform client of possible causes of an enlarged ovary
Biopsy	› Presence of cancer cells	› Inform client that biopsy is usually performed during surgery to remove the tumor.
Genetic testing	› BRCA1 and BRCA2 – Presence of gene mutation increases breast cancer risk. › HER2 – Presence of excess HER2 (normal gene that causes cell replication) indicates the need for targeted therapy.	› Recommend genetic testing for BRCA1 and BRCA2 to clients at risk (two first-degree relatives diagnosed with breast cancer prior to age 50 or family history of breast and ovarian cancer).
Tumor markers	› Alpha fetoprotein (AFP) – elevated › Cancer antigen-125 (CA-125) – elevated (greater than 35 units/mL).	› Inform client that unexpected AFP findings indicate probability of cancer (false positive – cirrhosis, hepatitis) › Inform client that unexpected CA-125 findings indicate possible cancer (false positive – endometriosis, pregnancy, fibroids).

  - ▪ Staging of ovarian cancer is determined at the time of the hysterectomy or exploratory laparotomy when the tumor is removed and examined by the pathologist.

Patient-Centered Care

- Therapeutic Procedures
  - ○ Chemotherapy (traditional or intraperitoneal)
    - ▪ Chemotherapy is always given for ovarian cancer, even if surgery was performed. Cisplatin and carboplatin are the most common chemotherapeutic medications used for ovarian cancer.
    - ▪ Intraperitoneal therapy with dwell time, a form of intracavitary chemotherapy, may be used.
    - ▪ Nursing Actions – Instruct the client to report findings of infection, including peritonitis.
  - ○ Pelvic or abdominal irradiation is only used if the disease is localized to a small area or if palliative treatment of tumors is the goal.

- Surgical Interventions
  - A total abdominal hysterectomy with bilateral salpingectomy and oophorectomy (TAH with BSO) is the usual treatment for ovarian cancer.
    - A TAH with BSO also helps determine the extent of the disease as well as local and distant metastases. Staging of the cancer is done at this time.
    - Nursing Actions
      - Observe for urinary retention and difficulty voiding.
      - Assess bowel sounds. Paralytic ileus may be more common due to manipulation of the bowel during surgery.
      - Discuss sexuality, surgically induced menopause, and other self-image issues with the client.
    - Client Education
      - Instruct the client to avoid straining, driving, lifting more than 5 lb, douching, and participating in sexual intercourse until the provider gives release.
      - Instruct the client to immediately report evidence of infection, as well as vaginal discharge that is excessive or has a foul odor.

Complications

- Abdominal ascites and intestinal obstruction

UTERINE (ENDOMETRIAL) CANCER

Overview

- Uterine (endometrial) cancer is the fourth most common cancer in women.
- Endometrial cancer is the most common gynecological cancer.
- Endometrial cancer is more common in older adult women (related to prolonged exposure to estrogen).
- Estrogen therapy in postmenopausal women who have a uterus should include progesterone to decrease the risk of endometrial cancer.

Health Promotion and Disease Prevention

- Avoid the use of unopposed estrogen when considering postmenopausal hormone replacement therapy.

Assessment

- Risk Factors
  - Genetic mutation for hereditary nonpolyposis colon cancer (HNPCC)
  - Over 55 years of age
  - Obesity (due to fat cell production of estrogen)

- ○ Unopposed estrogen hormone replacement therapy
- ○ Nulliparity
- ○ Use of tamoxifen to prevent/treat breast cancer
- ○ Late menopause (longer-term exposure to significant estrogen levels)
- Subjective Data
  - ○ Irregular and/or postmenopausal bleeding
- Objective Data
  - ○ Screening and Diagnostic Procedures

METHOD	EXPECTED FINDINGS	NURSING ACTIONS
Biopsy	› Endometrial biopsy – presence of carcinoma	› Inform client that biopsy is usually performed through transvaginal ultrasound.
Pathology testing for staging	› Extent, size of tumor, and metastasis	› Inform client that this occurs after exploratory laparotomy or hysterectomy following tumor removal.
Genetic testing	› HNPCC testing – presence of the gene	› Inform client that presence of HNPCC increases the risk of carcinoma.
Tumor markers	› Alpha fetoprotein (AFP) – elevated › Cancer antigen-125 (CA-125) – positive	› Inform client that results indicate some type of carcinoma.

Patient-Centered Care

- Therapeutic Procedures
  - ○ Radiation therapy is given as adjuvant therapy, usually after a hysterectomy.
    - ▪ Brachytherapy and external radiation therapy may be options for cancer that is no longer limited to the uterus.
  - ○ Chemotherapy is useful in palliative care of endometrial cancer.
- Surgical Interventions
  - ○ Total hysterectomy with bilateral salpingectomy/oophorectomy is the standard treatment. The vagina is spared, allowing for sexual intercourse to continue.
    - ▪ An open, laparoscopic, or vaginal approach may be used.
    - ▪ Peritoneal fluid sampling during this procedure allows for testing of metastasis to the peritoneal cavity.
  - ○ Nursing Actions
    - ▪ Observe for urinary retention and difficulty voiding due to proximity to the urethra (more common after vaginal hysterectomy).
    - ▪ Monitor bowel sounds for paralytic ileus (more common due to manipulation of the bowel during surgery).
    - ▪ Discuss sexuality, surgically induced menopause, and other self-image issues with the client.

○ Client Education

- Instruct the client to avoid straining, driving, lifting more than 5 lb, douching, and sexual intercourse until the provider gives release.

- Instruct the client to immediately report evidence of infection, excess vaginal discharge, or foul-smelling drainage.

- Discuss hormone replacement therapy options with the client if she is premenopausal.

Complications

- Anemia and uterine perforation

CERVICAL CANCER

Overview

- Cervical cancer is a slow-growing cancer. With proper screening, it may be detected early and treated with good results.
- The incidence of cervical cancer is increasing and affecting a younger population than in the past.
- Early cervical cancer is often undetected. Manifestations do not occur until the cancer has become invasive.

Health Promotion and Disease Prevention

- Vaccination with human papilloma virus (HPV) vaccine (Gardasil, Cervarix) between 9 and 26 years of age.
- Limit the number of sexual partners.
- Use condoms during sexual intercourse.

Assessment

- Risk Factors
  ○ Infection with HPV, which is associated in 90% of cases
  ○ Chronic cervical inflammation/infections
  ○ Infection with HIV or other immunosuppressive disorder
  ○ History of sexually transmitted infections
  ○ Early sexual activity (before 18 years of age)
  ○ Client and/or male partner has had multiple sexual partners
  ○ Male partner who had a female partner with cervical cancer
  ○ Low economic status
  ○ Family history of cervical cancer
  ○ African American
  ○ Cigarette smoking

- Subjective Data
  - Painless vaginal bleeding between menses
  - Watery, blood-tinged vaginal discharge
  - Unexplained weight loss
  - Pelvic pain
  - Pain during and after vaginal sexual intercourse
- Objective Data
  - Screening and Diagnostic Procedures

METHOD	EXPECTED FINDINGS	NURSING ACTIONS
Biopsy	› Abnormal cells (follow-up to Pap test)	› Provide diagnosis-specific information to the client.
HPV typing – DNA test	› Presence of HPV on cervical cells	› Inform client that HPV increases the risk of cervical cancer.
Papanicolaou (Pap) test	› Abnormal cells	› Instruct client to begin Pap screening by 21 years of age (or 3 years following first sexual intercourse). Frequency of screening depends on many factors (age, results, presence of a cervix).

  - Simultaneous PAP smear and HPV testing improves the accuracy of the reading.

Patient-Centered Care

- Nursing Care – Administer antibiotics for pelvic, vaginal, or urinary tract infections.
- Therapeutic Procedures
  - Removal of the lesion by conization, cryotherapy, laser ablation, hysterectomy, or a loop electrosurgical excision procedure.
    - Client Education
      - Teach the client to report heavy vaginal bleeding, foul-smelling drainage, or fever to the provider. Vaginal discharge is normal.
      - Teach the client to avoid heavy lifting, vaginal penetration, douches, and tampons for the prescribed time (typically 3 weeks).
  - Radiation
    - Brachytherapy and external radiation therapy may be options for cancer that is no longer limited to local invasion.
    - Nursing Actions – Monitor the client for skin damage, especially in the perineal area.
    - Chemotherapy may be used along with radiation.

- Surgical Interventions
  - Clients who have early stage cervical cancer may require a simple hysterectomy (one that removes the uterus and cervix) or a radical hysterectomy (one that removes the uterus, upper third of the vagina, uterosacral uterovesical ligaments, and pelvic nodes). The choice to have a hysterectomy is guided by the client's condition and desire for future childbearing.
  - Clients who have more extensive cancer may require a more extensive pelvic surgery called exenteration.
    - Anterior exenteration involves removal of the uterus, cervix, fallopian tubes, vagina, ovaries, bladder, urethra, and pelvic lymph nodes. An ileal conduit is established for urinary diversion.
    - Posterior exenteration involves removal of the uterus, cervix, fallopian tubes, vagina, ovaries, anal canal, rectum, and descending colon. A colostomy is established for bowel diversion.
    - A total exenteration involves removal of all of the above organs and establishment of both urinary and bowel diversions.
    - Nursing Actions
      - Manage drains as well as urinary and bowel diversions.
      - Assess for body image disturbance and encourage the client to speak openly about it.
    - Client Education
      - Teach the client about findings of wound infection and how to care for drains that may remain after discharge.
      - Instruct the client about how to care for urinary and bowel diversion.
      - Instruct the client about how to care for perineal wounds and expectations regarding discharge.

Complications

- Fistula development can occur after pelvic exenteration.
- Kidney infections are also common secondary to the urinary diversion.

TESTICULAR CANCER

Overview

- Testicular cancer is the most common reproductive malignancy in men.
- The cause of testicular cancer is unknown.
- There are two categories of testicular cancer:
  - Germ cell (sperm-producing cells) – classified as seminomas or nonseminomas. Seminomas are the more common type of testicular carcinoma and have the better prognosis.
  - Non-germ cell – classified as interstitial cell tumors or androblastomas. Androblastomas can secrete estrogen.
- Primary testicular cancer is usually unilateral. Bilateral tumors typically indicate metastasis from another primary site.
- Sperm banking options should be discussed with the client soon after diagnosis. Semen must be stored prior to intervention (surgery, chemotherapy, or radiation).

Health Promotion and Disease Prevention

- Consume a healthy diet and exercise regularly.
- Testicular cancer rarely affects sexual function, but may affect fertility.

Assessment

- Risk Factors
  - Human immune deficiency virus (HIV) infection
  - Undescended testis (cryptorchidism)
  - Genetic disposition
  - Metastases
  - Age 20 to 54 (but can occur at any age)
- Subjective Data
  - Lumps and/or swelling of testes
  - Feeling of heaviness in the testicles
  - Evidence of metastasis (abdominal masses, gynecomastia, back pain)
- Objective Data
  - Enlarged testes without pain
  - Palpable lump (assessed by the provider)
  - Swelling of lymph nodes in the groin
  - Screening and Diagnostic Procedures

METHOD	EXPECTED FINDINGS	NURSING ACTIONS
Biopsy (open or fine-needle)	› Presence of cancer cells (definitive diagnosis)	› Provide diagnosis-specific information to the client.
Ultrasound	› Visualization of tumor composition (solid or fluid-filled)	› Prepare client for imaging.
Tumor markers	› Alpha fetoprotein (AFP) – elevated › Beta human chorionic gonadotropin (hCG) – elevated › Lactate dehydrogenase (LDH) – elevated	› Inform client that tumor markers indicate some type of carcinoma.
Testicular self-exam (TSE)	› Presence of a lump; change in size, shape, or consistency of testes	› Instruct client to perform TSE monthly beginning at age 15. › After showering or bathing, use a mirror to observe scrotal sac and then feel testes by rolling them between the thumbs and forefingers.

METHOD	EXPECTED FINDINGS	NURSING ACTIONS
Testosterone	› Levels increased (non-germ cell Leydig cancer)	› Assess client history for factors that may also increase testosterone levels (alcohol consumption, taking antiepileptic medications).
Sperm count	› Low (oligospermia) or absent (azoospermia) due to increased testicular temperature which may indicate cancer	› Discuss other reasons for altered sperm count with the client (occupation, clothing).

Patient-Centered Care

- Therapeutic Interventions
  - Chemotherapy or radiation may be prescribed depending on the type of tumor and stage of cancer.
    - External beam radiation therapy (EBRT) is used with precaution to protect the remaining testis.
- Surgical Interventions
  - Orchiectomy – removal of the affected testis with placement of prosthesis. This is the treatment of choice for testicular cancer.
    - Abdominal exploration with retroperitoneal lymph node dissection can require a large incision extending from the xiphoid process to the pubis. Provide routine care for postoperative abdominal surgery for these clients.
    - Minimally invasive laparoscopic surgery is possible for some clients.
    - Nursing Actions
      - Preoperative
        - ▸ Discuss the client's concerns about sexual function and childbearing.
        - ▸ Instruct the client on what to expect in relation to incisions and pain.
      - Postoperative
        - ▸ Monitor functioning of urinary catheter and nasogastric tube (open surgery).
        - ▸ Assess and treat pain (administer analgesia, provide cold therapy).
        - ▸ Observe incisions for evidence of infection.
    - Client Education
      - Instruct the client who has open orchiectomy that a stay in intensive care is usually required postoperatively.
      - Instruct the client to report manifestations of infection.
      - Instruct the client to avoid heavy lifting and strenuous activity as prescribed (several weeks for open orchiectomy).
      - Instruct the client to wear a scrotal support for several days.
      - Teach client to prevent irritation of scrotum by wearing a dry dressing and loose clothing.
      - Instruct the client to continue TSE and promptly report unexpected findings.

Complications

- Paralytic ileus

PROSTATE CANCER

Overview

- Prostate cancer is a slow-growing cancer. Conservative treatment may be the treatment of choice for a client, based on how fast the cancer is growing, if the cancer has spread, and the client's age and life expectancy.

- The posterior lobe or outer gland epithelium are sites of origin for most prostate cancer. It is usually slow-growing in response to androgen (testosterone and dihydrotestosterone [DHT]).

- Conservative treatment is preferred, dependent on several client factors (rate of cancer growth and spread, age, life expectancy). Treatment may be delayed up to 10 years following diagnosis.

- Manifestations are often similar to those of benign prostatic hyperplasia (BPH).

Health Promotion and Disease Prevention

- Consume a diet low in animal fat and high in omega-3 fatty acids (fish), fruits, and vegetables.

- Engage in regular exercise.

Assessment

- Risk Factors
  - History of vasectomy
  - Age greater than 65 years (risk increases with age)
  - Family history
  - African-American heritage
  - High-fat diet
  - BRCA2 mutation may be associated with an increased risk
  - Rapid growth of the prostate (benign high-grade prostatic intraepithelial neoplasia [PIN])
- Subjective Data
  - Urinary hesitancy and weak stream
  - Recurrent bladder infections
  - Urinary retention
  - Blood in urine and semen (late manifestation)
  - Painful ejaculation
- Objective Data
  - Significant residual urine after voiding a small amount of urine
  - Screening and Diagnostic Procedures

METHOD	EXPECTED FINDINGS	NURSING ACTIONS
Digital rectal examination (DRE)	› Hard prostate with palpable irregularities	› Instruct client to discuss prostate screening after age 50.
Biopsy	› Presence of cancer	› Provide diagnosis-specific information to the client.
Genetic testing	› BRCA2 – positive	› Inform client that presence of the gene increases cancer risk.
Prostate specific antigen (PSA)	› Elevation (greater than 4 ng/mL) indicates possible prostate disease (not specific to carcinoma).	› Instruct client to discuss prostate screening after age 50. › Insure that the client's PSA is assessed prior to DRE to promote accuracy of results.
Early prostate cancer antigen (EPCA-2)	› Positive (possible serum maker for prostate cancer)	› Inform client that positive results are highly indicative for prostate cancer.
Other laboratory testing	› BUN, serum creatinine – elevated (renal damage)	› Explain unexpected findings to the client.
Transrectal ultrasonography (TRUS)	› Visualization of lesions	› Inform client an enema will be administered prior to procedure.
Urinalysis	› Hematuria, bacteriuria	› Inform client about causes of hematuria and bacteriuria.

- Regular screening may begin as early as age 40 for individuals with high risk.
- PSA levels should reduce within a few days postoperatively.
- EPCA-2 is highly sensitive; if positive, biopsy may be excluded.

Patient-Centered Care

- Medications
  - Hormone therapy
    - Leuprolide acetate (Lupron) – gonadotropin-releasing hormone (GnRH)
      - Used in advanced prostate cancer to produce chemical castration.
      - Client Education
        - Warn the client that hot flashes are an adverse effect.
        - Tell the client that impotence and decreased libido may also be adverse effects.
        - Inform the client that he should be monitored for osteoporosis, which can occur due to testosterone suppression.
    - Flutamide (Eulexin) – androgen receptor blocker
      - Used in conjunction with a GnRH.
      - Client Education
        - Alert the client that gynecomastia is an adverse effect.
        - Inform the client that liver function tests should be periodically monitored.
    - If primary medications are not successful, high dose ketoconazole (Nizoral); an antifungal that blocks androgen production, or estrogen (diethylstilbestrol) can be given.

○ Chemotherapy may be used on clients whose cancer has spread or who have had minimal improvement with other therapies.

▪ Docetaxel (Taxotere) – usually used to treat breast cancer.

▫ Client Education – Have routine blood tests performed to monitor for neutropenia, leukopenia, thrombocytopenia, and anemia.

- Therapeutic Procedures

○ Radiation therapy – external beam radiation therapy or brachytherapy

- Surgical Interventions

○ Radical prostatectomy is the treatment of choice.

▪ Involves the removal of the prostate gland, along with the seminal vesicles, the cuff at the bladder neck, and the regional lymph nodes.

▪ Open or laparoscopic surgery may be done using a suprapubic, perineal, or retropubic approach.

▪ Perineal nerves are seldom disrupted, so the client should not experience sexual dysfunction.

▪ Nursing Actions

▫ Preoperatively – Ensure the client understands the procedure and what to expect postoperatively.

▫ Postoperatively

▸ Provide care that is consistent with other types of abdominal surgery.

▸ Manage pain with analgesics and cold therapy.

▸ Observe for evidence of infection.

▸ If the client has a suprapubic surgical approach, a suprapubic catheter is inserted (in addition to the urethral catheter).

▹ Provide catheter care and administer bladder antispasmodics to the client as prescribed.

▹ Monitor the client's suprapubic catheter output (usually removed when residual urine measurements are less than 75 mL).

▪ Client Education

▫ Instruct the client to report manifestations of infection.

▫ Teach catheter care if the client is home with one in place.

▫ Tell the client to avoid heavy lifting (up to 6 weeks) and strenuous activity (up to 12 weeks) as prescribed.

▫ Instruct the client to avoid tub baths for at least 2 to 3 weeks (open radical surgery).

▫ Teach the client Kegel exercises to reduce urinary incontinence.

○ Some clients may have a transurethral resection of the prostate (TURP) if obstruction occurs in the early stages of cancer before treatment is initiated.

○ Bilateral orchiectomy can slow the rate of tumor growth (decreases testosterone levels).

Complications

- Urinary incontinence
- Erectile dysfunction
- Radiation cystitis or proctitis

APPLICATION EXERCISES

1. A nurse is caring for a client who has leukemia and has developed thrombocytopenia. Which of the following is the priority nursing intervention?

    A. Plan rest periods throughout the day.

    B. Encourage cough, turn, and deep breathing every 2 hr.

    C. Assess temperature every 4 hr.

    D. Monitor platelet counts.

2. A nurse is reviewing the health record of a client who has suspected ovarian cancer. Which of the following findings supports this diagnosis? (Select all that apply.)

    _____ A. Previous treatment for endometriosis

    _____ B. Family history of colon cancer

    _____ C. First pregnancy at age 24

    _____ D. Report of scant menses

    _____ E. Use of oral contraceptives for 10 years

3. A nurse is caring for a client who is 24 hr postoperative liver lobectomy for hepatocellular carcinoma. Which of the following laboratory reports should the nurse monitor?

    A. Urine specific gravity

    B. Blood glucose

    C. Serum amylase

    D. D-dimer

4. A nurse is providing education regarding colon cancer to a group of women ranging from 45 to 65 years of age. Which of the following is an appropriate statement by the nurse?

    A. "Colonoscopies for individuals with no family history of cancer should begin at age 40."

    B. "A sigmoidoscopy is recommended every 5 years beginning at age 60."

    C. "Fecal occult blood tests should be done annually beginning at age 50."

    D. "An endoscopy provides a definitive diagnosis of colon cancer."

5. A nurse is caring for a client who has multiple types of skin lesions. Which of the following skin lesions are suggestive of a malignant melanoma? (Select all that apply.)

_____ A. Diffuse vesicles

_____ B. A uniformly colored papule

_____ C. Area with asymmetric borders

_____ D. A rough, scaly patch

_____ E. Irregular colored mole

6. A nurse is teaching a client who has a new diagnosis of prostate cancer. What should be included in the teaching? Use the Active Learning Template: Systems Disorder to complete this item to include the following sections:

A. Medications: Describe at least four medications and their uses.

B. Surgical Interventions: Describe a prostatectomy.

C. Nursing Interventions: Describe at least three.

APPLICATION EXERCISES KEY

1. A. INCORRECT: This is an appropriate intervention but not the priority intervention.

    B. INCORRECT: This is an appropriate intervention but not the priority intervention.

    C. INCORRECT: This is an appropriate intervention but not the priority intervention.

    D. **CORRECT:** The greatest risk to the client who has thrombocytopenia is bleeding. Bleeding precautions are generally implemented for platelet counts less than 50,000/mm³.

     NCLEX® Connection: Safety and Infection Control, Standard Precautions/Transmission-Based Precautions/Surgical Asepsis

2. A. **CORRECT:** Endometriosis is a risk factor for ovarian cancer.

    B. **CORRECT:** A family history of breast, ovarian, or colon cancer is a risk factor for ovarian cancer.

    C. INCORRECT: A first pregnancy after 30 years of age or nulliparity is a risk factor for ovarian cancer.

    D. INCORRECT: Dysmenorrhea or heavy bleeding is a risk factor for ovarian cancer.

    E. INCORRECT: Birth control pills offer protection against ovarian cancer.

     NCLEX® Connection: Health Promotion and Maintenance, Health Promotion/Disease Prevention

3. A. INCORRECT: Alterations in urine specific gravity following a liver lobectomy are not expected.

    B. **CORRECT:** Blood glucose should be monitored during the first 24 to 48 hr following a liver lobectomy due to decreased gluconeogenesis and stress to the liver from surgery.

    C. INCORRECT: Alterations in serum amylase following a liver lobectomy are not expected.

    D. INCORRECT: Alterations in the D-dimer following a liver lobectomy are not expected.

     NCLEX® Connection: Physiological Adaptations, Alterations in Body Systems

4. A. INCORRECT: A colonoscopy is recommended every 10 years beginning at age 50 for a client who has no family history of cancer.

    B. INCORRECT: A sigmoidoscopy is recommended every 5 years beginning at age 50.

    C. **CORRECT:** Fecal occult blood tests should be done annually by clients ages 50 to 75.

    D. INCORRECT: A biopsy performed during an endoscopic procedure confirms this diagnosis.

    Ⓝ NCLEX® Connection: Health Promotion and Maintenance, Aging Process

5. A. INCORRECT: Diffuse vesicles are consistent with an allergic reaction.

    B. INCORRECT: A uniformly colored papule is consistent with a birthmark or skin injury.

    C. **CORRECT:** A lesion with asymmetric borders is considered suspicious for a melanoma.

    D. INCORRECT: A rough, scaly patch is consistent with skin irritation due to friction.

    E. **CORRECT:** A lack of uniformity of pigmentation of a mole is considered suspicious for a melanoma.

    Ⓝ NCLEX® Connection: Physiological Adaptations, Pathophysiology

6. *Using the Active Learning Template: Systems Disorder*

    A. Medications

    - Hormone therapy: gonadotropin-releasing hormone (GnRH) – leuprolide acetate (Lupron)
    - Androgen receptor blocker – flutamide (Eulexin)
    - Chemotherapy – docetaxel (Taxotere)
    - Antifungal – ketoconazole (Nizoral)
    - Estrogen – diethylstilbestrol

    B. Surgical Interventions

    - Prostatectomy is the surgical removal of the prostate gland, seminal vesicles, bladder cuff, and regional lymph nodes. It may be done by an open surgery or laparoscopic approach in the suprapubic, perineal, or retropubic area. Perineal nerves are usually not disrupted, so the client should not experience sexual dysfunction.

    C. Nursing Interventions

    - Provide preoperative teaching.
    - Implement care consistent with abdominal surgery.
    - Monitor pain; administer analgesics and cold therapy.
    - Monitor for evidence of infections.
    - Provide catheter care (suprapubic or urethral); administer bladder antispasmodics.

    Ⓝ NCLEX® Connection: Physiological Adaptations, Pathophysiology

chapter 94

Overview

- Management of cancer pain is necessary to optimize quality of life for a person who has cancer.

- Not all clients who have cancer have pain.

- Cancer pain may be caused by the tumor or may be a result of the cancer treatment.

  - Direct cancer pain is caused by tumor pressure or cell invasion and can include tissue, bone, and nerve pain.

  - Pain due to cancer treatment can be caused by surgery, radiation, chemotherapy, or inactivity.

Definition of Pain

- Pain is subjective and can be indicative of tissue injury or impending tissue injury.

- Pain can have physical and emotional components.

- The reaction to pain varies from person to person and can be influenced by the age, gender, and culture.

- Pain can be acute or chronic.

  - Acute pain occurs suddenly and is short-term. Acute cancer pain can be the result of surgery.

  - Chronic results from nerve changes and lasts longer than 3 months. Chronic cancer pain is usually caused by tumor growth and the effects on surrounding tissue (destruction or pressure).

- Type of pain

  - Neuropathic – due to nerve damage; described as numb, tingling, shooting, burning, or radiating pain

  - Visceral/Deep – occurs in internal organs; may be difficult to identify; characterized by deep, sharp pain

  - Somatic – occurs in bone or connective tissues; may be described as throbbing or dull

Assessment of Cancer Pain

- The most reliable indicator of pain is verbal expression of pain from the client.
- The nursing assessment should be performed using standard pain measures (location, quality, intensity, timing, setting, associated symptoms, aggravating/relieving factors).
- Pain assessment also involves observing and documenting nonverbal indicators and physiological changes.
  - Nonverbal indicators of acute pain
    - Agitation and grimacing
    - Elevated heart rate, respiratory rate, and/or blood pressure
    - Diaphoresis and pupil dilation
    - Splinting of a certain area
  - Nonverbal indicators of chronic pain
    - Depression
    - Lethargy
    - Anger
    - Weakness
- Barriers to effective pain management
  - Inadequate pain assessment
  - Inadequate education of the client related to proper analgesic use
  - Knowledge of the health care professional regarding pharmacological pain management
    - Reluctance by the client to report pain
    - Client fears addiction leading to noncompliance
    - Inadequate dosing

Management of Cancer Pain

- Palliative cancer pain management is intended to provide comfort and reduce pain rather than to cure the cancer.
- The goal of palliative pain management is to reduce pain to improve quality of life while maintaining dignity and mental clarity.
- Methods of pain management – Surgery, chemotherapy, and radiation therapy may reduce pain by removing the tumor or reducing its size, which can alter pressure on adjacent tissues or organs.
- Nursing Actions – specific to each surgery or procedure
  - Client and family education
    - Include information regarding the specific procedure or treatment.
    - Include the family in care and management.
    - Provide information about support groups, such as the American Cancer Society.
    - Radiation – Instruct the client about specific skin care and to avoid sun exposure.
    - Chemotherapy – Include information about avoiding infection and managing other adverse effects.

Medications

- Pharmacological management of pain includes NSAIDs, opioids, antidepressants, anticonvulsants, steroids, and local anesthetics. Some clients who have cancer pain may require regular use of analgesics for pain control.

NONOPIOID MEDICATIONS AND NONSTEROIDAL ANTI-INFLAMMATORY MEDICATIONS	
Therapeutic Intent	› For mild to moderate pain
Medication	› Acetaminophen (Tylenol)
	› Ketorolac (Toradol)
	› Aspirin (acetylsalicylic acid)
	› Ibuprofen (Motrin)
	› Celecoxib (Celebrex)
Nursing Considerations	› Monitor for gastrointestinal (GI) bleeding, such as bloody stools or emesis that looks like coffee grounds.
	› Monitor for bruising and bleeding.
	› Do not administer acetaminophen to clients who have liver disease.
	› Monitor for tinnitus and hearing loss if NSAIDs are prescribed
Client Education	› Take with food to prevent GI upset.
	› Be alert to GI or other bleeding and bruising.
	› Do not crush or chew enteric-coated products.

OPIOIDS	
Therapeutic Intent	› For moderate to severe pain
	› For breakthrough pain
Medication	› Morphine sulfate
	› Meperidine (Demerol)
	› Hydromorphone (Dilaudid)
	› Oxycodone (Oxycontin)
	› Fentanyl (Sublimaze) available for transdermal use
Nursing Considerations	› Use with caution in older adult clients.
	› Monitor for respiratory depression.
	» Have naloxone (Narcan) available to reverse effects.
	› Administer stimulant laxatives to prevent opioid-induced constipation.
Client Education	› Use medication as directed.
	› Prevent constipation with diet changes and stool softeners if needed.
	› Be aware that nausea may subside after a few days.

ANTIDEPRESSANTS

Therapeutic Intent	› Reduce associated depression, promote sleep, and increase serotonin levels that may improve feelings of well-being › May decrease neuropathic pain
Medication	› Amitriptyline (Elavil) › Desipramine (Norpramin) › Imipramine (Tofranil)
Nursing Considerations	› Use with caution in older adult clients. › Do not administer to clients who have seizure disorders or a history of cardiac problems. › Use with caution in young adult clients or clients who are at risk for suicide, because antidepressants may increase suicide risk.
Client Education	› Notify provider if depression increases or if thoughts of suicide occur. › Be aware that therapeutic effects may take 2 to 3 weeks to become established.

ANTICONVULSANTS

Therapeutic Intent	› Treat neuralgia or neuropathic-type pain
Medication	› Gabapentin (Neurontin) › Valproic acid (Depakene) › Pregabalin (Lyrica) › Carbamazepine (Tegretol)
Nursing Considerations	› Monitor electrolytes. › Monitor medications levels. › Monitor for tremors. › Monitor for rash (life-threatening)
Client Education	› Avoid the use of alcohol. › Do not drive at the start of therapy. › Notify provider if rash or tremors occur.

STEROIDS

Therapeutic Intent	› May reduce pain by reducing swelling
Medication	› Prednisolone (Prelone) › Dexamethasone (Decadron)
Nursing Considerations	› Reduce dosage gradually. › Monitor for muscle weakness, joint pain, or fever. › Monitor serum glucose.
Client Education	› Use only as directed. › Do not discontinue suddenly. › Take with food.

ADJUNCTIVE AGENTS: SYMPATHOLYTIC AGENTS

Therapeutic Intent	› Treat neuropathic pain » Used in conjunction with bupivacaine in epidural or other local infusions.
Medication	› Clonidine (Catapres)
Nursing Considerations	› Monitor for hypotension.
Client Education	› Change positions slowly, because these medications may cause postural hypotension.

ADJUNCTIVE AGENTS: SKELETAL MUSCLE RELAXANTS

Therapeutic Intent	› May be used along with other pain medications for muscle spasms associated with cancer pain
Medication	› Baclofen (Lioresal)
Nursing Considerations	› Monitor for seizure activity.
Client Education	› Take with food. › Use caution when driving or operating machinery. › These medications can cause drowsiness and dizziness.

SYSTEMIC LOCAL ANESTHETICS

Therapeutic Intent	› May be administered via an infusion pump directly into the area of pain (intrathecal, intra-articular, intrapleural) to provide pain relief
Medication	› Lidocaine (Xylocaine) › Bupivacaine (Marcaine) › Ropivacaine (Naropin)
Nursing Considerations	› Monitor for hypotension. › Monitor for evidence of infection at the catheter insertion site. › Evaluate pain status. › Monitor for motor impairment and level of sedation. › Can be used in combination with a narcotic or another medication, such as clonidine (Catapres).
Client Education	› Monitor the infusion site for evidence of infection, such as redness or swelling. › Monitor for fever. › Notify provider of increased pain or decreased movement that may indicate a motor block. › Care for and protect the external catheter.

TOPICAL ANESTHETICS	
Therapeutic Intent	› Treat oral ulcers that may be caused by radiation or chemotherapy and neuropathic pain, such as in postmastectomy axillary pain
Medication	› Lidocaine HCl (Lidoderm patch) › Eutectic mixture of local anesthetic (EMLA) cream
Nursing Considerations	› Monitor for pain relief and local skin reaction.
Client Education	› Use as directed. › Use only on intact skin.

ADMINISTRATION METHOD	DESCRIPTION
Oral	› First choice for administration › Long-acting formulations available
Transdermal – Fentanyl (Sublimaze)	› Easy to administer › Slow onset, consistent dosing › Long duration (48 to 72 hr)
Rectal	› Contraindicated for clients who have decreased WBC or platelet count
Subcutaneous infusion – morphine or hydromorphone	› Slow infusion rate (2 to 4 mL/hr) › Requires nursing support › Risk of infiltration › Rapid onset
Intravenous	› Requires nursing support › Risk of infiltration › Rapid onset
Epidural or intrathecal	› Risk of infection, pruritus, and urinary retention › Requires nursing care to monitor, especially with increase in dosage › More effective than IV analgesia during immediate postoperative period

Anesthetic Interventions

- Regional nerve blocks
  - An anesthetic agent, such as bupivacaine, and/or a corticosteroid is injected directly into a nerve root to provide pain relief.
    - Used to identify or treat an isolated area of pain
      - For example, an intercostal nerve block may be used to treat chest or abdominal wall pain.
    - The procedure may take from 15 min to 1 hr, depending upon the area receiving the block.
  - Nursing Actions
    - Obtain baseline vital signs. Monitor blood pressure and vital signs during the procedure and for at least 1 hr following the procedure (follow established guidelines).
    - Establish IV access before the procedure.

- Monitor for manifestations of systemic infusion (metallic taste, ringing in ears, perioral numbness, seizures).

- Assess the insertion site for redness and swelling.

- Assess level of nerve block and pain.

- Protect area of numbness from injury.

- Client Education

  - Advise client to monitor the injection site for swelling, redness, or drainage.

  - Advise client to protect the area of numbness from injury and to notify the provider of increased pain or manifestations of systemic infusion (metallic taste, ringing in ears, perioral numbness, seizures).

- Epidural or intrathecal catheters

  - A local anesthetic or analgesic is injected into the epidural space (the area outside the dura mater of the spinal cord) or intrathecal space (the subarachnoid area within the spinal cord sheath that contains cerebrospinal fluid).

    - An external catheter is surgically placed under the skin with an external port for long-term use.

      - Used for chronic pain management

      - May be attached to a continuous infusion or injected as needed

      - Used for upper abdominal pain, thoracic pain, and pain located below the umbilicus

  - Nursing Actions

    - Monitor during insertion/injection and for at least 1 hr following insertion/injection (follow established guidelines) for hypotension, anaphylaxis, seizures, and dura puncture.

    - Monitor for respiratory depression and sedation.

    - Monitor the insertion site for hematoma and evidence of infection.

    - Assess the level of sensory block.

    - Evaluate leg strength prior to ambulating.

    - Local anesthetics block the sympathetic nervous system, causing peripheral vasodilation and hypotension. This can cause reduced stroke volume, cardiac output, and peripheral resistance. IV fluids may need to be increased to compensate for the sympathetic blocking effects of regional anesthetics.

  - Client Education

    - Advise the client to notify the provider of manifestations of infection (fever, swelling and redness, increase in pain or severe headache, sudden weakness to lower extremities, decrease in bowel or bladder control).

    - Notify the provider of manifestations of systemic infusion (metallic taste, ringing in ears, perioral numbness, seizures).

    - Long-term reactions may include sexual dysfunction or amenorrhea.

Other Invasive Techniques

- Neurolytic ablation
  - ○ Involves interrupting the nerve pathway or destroying the nerve roots that are causing pain; usually involves a CT-guided probe and injection of chemicals, such as phenol or ethanol.
    - ▪ For example, celiac plexus nerve ablation can be effective for pancreatic, stomach, abdominal, small bowel, and proximal colon pain.
    - ▪ The procedure is considered irreversible. However, nerve ablation can provide relief for several months until nerve fibers regenerate.
    - ▪ Nerve ablation can cause loss of sensory, motor, and autonomic function.
    - ▪ Use only when noninvasive methods are ineffective.
- Radiofrequency ablation
  - ○ Electrical current creates heat on a probe that is guided to the tumor or nerves and is used to destroy cancer cells or ablate nerve endings. This is often used for lung and bone tumors.
- Cryoanalgesia
  - ○ Uses a needlelike probe to deliver extreme cold to interfere with pain conduction via nerve pathways
  - ○ Nursing Actions
    - ▪ Monitor vital signs, especially blood pressure, during and for at least 1 hr following the procedure (follow established guidelines).
    - ▪ Monitor for manifestations of bleeding, such as tachycardia and hypotension.
    - ▪ Monitor for skin irritation.
    - ▪ Monitor for other effects such as diarrhea, loss of bladder or bowel control, or extremity weakness.
    - ▪ Assess pain relief.
  - ○ Client Education
    - ▪ Instruct the client to apply cold if needed for pain at the insertion site.
    - ▪ Continue to use pain medications as directed if needed.
    - ▪ Notify the provider of an increase in pain or weakness of extremities.

Alternative Approaches

- Alternative approaches to pain management may be used in addition to pain medications or other techniques. Many of these provide some pain reduction with minimal side/adverse effects.
  - ○ Transcutaneous electrical nerve stimulation (TENS)
    - ▪ Low-voltage electrical impulses are transmitted through electrodes that are attached to the skin near or over the area of pain. This is usually used in conjunction with analgesics. It changes the brain's perception of pain and may cause a release of endorphins.
    - ▪ Nursing Actions
      - □ Use with conductive gel.
      - □ Monitor electrode sites for burns or rash.
      - □ Offer other pain medications if indicated.
      - □ Do not use on clients who have pacemakers, infusion pumps, or cardiac dysrhythmias.

- Client Education
  - Instruct client to place the electrodes on clean, intact skin.
  - Advise client to inspect the skin under the electrodes to monitor for burns or irritation.
  - Advise client not to use if pregnant.
  - Advice client not to use near the head or over the heart.

○ Relaxation techniques and imagery

- Useful during a procedure or a period of increased pain.
- Relaxation techniques include deep breathing, progressive relaxation, and meditation.
- Positive imagery involves visualizing a peaceful image and may be used with audiotapes.
- Relaxation and imagery may reduce anxiety, stress, and related pain, and they can assist the client to feel more in control of the pain.

○ Distraction

- Music, television, exercise, and family and friends can be effective distractions from pain and stress. Other distractions include repetitive actions or movements, focused breathing, or use of a visual focal point. A change of scenery can offer a distraction from pain.

○ Application of heat or cold, pressure, massage, or vibration

- Heat increases blood flow, relaxes muscles, and reduces joint stiffness. Cold decreases inflammation and causes local analgesia.
  - Do not use heat or cold directly on skin that is damaged by radiation.
- Massage and vibration can cause relaxation, distraction, and increased surface circulation.

○ Acupuncture

- Acupuncture is a technique that involves the use of small needles inserted into the skin at different depths to stimulate and alter nerve pathways. May also increase the client's pain threshold.

○ Hypnosis

- Hypnosis involves using an altered state of awareness to redirect a client's perception of pain. It can be helpful to induce positive imagery, reduce anxiety, and improve coping.

○ Peer group support

- A support group helps provide emotional support for the client and family. Other benefits include the presence of a social network, availability of information, and help in strengthening coping skills.

APPLICATION EXERCISES

1. A nurse is caring for a client who has cancer pain. Which of the following is the most reliable indicator of the client's pain?

    A. Change in pulse rate

    B. Facial expression of pain

    C. Verbal report of pain

    D. Massaging an area of pain

2. A nurse is caring for a client who has chronic cancer pain and has a permanent epidural catheter for administration of a fentanyl/bupivacaine solution. The nurse should monitor the client for which of the following findings? (Select all that apply.)

    _____ A. Respiratory depression

    _____ B. Hypotension

    _____ C. Sedation

    _____ D. Muscle spasticity

    _____ E. Motor blockage

3. A nurse is caring for a client who is to undergo neurolytic ablation. The nurse should recognize that this treatment is used only when other measures have failed due to the risk of

    A. irreversible nerve damage.

    B. increased pain.

    C. myelosuppression.

    D. thrombocytopenia.

4. A nurse is caring for a client who has cancer. The goal of palliative pain management is to increase which of the following? (Select all that apply.)

    _____ A. Mental acuity

    _____ B. Physical mobility

    _____ C. Time spent at home

    _____ D. Quality of life

    _____ E. Bowel function

5. A nurse is planning care for a client who has cancer and is to undergo cryoanalgesia. Which of the following interventions should be included in the plan of care?

    A. Monitor oxygen saturation during the procedure.

    B. Instruct client to apply heat to the insertion site.

    C. Assess for irritated oral mucous membranes following the procedure

    D. Evaluate bladder control after the procedure.

6. An oncology clinical nurse specialist is leading a discussion with a group of nurses on the oncology unit regarding alternative approaches to pain management. What should the nurse specialist include in the discussion? Use the ATI Active Learning Template: Basic Concept to include the following:

    A. Related Content:
- Describe four approaches that can be used.
- Describe two nursing interventions for each approach.
- Describe one teaching point for each approach.

APPLICATION EXERCISES KEY

1. A. INCORRECT: Physiologic changes can indicate the presence of pain, but they are not the most reliable indicators.

    B. INCORRECT: Nonverbal indicators can support the presence of pain, but they are not the most reliable indicator.

    C. **CORRECT:** A client's verbal report of pain in the most reliable indicator of pain.

    D. INCORRECT: Nonverbal indicators can support the presence of pain, but they are not the most reliable indicator.

    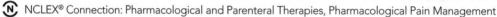 NCLEX® Connection: Pharmacological and Parenteral Therapies, Pharmacological Pain Management

2. A. **CORRECT:** Respiratory depression is an adverse effect of epidural analgesic and should be monitored.

    B. **CORRECT:** Hypotension is an adverse effect of epidural analgesic which can be corrected by administration of fluids and should be monitored.

    C. **CORRECT:** Sedation is an adverse effect of epidural analgesic and should be monitored.

    D. INCORRECT: Muscle weakness, not spasticity, is an adverse effect of epidural analgesic and should be monitored.

    E. **CORRECT:** Motor blockage is an adverse effect of epidural analgesic and should be monitored.

    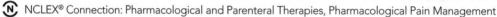 NCLEX® Connection: Pharmacological and Parenteral Therapies, Pharmacological Pain Management

3. A. **CORRECT:** Neurolytic ablation causes permanent nerve destruction and is used only after other methods have been unsuccessful.

    B. INCORRECT: Increased pain is not related to neurolytic ablation.

    C. INCORRECT: Myelosuppression is not related to neurolytic ablation.

    D. INCORRECT: Thrombocytopenia is not related to neurolytic ablation.

    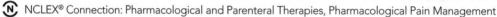 NCLEX® Connection: Reduction of Risk Potential, Therapeutic Procedures

4. A. INCORRECT: Maintaining mental clarity, rather than increasing it, is a goal of palliative therapy.

    B. **CORRECT:** Improved physical mobility occurs as a result of effective palliative pain management.

    C. **CORRECT:** Increased time in the home setting occurs as a result of effective palliative pain management.

    D. **CORRECT:** An increase in the quality of life occurs as a result of effective palliative pain management.

    E. INCORRECT: Effective pain management may alter or reduce bowel function as an adverse effect of the medication.

    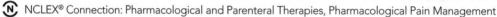 NCLEX® Connection: Basic Care and Comfort, Non-Pharmacological Comfort Interventions

5. A. INCORRECT: Blood pressure is the focus of vital sign monitoring to identify hypotension during and after cryoanalgesia.

   B. INCORRECT: The client should be instructed to apply cold to the insertion site for pain after cryoanalgesia.

   C. INCORRECT: The client's skin should be monitored for irritation following cryoanalgesia.

   D. **CORRECT:** Loss of bladder or bowel control is an effect of cryoanalgesia.

   Ⓝ NCLEX® Connection: Reduction of Risk Potential, Potential for Alterations in Body Systems

6. *Using the ATI Active Learning Template: Basic Concept*

   A. Related Content
   - Transcutaneous electrical nerve stimulation (TENS)
     - Use with conduction gel. Monitor electrode sites for burns or rash, offer pain medications if indicated. Do not use on clients who have pacemakers, infusion pumps, or dysrhythmias.
     - Place electrodes on clean, intact skin. Inspect skin under electrodes for burns or irritation. Do not use if pregnant. Do not use near the head or over the heart.
   - Relaxation and imagery
     - Use during a procedure or during a period of increased pain. Encourage deep breathing, progressive relaxation, meditation, or a focus on a peaceful image.
     - Can be used with audiotapes. Reduces stress, anxiety, and related pain, and promotes a feeling of control of the pain.
   - Application of heat or cold, pressure, massage or vibration
     - Apply heat to increase blood flow, relax muscles, and reduce joint stiffness. Apply cold to decrease inflammation and produce local analgesia. Massage can cause relaxation, distraction, and increased surface circulation.
     - Do not apply heat or cold directly to skin that is damaged by radiation. Avoid further skin irritation with excessive massage or vibration.
   - Distraction
     - Offer music. Encourage watching television, exercise, and activity with family and friends.
     - Use repetitive actions or movements, focused breathing, a visual focal point, and a change of scenery.
   - Acupuncture
     - Offer approach to increase the client's pain threshold. Make referral to appropriate community resource.
     - Small needles are inserted into the skin at different depths to stimulate and alter nerve pathways. This affects the pain threshold.
   - Hypnosis
     - Helps redirect client's perception of pain. Make referral to appropriate community resource.
     - Use to induce positive imagery, reduce anxiety, and improve coping.
   - Peer Group
     - Make referral to appropriate community resource. Encourage family participation as needed.
     - Provides emotional support for family members as well as client; offers the presence of a social network, availability of information, and strengthens coping skills.

   Ⓝ NCLEX® Connection: Basic Care and Comfort, Non-Pharmacological Comfort Interventions

UNIT 14   Nursing Care of Perioperative Clients

CHAPTERS

› Anesthesia and Moderate Sedation
› Preoperative Nursing Care
› Postoperative Nursing Care

NCLEX® CONNECTIONS

When reviewing the chapters in this unit, keep in mind the relevant sections of the NCLEX® outline, in particular:

Client Needs: Reduction of Risk Potential	Client Needs: Physiological Adaptation
› Relevant topics/tasks include: » Potential for Complications from Surgical Procedures and Health Alterations › Evaluate the client's response to postoperative interventions to prevent complications. » Therapeutic Procedures › Provide pre and/or postoperative education. › Provide preoperative care. › Provide intraoperative care. › Manage the client during and following a procedure with moderate sedation.	› Relevant topics/tasks include: » Alterations in Body Systems › Provide postoperative care.

chapter 95

Overview

- An anesthetic is a chemical agent that is administered prior to a surgical procedure to induce loss of consciousness, amnesia, and/or analgesia.
- Moderate sedation is a type of anesthesia. A client does not lose consciousness, but induction of amnesia and analgesia is still achieved.
- There are different types of anesthesia used in the surgical setting, and the nurse should be familiar with their side effects.

ANESTHESIA

Overview

- Anesthesia is a state of depressed CNS activity, marked by depression of consciousness, loss of responsiveness to stimulation, and/or muscle relaxation.
- Anesthesia is classified as general or local.
  - General anesthesia causes loss of sensation, consciousness, and reflexes. It is the method used when a client is undergoing major surgery, or one that will require complete muscle relaxation.
  - Local anesthesia causes loss of sensation without loss of consciousness. Local anesthetics block transmission along nerves. In turn, this provides for loss of autonomic function and muscle paralysis in a specific area of the body.

Risk Factors

- General anesthesia
  - Family history of malignant hyperthermia
  - Respiratory disease (hypoventilation)
  - Cardiac disease (dysrhythmias, altered cardiac output)
  - Gastric contents (aspiration)
  - Alcohol or drug use disorder
- Local anesthesia complications
  - Allergy to ester-type anesthetics
  - Alterations in peripheral circulation
- ⓖ Older adult clients are more susceptible than any other population to anesthetic agents.
  - Medications need to be titrated carefully to better control the incidence of unwanted effects.
  - Airway patency is the main priority in all situations, but cardiac problems can arise much more quickly in older adult clients.
  - The nurse should pay special attention when an older adult is undergoing a procedure, because the client's condition can deteriorate quickly.

General Anesthesia

- The phases of general anesthesia are

  ○ Induction – IV lines initiated, preoperative medications given, airway secured

  ○ Maintenance – surgery performed, airway maintenance

  ○ Emergence – surgery completed, removal of assistive airway devices

- Anesthetics used during general anesthesia are classified as either injectable or inhaled. Inhaled anesthetics are volatile gases or liquids that are dissolved in oxygen. Injectable anesthetics are given intravenously (IV).

  ○ Examples of inhalation anesthetic agents include halothane (Fluothane), isoflurane (Forane), and nitrous oxide in combination with oxygen.

  ○ Examples of IV anesthetic agents include benzodiazepines, etomidate (Amidate), propofol (Diprivan), ketamine (Ketalar), and short-acting barbiturates such as methohexital (Brevital) and thiopental (pentothal).

    ▪ Propofol is the most commonly used anesthetic agent.

    ▪ Propofol can be used while clients are on mechanical ventilation, during radiation therapy, and having a diagnostic procedure.

    ▪ Do not administer propofol if client has an allergy to eggs or soybean oil.

  ○ Inhalation anesthetics are eliminated predominantly through exhalation. The rate of elimination depends upon pulmonary ventilation and blood flow to the lungs. Postoperative administration of oxygen and encouraging the client to take deep breaths are important interventions.

- During administration of anesthetics, adjunct medications also are given. These substances are used to achieve further reactions as listed below:

OPIOIDS FENTANYL (SUBLIMAZE), SUFENTANIL (SUFENTA), ALFENTANIL (ALFENTA)	
Uses	› Sedation
	› Analgesic to relieve preoperative and postoperative pain
Adverse Effects	› Depresses the central nervous system, resulting in respiratory depression or distress
	› Delays awakening following surgery or a procedure
	› Can result in postoperative constipation and urinary retention
	› Can trigger nausea and vomiting
BENZODIAZEPINES DIAZEPAM (VALIUM), MIDAZOLAM (VERSED)	
Uses	› Reduce anxiety preoperative
	› Promote amnesia
	› Produce mild sedation (unconsciousness) with moderate to very little respiratory depression when titrated
Adverse Effects	› Can result in cardiac and respiratory arrest if not administered slowly or if doses are administered without waiting for the full effect to develop

ANTIEMETICS ONDANSETRON (ZOFRAN), METOCLOPRAMIDE (REGLAN), PROMETHAZINE (PHENERGAN)	
Uses	› Decrease post-anesthetic nausea and vomiting › Metoclopramide enhances gastric emptying › Promethazine induces sedation › Decrease the risk for aspiration
Adverse Effects	› Dry mouth › Dizziness › Use metoclopramide with caution if client has Parkinson's disease, asthma › Promethazine can cause respiratory depression and apnea
ANTICHOLINERGICS ATROPINE (ATROPAIR), GLYCOPYRROLATE (ROBINUL)	
Uses	› Decrease risk of bradycardia during surgery and, at times, vagal slowing of the heart due to parasympathetic response to surgical manipulation › Block muscarinic response to acetylcholine by decreasing salvation, bowel movement, gastrointestinal secretions › Slow mobility of the gastrointestinal tract › Decrease saliva, perspiration, and gastric and pancreatic secretions › Decrease risk for aspiration
Adverse Effects	› Urinary retention or difficulty starting urination › Tachycardia › Dry mouth › Decreased levodopa effects › Contraindicated with glaucoma or urinary problems
SEDATIVES PENTOBARBITAL (NEMBUTAL), SECOBARBITAL (SECONAL)	
Uses	› Sedative effect for preanesthesia sedation or amnesia effect › Induction of general anesthesia
Adverse Effects	› Avoid giving within 14 days of starting or stopping an MAO inhibitor › Respiratory depression
NEUROMUSCULAR BLOCKING AGENTS SUCCINYLCHOLINE (ANECTINE), VECURONIUM (NORCURON)	
Uses	› Skeletal muscle relaxation for surgery › Airway placement › In conjunction with IV anesthetic agents (propofol, opioids, benzodiazepines)
Adverse Effects	› Total flaccid paralysis › Requires mechanical ventilation because blocks contraction of all muscles, including the diaphragm and respiratory system

- Nursing Actions
  - Ensure that consent has been signed by the client, because legal consent cannot be given by a adult who is medicated.
  - Have the client void before the medication is administered so he will not need to get out of bed.
  - Ensure that the bed is in the low position and that the side rails are raised for safety.
  - Monitor airway and oxygen saturation.
  - Monitor and report laboratory values (ABGs, CBC, and electrolytes) as appropriate.
  - Monitor cardiac status (rhythm, heart rate, blood pressure).
  - Monitor temperature.
  - Monitor drains, tubes, catheters, and IV access throughout anesthesia and surgery.
  - Assess level of sedation and anesthesia (level of consciousness, vital signs).
  - If hypotension occurs as an adverse effect of medication or dehydration, lower the head of bed, administer a prescribed IV fluid bolus, and monitor.
  - Notify the surgeon and anesthesiologist if abnormalities are noted.

COMPLICATIONS OF GENERAL ANESTHESIA

MALIGNANT HYPERTHERMIA (MH)

Clinical Manifestations	› Acute life-threatening medical emergency.
	› Inherited muscle disorder, chemically induced by anesthetic agents.
	› Triggering agents include inhalation anesthetic agents, and the muscle relaxant succinylcholine
	› Hyper metabolic condition causing an alteration in calcium activity in muscle cells (muscle rigidity, hyperthermia, and damage to the central nervous system).
	› Tachycardia is a first manifestation, dysrhythmias, muscle rigidity, hypotension, tachypnea, skin mottling, cyanosis and protein in urine (myoglobinuria).
	› Elevated temperature is a late manifestation – rising 1° to 2° C (2° to 4° F) every 5 min.
Treatment	› Terminate surgery
	› Dantrolene (Dantrium) is a muscle relaxant to treat the condition
	› 100% oxygen, arterial blood gases
	› Infuse iced IV 0.9% sodium chloride
	› Apply a cooling blanket, ice to axillae, groin, neck and head, iced lavage

OVERDOSE OF ANESTHETIC

Clinical Manifestations	› Anesthetic and prescribed medication may cause complication related to the metabolize and interaction of the medication with the anesthetic.
	› May occur in an older client who has preexisting conditions
	› Occur in a client who has poor liver or kidney function
Treatment	› The nurse should complete pre-operative screening, documentation, and inform the provider or surgeon of pre-existing medical conditions and prescribed medications and allergies.

COMPLICATIONS OF GENERAL ANESTHESIA	
UNRECOGNIZED HYPOVENTILATION	
Clinical Manifestations	› Cardiac arrest, hypoxia and damage to the brain, and death may occur because of failure to adequately provide oxygen and exchange gases to the client during the surgery.
Treatment	› Monitor the end-tidal carbon dioxide levels of the client's expirations.
	› Check for malfunction of equipment and manually ventilate the client.
INTUBATION PROBLEMS	
Clinical Manifestations	› Injury to teeth, lips, and vocal cord during intubation may occur because the client's mouth is too small, inability to open the client's mouth wide, and mouth tumors.
	› Neck injury from improper neck extension during intubation may occur.
	› Sore throat
Treatment	› Nurse assist anesthesiologist with the intubation
	› Have available tracheostomy set-up.

Local Anesthesia

- There are three main methods of administration of local anesthesia
  - Topical – Applied directly to the skin or mucous membranes
  - Local infiltration – Injected directly into tissues through which a surgical incision is to be made.
  - Regional nerve block – Injected into or around specific nerves: four types of regional nerve blocks:
    - Spinal – Anesthetic is injected into the cerebral spinal fluid (CSF) in the subarachnoid space to provide autonomic, sensory, and motor blockade to the body below the level of innervation.
    - Epidural – Anesthetic is injected into the epidural space in the thoracic or lumbar areas of the spine, where sensory pathways are blocked, but motor function remains.
    - Nerve block – Injection of anesthetic around or into an area of nerves to block sensation. Often used for surgery to an extremity or for chronic pain.
    - Field block – Injection of anesthetic around the operative field commonly used for procedures of the chest, plastic surgery, dental, and hernia repairs.
    - Peripheral – injection of anesthetic into a specific nerve for analgesic and anesthetic use.
- Examples of local anesthetic agents include procaine (Novocain) and lidocaine (Xylocaine).
- Concurrent administration of a vasoconstrictor, usually epinephrine, is often used with local anesthetic administration to prolong the effects and to decrease the risk of systemic toxicity. This practice is avoided for distal injuries (finger) due to decreased circulation. Prolonged vasoconstriction could lead to tissue necrosis.
- Complications and Nursing Actions
  - Observe the client for systemic toxic reaction due to central nervous system (CNS) stimulation (headache, blurred vision, metallic taste). If untreated leads to unconsciousness, low blood pressure, apnea, cardiac arrest, and death.
    - Establish the client's airway, apply oxygen, and monitor oxygen saturation. Then notify the anesthesiologist and inform the surgeon.
    - Prepare to monitor client following anesthesiologist administering a fast-acting barbiturate such as thiopental (Pentothal) or methohexital (Brevital).
    - Monitor and report laboratory values (ABGs, CBC, and electrolytes) as appropriate.

- Monitor cardiac status (rhythm, heart rate, blood pressure).
- Monitor drains, tubes, catheters, and IV access throughout anesthesia and surgery
- Assess motor function to ensure paralysis does not ensue (movement returns first, then sense of touch, pain, warmth, and sensation of cold).
- Monitor for autonomic nervous system blockade (epidural and spinal) to include hypotension, bradycardia, nausea, and vomiting.
  - Lower head of bed, increase IV fluid if no restrictions, and frequently monitor vital signs.
- CSF leakage (spinal and epidural) manifests with a severe headache when head of bed is elevated.
  - Keep head of bed flat to promote the dura tear to seal.
  - Provide a quiet environment.
  - Keep the client well hydrated to help replace CSF loss.

MODERATE SEDATION

Overview

- Moderate sedation is the administration of sedatives and/or hypnotics to the point where the client is relaxed enough that minor procedures can be performed without discomfort, yet the client can respond to verbal stimuli, retains protective reflexes (gag reflex), is easily arousable, and, most importantly, independently maintains a patent airway.
- Only a qualified provider can administer moderate sedation. These include anesthesiologists, certified registered nurse anesthetists (CRNAs), attending providers, or RNs who are certified in advanced cardiac life support (ACLS) and are under the supervision of one of the previously mentioned providers.
- Continuously monitor a client who is undergoing moderate sedation. During the procedure, an RN must be present to monitor the client, with no other responsibilities at that time. This nurse is to remain with the client at all times before, during, and immediately after the procedure.
- Procedures that may require moderate sedation include:
  - Minor surgical procedures (dental, podiatric, plastic, and ophthalmic procedures).
  - Diagnostic procedures (various types of endoscopy, bone marrow aspiration, lumbar puncture).
  - Cardioversion.
  - Wound care (suturing, dressing changes, incision and drainage of abscesses, burn debridement).
  - Reduction and immobilization of fractures.
  - Placement and removal of implanted devices, catheters, and tubes.

Medications

- Medications used during moderate sedation
  - Opioids – morphine, fentanyl (Sublimaze), alfentanil (Alfenta)
  - Anesthetics – propofol (Diprivan)
  - Benzodiazepines – midazolam (Versed), diazepam (Valium), lorazepam (Ativan)

- Dosages required for "light sedation" are highly individualized and require careful titration.
- When a client receives moderate sedation, naloxone hydrochloride (Narcan) is used, if needed, to reverse the adverse effects of the opioid. If needed, flumazenil (Romazicon) is administered to reverse the adverse effects of the benzodiazepines.

Risk Factors

- Older adult clients are at a greater risk of adverse reactions to sedation medications because of decreased liver and kidney function that occurs with aging.
- Older adult clients have less physiologic reserve than younger clients, which may cause decreased immune system response and decreased wound healing.
  - Reduction of muscle mass and the amount of body water places the older adult client at risk for dehydration.
- Be aware and maintain a safe environment for older adult clients, due to sensory limitations.
- Pay careful attention to cardiac and respiratory status in the older adult clients, as problems may arise more quickly.

Nursing Actions

- Preprocedure
  - Obtain a full history from the client, including allergies, medication usage, and pre-existing medical conditions (pulmonary disease). Any previous experiences with sedation or anesthesia should to be reported, especially any adverse reactions. Note the last dose of each of the client's prescribed medications, especially if it could alter the client's response (diuretic, antihypertensive, narcotic).
  - Provide education about the procedure and the medications to be used.
  - Perform a full assessment on the client, including baseline vital signs, cardiac rhythm, and level of consciousness.
  - Determine the last time the client ate or drank (generally NPO for 6 hr or more before the procedure).
    - The client may have clear liquids up to 2 hr before the surgery or procedure.
    - Instruct the client to adhere to the instructions to remain NPO, or the surgery or procedure may be cancelled.
  - Establish IV access and administer fluids as prescribed.
  - Verify that the client signed the informed consent.
  - Attach monitoring equipment to the client.
  - Remove dentures (in case intubation would become necessary).
- Intraprocedure
  - Remain with the client at all times. Allow other staff to assist the provider with the procedure, if indicated.
  - Continually assess and monitor level of consciousness (Glasgow coma scale score), cardiac rhythm, respiratory status, and vital signs.
  - Maintain a safe environment for the older adult client due to sensory limitations.

○ Pay careful attention to cardiac and respiratory status for older adult clients, as problems can arise more quickly.

○ During the procedure, the following equipment must be present within immediate reach for routine monitoring and in case deep sedation with respiratory depression occurs.

▪ Fully equipped emergency cart that includes emergency medications, airway and ventilatory equipment, defibrillator, and IV supplies

▪ A 100% oxygen source and administration supplies, airways, manual resuscitation bag, and suction equipment

▪ ECG monitor/display, noninvasive blood pressure monitor, pulse oximeter, thermometer, and stethoscope

• Postprocedure

○ The nurse who is monitoring should continue to record vital signs and level of consciousness until the client is fully awake and all assessment criteria return to presedation levels. Only then can the nurse remove the monitor and all emergency equipment from the bedside.

○ Typical discharge criteria

▪ Level of consciousness as on admission

▪ Vital signs stable for 30 to 90 min

▪ Ability to cough and deep breathe

▪ Ability to tolerate oral fluids

▪ Ability to void

▪ Absence of nausea, vomiting, shortness of breath, or dizziness

Complications and Nursing Actions

• Before, during, and after the procedure, emergency equipment is to remain at the client's bedside. Some complications that can arise from moderate sedation include:

○ Airway obstruction, respiratory depression (administer reversal agents and oxygen), cardiac arrhythmias, hypotension, and anaphylaxis

▪ Insert airway and suction.

○ Respiratory depression

▪ Administer oxygen and reversal agents, such as naloxone (Narcan) and flumazenil (Romazicon).

○ Cardiac arrhythmias

▪ Set up a 12-lead ECG and provide antidysrhythmics and fluids.

○ Hypotension

▪ Provide fluids and vasopressors.

○ Anaphylaxis

▪ Administer epinephrine.

• Most hospitals and facilities require that for moderate sedation an RN is certified in ACLS or pediatric advanced life support (PALS) in case of an emergency. In all instances of complications, the sedation needs to be stopped and care given to the client to alleviate the problem.

APPLICATION EXERCISES

1. A nurse has administered midazolam (Versed) IV bolus to a client before a procedure. The client's blood pressure is 86/40 mm Hg and pulse is 134/min. Which of the following is an appropriate action by the nurse?

    A. Administer naloxone (Narcan) IV.

    B. Administer morphine IV.

    C. Administer 0.9% sodium chloride IV bolus.

    D. Administer atropine IV.

2. A nurse is assisting an anesthesiologist in the delivery of nitrous oxide per face mask to a client during the induction of anesthesia. Which of the following is a priority nursing action?

    A. Assess oxygen saturation.

    B. Obtain blood pressure.

    C. Palpate heart rate.

    D. Check temperature.

3. A nurse is providing information to a group of surgical nurses for the treatment of malignant hyperthermia. Which of the following should the nurse include in the information?

    _____ A. Infuse iced IV fluids.

    _____ B. Provide 100% oxygen.

    _____ C. Place on a cooling blanket.

    _____ D. Treat the condition while continuing surgery.

    _____ E. Administer IV dantrolene (Dantrium).

4. A nurse is caring for a client who displays systemic toxic reaction following a regional block. Which of the following actions by the nurse is appropriate?

    A. Monitor serum creatinine levels.

    B. Prepare to administer IV thiopental (Pentothal).

    C. Turn client to the right side.

    D. Administration 0.9% sodium chloride 500 mL IV bolus.

5. A nurse is caring for a client who reports a headache following an epidural regional nerve block. Which of the following is an appropriate nursing action?

    A. Decrease the client's fluid intake.

    B. Apply pressure to the puncture site.

    C. Place the client's head of bed flat.

    D. Instruct the client to lie prone.

6. A nurse is preparing to administer moderate sedation to a client who is to have a colonoscopy. What considerations should the nurse plan to prepare in the care of the client? Use the ATI Active Learning Template: Basic Concept to complete this item to include the following:

    A. Related Content: List three medications and classifications used for moderate sedation.

    B. Underlying Principles: Define the purpose of moderate sedation.

    C. Nursing Interventions: List two interventions for each: preprocedure, intraprocedure, and postprocedure.

APPLICATION EXERCISES KEY

1. A. INCORRECT: Naloxone is administered for respiratory depression caused by an opioid medication. This is not an appropriate action by the nurse.

    B. INCORRECT: Morphine sulfate is administered for pain and can cause hypotension and respiratory depression. This is not an appropriate action by the nurse.

    C. **CORRECT:** An IV fluid bolus should increase the client's hypotension and tachycardia to promote adequate cardiac output and tissue perfusion.

    D. INCORRECT: Atropine sulfate is administered for bradycardia. This is not an appropriate action by the nurse.

     NCLEX® Connection: Physiological Adaptations, Unexpected Response to Therapies

2. A. **CORRECT:** The greatest risk for the client is injury from hypoxia. The first action is to assess the client's oxygen saturations.

    B. INCORRECT: Obtaining blood pressure is important but is not the priority action by the nurse.

    C. INCORRECT: Palpating heart rate is important but is not the priority action by the nurse.

    D. INCORRECT: Checking temperature at the time of induction is not the priority action by the nurse.

     NCLEX® Connection: Reduction of Risk Potential, Therapeutic Procedures

3. A. **CORRECT:** Infusing iced IV fluids should help lower the client's rapidly rising temperature.

    B. **CORRECT:** Providing 100% oxygen will help to prevent hypoxia due to muscle tremors and rigidity from increased lactic acid.

    C. **CORRECT:** Placing the client on a cooling blanket will help lower the rapidly rising temperature.

    D. INCORRECT: Terminating surgery should occur as soon as malignant hyperthermia is suspected.

    E. **CORRECT:** Dantrolene IV is a muscle relaxant used to treat malignant hyperthermia.

     NCLEX® Connection: Physiological Adaptations, Medical Emergencies

4. A. INCORRECT: ABGs, CBC, and electrolytes, not serum creatinine levels, are monitored for systemic toxic reaction to a regional block

    B. **CORRECT:** Thiopental is a fast-acting barbiturate administered by an anesthesiologist for treatment of systemic toxic reaction to a spinal block.

    C. INCORRECT: Turning the client to the right side is not indicated as a treatment for systemic toxic reaction to a regional block.

    D. INCORRECT: Clinical manifestations of systemic toxic reaction include hypertension. Administration of a 500 mL IV bolus would exacerbate the problem.

     NCLEX® Connection: Physiological Adaptations, Medical Emergencies

5. A. INCORRECT: Increase fluid intake to keep the client well-hydrated and to help replace the cerebral spinal fluid.

    B. INCORRECT: Applying pressure to the puncture site is not an appropriate nursing action and will not relieve the headache from cerebral spinal fluid leakage.

    C. **CORRECT:** Placing the client's head of bed flat will decrease the intensity of the headache and decrease cerebral spinal fluid leakage.

    D. INCORRECT: Instructing the client to lie prone is not an appropriate action by the nurse in the treatment of a headache caused from cerebral spinal fluid leakage.

    (N) NCLEX® Connection: Reduction of Risk Potential, Potential for Complications of Diagnostic Tests/ Treatments/Procedures

6. *Using the ATI Active Learning Template: Basic Concept*

    A. Related Content
    - Fentanyl (Sublimaze) – opioid
    - Propofol (Diprivan) – anesthetic
    - Midazolam (Versed) – benzodiazepine

    B. Underlying Principles
    - The purpose of moderate sedation is to relax the client to a point where discomfort is not felt, yet the client is able to respond to verbal stimuli, retains reflexes (gag reflex), and is easily aroused.

    C. Nursing Interventions
    - Preprocedure
      - Instruct the client to be NPO for 6 hr before the procedure.
      - Attach monitor equipment.
      - Start IV access.
      - Verify informed consent.
    - Intraprocedure
      - Assess the level of consciousness.
      - Monitor cardiac and respiratory status.
      - Have emergency cart and equipment available in the room.
      - Have oxygen and suction equipment ready and available if needed.
    - Postprocedure
      - Continue to monitor vital signs and consciousness.
      - Determine ability to cough, deep breathe, and swallow.
      - Assess for nausea, vomiting, shortness of breath, or dizziness before discharge.

    (N) NCLEX® Connection: Reduction of Risk Potential, Therapeutic Procedures

chapter 96

Overview

- Surgery can take on many forms, including curative, palliative, cosmetic, and functional.
- Inpatient surgical procedures are performed by three categories: emergent, urgent, or elective type surgery.
- Outpatient or ambulatory surgery generally is an elective surgery that is not considered acute (cataract removal, hernia repair).
- Preoperative care takes place from the time a client is scheduled for surgery until care is transferred to the operating suite.
- Assessment of risk factors is one of the major aspects of preoperative care. Preoperative care includes a thorough assessment of the client's physical, emotional, and psychosocial status prior to surgery.

Risk Factors

- Surgery
  - Infection (risk of sepsis)
  - Anemia (malnutrition, oxygenation, healing impact)
  - Hypovolemia from dehydration or blood loss (circulatory compromise)
  - Electrolyte imbalance through inadequate diet or disease process (dysrhythmias)
  - Age (older adults are at greater risk because of decreased liver and kidney function due to age, and the use of multiple prescribed medications)
  - Pregnancy (fetal risk with anesthesia)
  - Respiratory disease (COPD, pneumonia, asthma)
  - Cardiovascular disease (cerebrovascular accident, heart failure, myocardial infarction, hypertension, dysrhythmias)
  - Diabetes mellitus (decreased intestinal motility, altered blood glucose levels, delayed healing)
  - Liver disease (altered medication metabolism and increased risk for bleeding)
  - Kidney disease (altered elimination and medication excretion)
  - Endocrine disorders (hypo/hyperthyroidism, Addison's disease, Cushing's syndrome)
  - Immune system disorders (allergies, immunocompromised)
  - Coagulation defect (increased risk of bleeding)
  - Malnutrition (delayed healing)
  - Obesity (pulmonary complications due to hypoventilation, impact on anesthesia, elimination, and wound healing)
  - Certain medications (antihypertensives, anticoagulants, NSAIDs, tricyclic antidepressants, herbal medications, over-the-counter medications)
  - Substance use (tobacco, alcohol)
  - Family history (malignant hyperthermia)

- ○ Allergies (latex, anesthetic agents)
- ○ Cancer of the oral cavity
- ○ Inability to cope, lack of support system
- ○ Disease processes involving multiple body systems
- ○ Older adult clients:
  - Are at a greater risk of adverse reactions to preoperative medications.
  - Have less physiologic reserve than younger clients, which may cause decreased immune system response and decreased wound healing.
  - Reduction of muscle mass and the amount of body water places the older adult client at risk for dehydration.
  - Can have sensory limitations (poor eyesight, hearing loss), so the nurse must be alert to maintaining a safe environment.
  - Can have oral alterations (dentures, bridges, loose teeth) that pose problems during intubation.
  - Perspire less, which leads to dry, itchy skin that becomes fragile and easily abraded. Precautions need to be taken when moving and positioning these clients.
  - Have decreased subcutaneous fat, which makes them more susceptible to temperature changes.

Diagnostic Procedures

- Urinalysis – ruling out of infection
- Blood type and cross match – transfusion readiness
- CBC – infection/immune status
- Hgb and Hct – fluid status, anemia
- Pregnancy test – fetal risk of anesthesia
- Clotting studies (PT, INR, aPTT, platelet count)
- Electrolyte levels – electrolyte imbalances
- Serum creatinine and BUN – renal status
- ABGs – oxygenation status
- Chest x-ray – heart and lung status
- 12-lead ECG – baseline heart rhythm, dysrhythmias, history of cardiac disease, performed on all clients older than 40 years

Preoperative Assessment

- Preoperative nursing assessments
  - ○ Detailed history (including medical history, medication use, substance use, psychosocial history, and cultural considerations)
  - ○ Allergies to medications, latex related to a sensitivity to bananas and other fruits, betadine related to an allergen to shellfish, propofol related to an allergy to eggs or soybean oil.
  - ○ Anxiety level regarding the procedure, support systems, and coping mechanisms.
    - Older adult clients may be more fearful due to financial concerns and lack of social support.
  - ○ Laboratory results
  - ○ Head-to-toe assessment, vital signs, and oxygen saturations to obtain baseline data.

Nursing Actions

- Informed consent
  - Once surgery has been discussed as treatment with the client and significant other, family member, or friend, it is the responsibility of the primary care provider to obtain consent after discussing the risks and benefits of the procedure. The nurse is not to obtain the consent for the provider in any circumstance.
  - The nurse can clarify any information that remains unclear after the provider's explanation of the procedure. The nurse may not provide any new or additional information not previously given by the provider.
  - The nurse's role is to witness the client's signing of the consent form after the client acknowledges understanding of the procedure.
  - The nurse should determine if the client is:
    - 18 years of age.
    - Mentally capable of understanding the risks, reason, and options for surgery and anesthesia.
    - Under the influence of medication that affects decision-making or judgment (opioids, benzodiazepines, sedatives). Do not have the client sign the informed consent if medications have been administered.
  - A legal guardian may need to sign the surgical consent form if the client is not capable of providing consent or if there is no family.
  - Two witnesses are required if the client is able to only sign with an "X", blind, deaf, or English is a second language.
  - Informed consent is required for surgical procedures, invasive procedures (biopsy, paracentesis, scopes), and any procedure requiring sedation or anesthesia, or involving radiation.

RESPONSIBILITIES FOR INFORMED CONSENT		
Provider: Obtains informed consent	› To obtain informed consent, the provider must give the client:	
	» A complete description of the treatment/procedure.	» A description of the potential harm, pain, and/or discomfort that may occur.
	» A description of the professionals who will be performing and participating in the treatment	» Options for other treatments.
		» The right to refuse treatment.
	» Information on the risks of anesthesia.	
Client: Gives informed consent	› To give informed consent, the client must:	
	» Give it voluntarily (no coercion involved).	» Be competent and of legal age or be an emancipated minor. When the client is unable to provide consent, another authorized person must give consent.
	» Receive enough information to make a decision based on an understanding of what is expected.	
Nurse: Witnesses informed consent	› To witness informed consent, the nurse must:	
	» Ensure that the provider gave the client the necessary information.	» Have the client sign the informed consent document.
	» Ensure that the client understood the information and is competent to give informed consent.	» The nurse documents questions the client has and notifies the provider. The nurse also documents any additional reinforcement of teaching.
	» Notify the provider if the client has more questions or appears to not understand any of the information provided. (The provider is then responsible for giving clarification.)	» Provide a trained medical interpreter (not a family member or friend) and record the use of an interpreter in the client's medical record.

- Preoperative teaching
  - Postoperative pain control techniques (medications, immobilization, patient-controlled analgesia pumps, splinting)
  - Demonstration and importance of splinting, coughing, and deep breathing
  - Demonstration and importance of range-of-motion exercises and early ambulation for prevention of thrombi and respiratory complications
  - Purpose of antiembolism stockings and pneumatic compression devices to prevent deep-vein thrombosis
  - Invasive devices (drains, catheters, IV lines)
  - Postoperative diet
  - Use of the incentive spirometer

 View Video: Incentive Spirometer

  - Preoperative instructions (avoid cigarette smoking for 24 hr preoperatively, medications to hold, bowel preparation)
    - Clients who are taking acetylsalicylic acid (Aspirin) should stop taking it for 1 week before an elective surgery to decrease the risk of bleeding.
    - Clients who take herbal medications (e.g., ginkgo biloba, ginseng, feverfew) should stop taking them 2 to 3 weeks before surgery to prevent hemorrhage or adverse affects to the anesthetic.
    - Medications for cardiovascular disease, pulmonary disease, seizures, and diabetes mellitus, certain antihypertensive medications, and eye drops for glaucoma may be taken prior to surgery or a procedure.
    - Teach the client how to use a pain scale to rate pain level postoperative.
  - Care and restrictions relative to surgical procedure performed
- Preoperative nursing actions
  - Verify that the informed consent is accurately completed, signed, and witnessed.
  - Administer enemas and/or laxatives the night before and/or the morning of the surgery for clients undergoing bowel surgery.
  - Regularly check the client's scheduled medication prescriptions. Some medications (antihypertensives, anticoagulants, antidepressants) may be held until after the procedure.

  - Ensure that the client remains NPO for at least 6 hr for solid foods and 2 hr for clear liquids before surgery with general anesthesia, and 3 to 4 hr with local anesthesia to avoid aspiration. Note on the chart the last time the client ate or drank.
  - Perform skin preparation, which may include cleansing with antimicrobial soap. If absolutely necessary, use electric clippers or chemical depilatories to remove hair in areas that will be involved in the surgery.
  - Ensure that jewelry, dentures, prosthetics, makeup, nail polish, and glasses are removed. These items can either be given to the family or stored safely.
  - Cover the client with lightweight cotton blanket heated in a warmer to prevent hypothermia.
    - Hypothermia increases the chance for surgical wound infections, alters metabolism of medication, and causes coagulation problems and cardiac dysrhythmias.

- ○ Establish IV access using a large-bore (18-gauge) catheter for easier infusing of IV fluids or blood products.
- ○ Administer preoperative medications (prophylactic antimicrobials, antiemetics, sedatives) as prescribed.
  - ▪ Prophylactic antibiotics are administered 1 hr prior to surgical incision.
  - ▪ If the client previously took a beta-blocker, administer a beta-blocker prior to surgery to prevent a cardiac event and mortality.
  - ▪ Have the client void prior to administration.
  - ▪ Monitor the client's response to the medications.
  - ▪ Raise side rails following administration to prevent injury.
- ○ Ensure that the preoperative checklist is complete.

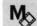 View Image: Preoperative Checklist

- ○ Confirm and verify the correct surgical site with the client and all health care team members before clearly marking the surgical site.

Complications

- • Complications during the postoperative period usually are related to the medications given preoperatively. These medications and their possible complications are as follows:

MEDICATION CLASS	POSSIBLE COMPLICATIONS
› Sedatives (benzodiazepines, barbiturates)	› Respiratory depression, drowsiness, dizziness
› Opioids	› Respiratory depression, drowsiness, dizziness, constipation, urinary retention
› IV infusions (0.9% NaCl, lactated Ringer's)	› Fluid overload, hypernatremia
› Gastrointestinal medications (antiemetics, antacids, H_2 receptor blockers)	› Alkalosis, cardiac abnormalities (certain H_2 receptor blockers), drowsiness

- • For clients encountering severe anxiety and panic, reassurance will be necessary and sedation medications may be given.
  - ○ Nonpharmacological interventions, such as distraction, imagery, and music therapy, can be initiated.
- • Ensure that measures are taken to prevent deep-vein thromboembolism postoperative by continuing anticoagulation therapy and/or antiembolism stockings, pneumatic compression device, and range-of-motion exercises.
- • Be alert for any allergic reactions the client has to medications.

APPLICATION EXERCISES

1. A nurse in the preoperative unit is assessing a client's laboratory values before surgery. Which of the following should the nurse report to the provider? (Select all that apply.)

_____ A. Potassium 3.9 mEq/L

_____ B. Sodium chloride 145 mEq/L

_____ C. Creatinine 2.8 mg/dL

_____ D. Blood glucose 235 mg/dL

_____ E. WBC 17,850/uL

2. A nurse is caring for a client who is scheduled for an exploratory laparotomy. The client's temperature is 39° C (102.2° F) orally. Which of the following is an appropriate action by the nurse?

A. Inform the surgeon of the elevated temperature.

B. Transfer the client to the preoperative unit.

C. Apply ice packs to the client's groin.

D. Encourage the client to increase intake of clear liquids.

3. A nurse is obtaining informed consent for a client who is having a paracentesis. Which of the following are appropriate nursing actions? (Select all that apply.)

_____ A. Explain to the client the purpose of having the procedure.

_____ B. Inform the client of risks to having the procedure.

_____ C. Ensure the client understood the information about the procedure.

_____ D. Witness the client signing the informed consent form.

_____ E. Determine if the client is mentally capable of understanding the reason for the procedure.

4. A nurse is preoperative teaching a client scheduled for abdominal surgery. Which of the following statements by the nurse are appropriate? (Select all that apply.)

_____ A. "Take your blood pressure medication with a sip of water before surgery."

_____ B. "Splint the abdominal incision with a pillow when coughing and deep breathing."

_____ C. "Bedrest is recommended for the first 48 hr."

_____ D. "Antiembolism stocking are applied before surgery."

_____ E. "You may eat solid foods up to 4 hr before surgery."

5. A preoperative nurse is caring for a client who is having a colon resection. Which of the following is an appropriate nursing action?

  A. Encourage the client to void after medication administration.

  B. Administer antibiotics 30 min prior to surgical incision.

  C. Remove hair using a manual razor.

  D. Remove nail polish on fingers and toes.

6. A preoperative nurse is planning preventative care for a client who is having a surgical procedure. What potential complications should the nurse include in the preventive plan of care? Use the ATI Active Learning Template: Basic Concept to complete this item to include the following:

  A. Related Content: List three preventions for potential complications.
   • Underlying Principles: Explain the related cause of each potential complication.
   • Nursing Interventions: Include one intervention for each potential complication.

APPLICATION EXERCISES KEY

1. A. INCORRECT: The potassium level is within the expected reference range.

   B. INCORRECT: The sodium chloride is within the expected reference range.

   C. **CORRECT:** The nurse should report an elevated creatinine level, which may indicate kidney failure, to the provider before surgery.

   D. **CORRECT:** The nurse should report an elevated blood glucose, which needs treatment prior to surgery.

   E. **CORRECT:** The nurse should report an elevated WBC count, which indicates a need for antibiotic therapy before surgery.

   Ⓝ NCLEX® Connection: Reduction of Risk Potential, Laboratory Values

2. A. **CORRECT:** An appropriate action by the nurse is immediately notifying the surgeon of the elevated temperature to determine if cancelling the surgery is necessary due to an underlying infection.

   B. INCORRECT: Transferring the client to the preoperative unit is not an appropriate nursing action when there is a possible underlying infection.

   C. INCORRECT: Applying ice packs to the client's groin is not an appropriate action by the nurse for a temperature of 39° C (102.2° F). Instead, administer acetaminophen (Tylenol).

   D. INCORRECT: Increasing intake of clear liquids is not an appropriate action by the nurse because the client should be NPO for at least 2 hr before surgery.

   Ⓝ NCLEX® Connection: Reduction of Risk Potential, Therapeutic Procedures

3. A. INCORRECT: The provider should explain the purpose of the procedure.

   B. INCORRECT: The provider should inform the client of risks to having the procedure.

   C. **CORRECT:** Ensuring the client understood the information about the procedure is an appropriate nursing action.

   D. **CORRECT:** Witnessing the client signing the informed consent is an appropriate nursing action.

   E. **CORRECT:** Determining if the client is mentally capable to sign the informed consent is an appropriate nursing action.

   Ⓝ NCLEX® Connection: Reduction of Risk Potential, Therapeutic Procedures

4. A. **CORRECT:** The nurse should teach the client to take certain antihypertensive and other medications as prescribed with a sip of water before surgery.

　　B. **CORRECT:** The nurse should teach the client how to splint with a pillow to support the incision when coughing and deep breathing postoperatively.

　　C. INCORRECT: The nurse should teach the client the importance of early ambulation following abdominal surgery to prevent complications.

　　D. **CORRECT:** The nurse should inform the client of the application of antiembolism stockings to prevent deep-vein thrombosis.

　　E. INCORRECT: The nurse should inform the client to stop eating solid food for 6 hr or more before surgery.

　　Ⓝ NCLEX® Connection: Reduction of Risk Potential, Therapeutic Procedures

5. A. INCORRECT: The client should void before administration of medication for relaxation or sedation to prevent the risk for falls.

　　B. INCORRECT: The nurse should administer antibiotics 1 hr prior the surgical incision as a prophylactic measure to prevent infection.

　　C. INCORRECT: The nurse should remove the client's hair at the surgical site with electric clippers or use a chemical depilatory to prevent traumatizing the skin and increasing the risk for infection.

　　D. **CORRECT:** The nurse should ensure the nail beds are visible for color and circulation by removing nail polish before surgery.

　　Ⓝ NCLEX® Connection: Reduction of Risk Potential, Therapeutic Procedures

6. *Using the ATI Active Learning Template: Basic Concept*

　　A. Related Content

- Prevent respiratory depression
  - Caused by overmedication with benzodiazepines, barbiturates, or opioids.
  - Administer a reversal agent, and monitor closely.
- Prevent fluid overload
  - Caused by too much IV fluids and inability to readily excrete the fluids.
  - Obtain a preoperative cardiac and pulmonary history, monitor I&O closely, slow the rate of IV fluids, and administer a prescribed diuretic.
- Prevent deep-vein thrombosis
  - Caused by blood stasis in lower extremities due to absent muscle contractility.
  - Apply antiembolism stocking and pneumatic compression device, administer prescribed anticoagulants, and teach range-of-motion exercises.
- Prevent infection
  - Caused by microorganisms contaminating the surgical wound.
  - Administer a prophylactic antibiotic 1 hr before the surgical incision is made.

　　Ⓝ NCLEX® Connection: Reduction of Risk Potential, Potential for Complications from Surgical Procedures and Health Alterations

chapter 97

Overview

- Transferring a client who is postoperative from the operating suite to the postanesthesia care unit (PACU) is the responsibility of the anesthesia provider who is either an anesthesiologist or a certified registered nurse anesthetist (CRNA). The circulating nurse will give the verbal "hand-off" report to the PACU nurse.

- Postoperative care is usually provided initially in the PACU, where skilled nurses who are certified in advanced cardiac life support (ACLS) can monitor a client's recovery from anesthesia.

- In some instances a client is transferred from the operating suite directly to the intensive care unit. Initial postoperative care involves making assessments, administering medications, managing the client's pain, preventing complications, and determining when a client is ready to be discharged from the PACU.

- During the immediate postoperative stage, maintaining airway patency and ventilation and monitoring circulatory status are the priorities for care.

- Postoperative clients who receive general anesthesia require frequent assessment of their respiratory status. Postoperative clients who receive epidural or spinal anesthesia require ongoing assessment of motor and sensory function.

- A client who is stable and able to breathe spontaneously is either discharged to a postsurgical unit or to home if an outpatient surgical procedure was performed. A client discharged home must demonstrate the ability to swallow and safely ambulate to the bathroom and wheelchair with assistance. A client who had an outpatient surgery should be accompanied by a significant other, family member, or other caregiver who can receive the discharge instructions and transport the client home.

Risk Factors for Postoperative Complications

- Immobility (respiratory compromise, thrombophlebitis, pressure ulcer)
- Anemia (blood loss, inadequate/decreased oxygenation, and healing factors)
- Hypovolemia (tissue perfusion)
- Hypothermia (risk of surgical wound infection, altered absorption of medication, coagulopathy, and cardiac dysrhythmia)
- Cardiovascular diseases (fluid overload, deep-vein thrombosis, arrhythmia)
- Respiratory disease (respiratory compromise)
- Immune disorder (risk for infection, delayed healing)
- Diabetes mellitus (gastroparesis, delayed wound healing)
- Coagulation defect (increased risk of bleeding)

- Malnutrition (delayed healing)

- Obesity (wound healing, dehiscence, evisceration)

Ⓖ • Age-related respiratory, cardiovascular, and renal changes necessitate special attention to the postoperative recovery of older adults.

   ○ Older adult clients are more susceptible to cold temperatures, so additional warm blankets in the PACU may be required.

   ○ Responses to medications and anesthetics may delay return of orientation postoperatively.

   ○ Age-related physiologic changes (decreased liver and kidney function) can affect response to and elimination of postoperative medications. Monitor the client for appropriate response and possible adverse effects.

     ▪ Older adults perspire less, which leads to dry, itchy skin that becomes fragile and easily abraded. The use of paper tape for wound dressings may be appropriate, as well as lifting precautions.

     ▪ Older adults may be at risk for delayed wound healing because of possible compromised nutrition.

Diagnostic Procedures

- CBC (infection/immune status)

- Hgb and Hct (fluid status, anemia)

- Serum electrolytes (electrolyte balance)

- Serum creatinine and BUN (kidney function)

- ABGs (oxygenation status)

- Additional laboratory tests (serum glucose, prothrombin time, INR) based on procedure and associated health problems

PACU Assessments and Nursing Interventions

- Upon receiving a client from the operating suite, the unit nurse should immediately perform a full body assessment with priority given to airway, breathing, and circulation.

- Nursing monitoring and management

   ○ Airway

     ▪ An artificial airway (endotracheal tube, nasal trumpet, or oral airway) is left in place until a client can maintain an open airway without support.

     ▪ Assess blood oxygen saturation levels continuously (greater than 92% or at preoperative status).

     ▪ Assess the respiratory pattern, rate, and depth to determine adequacy of oxygen exchange.

     ▪ Assess for symmetry of breath sounds and chest wall movement.

       □ Absent breath sounds on the left may indicate the endotracheal tube has migrated down the right mainstem bronchus or there is a pneumothorax.

       □ Snoring or stridor (a high pitch crowing type sound) may indicate poor oxygen exchange.

- Auscultate lung sounds.
- Administer humidified oxygen.
- Suction accumulated secretions if the client is unable to cough with a Yanhauer suction for thick oral secretions or a large French suction catheter for nasopharyngeal or nasotracheal secretions.
  - □ Retained neuromuscular blocking agents may hinder the client's ability to cough and eliminate secretions.
  - □ Extubation of endotracheal tube is based on client's response to commands, ability to elevate head, and use of thoracic breathing.
  - □ As soon as the client follows commands, encourage coughing and deep breathing, and the use of the incentive spirometer.
- ○ Circulation
  - Observe for internal bleeding (abdominal distention, visible hematoma under/near the surgical site, tachycardia, hypotension, increased pain) and external bleeding.
  - Assess for hypervolemia and hypovolemia.
  - Assess skin color, temperature, sensation, and capillary refill.
  - Check mucous membranes, lips, and nail beds for cyanosis.
  - Assess and compare peripheral pulses for impaired circulation, deep-vein thrombosis.
    - □ Continue with preventative deep vein thrombosis measures – sequential compression devices, antiembolism stockings, prescribed anticoagulants or antiplatelet medications.
  - Monitor ECG readings and apical pulse to determine a pulse deficit, which can indicate a dysrhythmia.
  - Monitor fluid and electrolyte balance.
- ○ Vital signs
  - Per agency protocol, obtain vital signs until stable (every 15 min) and assess for trends.
  - Provide heated blankets when the client arrives after a temperature is obtained and reapply if the client is hypothermic.
    - □ Causes of hypothermia include decreased body fat, age-related changes in the hypothalamus that regulates body temperature, and decreased environmental temperature in the surgical suite.
- ○ Positioning
  - Position the client who is responding to verbal stimuli with head of bed gradually elevated to semi-Fowler's position if not contraindicated to facilitate chest expansion.
  - Maintain lateral position (right or left side) if unresponsive or unconscious (risk of aspiration).
  - Do not elevate legs higher than placement on a pillow if the client has received spinal anesthesia.
  - Avoid placing a pillow under the knees or engaging the knee gatch of the bed, which can decease venous return.
  - Elevate legs and lower the head of the bed if hypotension or shock develops.

- ○ Response to anesthesia (sedation, nausea and/or vomiting)
  - Monitor level of consciousness (weakness, restlessness, agitation, somnolence, irritability, change in orientation).
  - Assess for movement of and sensation in extremities.
    - □ Sensory function and voluntary movement of the extremities following a regional block should occur before transfer to another unit.
  - Administer an antiemetic for nausea and vomiting after checking bowel sounds.
- ○ I&O
  - Monitor fluid and electrolyte balance following surgery.
    - □ Review postoperative laboratory findings (potassium, sodium, creatinine and BUN, hemoglobin and hematocrit).
    - □ Assess skin turgor, diaphoresis.
    - □ Review I&O during surgery and in PACU (emesis, drains, nasogastric (NG) tube, urine, IV fluids, blood products).
    - □ Administer isotonic IV fluids (0.9% sodium chloride, lactated Ringer's, dextrose 5% in lactated Ringer's) to maintain adequate cardiac output and fluid and electrolyte balance.
    - □ Administer prescribed blood products to treat hypovolemia (autologous blood, intraoperative blood salvage using a cell saver device, packed cells, fresh frozen plasma, albumin, platelets).
  - Palpate bladder for distention.
  - Monitor urinary catheters for patency.
  - Observe the color, consistency, odor, and amount of urine.
    - □ Urine output less than 30 mL/hr may indicate hypovolemia.
- ○ Surgical wound, incision site, and/or dressing
  - Observe drainage tubes for patency and proper function.
  - Check the client's dressings for excessive drainage and reinforce as needed. Report excess drainage to the surgeon.
- ○ Pain
  - Administer pain medication as appropriate, secondary to recovery status.
  - Observe for respiratory depression and decreased oxygen saturation.

- Monitor recovery from anesthesia by using the Aldrete scoring system. Each of the following five factors is given a score based upon the nurse's observations of the client. The five scores are totaled to determine the client's Aldrete Score.

MODIFIED ALDRETE SCORING SYSTEM		
FACTOR	ASSESSMENT/OBSERVATION	SCORE
Activity	› Able to move 4 extremities	2
	› Able to move 2 extremities	1
	› Able to move 0 extremities	0
Consciousness	› Fully awake	2
	› Arousable	1
	› Unarousable	0
Respiration	› Breathe deeply and cough	2
	› Dyspnea, hypoventilation	1
	› Apneic	0
O_2 Saturation	› O_2 Saturation maintained at 92% (minimum) on room air	2
	› Inhaled oxygen is necessary to maintain O_2 saturation level at 92% (minimum)	1
	› O_2 saturation level is below 90% even though inhaled oxygen is being given	0
Circulation	› Blood pressure is within 20% of preanthesia level	2
	› Blood pressure is within 21% to 49% of preanthesia level	1
	› Blood pressure is within 50% of preanthesia level	0

- Criteria indicating readiness for discharge from the PACU
  - Aldrete Score of 8 to 10
  - Stable vital signs
  - No evidence of bleeding
  - Return of reflexes (gag, cough, swallow)
  - Minimal to absent nausea and vomiting
  - Wound drainage that is minimal to moderate
  - Urine output of at least 30 mL/hr
- The anesthesiologist must sign out the client before transfer to another unit or discharged to home.

Unit Assessments and Nursing Interventions

- Upon receiving the client from the PACU, the unit nurse should immediately perform a full body assessment with priority given to airway, breathing, and circulation. This assessment serves as a baseline to identify changes in the client's postoperative status.
- Nursing monitoring and management
  - Airway
    - Monitor the oxygen saturation using a pulse oximeter.
    - Assist with coughing and deep breathing at least every 2 hr, and provide a pillow or folded blanket so the client can splint as necessary for abdominal incision.

- Assist with the use of an incentive spirometer at least every 2 hr to encourage expansion of the lungs and prevent atelectasis.

- Reposition every 2 hr and ambulate early and regularly.

○ Positioning

  - Do not put pillows under knees or elevate the knee gatch on the bed (decreases venous return).

  - Encourage early ambulation with adequate rest periods to prevent cardiovascular disorders, deep-vein thrombosis, and pulmonary complications.

○ Fluid status and oral comfort

  - A client who returns to the medical surgical unit is usually given IV solution of dextrose 5% in 0.45% sodium chloride, or prescription fluids based on the client's needs (hydration, electrolytes).

  - Encourage ice chips and fluids as prescribed/tolerated.

  - Provide frequent oral hygiene.

○ Pain

  - If prescribed, provide continuous pain relief through the use of a patient-controlled analgesia (PCA) pump. Epidural and intrathecal infusions are also available.

  - Assess pain level frequently, using a standardized pain scale.

  - Encourage the client to ask for pain medication before the pain gets severe.

  - Assess for manifestations of pain, such as an increased pulse, respirations, or blood pressure; restlessness; and wincing or moaning during movement.

  - Monitor for adverse effects of opioids, such as nausea (encourage the client to change positions slowly), respiratory depression, urinary retention, and constipation.

  - Provide analgesia 30 min before ambulation or other painful procedures.

○ Kidney function (output should equal intake)

  - Monitor and report urinary outputs of less than 30 mL/hr.

  - Palpate bladder following voiding to assess for distention.

  - Consider using a bladder scan to assess suspected retention of urine.

○ Bowel function

  - Maintain the client NPO until return of the gag reflex (risk of aspiration) and peristalsis (risk of paralytic ileus).

  - Irrigate NG suction tubes with saline as needed to maintain patency. Do not move the NG tubes in clients who are postoperative gastric surgery as ordered by the surgeon (risk to incision).

  - Monitor bowel sounds in all four quadrants as well as ability to pass flatus.

  - Advance diet as prescribed and tolerated (clear liquids to regular).

- Prevent and monitor for thromboembolism

  ○ Apply pneumatic compression stockings and/or elastic stockings.

  ○ Reposition every 2 hr and ambulate early and regularly.

  ○ Administer prescribed anticoagulants or antiplatelet medications.

  ○ Monitor extremities for calf pain, warmth, erythema, and edema.

- Monitor incisions and drain sites for bleeding and/or infection.

  ○ Monitor drainage (should progress from sanguineous to serosanguineous to serous).

  ○ Monitor the incision site (expected findings include pink wound edges, slight swelling under sutures/staples, slight crusting of drainage). Report any evidence of infection, including redness, excessive tenderness, and purulent drainage.

  ○ Monitor wound drains (with each vital sign assessment). Empty as often as needed to maintain compression. Report increases in drainage (possible hemorrhage).

M⬙ View Images

  › Penrose Drain   › Jackson-Pratt Drain

  › Hemovac Drain

  ○ In most instances, the surgeon will change the dressing the first time. Subsequent dressing changes may be performed by the nurse using surgical aseptic technique.

  ○ Use an abdominal binder for clients who are obese or debilitated, as prescribed.

  ○ Encourage splinting with position changes and cough and deep breathing.

  ○ Administer prophylactic antibiotics as prescribed.

  ○ Remove sutures or staples in 6 to 8 days as prescribed.

- Promote wound healing.

  ○ Encourage the client to consume a diet that is high in calories, protein, and vitamin C.

  ○ If the client has diabetes mellitus, maintain appropriate glycemic control.

- Provide discharge teaching.

  ○ Medications (purpose, administration guidelines, adverse effects)

  ○ Activity restrictions (driving, stairs, limits on weight lifting, sexual activity)

  ○ Dietary guidelines, if applicable

  ○ Special treatment instructions (wound care, catheter care, use of assistive devices)

  ○ Emergency contact information and findings to report

Complications

- Airway obstruction

  ○ The tongue can fall back in the nasopharynx, causing airway obstruction.

  ○ Stridor or laryngeal spasm caused from swelling or mucous secretion on the vocal cords results in airway obstruction and difficult oxygen exchange.

  ○ Nursing Actions

    ▪ Monitor for choking, noisy, irregular respirations, decreased oxygen saturation values, and cyanosis. Intervene accordingly.

    ▪ Keep emergency equipment at the bedside in the PACU (resuscitation bag, suction equipment, airways).

    ▪ Notify the anesthesiologist, elevate head of bed if not contraindicated, provide humidified oxygen, and plan for reintubation with endotracheal tube.

- Hypoxia
  - Hypoxia is evidenced by a decrease in oxygen saturation.
  - Nursing Actions
    - Monitor oxygenation status and administer oxygen as prescribed.
    - Encourage cough and deep breathing to prevent atelectasis.
    - Position client with head of bed elevated and turn every 2 hr to facilitate chest expansion.
- Hypovolemic shock
  - Postoperative shock can result from a massive loss of circulating blood volume.
  - Nursing Actions
    - Monitor for decreased blood pressure and urinary output, increased heart rate, and slow capillary refill.
    - Administer IV fluids and vasopressors as indicated.
- Paralytic ileus
  - Can occur due to the absence of gastrointestinal peristaltic activity caused by abdominal surgery or other physical trauma
  - Nursing Actions
    - Monitor bowel sounds, encourage ambulation, advance the diet as tolerated when bowel sounds are present, may have NG tube inserted to empty stomach contents, and administer prokinetic agents, such as metoclopramide (Reglan), as prescribed.
- Wound dehiscence or evisceration
  - Caused by spontaneous opening of the incisional wound (dehiscence), and can progress to the protrusion of the intestine through the incision (evisceration)
  - Nursing Actions
    - Monitor risk factors (obesity, coughing, moving without splinting, diabetes mellitus, infection, hematoma).
    - If wound dehiscence or evisceration occurs, call for help, stay with the client, cover the wound with a sterile towel or dressing that is moistened with sterile saline, do not attempt to reinsert organs, place in supine position with hips and knees bent, monitor for shock, and notify the provider immediately.

 View Video: Wound Evisceration

- Deep-vein thrombosis
  - Caused by dehydration, stress response that leads to hypercoagulability of the blood, obesity, trauma, malignancy, history of thrombosis, hormones, and use of indwelling venous catheter
    - Nursing Actions: Prophylactic measures include administration of lower-molecular-weight or low-dose heparin or low-dose warfarin (Coumadin), antiembolism stockings, pneumatic compression devices, range of motion exercises, and early ambulation.
    - Avoid any form of pressure behind the knee with a pillow or blanket, which can cause constriction of blood vessels and decreased venous return.
    - Avoid dangling client for long periods of time.
    - Provide adequate hydration by administering IV fluids or encouraging increased oral fluid intake.

APPLICATION EXERCISES

1. A nurse is reviewing the health records of several clients in the postanesthesia care unit (PACU) to identify risk factors that can lead to postoperative complications. Which of the following clients are at risk for complications? (Select all that apply.)

_____ A. A client who has a WBC of 22,500/uL

_____ B. A client who uses an insulin pump

_____ C. A client taking warfarin (Coumadin) daily

_____ D. A client who had a bowel prep

_____ E. A client who has a BMI of 26

2. A nurse is caring for a female client who manifests indications of hypovolemia while in the PACU. Which of the following findings requires action by the nurse? (Select all that apply.)

_____ A. Urine output less than 25 mL/hr

_____ B. Hematocrit 48%

_____ C. BUN 24 mg/dL

_____ D. Tenting of skin over the sternum

_____ E. Apical pulse rate 62/min

3. A nurse is caring for a client who arrived in the PACU following a total hip arthroplasty. The client is not responding to verbal stimuli. Which of the following actions should the nurse perform first?

A. Compare and contrast the peripheral pulses.

B. Apply a warm blanket.

C. Assess the client's dressings.

D. Place the client in a lateral position.

4. A nurse is planning care for a client to prevent postoperative atelectasis. Which of the following interventions should the nurse include in the plan of care? (Select all that apply.)

_____ A. Encourage the use of the incentive spirometer every 2 hr.

_____ B. Instruct to splint incision when coughing and deep breathing.

_____ C. Reposition the client every 2 hr.

_____ D. Administer antibiotic therapy.

_____ E. Assist with early ambulation.

5. A nurse is caring for a client who reports nausea and vomiting 2 days postoperative after hysterectomy. Which of the following actions should the nurse perform first?

    A. Assess bowel sounds.

    B. Administer antiemetic medication.

    C. Restart prescribed IV fluids.

    D. Insert a prescribed nasogastric tube.

6. A nurse is reviewing the health records of several clients to identify postoperative complications. What information should the nurse expect to find in this review? Use the ATI Active Learning Template: Basic Concept to complete this item to include the following:

    A. Related Content:
- List three possible complications.
- Describe one cause for each complication.
- List one intervention for each complication.

APPLICATION EXERCISES KEY

1. A. **CORRECT:** An increased WBC indicates an underlying infection and places the client at risk for postoperative complications.

    B. **CORRECT:** An insulin pump indicates the client has type 1 diabetes mellitus and places the client at risk of postoperative complications.

    C. **CORRECT:** A client who takes warfarin daily is at risk for bleeding and postoperative complications.

    D. **CORRECT:** Receiving a bowel prep to cleanse the colon can cause dehydration and places the client at risk for complications.

    E. INCORRECT: A BMI of 26 is within the expected reference range and does not place the client at risk for postoperative complications.

    Ⓝ NCLEX® Connection: Reduction of Risk Potential, Potential for Complications of Diagnostic Tests/Treatments/Procedures

2. A. **CORRECT:** Urine output less than 25 mL/hr is a manifestation of hypovolemia and requires intervention by IV fluid therapy.

    B. **CORRECT:** Hematocrit of 48% indicates concentrated blood volume and is a manifestation of hypovolemia, requiring intervention by IV fluid therapy.

    C. **CORRECT:** BUN of 24 mg/dL indicates decreased kidney function and can be a manifestation of hypovolemia, requiring intervention with IV fluid therapy.

    D. **CORRECT:** Tenting of skin indicates decreased or absent skin turgor due to dehydration, requiring intervention with IV fluid therapy.

    E. INCORRECT: An apical pulse rate of 62/min is not a manifestation of hypovolemia.

    Ⓝ NCLEX® Connection: Physiological Adaptations, Medical Emergencies

3.   A. INCORRECT: Comparing and contrasting the client's peripheral pulses is important but is not the first nursing action.

     B. INCORRECT: Applying warm blankets to prevent hypothermia is important but is not the first nursing action.

     C. INCORRECT: Assessing the client's dressings for drainage is important but is not the first nursing action.

     D. **CORRECT:** The greatest risk to the client is injury from aspiration. The first action is to position the client laterally.

      NCLEX® Connection: Reduction of Risk Potential, Potential for Complications of Diagnostic Tests/ Treatments/Procedures

4.   A. **CORRECT:** The use of the incentive spirometer every 2 hr expands the lungs and prevents atelectasis.

     B. **CORRECT:** Incisional splinting with a pillow or blanket supports the incision during coughing and deep breathing which prevents atelectasis.

     C. **CORRECT:** Repositioning the client every 2 hr will cause the client to deep breathe and expand the lungs to prevent atelectasis.

     D. INCORRECT: Antibiotic therapy is used to prevent/treat infection and does not prevent atelectasis.

     E. **CORRECT:** Early ambulation expands the lungs through deep breathing and prevents atelectasis.

      NCLEX® Connection: Physiological Adaptations, Alterations in Body Systems

5.   A. **CORRECT:** Using the nursing process, the first step is to assess the client. Assessing bowel sounds is the correct action by the nurse.

     B. INCORRECT: Administer an antiemetic medication may alleviate the nausea and vomiting but is not the first nursing action.

     C. INCORRECT: Restarting the prescribed IV fluids will prevent dehydration but is not the first nursing action.

     D. INCORRECT: Inserting a prescribed nasogastric tube can alleviate nausea and vomiting but is not the first nursing action.

      NCLEX® Connection: Basic Care and Comfort, Elimination

6. *Using the ATI Active Learning Template: Basic Concept*

    A. Related Content

    -   Paralytic ileus

        ○ Caused by abdominal surgery or other physical trauma and absent gastrointestinal peristaltic activity.

        ○ Monitor bowel sounds, encourage ambulation, insert nasogastric tube to empty stomach contents.

    -   Wound evisceration

        ○ Protrusion of the intestines through the incisional wound of the abdominal cavity, caused by failure to splint when moving or coughing, delayed healing due to obesity or diabetes mellitus.

        ○ Call for help, cover wound with sterile saline soaked dressings or towel, position client in semi Fowler's position with hips and knees bent.

    -   Airway obstruction

        ○ Stridor caused by trauma to the vocal cords due to intubation resulting in reduced oxygen exchange.

        ○ Notify the anesthesiologist, provide humidified oxygen, elevate the head of the bed if not contraindicated, plan for reintubation of the endotracheal tube.

    -   Hypovolemic shock

        ○ Caused by blood loss.

        ○ Administer IV fluids and vasopressors, monitor for decreased blood pressure, tachycardia, and urinary output.

(N) NCLEX® Connection: Physiological Adaptations, Unexpected Response to Therapies

REFERENCES

Berman, A. J., & Snyder S. (2012). *Fundamentals of nursing: Concepts, process, and practice* (9th ed.). Upper Saddle River, NJ: Prentice-Hall.

Burke, K., LeMone, P., & Mohn-Brown, L. (2011). *Medical-surgical nursing care* (3rd ed.). Upper Saddle River, NJ: Prentice-Hall.

Dudek, S. G. (2010). *Nutrition essentials for nursing practice* (6th ed.). Philadelphia: Lippincott Williams & Wilkins.

Eliopoulos, C. (2014). *Gerontological nursing* (8th ed.). Philadelphia: Lippincott Williams & Wilkins.

Ford, S. M., & Roach, S. S. (2013). *Roach's introductory clinical pharmacology* (10th ed.). Philadelphia: Lippincott Williams & Wilkins.

Grodner, M., Roth, S. L., & Walkingshaw, B. C. (2012). *Nutritional foundations and clinical applications: A nursing approach* (5th ed.). St. Louis, MO: Mosby.

Ignatavicius, D. D., & Workman, M. L. (2013). *Medical-surgical nursing* (7th ed.). St. Louis, MO: Saunders.

Lehne, R. A. (2013). *Pharmacology for nursing care* (8th ed.). St. Louis: Saunders.

Lilley, L. L., Harrington, S., & Snyder, J. S. (2014)). *Pharmacology and the nursing process* (7th Ed.). St. Louis, MO: Mosby.

Lowdermilk, D. L., Perry, S. E., Cahsion, M. C., & Aldean, K. R. (2012). *Maternity & women's health care* (10th ed.). St. Louis, MO: Mosby.

Potter, P. A., Perry, A. G., Stockert, P., & Hall, A. (2013). *Fundamentals of nursing* (8th ed.). St. Louis, MO: Mosby.

Smeltzer, S. C., Bare, B. G., Hinkle, J. L., & Cheever, K. H. (2010). *Brunner and Suddarth's textbook of medical-surgical nursing* (12th ed.). Philadelphia: Lippincott Williams & Wilkins.

Touhy, T. A., & Jett, K. F. (2012) *Ebersole & Hess' toward healthy aging: Human needs and nursing response* (8th ed.). St. Lois, MO: Mosby.

Townsend, M. C. (2011). *Essentials of psychiatric mental health nursing: Concepts of care in evidence-based practice* (5th ed.). Philadelphia: F. A. Davis.

Varcarolis, E. M., Carson, V. B., & Shoemaker, N. C. (2010). *Foundations of psychiatric mental health nursing: A clinical approach* (6th ed.). St. Louis, MO: Saunders.

Wilson, B. A., Shannon, M. T., & Shields, K. M. (2013). *Pearson nurse's drug guide 2013*. Upper Saddle River, NJ: Prentice Hall.

| APPENDIX | ACTIVE LEARNING TEMPLATES |
| TEMPLATE | Basic Concept |

CONTENT_____ REVIEW MODULE CHAPTER _____

TOPIC DESCRIPTOR_____

Related Content
(e.g. delegation, levels of
prevention, advance directives)

Underlying Principles

Nursing Interventions
› Who?
› When?
› Why?
› How?

Appendix

CONTENT_____ REVIEW MODULE CHAPTER _____

TOPIC DESCRIPTOR_____

DESCRIPTION OF PROCEDURE:

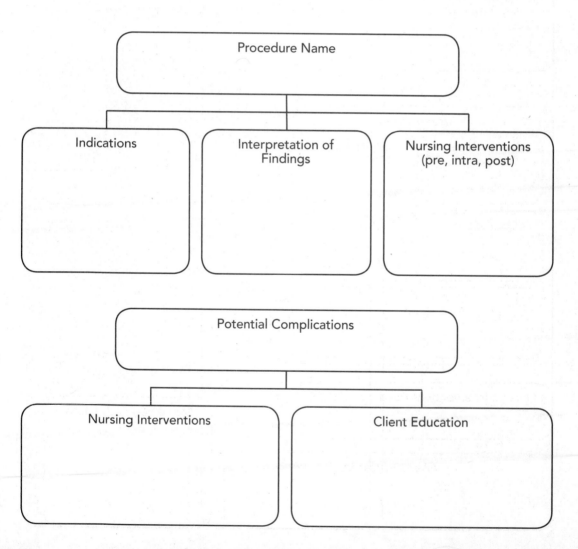

Procedure Name

Indications

Interpretation of Findings

Nursing Interventions (pre, intra, post)

Potential Complications

Nursing Interventions

Client Education

Appendix

CONTENT _____ REVIEW MODULE CHAPTER _____

TOPIC DESCRIPTOR _____

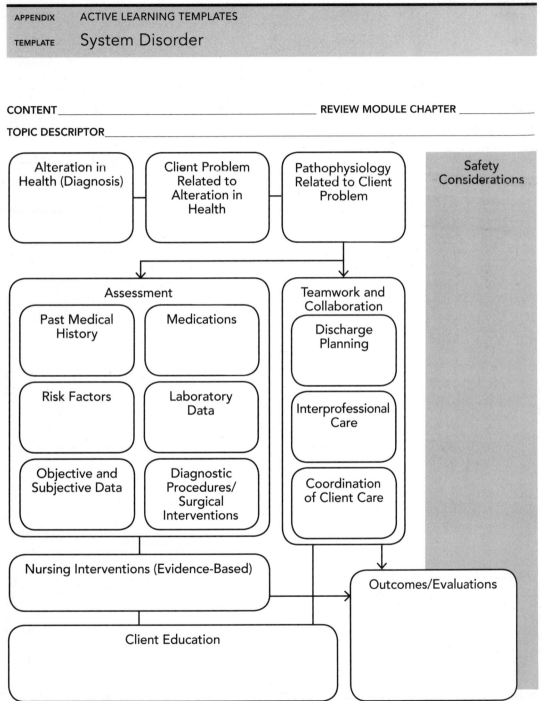

| Alteration in Health (Diagnosis) | Client Problem Related to Alteration in Health | Pathophysiology Related to Client Problem | Safety Considerations |

Assessment
- Past Medical History
- Medications
- Risk Factors
- Laboratory Data
- Objective and Subjective Data
- Diagnostic Procedures/ Surgical Interventions

Teamwork and Collaboration
- Discharge Planning
- Interprofessional Care
- Coordination of Client Care

Nursing Interventions (Evidence-Based)

Outcomes/Evaluations

Client Education

Appendix

CONTENT _____ REVIEW MODULE CHAPTER _____

TOPIC DESCRIPTOR _____

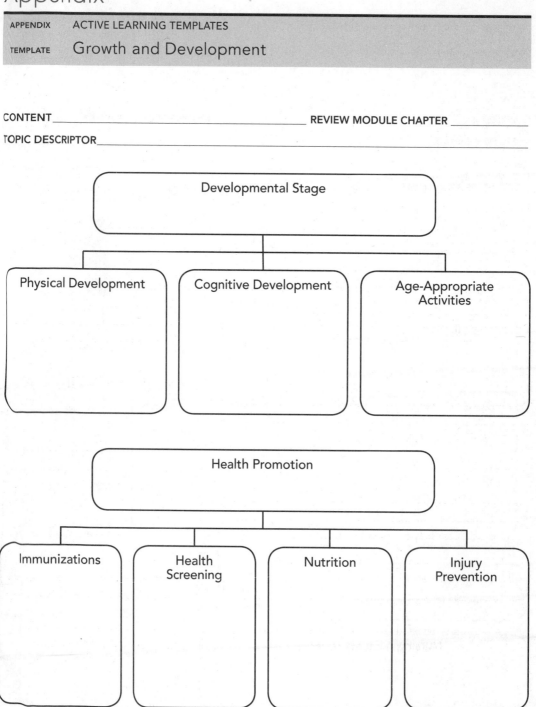

Developmental Stage

Physical Development

Cognitive Development

Age-Appropriate Activities

Health Promotion

Immunizations

Health Screening

Nutrition

Injury Prevention

APPENDIX	ACTIVE LEARNING TEMPLATES
TEMPLATE	Medication

CONTENT _____ REVIEW MODULE CHAPTER _____

TOPIC DESCRIPTOR_____

MEDICATION _____

EXPECTED PHARMALOGICAL ACTION:

```
┌─────────────────────────────────────────┐
│            Therapeutic Uses               │
│                                           │
└─────────────────────────────────────────┘
```

```
┌──────────────────────┐        ┌──────────────────────┐
│    Adverse Effects    │        │  Nursing Interventions │
│                       │        │                        │
│                       │        │                        │
└──────────────────────┘        │                        │
                                 └──────────────────────┘
┌──────────────────────┐
│   Client Education    │
│                       │        ┌──────────────────────┐
│                       │        │    Client Education   │
└──────────────────────┘        │                       │
                                 │                       │
┌──────────────────────┐        │                       │
│ Medication/Food       │        └──────────────────────┘
│ Interactions          │
│                       │
└──────────────────────┘
```

```
┌──────────────────────┐        ┌──────────────────────┐
│ Nursing Administration │        │ Evaluation of Medication│
│                       │        │      Effectiveness     │
│                       │        │                        │
└──────────────────────┘        └──────────────────────┘
```

Appendix

CONTENT_____ REVIEW MODULE CHAPTER _____

TOPIC DESCRIPTOR_____

DESCRIPTION OF SKILL:

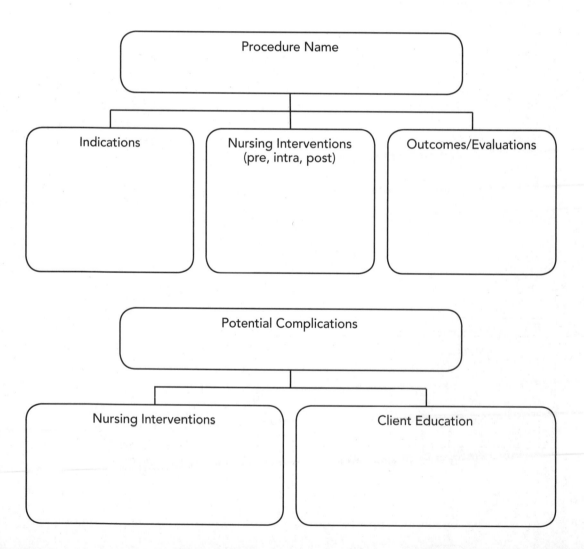

Appendix

CONTENT_____ REVIEW MODULE CHAPTER _____

TOPIC DESCRIPTOR_____

DESCRIPTION OF PROCEDURE:

```
                          ┌─────────────────────────────┐
                          │       Procedure Name        │
                          │                             │
                          └─────────────────────────────┘
                ┌──────────────────┼──────────────────┐
    ┌───────────────┐   ┌───────────────────┐   ┌───────────────────┐
    │               │   │ Nursing Interventions │   │                   │
    │  Indications  │   │  (pre, intra, post)   │   │ Outcomes/Evaluations │
    │               │   │                       │   │                   │
    └───────────────┘   └───────────────────┘   └───────────────────┘
```

Procedure Name

Indications

Nursing Interventions (pre, intra, post)

Outcomes/Evaluations

Potential Complications

Nursing Interventions

Client Education